Nutrition and diet therapy

Sue Rodwell Williams

M.R.Ed., M.P.H.

*Instructor in Nutrition and Clinical Dietetics,
Kaiser Foundation School of Nursing; Nutrition
Consultant and Program Coordinator, Health Education
Research Center, Permanente Medical Group, Oakland,
California; Field Faculty, M.P.H.-Dietetic Internship
Program, University of California, Berkeley, California*

With 117 illustrations, including original drawings by
George Straus

Saint Louis

The C. V. Mosby Company

1969

Nutrition
and
diet therapy

To my husband

Luke

minister, helpmate, "my other self";
and to our children

Jim, Mary, Ruth

whose constant support and encouragement
never cease to sustain me

Foreword

In this book Mrs. Williams shows her great understanding of the field of nutrition. She demonstrates strongly the concept that all of us—the nurse, the nutritionist, and the physician, that is, all who are associated with the care of our fellow human beings—work as a team. In this concept, care of the patient is the primary objective of all members of the team. Mrs. Williams stresses the role, obligations, and importance of the nurse in this total picture. She emphasizes the fact that change in environment, affected by the scientific advances of our times, must be accepted and that "health is a relative concept in any culture."

Mrs. Williams has conscientiously laid out her philosophy relating to nutrition and has masterfully organized her book to focus on the needs of the nurse. It is also apparent that this book is of value to others in the health sciences and is worthy of the author's effort.

A. J. Sender, M.D.

Physician in Chief,
Oakland Division,
Permanente Medical Group

This most interestingly written book meets a very important need for an up-to-date, comprehensive, and authoritative text on nutrition as related to nursing and patient care. The reader will be quickly aware that Mrs. Williams is a highly able and dedicated person. She has a unique ability to make the subject matter actually live for the student, almost as though she were teaching the material personally to each reader.

Sufficient basic information about nutrition is provided to enable the student to become knowledgeable about the subject and to recognize and refute food faddism, which often creeps into patient care from one source or another. Nursing students will become very aware of the great importance of nutrition in the care of patients of all ages.

The inclusion of a nutrition course in nursing education programs is extremely important. I decry the recent practice in some nursing curricula of removing or curtailing the subject because of the pressures from other topics. A study of the contents of this book should provide proof of nurses' need for nutritional education; this need is demonstrated by the vital interrelationships of nutrition to disease, patient care and well-being, and good health.

I highly recommend this textbook, not only for nurses but also for other professional workers interested in patient care as it relates to nutrition.

George M. Briggs

Department of Nutritional Sciences,
University of California,
Berkeley, California

Preface

This book is concerned with nutrition and human health. A careful reading of Chapter 1 will reveal its tone, its focus, and its form.

This is a new book. It is the result of many years of teaching and clinical practice and is born of two deep feelings: my concern for students and my concern for people—or, more rightly, I should say persons, for we relate to individual persons, not to masses of people. Through these pages I have tried to reach not only the students' minds and intellects, but also their hearts by seeking to stimulate deeper dimensions of caring for persons and their individual health needs. For this I make no apology. Learning itself involves by necessity not only the intellect but also the emotion and the will. I realize that I may have challenged some old ideas and ritualistic practices. But at the same time I hope that I may have caused some new thinking and initiated some new approaches, which are demanded of us in these rapidly changing times, to pressing human needs, to the basic role of nutrition in meeting these needs, and to the vital teaching-learning process.

In these days of burgeoning scientific knowledge and booming population growth, we are beginning to hear an increased number of concerned cries for more comprehensive, less fragmented patient care, for greater awareness of individual need, of concern for the "whole man." As health professionals in the midst of this rapidly changing world, we are at one and the same time charged with two responsibilities—to know our subject and to know our patient. Sound knowledge must be our tool; genuine concern for human need must be our motive. Furthermore, the realities of life must be the context of the practice of our art.

For whom, then, do I write this book? You will see that I focus primarily upon nutrition in nursing, seeking to provide a textbook for professional nursing students and their teachers. However, other health team members, all those concerned with the integration of nutritional needs in the care of patients and families, will find here useful, practical information and direction. The book may well serve as a tool of learning for students in dietetics and other health fields, as well as a helpful resource to busy clinicians and practitioners—physicians, nurses, nutritionists, dietitians, dentists, dental hygienists, public health workers, health educators, physical therapists, home economists, and others.

In decisions concerning organization of material, one idea has remained uppermost in my mind. I suppose the word *life* describes it best. I wanted to provide "meat" for my subject, to give it "bone and blood and sinew," to make a subject too long lifeless and colorless and irrelevant in the experience of many nurses come alive with new meaning. I wanted to help them view nutrition in terms of the very throbbing, pulsating "stuff of life" which it provides, and to see it applied to living persons in real life situations of daily living as well as in times of stress. To this end, two basic objectives have prevailed: *clarity of content* and *person-centered focus*. To achieve greater clarity of content, scientific and philosophical concepts are developed in more depth through discussion of key terms and relationships as well as through visual diagrams, illustrations, questions raised for study, outlines, boxes giving further background, and summary glossaries. To achieve a greater degree of person-centered focus, clinical application is made of all scientific principles and increased emphasis is given to the role of nutrition in public health, in the basic nursing specialties, and in clinical management of disease—all in the context of human need. The book is divided, therefore, into four parts: I, Foundations of Nutrition; II, Applied Nutrition in Public Health; III, Nutrition in the Nursing Specialty; IV, Nutrition in Medical-Surgical Nursing.

To facilitate the use of the book, several reference tools are used. There is considerable cross-reference throughout the text to relate similar or needed material. Appendixes provide the basic tables for simple calculations. An index provides ready access to desired material. If anything, I may have erred on the side of overindexing. Perhaps this results from my own personal irritation with a book in whose index I have to search in vain through a series of related words for reference to some needed bit of information. One thing, however, I have not included. Those looking for recipes among the references will be disappointed. I do not think that a student comes to nursing school to learn to cook.

A book of this nature emerges gradually from the work of many people. I am deeply indebted to all those persons who have helped to make this one become a reality. I owe much to Ruth Straus, scientific editor, writer, craftsman, and friend, for her constant encouragement, her sharp and discerning eye to editorial details, and sympathetic feeling for student and patient alike. Many times her probing questions led to greater clarification of the writing. Also I am grateful to George Straus for bringing further clarification and sheer beauty to scientific concepts through his diagrammatic illustrations. In these illustrations he has contributed a freshness of view, a precision of content, and a rare artistry. The book is a better book because of the loving efforts of these dear friends.

I am also particularly indebted to my esteemed teacher and friend, George M. Briggs, Chairman of the Department of Nutritional Sciences at the University of California, Berkeley, who counseled with me at the outset when the book was only the germ of an idea, who helped the idea to grow and gave me the courage to undertake the enormous effort to develop the material which nourished it. I am grateful for his careful reading of the manuscript's first basic science section, his discussions with me of many interesting points, and his writing of part of the book's foreword.

Many other persons made valuable contributions that shaped the course of the book. To each of the following I give my deep appreciation: the fine faculty of nurse-educators with whom I, a nutritionist, am privileged to teach, and in whom I have found the highest ideal of nursing, and especially to those among them who have read various portions of the manuscript and offered helpful suggestions—Clair Lisker, Elizabeth Bridston, Betty Smith, and Marion Yeaw; my colleagues in the California Bay Area Dietetic Association, especially those close friends and fellow teachers who have encouraged my effort, reviewed material, and influenced my thinking—Claire Fry, Natalie Calhoun, Phyllis Howe, Mildred Bennett, Leona Shapiro, and Sylvia Mitchell; Pat Collins and Mary Williams of Agricultural Extension Service, University of California, for aiding in early explorations for direction and for giving many practical guides for community application; my teachers, whose examples inspired my own effort—Ruth Huenemann, Harold Harper, and Sheldon Margen; my students—past, present, and future—who always teach me much and some of whom will find familiar words on many pages; the physicians with whom I work, all of whom have contributed much to my own learning and given to me a model of professional practice, especially to Dr. A. J. Sender, our physician-in-chief, who reviewed clinical sections of the manuscript and wrote part of the foreword; my dietetic interns, who stimulate and challenge my thinking, and especially to Mary Blackburn and Marni Miller, who helped teach me what human need means; the many authors, publishers, companies, government agencies, and world health organizations—at home and abroad—who have generously permitted me to use their materials and provided resources, illustrations, and personal encouragement; the patients and staff in our hospital and in the public health department who graciously served as models for our photographs; the typists whose unfailing assistance at various stages of the writing produced the final typescript—Aileen Simpson, Elin Carlson, and Lorraine Satterthwaite.

And finally, but certainly not least, to my family I give my love and my deepest gratitude—to my patient husband who helped to develop my insight at numerous points, to my Peace Corps son teaching in Africa whose standards of scholarship and personal example of concern for human need have helped to open my own eyes of understanding, to my alert and sensitive daughters whose keen awareness and warm encouragement have lighted my way, and to Bob, who is like a son and whose creative talents have inspired my own efforts. All of these persons close to me have stimulated me enormously and have never ceased to share in this family project—"the book!"

S. R. W.
Oakland, California

Contents

Chapter 27

Diseases of the liver and gallbladder, 514

Chapter 28

Cardiovascular diseases, 523

Chapter 29

Renal disease, 542

Chapter 30

Care of the surgery patient, 568

Appendixes

FOUNDATIONS
OF
NUTRITION

CHAPTER 1

The study of nutrition

The thoughtful student of nursing may well ask, "What place does a knowledge of nutrition have in the practice of my profession?" This is a significant question, for ideas concerning nutrition are currently undergoing tremendous change in America as well as throughout the world. Nutrition as a part of nursing must be viewed in the context of human need if the study of nutrition is to have relevancy and meaning. The focus of this book is man and his needs—patient-centered care.

NUTRITION AND NURSING

The relationship between nutrition and nursing is evident in the words themselves since both come from a common Latin root, *nutr-*. The English words nurse (Latin, *nutrix*), to nourish or to nurture (L. *nutrire*), and several other closely related words all have this common base. Several related ideas are bound up in these words. To be a *nurse* is to give attendance and service; to *nourish* is to provide whatever is needed for growth and development, and to *nurture* is to provide a safe environment for growth and development. Both nutrition and nursing convey the idea of nourishing: to nurse, at least in one sense, is to nourish.

Nourishment is that which sustains life. Nursing and the science of human nutrition both focus upon nourishing human life. They do this in many ways. Man breathes, works, rests, plays, sleeps, and so on, all of which require energy. Man must replenish that energy with food to sustain physical life. This need for food is basic to survival and is a fundamental concern of nutrition.

However, man is much more than a mere biological organism, and food has many meanings for him other than simply physical sustenance. The nurse must have a broad range of knowledge, understanding, and skills which will enable her to meet human needs. The patient needs care that helps to heal both body and spirit, and the nurse must be concerned with the patient's physical and emotional needs if she is to provide total care.

Physical needs. Physiologic health depends upon certain essential chemicals and their intricate biological interrelationships in the body's cells and tissues. These basic chemicals are supplied by, or derived from, food. A person is, quite literally, what he eats.

Emotional needs. Psychologic health depends upon certain personal, social, and cultural factors which exert strong influences on each individual. Unmet needs may bring about actual physical illness. Medical experts generally agree that there is a psychologic component in almost all disease.

The relationship between the physical and emotional aspects of health and the pertinent functions of nutrition and nursing, may be seen by applying the four functions of nutrition (to sustain life, to promote growth, to replace loss, and to provide energy) to the concept of nursing as the nurturing and healing of patients, both physically and emotionally.

Functions of nutrition	Related emotional functions of nursing
1. To sustain life	1. To sustain and support persons through times of dependence and need
2. To promote growth	2. To promote personal growth and restore health
3. To replace loss	3. To replace the loss of self-care ability and help maintain a sense of personal wholeness
4. To provide energy	4. To help provide emotional strength to cope with the total experience of illness

All of these ideas are part of the evolving concepts of nutrition and nursing.

CHANGING CONCEPTS OF DISEASE AND HEALTH

Since nutrition and nursing are both a part of health care, the changes in the concepts of disease and health that are taking place today have profound effects on the practice of these professions.

In primitive societies disease was associated with evil spirits, mysterious supernatural powers which had to be driven out by some means. Treatment of disease, therefore, was in the hands of the religious leader of the group, the shaman who acted as both priest and doctor. Gradually, as scientific knowledge increased the biologic basis for disease became well established. Consequently, public and personal hygiene improved, treatment for specific diseases became more scientific and skilled, and many of the most lethal childhood diseases were eliminated.

Faced now with the so-called gift of longer life, man began to view health increasingly in qualitative terms. Health concepts are moving from the wholly negative view of absence of disease (the curative approach), to a more positive view of optimum productivity (the preventive approach). This positive view was written into the preamble to the World Health Organization constitution in 1946: "Health is a state of complete physical, mental, and social well-being, and not merely the absence of disease or infirmity."

On the face of it, this is a noble goal for men of all nations, but it is not totally realistic. Is such a complete state of health possible, and if it is possible, is it consistent with a state of social well-being? Such a goal is neither possible or attainable, or, perhaps, even desirable. In reality, man has health goals in two categories. (1) At any given time, an individual may have an obvious, specific health need. (For example, he may need to have a broken bone set so that it will heal in good alignment, or he may need an antibiotic to help him overcome a specific disease.) (2) At the same time, whether he is aware of it or not, he has other needs. In some instances these other needs may even be in conflict with the need for restoration of physical health.

An example of such a conflict would be two men who have each had a stroke. One is a wealthy retired financier who can readily afford to spend a year or two in a rehabilitation center, and may learn to be relatively contented when he has regained sufficient function to enable him to manage his own physical care. The other man is a forty-five-year-old engineer with three chidren in school. This man must choose between prolonged rehabilitation therapy, while earning nothing, and returning to a job offered by his employer at half his former salary—barely enough to maintain his family.

Health is a relative concept in any culture, and it must be viewed in relation to man's total wants and needs. Health competes with other values and is relative to a culture's way of life. The kind and degree of physical health required for success as an accountant in New York differs from the kind and degree of physical health needed to succeed as a Maori hunter. This recognition of the difference in needs extends the concepts of health to include moral, religious, and philosophical dimensions.

Perhaps a more realistic goal for world health efforts would be a level of physical and mental health that would make for social well-being within the social system in which the individual must live, and that would provide opportunity for personal productivity and self-fulfillment. Health workers, therefore, work at three levels: (1) personal health care, (2) control of devastating epidemics, and (3) promotion and maintenance of general health levels adequate to enable individuals to achieve self-fulfillment.

Causes of change in concepts of disease and health

A number of factors in this rapidly evolving society have contributed to changes in health values and practices.

Scientific knowledge explosion. The accelerated pace of expansion of scientific knowledge challenges the medical profession's capacity to integrate and use it. Cures for specific diseases, a wide variety of therapeutic techniques, a panoply of pharmaceutical agents, constantly increasing knowledge of the body's intricate chemistry, and use of many delicate electronic and other instruments in diagnostic and therapeutic procedures have all become a regular part of medical care. This burgeoning knowledge in each field means that few persons can gain an adequate comprehension of more than one specialty. The benefits that specialization provide are obvious. However, as anyone who has ever visited a large clinic is aware, specialization (which from the point of view of the medical worker is necessary) means to the patient that services are fragmented. He feels further and further removed from his doctor and from allied workers in the health professions. He feels that no one member of the health team sees him as a total person. To the medical worker, the patient often becomes the forgotten man.

Population explosion. Already in some parts of the world, the population has increased beyond the available food supply. In their disturbing new book, *Famine— 1975!*, William and Paul Paddock[1] write of the inevitability of famine because of the rapid increase in world population and the decrease in food production resources. They show why famine cannot be evaded in underdeveloped nations, and they point out the critical questions that the affluent nations must consider concerning the use of resources.

Sociologist Kingsley Davis,[2] reports that the approximately 3.5 billion people of the world are multiplying so fast that, if the present rate continues, the population will double about every thirty years. Within 200 years, according to Davis, the world population would be approximately 230 billion—nearly 70 times the present total.

In America, this population increase has been reflected not only in total numbers, but also in percentage shifts in age and location. For example, there is an increasing percentage of older people and there is greater overall mobility. Urban-suburban trends have created changes in individual psychologic patterns, in family patterns, and in community and national social patterns. All of these changes affect health needs and social values.

Social revolution. Radical changes in family and community patterns have come with the development of the urban-suburban complex in a highly industrialized society. Crowded, low-income housing in the cities contrasts with sprawling, affluent suburbs which consume, at an alarming rate, open land that was once used for agriculture. While the food-eating population grows, the food-bearing potential of the land is being rapidly destroyed. Economic affluence, higher costs of living, and more emphasis on higher education, (all in the face of poverty pockets in urban and some rural areas) have changed human goals, health values, and medical care programs.

Development of the social sciences. The behavioral sciences (psychology, sociology, and anthropology) are contributing insights concerning human behavior and response to illness, and there is a new effort within the health professions to understand and help the total patient. More time is devoted to analysis of the impact of social and cultural factors upon human life. The functional illness is recognized as a very real phenomenon and the medical profession is beginning to realize that an individual's life situation and his reaction to stress must be considered if his total health needs are to be met.

However, the recognition that the social sciences are basic to medicine and nutrition is still in the course of a slow development. It is significant, however, that an increasing number of current texts emphasize this combined approach.[3]

EFFECT OF CHANGE AND DEVELOPMENT ON HEALTH CARE PRACTICES

Scientific and social developments, together with the changing attitudes toward health and disease, have produced some profound effects upon the kind of health services provided to the individual patient by physicians, dentists, nurses, nutritionists, social workers, and other health personnel. Two effects of these changes, particularly, touch the nurse and involve her application of nutritional sciences to her practice. The nurse must reconcile the possible conflict between the *science* and the *art* of nursing, and the nurse must function as a member of the *health team.*

The science and art of nursing

Science is a body of systematic knowledge, facts, and principles that shows the operation of natural law. The rapid advances in scientific knowledge have provided nursing and nutrition with a stronger basis on which to build professional practice. *Art* is an exceptional ability to conduct any human activity. Some writers believe there is conflict between the science and the art of professional nursing. One writer has labeled it a conflict between the roles of "mother surrogate" and "healer."[4] Do these two roles really conflict with one another? Or could they support one another? The nurse and the nutritionist must develop both aspects to the highest possible degree. Each must base her practice upon sound scientific knowledge and each must know and care about people and their needs. Scientific knowledge has little significance apart from application to human need. In each aspect of patient care, the nurse functions as the catalyst that brings scientific knowledge and human living together. She brings a particular knowledge and skill to bear upon the patient's need at a particular point in his life. Her role is shown diagrammatically in Fig. 1-1.

The health team approach

The health team approach has been devised as an attempt to meet some of the problems brought about by the rapid increase in population and the equally rapid expansion of scientific knowledge. It is based upon a recognition that two groups of persons are directly affected by these

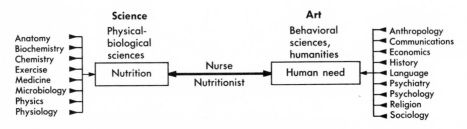

Fig. 1-1. The science and art of nutrition applied to human need.

developments—those in need of health care, and those who are trained to give health care.

The rapidly increasing number of people needing care has brought tremendous pressure upon community health resources. Physicians, charged with the major responsibility of medical care have felt this pressure most. They have realized that the time is long past when they can be all things to all people. The modern physician is usually interested in the building of an effective health care team.

The rapid advance of science has brought an increasing complexity to health care. The cooperation of a team of specialists is required, who share their special knowledge and learn from each other for the welfare of the patient. The care of the total patient also requires a wide range of facilities. Even the most elaborate facilities, however, are useless unless they are available to the people whom the health team seeks to serve.

Unique position of the nurse on the health team. Whether the nurse is functioning in the hospital, the clinic, or the community, she holds a position on the health team which places her in a unique relation to the patient. In certain respects, she is closest to the patient and his family. She has the opportunity to help determine many of the patient's needs, which include his basic nutritional requirements. She must coordinate services in his behalf. Often it is she alone who can help him understand and participate in his care. She has unparalleled opportunity to practice continuous, patient-centered care which treats the whole person. In carrying out the other aspect of her role, it will frequently be the nurse who reminds the entire health team that a person has emotional as well as physical needs, that he is part of a family whose members are also involved in his care, that he has an occupation, and that he lives in a specific community environment.

A number of leaders in nursing have defined the unique nature of nursing in these nurse-patient relationship terms. Joyce Travelbee has said, "Nursing needs are met by a nurse who possesses and uses a disciplined intellectual approach to patient problems combined with a therapeutic use of self."[5] Such a nurse knows and uses concepts and principles from the physical sciences as well as the social sciences. She can identify those principles that operate in a given nursing situation. She is concerned not merely with the *how* but also with the *why*. More pointedly still, she is concerned with the *who*, and realizes that her most therapeutic contribution is her genuine involvement and concern.

THE STUDY OF NUTRITION IN PROFESSIONAL NURSING EDUCATION

In the light of the preceding discussion the question, "What place does knowledge of nutrition have in the practice of my profession?" can be considered.

The answer to the question must be sought in the context of the ideas about what professional nursing entails that have been developed in this chapter. Food is fundamental to life and health, and a professional nurse is concerned with helping each person under her care to achieve his goals and to experience life and health to the fullest possible degree. The answer to the question lies in recognizing the evolving nature of professional nursing in a rapidly changing society. Since nutrition and nursing are integral parts of the health care professions, the nutritionist and the nurse must be sensitive to current and future health needs, and they must use these insights in setting their professional directions.

The plan of study

Basic objective. The basic objective of this book is twofold. The objective is to provide sound, relevant background knowledge in the science of human nutrition, and then to translate the scientific principles of nutrition into clear concepts with significant application to patient-centered nursing care.

In this person-centered approach, the science of nutrition is applied to individuals and their families in various situations, and in the stress situation of illness.

Method. Four areas of nutrition in nursing will be considered: (1) the scientific basis of nutrition, (2) nutrition as a part of public health, (3) the importance of nutrition in nursing specialties, such as maternity, obstetric, geriatric, and psychiatric nursing, and (4) the role of nutrition in clinical dietetics.

Unit I, "Foundations of Nutrition," presents the fundamental principles of nutrition as they relate to human life and growth, and emphasizes the scientific base of nutrition. In applying the scientific method to the study of man, the whole must be considered first and then each component part is studied in turn. This is the *analytical* method of scientific investigation. However, man exists not in parts, but as a coordinated whole. The attempt is therefore made in each case to achieve a *synthesis*, which will relate each part to the whole. Emphasis will be placed on the fact that the unity of the whole is maintained by means of interrelationships between all the chemical elements and functions in the body.

In the spirit of mutual and open inquiry, this unit will be concerned with the basic nutrients (carbohydrates, fats, proteins), their nature, their fate and function in the body, and with the regulatory roles of the accessory factors (vitamins and minerals). This unit will also be concerned with the way man secures energy for his many life needs. In addition, the vital balance between water and electrolytes, and the maintenance of the acid–base equilibrium will be discussed. Finally, the interrelationships in the overall process of digestion, absorption, and metabolism will be summarized.

Unit II, "Applied Nutrition in Public Health," applies the basic elements of nutritional science to man as he lives from day to day. This unit will deal with factors important in any nursing situation, but will present facts which are particularly applicable to public health nursing. Unit II will be concerned with the reasons for and the dangers of food faddism. It will also be concerned with the community food supply and how it is protected, and with cultural food patterns and the significant cohesive force they exert on man's community life. The cost of food and the wise use of the family food dollar, especially at low-income levels will be considered. The unit will also consider ways of teaching nutrition in community settings, the need for family counseling, the use of dietary guides, and the basic nutritional deficiency diseases.

Unit III, "Nutrition in the Nursing Specialty," applies nutritional knowledge to the various nursing specialties. The fundamental experience of birth and growth is the background for the Chapter on "Nutrition during Pregnancy and Lactation." This chapter considers the nutritional needs of the expectant mother and her newborn infant. The chapter on "Nutrition for Growth and Development" focuses upon the nutritional needs of the growing child. In special needs, such as toxemias of pregnancy and deficiency diseases of childhood, modifications or emphases of diet therapy are correlated with the specific condition. Other sections of Unit III are devoted to nutritional aspects of geriatric, psychiatric, and rehabilitation nursing.

Unit IV, "Nutrition in Medical-Surgical Nursing," applies basic nutritional science to the care of persons with specific diseases, on the premise that sound optimum nutrition is a primary consideration in any illness and that therapeutic diets should modify an adequate diet only so far as is necessary to meet a specific condition. The introductory section deals with the study and care of the hospitalized patient, and recognizes the stress that illness and hospitalization impose upon him. Other chapters deal with clinical diet therapy in medical-surgical nursing with emphasis upon the health teaching function of the nurse.

Tools for study

To aid and focus the overall study of nutrition and diet therapy, several learning devices will be used.

Concepts. Each idea is considered first from the point of view of basic principles, which are then applied to specific situations.

Terms. Words are important vehicles for communicating ideas. Many key words will be analyzed, and their derivations will be considered. To illustrate, the English word *concept* comes from a Latin root verb, *capere,* which means "to seize." The prefix *con-* is a derived form of the Latin word *cum,* meaning "with." Combining the two parts, the literal meaning of "concept" is "to seize with" which means that one idea is "seized" and put "with" other ideas to construct a mental image of the whole idea. Diagrams will also be used in this book to further illustrate concepts. At the end of some chapters there will be a glossary of the key terms that have been introduced in the chapter. These do not simply contain dictionary definitions, but have brief explanations of the concepts represented by the words. These glossaries should be useful tools for review.

Questions. When introducing basic material, salient questions will often be raised to stimulate the search for answers. A spirit of open inquiry is an important attitude to form in any scientific study. These questions will also serve as hooks on which to hang subsequent learning.

General and specific references. As a stimulus to still further inquiry and reading, references are given at the end of each chapter. These include basic texts in the subject area, articles of related interest in journals, bulletins, pamphlets, and reviews. Also, at various points there will be boxes entitled "To Probe Further." These offer additional material designed to take the curious student a step further with explanatory material or research on which theories are based.

Clinical application. Abstract theory is of little practical value. It finds meaning only as it is applied to real situations. Throughout this study, emphasis will be placed upon application of the nutritional science principles to specific clinical situations and individual needs. This book will look into the *why* of certain observations. The rationale for treatment and nursing care will be considered both in general terms and on an individual patient basis.

Results of this approach to study of nutrition. The nursing profession will be enriched as it outgrows the image of nutrition as a sterile, stereotyped, and often irrelevant set of diet lists and learns to take into consideration the fascinating subtleties of man's relationship to his food. The hospitalized patient looks forward to three events during each day—the doctor's visit, the visit of loved ones, and the food tray. Man's hunger and its fulfillment must be placed in proper perspective as basic to vital, patient-centered care. The nurse must realize that food bears the imprint of man's culture, and that it reflects the person's attitudes and the pattern of his social group. Nothing is more basic than food to an individual's physical existence and maintenance of health.

Recognizing the importance of food will deepen and facilitate patient care. It will help the nurse (1) to think of patients as individual, unique human beings with specific needs, (2) to think of nursing as a person-centered profession, and (3) to think of nutrition as a dynamic applied science which deals with both physical and psychosocial components. Nutrition as a science and an art is not applicable only to the patient on a special diet. It is a constant vital part of person-centered nursing care for every patient.

References
Specific
1. Paddock, W., and Paddock, P.: Famine—1975! America's decision: who will survive?, Boston, 1967, Little, Brown and Company.
2. Davis, K.: The world's population crisis. In Merton, R. K., and Nisbet, R. A., editors: Contemporary social problems, New York, 1966, Harcourt, Brace & World, Inc., p. 374.
3. Beland, I. L.: Clinical nursing: pathophysiological and psychosocial approaches, New York, 1965, The Macmillan Company.
4. Schulman, S.: Basic functional roles in nursing: mother surrogate and healer. In Jaco, E. G., editor: Patients, physicians, and illness, New York, 1958, The Free Press, p. 528.
5. Travelbee, J.: Interpersonal aspects of nurs-

ing, Philadelphia, 1966, F. A. Davis Company, p. 14.

General

American Journal of Public Health Vol. 57: No. 7, July 1967, Entire issue. Papers from 1966 meeting of the American Public Health Association, San Francisco, Special Sessions: Impact of recent federal legislation on personal health services.

American Public Health Association, Program Area Committee on Medical Care Administration: A guide to medical care administration. Vol. 1. Concepts and principles, New York, 1965.

Brown, E. L.: Newer dimensions of patient care. Part 3. Patients as people, New York, 1964, Russell Sage Foundation.

Bulletin of the New York Academy of Medicine, 1965 Health Conference: Closing the gaps in the availability and accessibility of health services, 41(12), 1965.

Bulletin of the New York Academy of Medicine, 1966 Health Conference: New directions in public policy for health care, 42(12), 1966.

Cassel, J.: Social and cultural implications of food and food habits, Amer. J. Public Health 47:732, 1957.

Folta, J. R., and Deck, E. S.: A sociological framework for patient care, New York, 1966, John Wiley & Sons, Inc.

Henderson, V.: The nature of nursing, New York, 1966, The Macmillan Company.

Katz, A. H., and Felton, J. S., editors: Health and the community, New York, 1965, The Free Press.

Knutson, A. L.: The individual, society, and health behavior, New York, 1965, Russell Sage Foundation.

Kron, T.: Nursing team leadership, Philadelphia, 1965, W. B. Saunders Co.

Lee, D.: Cultural factors in dietary choice, Amer. J. Clin. Nutr. **5:**166, 1957.

Macgregor, F. C.: Social science in nursing, New York, 1965, John Wiley & Sons, Inc.

Merton, R. K., and Nisbet, R. A., editors: Contemporary social problems, New York, 1966, Harcourt, Brace & World, Inc.

Morris, E.: How does a nurse teach nutrition to patients? Amer. J. Nurs. **60:**1, 1960.

Orlando, I. J.: The dynamic nurse-patient relationship, New York, 1961, G. P. Putnam's Sons.

Tao-Kim-Hai, A. M.: Orientals are stoic, *The New Yorker* Sept. 28, 1957. Reprinted in Macgregor, F. C.: Social science in nursing, New York, 1965, John Wiley & Sons, Inc., p. 313.

CHAPTER 2

Carbohydrates

Over the ages, of all the basic nutrients that sustain man, carbohydrates have been of prime importance. Four factors have contributed to this primacy.

Availability. Carbohydrates comprise a large part of the world's available food supply. They are widely distributed in such easily grown plants as grains, vegetables, and fruits. In fact, in some countries these carbohydrate foods make up almost the entire diet of the people. Even in America, where a greater dietary variety is available, about 50% of the total caloric intake is in the form of carbohydrates.

Low cost. As a result of their wide distribution and supply, carbohydrate foods are relatively inexpensive. If the general income level of a people or an individual family lowers, the proportion of carbohydrate foods consumed rises. This becomes a special concern for the nurse and the nutritionist dealing with low income families.

Ease of storage. Compared with other types of food, carbohydrate foods (grains and some fruits and vegetables) can be kept in dry storage for relatively long periods of time without spoilage. In many countries modern processing and packaging have extended the shelf life of carbohydrate products almost indefinitely. On the other hand, protein foods (such as meat and dairy products) must be kept under refrigeration.

Energy value. Because of the readily available glucose equivalent of carbohydrates, man depends upon them for a main fuel source. The body rapidly oxidizes starches and sugars to yield carbon dioxide and water; this process is a major source of body heat and energy.

GENERAL AND CHEMICAL DEFINITIONS OF CARBOHYDRATES

General definition. For practical purposes in the discussion of dietetics, carbohydrates are starches and sugars. Plants are the main source of carbohydrate in the human diet. These food materials are produced by *photosynthesis* from carbon dioxide and water in the presence of sunlight and the plant's chlorophyll. The carbohydrate product is then stored in the various plant parts such as root, pod, seed, fruit, stem, or leaf. From animals, a lesser source, come carbohydrates in such forms as lactose (milk sugar) and fructose (the sugar in honey).

Chemical definition. Carbohydrates may be further defined according to their chemical elements—carbon, hydrogen, and oxygen. The hydrogen and oxygen occur in the same 2 : 1 ratio as that found in water (2 hydrogen atoms to 1 oxygen atom; H_2O), although the chemical joining differs from that in water. The name, "carbo-hydrate," originally given to this group of food substances to indicate their basic chemical composition, fails to point out this different type of chemical joining.

The basic chemical structure of the simple sugars is a carbon chain, ranging from three to seven carbon atoms, with the hydrogen and oxygen atoms attached singly and in alcohol or aldehyde groups. The most common carbon chain length is the 6-carbon chain—hexose. Of the hexoses,

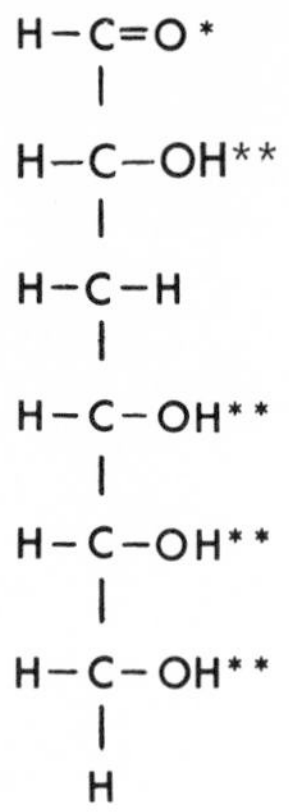

```
      H−C=O *
        |
      H−C−OH**
        |
      H−C−H
        |
      H−C−OH**
        |
      H−C−OH**
        |
      H−C−OH**
        |
        H
```

* Aldehyde group

** Alcohol group

Fig. 2-1. Chemical structure of d-glucose.

glucose $(C_6H_{12}O_6)$, the most common simple sugar, serves as a good example of the structure (Fig. 2-1).

CLASSIFICATION OF CARBOHYDRATES

Monosaccharides. The simplest form of carbohydrate is the *monosaccharide*, often called simple sugar (Gr. *monos,* single or alone; L. *saccharum,* sugar). The monosaccharides are grouped according to the number of carbon atoms in their basic chain structure:

Trioses—3 carbons
Tetroses—4 carbons
Pentoses—5 carbons
Hexoses—6 carbons
Heptoses—7 carbons

The *hexoses* are more important nutritionally and physiologically than all the others combined. The four monosaccharides in the hexose group are glucose, fructose, galactose, and mannose.

Glucose (also called dextrose because it is the *dextro*rotatory form of this molecule) is a moderately sweet sugar. It is found as preformed natural glucose in foods, or is formed in the body from starch digestion. In human metabolism, all other types of sugar are converted by the body into glucose. Glucose is the form in which sugar circulates in the blood stream and it is oxidized to give energy.

Fructose (also called levulose because it is the *levo*rotatory form of the molecule) is the sugar found in fruits and honey. It is the sweetest of the simple sugars. In human metabolism, it is converted to glucose for energy.

Galactose is not found free in foods, but is produced from lactose (milk sugar), and is then changed to glucose for energy. The

---

TO PROBE FURTHER
Monosaccharide combinations

Also of interest and importance in medicine and allied fields are combination forms of monosaccharide.

A *glycoside* is a monosaccharide plus a noncarbohydrate residue in the same molecule. Examples are the digitalis derivatives, which form drugs essential to cardiac therapy, and steroids, the adrenal hormones.

A *deoxy sugar* is a sugar with fewer oxygen than carbon atoms. An important and familiar example in physiology is *deoxyribose*, which occurs in nucleic acids such as *deoxyribonucleic acid* (DNA). DNA is the cellular substance that is believed to transmit genetic characteristics.

Amino sugars are sugars that contain an amino group (NH_2). An important example of their occurrence is in antibiotics such as the *mycin drugs.* The presence of these sugars is believed to give the antibiotic activity to such drugs.

reaction is reversible, and during lactation glucose may be reconverted to galactose, for the lactose component in breast milk is produced from galactose.

Mannose, a relative unimportant sugar in human nutrition, is not found free in foods, but is derived from certain gums.

Disaccharides. Disaccharides (Gr. *di-,* twice, double) are more complex sugars, made up of two monosaccharides. The three main disaccharides with their two component monosaccharides are:

sucrose = glucose + fructose
lactose = glucose + galactose
maltose = glucose + glucose

In each of these disaccharides glucose is one of the two components.

Sucrose (common table sugar) is the most prevalent dietary disaccharide, and it contributes about 25% of the total carbohydrate calories. It is found in many food sources, including cane and beet sugar, brown sugar, sorghum cane and molasses, maple syrup, pineapple, and carrot roots.

Lactose is the sugar in milk. It is formed in the body from glucose to supply the carbohydrate component of milk during lactation. It is the least sweet of the disaccharides, about one-sixth as sweet as sucrose. It is often used in high carbohydrate, high calorie liquid feedings when the needed quantity of sucrose cannot be tolerated. When milk sours, as in the initial stages of cheese making, the lactose is changed to lactic acid and separates in the liquid whey from the remaining solid curd. The curd is then processed for cheese. Therefore, although milk has a relatively

high carbohydrate content (lactose), one of its main products—cheese—has none.

Maltose occurs in malt products and in germinating cereals. As such, it is a negligible dietary carbohydrate. However, it is important as an intermediate product of starch digestion.

Relative sweetness of the sugars. With sucrose as a base for comparison given a value of 100, the general relative sweetness of the common sugars has been evaluated as follows:

Fructose	110 to 175
Sucrose	100
Glucose	75
Galactose	35 to 70
Lactose	15 to 30

Polysaccharides. Polysaccharides are even more complex carbohydrates, made up of many units of one monosaccharide.

Starch is the most significant polysaccharide in human nutrition. It is a compound made up of glucose chains, hence it yields only glucose upon hydrolysis or digestion. Starch granules vary in size and shape according to the source (Fig. 2-2). Potato granules, for example, are relatively large, while rice granules are small.

Starch is by far the most important source of carbohydrate, and accounts for approximately 50% of the total carbohydrate intake in the American diet. In other countries, where it is the staple food substance, it makes up an even higher proportion of the total diet. Major food sources include cereal grains, potatoes and other root vegetables, and legumes.

The cooking of starch not only improves

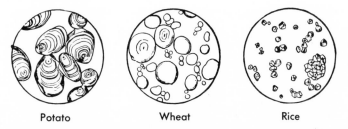

Potato   Wheat   Rice

Fig. 2-2. Starch granules of different sizes from different sources. (From Fearon, W. R.: An introduction to biochemistry, ed. 2, St. Louis, 1940, The C. V. Mosby Co.)

flavor, but also softens and ruptures the starch cells, which facilitates enzymatic digestive processes. The reason that starch mixtures thicken when cooked is that the amylopectin which encases the starch granules has a gel quality; this thickens in the same way that fruit pectin causes jelly to set.

Dextrins are polysaccharide compounds which are intermediate products of starch breakdown in the formation of maltose:

(ptyalin)
Starch + water → Soluble starch + maltose

(ptyalin)
Soluble starch + water → Erythrodextrins + maltose

(ptyalin)
Erythrodextrins + water → Achroodextrins + maltose

(ptyalin)
Achroodextrins + water → maltose

This breakdown is accomplished physiologically as a normal part of the body's digestion of starch (starch → dextrins → maltose → glucose), or commercially by a process of acid hydrolysis. Dextrins form a soluble, gummy carbohydrate which is used commercially as mucilage for envelopes and postage stamps or as sizing for adhesive tape. Dextri-Maltose, an infant formula preparation, is a combination of dextrins and maltose.

Cellulose is a form of polysaccharide that is resistant to the digestive enzymes in man. It remains in the digestive tract and contributes important bulk to the diet. This bulk helps to move the digestive food mass along and stimulates peristalsis. Cellulose forms the supporting framework of plants. The main sources are the stems and leaves of vegetables, seed and grain coverings, skins, and hulls.

Pectins are nondigestible, colloidal polysaccharides. They are found mostly in fruits, and possess a thickening quality. They are often used as a base for fruit jellies. This ability to solidify to a gel also makes them useful in cosmetics and drugs.

Glycogen is often called animal starch. It is formed from glucose and is stored in the liver and in muscle tissue. Chief food sources of glycogen are meat and seafood. Since it is formed from glucose, it yields only glucose upon digestion.

Inulin, a polysaccharide composed of fructose units, has little dietary significance. It is found only in a few common foods, such as onions, garlic, and artichokes. It is only partially digested, although further breakdown by bacteria may occur in the large intestine. Storage of inulin-containing foods also affects this carbohydrate. The fresh food may have much of its carbohydrate in this unavailable inulin form, however, upon storage much of the inulin may be converted to available sugar.

Although inulin is of small dietary significance, it is of interest and importance in medicine and nursing because it provides a test of renal function. Since inulin is filtered at the glomerulus, but neither secreted nor reabsorbed by the tubule, it can be used to measure glomerular filtration rate. This test is called the *inulin clearance test.*

FUNCTIONS OF CARBOHYDRATES IN THE BODY

Energy. The prime, overall function of carbohydrate in human nutrition is to provide energy. Although fat also is a fuel, it is primarily a storage form and the body may function without it. However, the body tissues require a constant dietary supply of carbohydrate to exist. The metabolic interrelationships involved are further discussed in this chapter in the section concerning the Krebs cycle (see pp. 23 and 24).

The amount of carbohydrate in the body is relatively small. A total of approximately 365 gm. is stored in the liver and the muscle tissues, and is present in circulating blood sugar. The following shows the breakdown of carbohydrate storage in the body of a man weighing 70 kg.

Liver glycogen	110 gm.
Muscle glycogen	245 gm.
Extracellular blood sugar	10 gm.
Total	365 gm.
	(1,460 calories)

The 365 gm. of glucose provide energy sufficient for only about thirteen hours of very moderate activity. Carbohydrates must be ingested regularly and at moderately frequent intervals to meet the energy demands of the body.

Of the total carbohydrate ingested, however, three general factors affect the amount that will be available for use, and the way that the body will use it:

1. The state of the mucous membrane of the digestive tract and the time the carbohydrate is held in contact with this absorbing surface affects the availability of carbohydrates. Intestinal diseases affecting the bowel lining or a hyperactive bowel (which causes rapid passage of food materials) greatly decreases the proportion of the total ingested carbohydrate that will be used by the body.

2. Endocrine function is also important in carbohydrate availability. Several hormones play important roles in the use of carbohydrate. Among these are insulin and the several insulin antagonists such as hormones secreted by the pituitary gland, steroids secreted from the adrenal glands, glucagon secreted by the pancreas, and epinephrine secreted by the adrenal medulla. Imbalance among these various regulatory agents can greatly affect the body's use of carbohydrate.

3. Vitamins must be present in adequate amounts. Vitamins of the B complex, especially, are involved in the metabolism of carbohydrate. Thiamine, niacin, riboflavin, and others perform key functions in the enzyme systems for the oxidation of carbohydrate.

Special functions of carbohydrates in vital organs. In addition to their overall function as the body's main energy source, carbohydrate also serves special functions in certain vital organs.

Liver. In the liver, carbohydrate is not only oxidized as fuel, but also serves two other important functions. First, it exerts a protective action by being present as glycogen, and by participating in specific detoxifying metabolic pathways. For example,

a glucose derivative, glucuronic acid, conjugates with certain toxic materials (drugs) to produce harmless forms for excretion.

Second, carbohydrate has a regulating influence on protein and fat metabolism. The presence of sufficient carbohydrate for energy demands prevents the channeling of too much protein for this purpose. This *protein-sparing action* of carbohydrate allows a major portion of protein to be used for its basic structural purpose of tissue building. The amount of carbohydrate present also determines how much fat will be broken down. Therefore, it affects the formation and disposal rates of ketones. Ketones are intermediate products of fat metabolism, which normally are broken down to fatty acids. However, in extreme conditions (such as starvation or uncontrolled diabetes) in which carbohydrate is inadequate or unavailable, the ketones accumulate and produce a condition called ketosis or acidosis (see p. 24). The *antiketogenic effect* of carbohydrate prevents a damaging excess of ketone formation and accumulation.

Heart. Heart action is a life-sustaining muscular exercise. The glycogen in cardiac muscle is an important emergency source of contractile energy. In a damaged heart, poor glycogen stores or a low carbohydrate intake may cause cardiac symptoms or angina.

Central nervous system. A constant amount of carbohydrate is necessary for the proper functioning of the central nervous system. Its regulatory center, the brain, contains no stored supply of glucose and is, therefore, especially dependent upon a minute-to-minute supply of glucose from the blood. Sustained and profound hypoglycemic shock may cause irreversible brain damage. In all nerve tissue carbohydrate is indispensable for functional integrity.

DIGESTION OF CARBOHYDRATE

The digestion of carbohydrate proceeds through the successive parts of the gastrointestinal tract, aided by both mechanical and chemical processes. The chemical processess involved are enzymatic in nature.

Table 2-1. Summary of carbohydrate digestion

Organ	Enzyme	Action
Mouth	Ptyalin	Starch → Dextrins → Maltose
Stomach	None	(Above action continued to minor degree)
Small intestine	Pancreatic	
	Amylopsin	Starch → Dextrins → Maltose
	Intestinal	
	Sucrase	Sucrose → Glucose + Fructose
	Lactase	Lactose → Glucose + Galactose
	Maltase	Maltose → Glucose + Glucose

An enzyme is a complex organic substance, produced in a living cell and capable of causing certain chemical changes in other organic materials by acting as a catalyst. These processes are explained in greater detail in Chapter 5.

Mouth. Mastication breaks the food into fine particles and mixes it with the saliva. During this process, a component enzyme of the saliva secreted by the parotid gland, *ptyalin,* acts upon starch to begin its breakdown into dextrins and maltose.

Stomach. Mechanical digestion is continued in the stomach by successive wavelike contractions of the muscle fibers of the stomach wall. This action, peristalsis, further mixes food particles with gastric secretions to allow the chemical activity of digestion to take place more readily. The gastric juice contains no specific enzyme for the breakdown of carbohydrate, and hydrochloric acid (HCl) in the stomach counteracts the alkaline activity of ptyalin. Mechanical digestion continues to bring the carbohydrate to the pyloric valve as part of the food mass, now a thick, creamy *chyme,* ready for emptying into the duodenum, the first portion of the small intestine.

Small intestine. Peristalsis continues to aid digestion in the small intestine by mixing and moving the chyme along the length of the tube. Chemical digestion of carbohydrate is completed in the small intestine by enzymes from two sources. (1) The *pancreatic juice,* which enters the duodenum through the common bile duct, contains an amylase, *amylopsin,* which continues the breakdown of starch to maltose. (2) The *intestinal juice* contains three disaccharidases, *sucrase, lactase,* and *maltase,* which act on their respective disaccharides to render the monosaccharides, glucose, galactose, and fructose, ready for absorption. Interestingly enough, these disaccharidases are almost exclusively *intracellular;* that is, they reside and carry on their activities within the cells of the mucosa (the inner layer of the intestinal wall). The digestion of disaccharides takes place, not in the lumen of the intestine, but within the intestinal mucosal cell.

A summary of the digestion of carbohydrate through these successive parts of the gastrointestinal tract is given in Table 2-1.

ABSORPTION OF CARBOHYDRATE INTO THE BLOODSTREAM

Carbohydrate is absorbed into the bloodstream as glucose, galactose, and fructose. The absorbing surface area of the small intestine is greatly enlarged by millions of villi, which are tiny, fingerlike projections of the mucous membrane. This large absorbing surface allows 90% of the digested food materials to be absorbed in the small intestine. Only water absorption remains to be accomplished in the large intestine.

By way of the capillaries of the villi, the simple sugars enter the portal circulation

TO PROBE FURTHER
The process of carbohydrate absorption

The process by which glucose and other monosaccharides are absorbed across the epithelial cells of the intestine is complex, and is another example of the specificity of the body's mechanisms. Classic research in the field of glucose absorption, synthesis to glycogen, and reconversion to glucose has been done by Drs. Carl and Gerty Cori* of Washington University School of Medicine. In 1947, they were awarded the Nobel Prize in Medicine for their work.

Their studies seem to indicate that the common hexose sugars are absorbed at a fixed, fairly rapid rate, which is independent of their concentration in the intestinal lumen, even against an osmotic gradient. Simple diffusion would be dependent solely upon the balance of osmotic forces on both sides of the cell wall. Therefore, it is evident that a mechanism other than diffusion is also operating here.

Moreover, the Coris' data indicate that the rates of absorption of the different monosaccharides are not alike. Giving glucose an absorption rate of 100, the comparative rates for the other main simple sugars are 110 for galactose and 43 for fructose. The work of other researchers† concerning glucose jejunal absorption bears out this relative rate. There seems, then, to be a *specific selectivity* in the absorption of these monosaccharides.

Two mechanisms apparently are involved in sugar absorption: (1) *simple diffusion,* dependent upon a greater sugar concentration within the intestinal lumen than in the mucosal cells and, in turn, in the blood plasma, and (2) *active transport* that requires energy, independent of the intestinal concentration (some sort of "pump"). This concept is further discussed in Chapter 10.

---

*Cori, C. F.: Mammalian carbohydrate metabolism, Physiol. Rev. **11**:143, 1931.
†Inglefinger, F. J.: Gastrointestinal absorption, Nutrition Today **2**:2, 1967.

and are transported to the liver. Here the fructose and galactose are converted to glucose, and the glucose is in turn converted to glycogen for storage. The glycogen is reconverted to glucose as needed by the body.

Factors influencing absorption

The absorption of digested carbohydrate is influenced by four factors.

1. The rate at which the carbohydrate enters the small intestine affects its absorption. This rate of entry depends upon the motility of the stomach and the control of the duodenal sphincter muscle, the pyloric valve.
2. The type of food mixture present in-fluences the degree of competition for absorbing sites and available carrier transport systems.
3. Absorption is also influenced by the condition of intestinal membranes and the time carbohydrate is held in contact with these membranes. Any abnormality of the mucosal tissue (enteritis, celiac disease), or an abnormally rapid movement of the carbohydrate along the intestine (diarrhea) will hinder absorption.
4. Normal endocrine activity of the anterior pituitary and the related functioning of the thyroid is necessary for normal absorption. In addition, the adrenal cortex hormones regulate the

TO PROBE FURTHER
Sodium-potassium pump

An interesting mechanism believed to be operative in glucose absorption demonstrates the principle of *intimate metabolic interrelatedness of the nutrients.* It has been called the sodium-potassium pump, because it controls the ratio of sodium to potassium ion concentrations outside and inside the cell (Fig. 2-3).

Current evidence indicates that the entrance of glucose into intestinal wall cells and hence into the blood is sodium-dependent. The work of R. K. Crane* has shown that a sodium deficiency inhibits glucose absorption. Moreover, when cells are incubated in a glucose-free environment, the pump is reversed: sodium and potassium leave the cell. When glucose is added, the pump reverts to its proper direction. This finely balanced homeostatic mechanism of active transport of glucose requires energy which is supplied by metabolic processes within the cell.

*Crane, R. K.: Intestinal absorption of sugars, Physiol. Rev. **40:**89, 1960; Hypothesis for mechanism of intestinal active transport of sugars, Fed. Proc. **21:**891, 1962.

body's sodium exchange, which indirectly influences the operation of the sodium pump.

METABOLISM OF CARBOHYDRATE

In this discussion and in those to follow concerning the other nutrients, a significant scientific principle will emerge. This principle may be stated as the *unity of the human organism.* The human organism is a whole made up of many parts and processes which possess unequalled specificity and flexibility. Intimate metabolic relationships exist between all the basic nutrients and metabolites, and it is impossible to understand any one of man's metabolic processes without viewing it in relationship to the others that comprise the whole.

Metabolism is the sum of the physical and chemical processes in a living organism by which protoplasm, the basic substance of cells and tissues, is produced, maintained, or destroyed; and by which energy is made available for the functioning of the organism. A *metabolite* is a product of a specific metabolic process.

Three terms of medical importance which

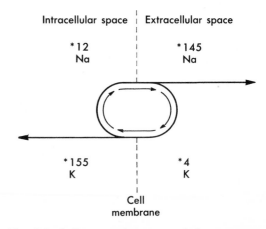

Fig. 2-3. Sodium-potassium pump. Active transport of ions across the cell membrane. (*Sodium and potassium concentration [mEq./L.] inside and outside the cell.)

relate to blood sugar levels should be clearly understood by the nurse who will constantly encounter them in clinical work. *Normoglycemic* refers to blood sugar levels within the range of normal; *hypoglycemic* indicates blood sugar levels below the normal range; *hyperglycemic* means blood sugar levels are above the normal range.

In cell nutrition, the most important end

product of the digestion of dietary carbohydrate is glucose since fructose and galactose are eventually converted to glucose. The liver is the major site of the fascinating metabolic machinery that handles glucose, and much of the chemical activity takes place there. However, other tissues such as adipose fat tissue, muscle tissue, and renal tissue play important roles, and energy metabolism in general goes on in all cells.

The answers to four basic questions concerning carbohydrate metabolism are important to understand how the body handles glucose:

1. What are the sources from which glucose enters the blood?
2. What happens to glucose in the blood and tissues?
3. What hormones control the metabolism of glucose?
4. How is energy produced from glucose?

Sources of blood glucose

The sources of blood glucose are divided into carbohydrate and noncarbohydrate substances.

Carbohydrate sources. Carbohydrate sources include dietary carbohydrate, glycogen, and products of intermediary carbohydrate metabolism.

Dietary carbohydrates are starches and sugars which are ingested, digested, and absorbed into the bloodstream. These form the major source of the body's glucose. *All* of these carbohydrate food materials are converted into glucose.

Glycogen (also called glucogen) is stored in the liver and is the second main source of blood glucose. The hydrolysis of glycogen to form glucose is called *glycogenolysis.*

Products of intermediary carbohydrate metabolism include lactic acid and pyruvic acid. These products are formed by reactions that may either proceed or return to their source material.

Noncarbohydrate sources. Protein and fat are the noncarbohydrate sources of glucose.

Certain *amino acids* are *glucogenic,* that is, they form glucose upon metabolic breakdown. After *deamination* (removal of the amino group, see p. 54), the remaining carbon chain forms the skeleton for glucose. This conversion process is catalyzed by adrenocortical steroids (such as cortisone). These steroids have, therefore, been called the S-hormones or sugar-forming hormones. About 58% of the protein in a mixed diet is composed of glycogenic amino acids. Therefore, it may be stated that more than half of the dietary protein, although it is consumed primarily for its tissue-building function, may ultimately be used for energy.

Fat is also converted into glucose. As will be seen later in greater detail in the discussion of fat metabolism (Chapter 3), after the breakdown of neutral fat into fatty acids and glycerol, the glycerol portion upon hydrolysis may be converted to glycogen in the liver, and made available for glucose formation. Since glycerol comprises only about 10% of the fat, it normally contributes very little available glucose. However, under abnormal conditions of carbohydrate metabolism, as in diabetes mellitus, fat assumes a much more significant role in the complicating condition of ketosis.

The production of glucose from protein, fat and the various intermediate carbohydrate metabolites is call *gluconeogenesis.*

Glucose in the blood and tissues

The body has several means of handling glucose. The blood sugar may be (1) burned for energy, (2) stored for reserve use, or (3) converted to other forms of nutrient. Together these uses of glucose serve to regulate the blood sugar to a normal range of 70 to 120 mg. per. 100 ml.

The primary function of glucose is to supply energy according to the body's demands. Various metabolic pathways are used to accomplish this task in a highly efficient manner. The two main oxidative

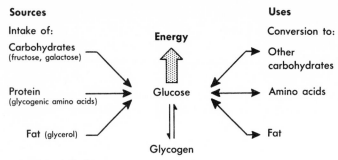

Fig. 2-4. Sources and uses of glucose.

pathways, the Embden-Meyerhof glycolytic pathway and the Krebs cycle, together form one continuous pathway (see pp. 22-25).

There are two major processes that convert glucose to storage forms. Glucose may be converted to glycogen and stored as such in the liver and in muscle tissue. This conversion process is called *glycogenesis.* The capacity for this type of storage is limited. Only a small supply of glycogen is present at any one time, and it may be depleted rapidly. After energy demands have been fulfilled by oxidation of glucose and a limited amount has been stored for circulation and emergency reserves, any excess glucose is converted to adipose tissue and stored as fat. This process of conversion to fat is called *lipogenesis.* The capacity for this type of storage seems to be unlimited, to judge from the everyday observation of some human beings!

Some glucose is used in the production of various compounds which are important to the total functioning of the body. A relatively small amount of glucose goes into other carbohydrate compounds which have significant roles in overall body metabolism. Examples of these are:

1. Ribose and deoxyribose, required for nucleic acids in the formation of DNA and RNA; believed to be key substances in genetic inheritance
2. Mannose, glucosamine, and galactosamine, required, for mucopolysaccharides and glycoproteins, such as heparin and blood group materials responsible for the major blood types
3. Glucuronic acid, involved in various

detoxification reactions by which the body excretes certain harmful substances

4. Galactose, required for glycolipids and for lactose during the lactation period

Certain amino acids that are synthesized in the body derive their carbon skeletons from glucose or its metabolites (see Chapter 4).

These sources and uses of glucose act as checks and balances to maintain the blood sugar within its normal range by adding sugar to the blood or removing it, so that the body maintains a fairly constant internal environment which enables it to meet changing demands and stresses. This is but one more example of the remarkable *homeostatic* mechanisms of the body, built in to sustain life and promote health (Fig. 2-4).

Hormones that control metabolism of glucose

A number of hormones directly and indirectly influence the metabolism of glucose and regulate the blood sugar level according to the body's need. These hormones may be classified according to whether they lower or raise the blood sugar level.

Hormone that lowers the blood sugar level. Insulin is the only hormone that lowers the blood sugar. This hormone is perhaps more widely known than all the others. Insulin is produced by beta cells of the pancreas, which are specialized for this purpose. The beta cells form "islands" in the pancreatic tissue, and are called the *islets of Langerhans,* named for the scientist who discovered and studied them.

Insulin fosters *glycogenesis* by conversion of glucose to glycogen in the liver, where the glycogen is then stored.

Insulin also fosters *lipogenesis,* which is the formation of fat. Glucose is converted to fat for storage in adipose (fat depository) tissue. This conversion takes place mainly in the adipose tissue itself, but some glucose is converted to fat in the liver (see pp. 37 and 38).

Insulin increases *cell permeability to glucose*, and allows glucose to pass from the extracellular fluids into the cells for oxidation to supply needed energy. The precise mechanism by which this is accomplished is not determined, but studies[1-4] indicate that a definite glucose-carrier system exists. Evidence demonstrates that in the presence of insulin, entry of sugar into cells is accelerated. Conversely, in the absence of insulin, sugar is prevented from entering. The cell wall presents a barrier to glucose and an active transfer system is necessary to carry it into the cells. Insulin in some way acts upon such a transfer system.

There is evidence that potassium as well as insulin is necessary for glucose entry into cells. When glucose enters the cell, potassium enters with it. Evidence for this association of potassium with glucose can be seen in the uptake of potassium in patients with diabetic acidosis who are treated with insulin. This makes replacement potassium an important part of treatment.

Apparently the cell's dependence upon insulin for glucose entry differs in various tissues. For example, studies[5] indicate that glucose uptake is unaffected by the absence of insulin in the brain, red blood cells, intestinal mucosa, kidney tubules, and probably the liver. Tissues dependent upon the presence of insulin for glucose uptake are skeletal muscle, adipose tissue, cardiac muscle, eye lens, the aqueous humor, leukocytes, and pituitary tissue.

Although some of the evidence may be inconclusive, insulin is also believed to influence *phosphorylation*. Phosphorylation is the initial and necessary phosphorus coupling step that allows glucose to enter the cell's metabolic pathway to produce energy. According to this theory[6,7] insulin acts upon antagonists to the reaction to prevent them from inhibiting the action of *glucokinase* (the specific hexokinase needed to catalyze glucose phosphorylation).

Much evidence[8] exists that insulin promotes *protein synthesis*. However, this may be an indirect result of the increase in energy available for tissue building, which has been facilitated by glucose oxidation.

Hormones that raise the blood sugar level. A number of hormones effectively raise the blood sugar. These include glucagon, steroid hormones, epinehprine, the growth hormone, ACTH, and thyroxine.

Glucagon is also produced by the islets of Langerhans in the pancreas. However, it is produced in the alpha cells and has an effect opposite to that of insulin. Glucagon raises the blood sugar level by increasing hepatic *glycogenolysis*, the breakdown of liver glycogen to glucose. It probably does this by activating the hepatic enzyme catalyst for this conversion, phosphorylase. Glucagon may well be an important factor in maintaining the blood sugar level during starvation.

The *steroid hormones* of the adrenal cortex raise the blood sugar level by stimulating *gluconeogenesis,* which releases glucose-forming carbon units from protein. The steroids also act as insulin antagonists and block the sugar-lowering effect of insulin.

Epinephrine, which is secreted by the adrenal medulla also raises the blood sugar level by stimulating *glycogenolysis*. Epinephrine is sometimes administered to diabetic patients in insulin shock to counteract severe hypoglycemia. Epinephrine causes a quick release of readily available glucose for immediate use. Apparently epinephrine also influences the resynthesis and reactivation of phosphorylase in liver and muscle.

Growth hormone (GH) and *adrenocorticotrophic hormone (ACTH)* are hormones

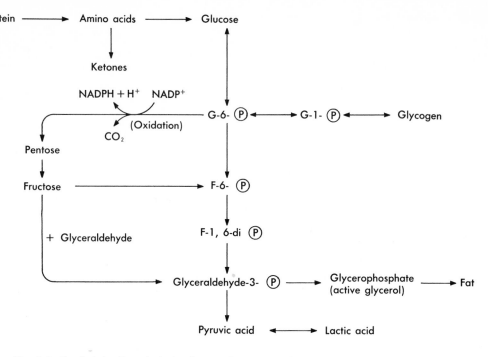

Fig. 2-5. The Embden-Meyerhof glycolytic pathway. F, fructose; G, glucose; P, phosphate; NADP, niacin adenine dinucleotide phosphate; NADPH, same as NADP, carrying H.

secreted by the anterior pituitary gland. They raise the blood sugar level by acting as insulin antagonists.

The principal hormone secreted by the thyroid gland, *thyroxine,* has an elevating effect on blood sugar, probably because it influences the rate of insulin destruction, increases glucose absorption from the intestine, and liberates epinephrine.

Energy production from glucose

Once in the cell, glucose must undergo a series of reactions to produce energy for the body's varied demands. Two major pathways, which together form one continuous overall route, are most commonly used. By this route, glucose is broken down into the end products of carbon dioxide and water. Large amounts of energy are generated in the process of breakdown.

Embden-Meyerhof pathway. Through this initial glycolytic pathway glucose is converted to glycogen and glycogen to glucose. Glucose is also carried to pyruvic

and lactic acids (Fig. 2-5). Several important steps along this pathway illustrate the principle of the metabolic interrelatedness of nutrients in human nutrition.

Initial phosphorylation is the first step in a series of reactions. This process adds phosphorus to glucose. The phosphorus traps the glucose in the cell and forms the compound glucose-6-phosphate which begins the series of reactions that constitute the Embden-Meyerhof pathway. Phosphate compounds are closely connected with the chemical energy bonds developed during the process of oxidation. An example is ATP (adenosine triphosphate), a compound with high energy bonds which stores the energy produced during glucose oxidation (p. 64). The phosphorylation reaction is catalyzed by the enzyme glucokinase, which is the glucose-specific hexokinase. This reaction is believed to be one of the key points at which insulin acts.

The reaction which forms *glycogen* is reversible. Glucose can be removed from the blood to be stored as glycogen, or gly-

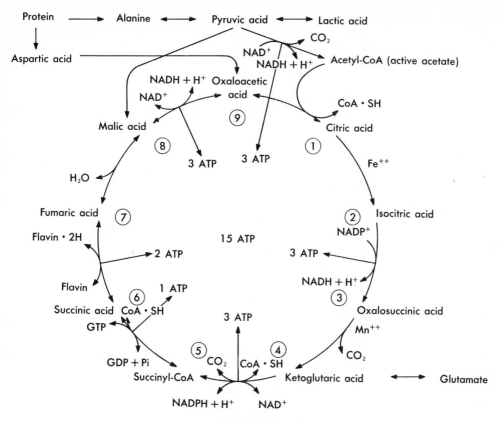

Fig. 2-6. The Krebs cycle. NAD, niacin adenine dinucleotide; NADP, niacin adenine dinucleotide phosphate; NADPH, same as NADP, carrying H; ATP, adenosine triphosphate.

cogen can be broken down to form blood glucose.

Glyceraldehyde-3-phosphate provides the active form of glycerol needed for *lipogenesis* (the synthesis of fat from carbohydrate).

The formation of *pyruvic acid*, together with its product, *lactic acid*, ends the glycolytic pathway. The formation of pyruvic acid is important as a junction point because (1) pyruvic acid is the gateway to the final common pathway, the Krebs cycle and, (2) it provides the vital acetyl CoA (active acetate), the metabolic step through which fatty acids (and in turn fat) are produced from glucose.

Krebs cycle. The Krebs (or citric acid) cycle is the final common pathway, which all nutrient metabolites involved in energy production finally enter in some form. It provides more than 90% of the body's

energy (Fig. 2-6). Several reaction products along this pathway demonstrate the interrelatedness of the nutrients.

Several B-complex vitamins are involved in the formation of *acetyl CoA* (active acetate). The compound itself contains pantothenic acid, which is one of the B vitamins. The formation of active acetate from pyruvic acid requires two other B vitamins, thiamine and lipoic acid, as coenzymes. The formation of active acetate is a major junction point which integrates carbohydrate, fat, and protein metabolism, for acetyl CoA can also be formed from fatty acids and certain amino acids.

Oxaloacetate (oxaloacetic acid) is formed from pyruvic acid as well as from certain amino acids. Active acetate reacts with oxaloacetate to form *citric acid*. Oxaloacetate is the necessary carbohydrate fuel to keep the process going, for with each complete cycle of reactions by which active acetate is broken down to produce carbon dioxide, water, and energy, another unit of oxaloacetate is produced which begins the process again. If there is not adequate oxaloacetate from carbohydrate to maintain the cycle efficiently, active acetate from fat cannot be handled properly and is diverted to form ketone bodies. Under usual circumstances, ketones may be considered normal intermediates of fat metabolism. However, when the amount of glucose available is insufficient to perpetuate this process, fat is broken down so rapidly that it cannot be used for fuel. Without the necessary carbohydrate to handle the fat properly the ketones accumulate, causing ketosis. These ketones are acids (acetoacetic acid, acetone, and beta-hydroxybutyric acid) and their accumulation upsets the normal acid-base balance in the body and acidosis results. Diabetic acidosis clearly demonstrates the interrelatedness of the nutrients and their metabolites. When glucose cannot be properly oxidized because insulin is lacking or unavailable, the oxaloacetate which is necessary to the maintenance of the Krebs cycle is not provided, and the active acetate from fat cannot be handled and instead is converted to ketones.

In summary, the Embden-Meyerhof pathway and the Krebs cycle serve several important metabolic functions:

1. They provide the body's major source of energy.
2. They provide glycogen formation and release.
3. They provide intermediates for fat formation (lipogenesis).
4. They provide intermediates for synthesis of some amino acids (protein synthesis).

The interrelationships between these pathways are shown in Fig. 2-7.

Alternate pathways. Alternate pathways open to glucose serve specific related functions.

The pentose shunt (also called the hexosemonophosphate shunt) of the Embden-

---

TO PROBE FURTHER
Energy output from glucose oxidation*

The major route of carbohydrate oxidation—the Embden-Meyerhof glycolytic pathway together with the Krebs cycle—is a tremendously efficient producer of energy. It has been credited with an overall efficiency rate of 42%, which results from its ability to produce and store large amounts of energy, while relatively little energy is expended in "running the machine." According to engineering standards, this efficiency rate is above that of many man-made machines.

The energy produced in this route of glucose oxidation is trapped as chemical energy in phosphorus-containing compounds, such as ATP, which store the energy until it is needed. The body's energy supply is conserved rather than dissipated all at once (this point is further discussed in Chapter 5).

It has been calculated that the oxidation if 1 mole of glucose through this efficient system produces 38 high energy phosphorus bonds—8 in the initial Embden-Meyerhof glycolytic pathway, and 30 in the final common Krebs cycle. This is equivalent to an energy output of 288,800 calories!

---

*Harper, H. A.: Review of physiological chemistry, Los Altos, Calif., 1967, Lange Medical Publications, p. 228.

Meyerhof pathway is a side channeling of glucose and it serves a number of physiologic ends (see Fig. 2-5). It produces an important enzyme factor—NADPH (reduced niacin adenine dinucleotide phosphate)—which is essential in the synthesis of fatty acids. (NADPH is another example of the integration of a B vitamin, niacin, in glucose metabolism.) Insulin's role in lipogenesis may be that of stimulating the operation of this shunt pathway. NADPH is also involved as a cofactor in steroid synthesis which makes the shunt active in the adrenal gland.

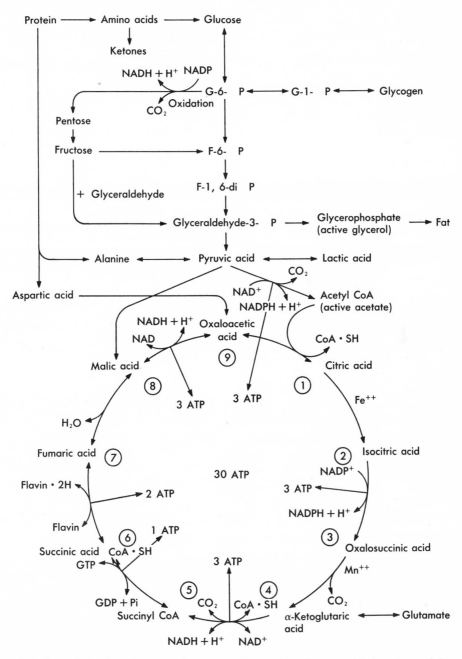

Fig. 2-7. Interrelationships between the two pathways for glucose oxidation—the Embden-Meyerhof pathway and the Krebs cycle.

The uronic acid pathway is a side pathway which changes some of the glucose into glucuronic acid. Glucuronic acid in turn combines with certain toxic materials (such as some drugs) to remove them from the body, which is an important detoxifying function.

SUMMARY

What is the significance of this overall picture of carbohydrate metabolism for students of nursing and nutrition? What does this all mean in the care of patients and the teaching of positive health principles? Certainly it is not important to remember all the details of metabolism—and only a very few have been presented here. This is the sort of information it is important to have only as reference knowledge. The complex and fascinating intricacies of body chemistry lie in the realm of the biochemist and the physiologist, whose imaginative research efforts have given the medical profession greater knowledge of the marvelous inner workings of the human body.

At least two basic concepts can be gained from this background knowledge: (1) the interrelatedness of nutrients, and (2) the relation of the separate chemical reactions of the body to the total process of metabolism. There is an intimate metabolic interrelatedness between the basic nutrients and their metabolites. No one substance exists or operates alone during metabolism. Rather, there is a tremendously significant interdependence among them all. From this fact, two practical conclusions may be drawn:
1. The emphasis in health teaching and in nutrition education should be on achieving a sound, balanced, normal nutritional basis for any dietary program.
2. It is entirely possible that some deficiency states may be iatrogenic, may have their origin in a fad, or may be caused by long-term, overzealous emphasis on one particular nutrient to the exclusion of other equally essential ones.

The general picture of carbohydrate metabolism can help one to understand more clearly how smaller segments, affecting a particular symptom or condition, relate ultimately and intimately to the whole process of metabolism. The serious student will translate this information clearly and simply to individual patients. Because she perceives the relationship of the part to the whole, she will be able to help the patient understand his needs and accept the treatment warranted by the specific situation.

GLOSSARY

disaccharides a class of compound sugars composed of two molecules of monosaccharide. The three common members are sucrose (table sugar), lactose (milk sugar), and maltose (grain sugar).

enzymes various complex organic substances produced by living cells which act independently of these cells. Enzymes are capable of producing certain chemical changes in other substances without themselves being changed in the process. Their action is therefore that of a catalyst. Digestive enzymes of the gastrointestinal secretions act upon food substances to break them down into simpler compounds, and greatly accelerate the speed of these chemical reactions. An enzyme is usually named according to the substance (substrate) on which it acts, with the common suffix -*ase: sucrase* is the specific enzyme for *sucrose*, and breaks it down to glucose and fructose.

glucagon a hyperglycemic factor (HGF) secreted by the alpha cells of the pancreas which stimulates glycogenolysis.

gluconeogenesis the formation of glucose from noncarbohydrate sources (protein or fat).

glycogen The polysaccharide of the animal body (animal starch). It is formed in the body from glucose and stored in the liver and in muscle tissue.

glycogenesis the general term for formation of glycogen from glucose. It is usually used interchangeably with the term *glucogenesis*.

glycogenolysis the specific term for conversion of glycogen into glucose in the liver. Glycogenolysis is the chemical process of enzymatic hydrolysis or breakdown by which this conversion is accomplished.

glycolysis catabolism of carbohydrate (glucose and glycogen) by enzymes with release of energy and production of pyruvic acid or lactic acid.

hexoses a class of simple sugar (monosaccharides)

that contain 6 carbon atoms ($C_6H_{12}O_6$). The most comomn members are glucose (dextrose), fructose (levulose), and galactose.

hormones various internally secreted substances from the endocrine organs, which are conveyed by the blood to another organ or tissue upon which they act to stimulate increased functional activity or secretion. The tissue or substance acted upon by a specific hormone is called its target organ or substance. For example, insulin, a hormone secreted by special cells of the pancreas (islets of Langerhans), acts to facilitate glucose metabolism.

metabolism the sum of all physical and chemical changes that take place within an organism, by which it maintains itself and produces energy for its functioning. Products of these various reactions are called *metabolites*. Interrelationships of substances in these processes are called *metabolic relationships*.

phosphorylation the combining of glucose with a phosphoric acid radical to produce glucose-6-phosphate as a first step in the cellular oxidation of glucose to produce enegry. This reaction is catalyzed by the enzyme glucokinase, the specific hexokinase for this purpose.

photosynthesis the process by which plants containing chlorophyll are able to manufacture carbohydrates by combining carbon dioxide from the air and water from the soil. Sunlight is used as energy and chlorophyll is a catalyst. The basic chemical reaction is:

$$6CO_2 + 6H_2O + energy \xrightarrow{\text{chlorophyll}} C_6H_{12}O_6 + 6H_2O$$

polysaccharides a class of complex sugars composed of many monosaccharide units. The common members are starch, dextrins, cellulose, pectins, and glycogen.

portal an entryway, usually referring to the portal circulation of blood through the liver. Blood is brought into the liver by the portal vein and out by the hepatic vein.

References
Specific

1. Levine, R.: Concerning the mechanisms of insulin action, Diabetes **10**:421, 1961.
2. Levine, R., Goldstein, M. S., Huddleston, B., and Klein, S. P.: Action of insulin on "permeability" of cells to free hexoses, as studied by its effect on distribution of galactose, Amer. J. Physiol. **163**:79, 1950.
3. Morgan, H. E., Regen, D. M., Henderson, M. J., Sawyer, T. K., and Park, C. R.: Regulation of glucose uptake in muscle. VI. Effects of hypophysectomy, adrenalectomy, growth hormone, hydrocortisone, and insulin on glucose transport and phosphorylation in the perfused rat heart, J. Biol. Chem. **236**:2162, 1961.
4. Morgan, H. E., Regen, D. M., and Park, C. R.: Identification of a mobile carrier-mediated sugar transport system in muscle, J. Biol. Chem. **239**:369, 1964.
5. Park, C. R., Johnson, L. H., Wright, J. H., Jr., and Batsel, H.: Effect of insulin on transport of several hexoses and pentoses into cells of muscle and brain, Amer. J. Physiol. **191**: 13, 1957.
6. Post, R. L., Morgan, H. E., and Park, C. R.: Regulation of glucose uptake in muscle. III. The interaction of membrane transport and phosphorylation in the control of glucose uptake, J. Biol. Chem. **236**:269, 1961.
7. Krahl, M. E.: The action of insulin on cells, New York, 1961, Academic Press.
8. Penhos, J. C., and Krahl, M. E.: Insulin stimulus of leucine incorporation into frog liver protein, Amer. J. Physiol. **203**:687, 1962.

General

Bogert, L. J., Briggs, G., and Calloway, D.: Nutrition and physical fitness, ed. 8, Philadelphia, 1966, W. B. Saunders Co.

Cantarow, A., and Trumper, M.: Clinical biochemistry, ed. 6, Philadelphia, 1962, W. B. Saunders Co.

Cereal enrichment in perspective, 1958. Prepared by the Committee on Cereals, Food and Nutrition Board, Washington, D. C., March, 1958, National Academy of Sciences, National Research Council.

Hardinge, M. G., Swarner, J. B., and Crooks, H.: Carbohydrates in foods, Amer. J. Diet. Ass. **46**:197, 1965.

Harper, H. A.: Review of physiological chemistry, ed. 11, Los Altos, Calif., 1967, Lange Medical Publications.

Jolliffe, N., editor: Clinical nutrition, ed. 2, New York, 1962, Harper and Row.

Krehl, W A.: The nutritional significance of the carbohydrates, Borden Rev. Nutr. Res. **16**:85, 1955.

Reviews: The role of carbohydrates in the diet, Nutr. Rev. **22**:102, 1964; Carbohydrate intake and respiratory quotient, Nutr. Rev. **22**:104, 1964; Digestion and absorption of disaccharides in man, Nutr. Rev. **20**:203, 1962.

Soskin, S., and Levine, R.: Carbohydrate metabolism, Chicago, 1952, University of Chicago Press.

Stefferud, A., editor: Food: the yearbook of agriculture, 1959, Washington, D. C., 1959, U. S. Department of Agriculture.

White, A., Handler, P., and Smith, E.: Principles of biochemistry, ed. 3, New York, 1964, McGraw-Hill Book Co.

Wohl, M., and Goodhart, R., editors: Modern nutrition in health and disease, ed. 4, Philadelphia, 1968, Lea & Febiger.

CHAPTER 3

Fats

Since recorded history, and probably before, man has used fats to supply light and heat for his shelter and lubrication for his tools. Man has even used fat for beautifying himself.

Man's major use of fat, however, has been as food. There seems to be no set quantitative requirement of fat in human nutrition. People of many different cultures exist on widely various amounts of fat in their diets. For example, the fat intake of Japanese soldiers in wartime probably accounted for as little as 3% of their total calories, whereas the general Japanese population consumed from 6 to 10% of their total calories as fat.[1] About 40% of the total caloric intake of Americans is from this source, which is an excessive quantity, according to some authorities. The Food and Nutrition Board of the National Research Council reports that an adequate intake of fat is about 25% of the total calories, with 1 to 2% as the essential fatty acid, linoleic acid. However, there is no basis for agreement on the required level of fat, and the human body appears to be able to function on a wide range of fat intake.

GENERAL AND CHEMICAL DEFINITIONS OF FATS

General definition. Fats may be defined as a group of organic substances—fats, oils, waxes, and related compounds—which are greasy to the touch and insoluble in water, but are soluble in alcohol or ether. Substances of this class are called *lipids* (Gr. *lipos,* fat). The food sources of fats are usually obvious to the consumer. The so-

called visible fats include butter, margarine, oil, salad dressings, bacon, and cream. Egg yolk, meat fats, olives, avocado, and nuts are the so-called hidden fats.

Chemical definition. Fats may be defined according to their basic structural elements: carbon, hydrogen, and oxygen. Although these are the same elements that comprise the carbohydrates, in fat the relative hydrogen content is higher than in carbohydrate. Fats are actual or potential esters of fatty acids. (An *ester* is a compound of an alcohol and an acid.) These fatty acids are utilized in the metabolism of living organisms.

CLASSIFICATION OF FATS

The commonly used classification of fats suggested by Bloor and Deuel[2] divides them into three main groups: simple lipids, compound lipids, and derived lipids.

Simple lipids. The simple lipids are neutral fats and waxes.

Neutral fats are esters of fatty acids with glycerol, in the ratio of three fatty acids to

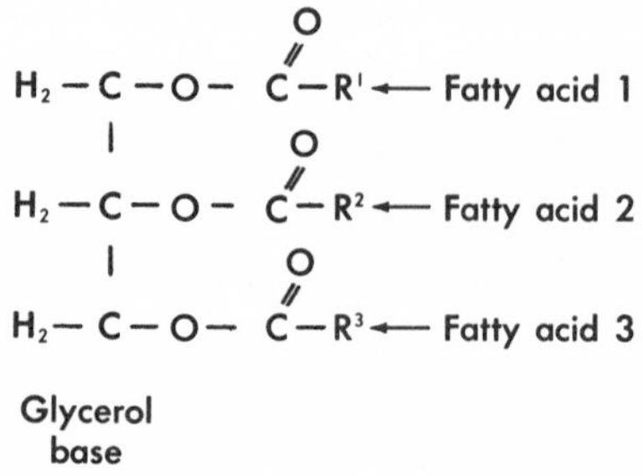

$$H_2-C-O-\overset{\overset{O}{\parallel}}{C}-R^1 \longleftarrow \text{Fatty acid 1}$$
$$H_2-C-O-\overset{\overset{O}{\parallel}}{C}-R^2 \longleftarrow \text{Fatty acid 2}$$
$$H_2-C-O-\overset{\overset{O}{\parallel}}{C}-R^3 \longleftarrow \text{Fatty acid 3}$$

Glycerol base

Fig. 3-1. Triglyceride.

each glycerol base. They are therefore called *triglycerides* (Fig. 3-1).

Waxes are esters of fatty acids with straight-chain alcohols. Generally, these substances are more solid than fats. They have little importance in human nutrition, but are used more extensively in commercial products.

Compound lipids. Compound lipids are various combinations of neutral fat with other components. Three types of compound lipid are important in human nutrition: phospholipids, glycolipids, and lipoproteins.

Phospholipids are compounds of neutral fat, a phosphoric acid, and a nitrogenous base. The largest group of phospholipids, *lecithins*, contain glycerol, two fatty acids, phosphoric acid, and choline. Other important phospholipids are *cephalins* and *lipositols,* which are like the lecithins except that they contain other factors in place of choline.

Glycolipids are compounds of fatty acids which are combined with carbohydrates and nitrogen. Because they are found chiefly in brain tissue, these substances are also called *cerebrosides.*

Lipoproteins are compounds of various lipids with protein. Studies indicate that the intimate relation between plasma lipids and certain parts of the plasma proteins provides the main transport form of lipid substances in the blood stream. These plasma lipoproteins contain cholesterol (free and esterified), phospholipids, neutral fat, unesterified (free) fatty acids, and traces of other related materials such as fat-soluble vitamins and the steroid hormones. Lipids always travel in the blood bound with protein in varying ratios. This illustrates again the intimate interrelationships among the various nutrients and their interdependent nature.

Derived lipids. Derived lipids are fat substances derived from simple and compound lipids by hydrolysis or enzymatic breakdown. Three important members of this group are fatty acids, glycerol, and steroids.

Fatty acids are the basic components of triglycerides (neutral fats), and they may be *saturated* or *unsaturated.*

Glycerol, the water soluble component of triglycerides, is interconvertible with carbohydrate, and therefore contributes to the total available glucose in the diet.

Steroids are a class of lipid substances that contain sterols, such as cholesterol and ergosterol (a precursor of vitamin D). Other important steroids are the bile salts, certain fat-soluble provitamins, and adrenal hormones.

FATTY ACIDS

Since fatty acids are the basic structural units of fats, a close study of them is important to an understanding of lipids. Terms applied to the fatty acids relate to their degree of chemical saturation, or to their synthesis and function in the body.

Saturated and unsaturated fatty acids

The state of saturation or unsaturation of fatty acids is an important chemical characteristic. This state results from the ratio of hydrogen atoms to carbon atoms in the basic carbon chain which forms the individual fatty acid. In terms of chemical combining power, carbon has a *valence* of 4, meaning that *four* other atoms may attach themselves to positions on the carbon atom when various carbon compounds are formed. In a given fatty acid, if all of the available valence bonds of a basic carbon chain are filled with hydrogen, the fatty acid is said to be completely *saturated with hydrogen.* However, if at one point along the carbon chain there are two fewer hydrogen atoms, the two involved carbon atoms take up their two available valence bonds to make one mutual bond. When this newly created mutual bond is added to the already existing bond between them, a double bond between the two carbon atoms is created. If only one such double bond occurs along the carbon chain, the fatty acid is called a *monounsaturated* fatty acid. If two or more double bonds occur along the carbon chain of the fatty

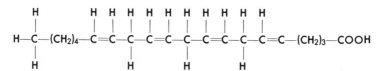

H H H
| | |
H—C—C—C—COOH
| | |
H H H

Saturated—butyric acid, as found in butter (4 carbons, no double bond)

H   H H
| | |
H—C—(CH₂)₇—C=C—(CH₂)₇—COOH
|
H

Monounsaturated—oleic acid, component fatty acid in olive oil (18 carbons, 1 double bond)

H   H H H H
| | | | |
H—C—(CH₂)₇—C=C—C—C=C—(CH₂)₄—COOH
| |
H   H

Polyunsaturated—found in various vegetable oils
Linoleic acid (18 carbons, 2 double bonds)

H   H H H H H H H
| | | | | | | |
H—C—(CH₂)₂—C=C—C—C=C—C—C=C—(CH₂)₇—COOH
| | |
H   H   H

Polyunsaturated linolenic acid (18 carbons, 3 double bonds)

H   H H H H H H H H H
| | | | | | | | | |
H—C—(CH₂)₄—C=C—C—C=C—C—C=C—C—C=C—(CH₂)₃—COOH
| | | |
H   H   H   H

Polyunsaturated arachidonic acid (20 carbons, 4 double bonds)

acid, it is called a *polyunsaturated* fatty acid. A comparison of the basic structure of representative examples of each form of fatty acid is shown above.

Food fats. From the preceding facts, the concept of degrees of saturation and unsaturation of fatty acids can be derived. Fig. 3-2 shows the general saturated—unsaturated spectrum of food fats. One would expect the more saturated food fats to be the more solid, hard ones. Usually this is the case. The more saturated food fats have a higher melting point (solidification point). The fats on the saturated end of the spectrum are animal fats, and the fats toward the center of the spectrum become softer in texture. The fats on the unsaturated end of the spectrum are of plant origin, and are usually free-flowing oils which do not solidify even at low temperatures.

Essential and nonessential fatty acids

The terms "essential" or "nonessential," when applied to fatty acids, refer to the twofold physiologic fact: (1) A fatty acid is essential if its absence will create a specific deficiency disease. For example, a type of eczema in infants is caused by a lack of linoleic acid in the diet. (2) A fatty acid is essential if the body cannot manufacture it and must obtain it from the diet. Either or both of these things may be true of a specific fatty acid.

The three polyunsaturated fatty acids—linoleic acid, linolenic acid, and arachi-

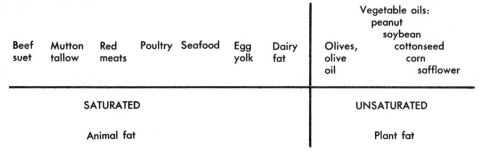

Beef suet	Mutton tallow	Red meats	Poultry	Seafood	Egg yolk	Dairy fat	Olives, olive oil	Vegetable oils: peanut soybean cottonseed corn safflower
		SATURATED						UNSATURATED
		Animal fat						Plant fat

Fig. 3-2. Spectrum of food fats according to degree of saturation of component fatty acids.

donic acid—have for many years been called the essential fatty acids, because they are essential for certain body functioning. Evidence also seemed to indicate that the body could not synthesize them. However, current research[1,3] indicates that *linoleic acid* may be considered the one essential fatty acid for two reasons. Linolenic acid has relatively little effect in relieving the skin lesions originally associated with a deficiency of the essential acids. Arachidonic acid can be synthesized by the body from linoleic acid, and therefore does not have to be supplied as such in the diet.

These three fatty acids, especially linoleic acid, serve important functions in the body:

1. They strengthen capillary and cell membrane structure, which helps prevent an increase in skin permeability. A deficiency of linoleic acid leads to a breakdown in skin integrity with resulting eczematous skin lesions.
2. They combine with cholesterol to form cholesterol esters. They are also part of the phospholipid and lipoprotein complexes.
3. They lower serum cholesterol. Some investigators suggest that linoleic acid may play a key role in the transport and metabolism of cholesterol, although just what this role may be is not known at this time.
4. They prolong blood clotting time and increase fibrinolytic activity.

The precise relationship between these fatty acids and the critical tissue change in coronary artery disease (atherosclerosis) has not been determined.

The monounsaturated acid, oleic acid, is not included as an essential acid as it can be readily synthesized in the tissues.

SOME COMMON CHEMICAL REACTIONS OF FATS

Certain common chemical reactions of fats have much dietary or commercial significance and should be clarified.

Hydrolysis. Hydrolysis is the process in which enzyme action by the lipases breaks down neutral fats in foods to their component fatty acids and glycerol (see the section on Digestion of Fats, pp. 32 and 33).

Saponification. Hydrolysis by an alkali breaks down fats into glycerol and the alkali salt of the fatty acids. The latter products are *soaps*. In certain abnormal states (for example, sprue), the body produces soaps.

Hydrogenation. The process of hydrogenation introduces hydrogen into the available double bond linkages of unsaturated fats. Industrially, nickel is used as a catalyst. The process is also known as "hardening." It has commercial value, as it converts liquid fats such as vegetable oils into a solid form for use as vegetable shortenings and margarines.

Rancidity. Rancidity is the result of chemical change in a fat caused by air exposure and age. The fat has an unpleasant odor and taste. Because oxygen in the air causes this chemical change, antioxidants are used in commercial food processing to prevent a fat from turning rancid.

FUNCTIONS OF FAT IN THE BODY

Fat serves two basic functions in the human body: (1) a primary metabolic function, to produce energy, and (2) a secondary mechanical or structural function, for example, the protection of vital organs.

Metabolic function. The primary function of fat in human nutrition is to supply the body's most concentrated source of energy. Fat has more than twice the fuel value concentration of either carbohydrate or protein. In colder climates and seasons, therefore, fat generally assumes a greater role in the diet to supply needed body heat.

Moreover, because of its concentration, high density, and low solubility, fat has value in the body as the storage form of energy. Carbohydrates and some proteins may also be converted to fat for storage as adipose fat tissue. The turnover of fats in adipose tissue is a dynamic, continuous process.

Mechanical or structural function. Fat provides a general padding for vital organs and nerves which holds them in place and helps to absorb shocks. Further protection for the entire body is provided by the subcutaneous layer of fat, which insulates the body against rapid temperature changes or excessive heat loss.

Function of fat-related compounds

Other important functions of fat are those associated with fat-related compounds. Phospholipids, for example, are vital constituents of all cells. Brain and nerve tissue are especially rich in phospholipids. Unlike neutral fats, these compounds are water soluble, and may therefore help facilitate the passage of neutral fats in and out of cells. Phospholipids probably also aid in the absorption of fats from the intestine. Cholesterol, another vital fat-related compound, is closely related chemically to the sex hormones and adrenal hormones.

DIGESTION OF FATS

Chemical digestion of fats takes place only in the small intestine; the general preparatory action occurs in the preceding parts of the gastrointestinal tract.

Mechanical digestion. Mechanical digestion of fats begins in the mouth. Mastication breaks the food up into fine particles and moistens it for passage into the stomach. In the stomach peristalsis continues the mechanical mixing of fats with the stomach contents. No significant enzyme specific for fats is present in the gastric secretions. As the gastric enzymes act upon specific nutrients, however, fat is separated from them and made more readily accessible to its own specific chemical breakdown in the small intestine.

Chemical digestion. It is not until fat reaches the small intestine that chemical digestion takes place. Agents from the *liver* and *gallbladder*, the *pancreas*, and the *small intestine* aid in this enzymatic breakdown of fats.

Bile salts from the liver and gallbladder. The presence of fat in the duodenum stimulates the secretion of *cholecystokinin* from glands in the walls of the intestine. Cholecystokinin provides the stimulus for the contraction of the gallbladder, relaxation of the sphincter, and subsequent secretion of bile salts into the intestine via the common bile duct. Bile is produced in the liver, and then is concentrated and stored in the gallbladder ready for use in the handling of fats. Its function is that of an emulsifier. Emulsification is an important first step in the preparation of fats for digestion by the enzymes. This emulsifying process has a twofold nature: (1) it breaks the fat into small particles or globules, which greatly enlarges the surface area available for action of the enzymes, and (2) this action also serves to lower the surface tension of the finely dispersed and suspended fat globules, thus allowing greater ease of penetration of the enzymes. This is similar to the wetting action of detergents. The bile also provides an alkaline medium for the action of lipase.

Table 3-1. Summary of triglyceride breakdown

$$\text{Triglyceride} + H_2O \xrightarrow{\text{lipase}} \text{Diglyceride} + 1 \text{ fatty acid}$$

$$\text{Diglyceride} + H_2O \xrightarrow{\text{lipase}} \text{Monoglyceride} + 1 \text{ fatty acid}$$

$$\text{Monoglyceride} + H_2O \xrightarrow{\text{lipase}} \text{Glycerol} + 1 \text{ fatty acid}$$

Table 3-2. Summary of fat digestion

Organ	Enzyme	Activity
Mouth	None	Mechanical; mastication
Stomach	None	Mechanical separation of fats as protein and starch digested out
Small intestine	Gallbladder	
	Bile salts (emulsifier)	Emulsifies fats
	Pancreatic	
	Lipase (steapsin)	Triglycerides to di- and monoglycerides in turn, then fatty acids and glycerol
	Cholesterol esterase	Free cholesterol + fatty acids to cholesterol esters
	Intestinal	
	Lecithinase	Lecithin to glycerol, fatty acids, phosphoric acid, choline

Enzymes from the pancreas. The pancreatic juice contains an enzyme for fat and an enzyme for cholesterol. The pancreatic *lipase* which acts upon fats is a powerful enzyme called *steapsin.* In a stepwise fashion, it breaks off one fatty acid at a time from the glycerol base of neutral fats. Thus, one fatty acid and diglyceride, then another fatty acid and monoglyceride, are produced in turn. Each succeeding step of this breakdown is effected with increasing difficulty. In fact separation of the final fatty acid from the remaining monoglyceride is such a slow process that less than one-third of the total fat present actually reaches complete breakdown. The final products of fat digestion are fatty acids, diglycerides, monoglycerides, and glycerol (Table 3-1).

The formation of cholesterol esters by the combination of cholesterol and fatty acids is an important step in the preparation of free cholesterol for absorption by the bloodstream from the intestine. *Cholesterol esterase* is an enzyme of the pancreatic juice which, along with bile salts, catalyzes this action.

Enzyme from the small intestine. The small intestine secretes an enzyme in the intestinal juice called *lecithinase.* It acts upon lecithin (a phospholipid) to break it down into its components of glycerol, fatty acids, phosphoric acid, and choline.

Large intestine. Some remaining fat may be secreted into the large intestine and eliminated as fecal fat.

A summary of fat digestion in the successive parts of the gastrointestinal tract is given in Table 3-2.

ABSORPTION OF FAT INTO THE BLOODSTREAM

Because of the increasing difficulty in breaking off the final fatty acid from original triglycerides, only about one-third of the triglycerides are completely digested in the lumen of the small intestine. The major end products of fat digestion in the gastrointestinal tract are monoglycerides, some diglycerides, glycerol, and fatty acids.

The absorbing surface of the small intestine, with its millions of small villi, handles these products of fat digestion in various ways.

Initial fat absorption

Triglyceride products. Because it is water soluble, glycerol is easily absorbed into the portal blood system and carried to the liver.

The term "free" fatty acid is a misnomer, since all fats and fat products travel in the plasma bound with some small amount of protein. The term "free" here means *unesterified.* The unesterified fatty acids (UFA) are usually short-chain fatty acids, which may be absorbed directly into the portal vein and carried to the liver.

The remaining monoglycerides, diglycerides, and fatty acids are less water soluble and require a wetting agent to facilitate their absorption. Bile salts perform this vital function and act as a ferry system to transport these products of fat digestion into the intestinal wall. With the monoglycerides and fatty acids, these bile acids form a micellar complex so fine that it is almost a clear solution, and the fat particles are about 1/100 the size of those that first entered the intestine. With the remaining unhydrolyzed triglycerides and diglycerides, bile forms an emulsion for absorption (Fig. 3-3).

Some electron microscopic observations suggest that the neutral fat complex may be absorbed by a process called *pinocytosis,* an engulfing of the globule directly by the cell membrane (see Fig. 9-3, p. 158).

Absorption of fat-related products. Cholesterol may be taken in as such in the diet (exogenous cholesterol), or it may be synthesized by the body (endogenous cholesterol). One of the major sites of cholesterol synthesis is intestinal tissue. Some cholesterol is absorbed with the aid of bile salts as free or unesterified cholesterol. Most of it, however, is esterified with fatty acids by the enzymatic action of cholesterol esterase and is absorbed as cholesterol esters.

The *phospholipids,* mainly lecithin, may also be taken in as such in the diet or synthesized in intestinal tissue. Some preformed dietary phospholipid, because of its *hydrophilic* nature (strong affinity for water), may be absorbed directly into portal blood. Other phospholipid synthesized in intestinal tissue becomes part of the lipoprotein complex (chylomicrons) that is absorbed into the lymphatic system. It then passes to the liver by way of the thoracic duct.

Subsequent steps in fat absorption carried out by the intestinal wall

A highly significant second stage of fat absorption takes place in the wall of the intestine. The mucosa does not act merely as passive tissue for a diffuse sort of entry and passage of fats. Rather, recent studies[4-6] have revealed it to be a dynamic metabolic tissue which is actively engaged in resynthesis of triglycerides and related fat products.

In the intestinal wall, bile salts are separated from the initial fatty acid complex absorbed from the intestinal lumen, and are returned to the liver by way of the portal blood. In the liver, the bile salts are then recirculated in the bile. This cycle, the *en-*

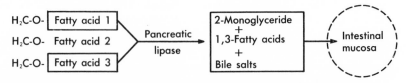

Fig. 3-3. Micellar complex of fats with bile salts for transport of fats into intestinal mucosa.

TO PROBE FURTHER
The enterohepatic circulation

The efficiency of the enterohepatic circulation of bile salts demonstrates the body's amazing ability to conserve materials needed for its basic functions. These built-in conservation systems, because they maintain their own balance, are called *homeostatic mechanisms.* They are designed to sustain life in a relatively stable state of equilibrium between the multitude of interdependent elements and subsystems that comprise the human organism.

For example, of the 20 to 30 gm. of needed bile acids circulated daily in the body, only about 0.8 gm. is lost in the feces. Therefore, only this small amount needs to be replaced daily by newly synthesized bile acids. After its tasks in digestion and absorption (emulsifying and transporting) are completed, the bile is separated from its fat complex, returned to the liver, and recirculated again and again (Fig. 3-4).

terohepatic circulation of bile salts, forms an efficient system for maintaining a constant supply as needed.

There is evidence[7] that an intestinal lipase (enteric lipase) exists within the cells of the intestine wall which continues the hydrolysis of the remaining triglycerides, diglycerides, and monoglycerides to fatty acids and glycerol. These fatty acids, together with those released from the initial bile salts—fatty acid complex, are activated and resynthesized with an activated glycerol. This glycerol is probably produced from the Embden-Meyerhof glycolytic pathway for glucose metabolism (see Chapter 2), and is not a new glycerol just produced by digestion. Resynthesized triglycerides are formed and are ready to be used by the tissues.

Final absorption and transport of fat

Through the metabolic action of the intestinal mucosa final fat products are formed. These include fatty acids, phospholipids, free cholesterol, cholesterol esters, and triglycerides. This complex of materials is then bound with small amounts of protein to form a lipoprotein complex called *chylomicrons.* These chylomicrons penetrate the intercellular spaces of the intestinal mucosa and enter the abdominal lacteals. The chylomicrons can apparently cross the cell wall intact. These lipoprotein particles are transported through the lymphatic system to the thoracic duct, where they enter the blood through the left subclavian vein. The various stages in the overall process of fat absorption are summarized in Fig. 3-5.

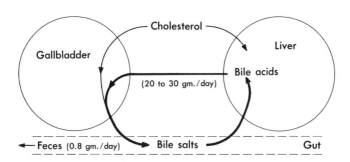

Fig. 3-4. Enterohepatic circulation of bile salts.

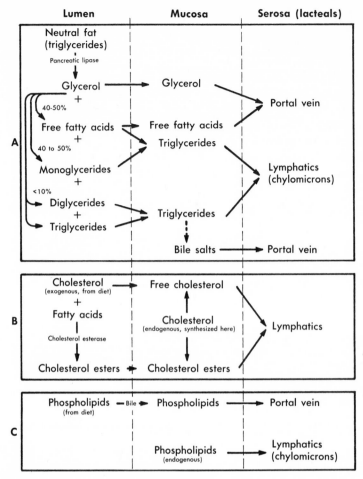

Fig. 3-5. Absorption of fat, cholesterol, and phospholipids.

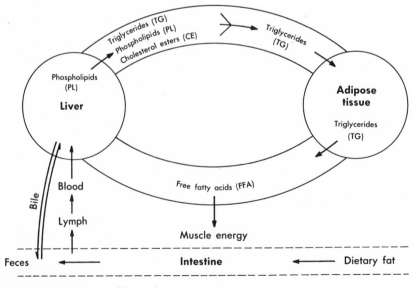

Fig. 3-6. Liver-adipose tissue axis of fat exchange.

TO PROBE FURTHER
Chylomicrons

Following a meal, lipoprotein particles of fat, related fat products, and protein accumulate in the lymphatic vessels and the plasma. These particles are called *chylomicrons*. The term chylomicrons refers to their composition and size. These fat droplets contain mostly triglycerides, but also small amounts of other fat products. Their approximate composition is:

Triglycerides	81%
Cholesterol (free and esters)	9%
Phospholipids	7%
Free fatty acids	1%
Protein	2%

The chylomicrons disappear rather quickly from the plasma into various tissues for oxidation or storage. The efficient clearing factor is an enzyme, *lipoprotein lipase*, which begins its action in the plasma, but continues it mainly in the tissue taking up the fat. It releases free (unesterified) fatty acids after their hydrolysis from depot fats. As one would expect, a large amount of the enzyme is present in adipose tissue, but none has been found in liver, where fat is not stored.

METABOLISM OF FATS

Five factors work together to control the level of plasma lipids: (1) diet, (2) synthesis of fat in the tissues, (3) mobilization of fat from the depots, (4) the rate of oxidation in the various body tissues, and (5) deposition of fat in adipose tissue and the liver.

The main sites of utilization of lipids are adipose tissue and the liver. This basic interdependent relationship has been called the "liver-adipose tissue axis" (Fig. 3-6). Fat metabolism may be considered in terms of the fat-related activities of these two organ tissues. These metabolic activities in adipose and liver tissue are twofold: (1) *lipogenesis* (synthesis and deposit of fat); and (2) *lipolysis* (mobilization and oxidation of fat). Although these functions are considered separately here, they do not exist apart form each other; rather, they are constantly interbalanced to maintain blood lipid levels and to help supply energy needs.

Adipose tissue metabolism

Adipose tissue is by no means the static storage reserve of fat it was once thought to be. It is now known to be one of the most metabolically active body tissues. It maintains a constant turnover, depositing and mobilizing fat. In the body's total fat metabolism picture, endogenous as well as exogenous fat must be considered.

Fat synthesis and deposit. The most active site of lipogenesis in the human body is adipose tissue. Triglycerides are formed from fatty acids and glycerol. Two sources supply the needed fatty acids: (1) degraded neutral fat or dietary fat, and (2) synthesized fatty acids from precursors such as carbohydrate and its metabolites (glucose, pyruvate, and active acetate). The synthesis of fatty acids from these precursors requires the presence of the niacin-containing coenzyme NADPH, which is produced by the pentose shunt of the Embden-Meyerhof glycolytic pathway (see pp. 24 and 25). Tissues active in lipogenesis, such as adipose tissue and the lactating mammary glands, also have a very active shunt pathway. This helps to explain why glucose and insulin are necessary for lipogenesis. The required coenzyme, NADPH, is produced by glucose oxidation through this shunt.

The glycerol used in lipogenesis must be an activated form (it must contain phosphorus), rather than be newly released free glycerol. Since adipose tissue lacks the activating enzyme *glycerokinase,* active glycerol (α-glycerophosphate) must come from the glycolytic pathway of glucose metabolism (see p. 22).

These two factors of fat metabolism again demonstrate the closely interdependent relationships of the basic nutrients, fat and carbohydrate, and indicate that adipose tissue is in fact one of the major sites of insulin activity.

The synthesized fat is deposited in three major body sites: (1) subcutaneous connective tissue, (2) abdominal cavity, (3) intermuscular connective tissue.

Fat mobilization and oxidation. Lipolysis also takes place in adipose tissue, since depot fat is constantly being mobilized by the body. The fat is again broken down into glycerol and fatty acids. The glycerol is released and subsequently converted in the liver to glycogen, and is eventually oxidized as glucose. The free (unesterified) fatty acids released are transported to various cells as needed to be oxidized for energy. The turnover rate of these free fatty acids is high. They are the metabolically active forms of lipids. All tissues can oxidize them completely to carbon dioxide and water. They are even the preferred form of fuel for some tissues such as the myocardium.

Liver metabolism

In the overall balanced axis of fat metabolism, the liver also functions in lipogenesis and lipolysis.

Fat synthesis and deposit. The liver also synthesizes fatty acids and triglycerides, but to a lesser extent than occurs in adipose tissue. Unlike adipose tissue, however, the liver normally does not store deposits of fat. Such deposits produce a "fatty liver," an abnormal, pathologic state. Several conditions may contribute to the abnormal deposit of fat in the liver:

1. Excess mobilization of fat as in starvation or uncontrolled diabetes which produces ketosis
2. Malnutrition, especially deficiencies in protein and key vitamins related to carbohydrate and fat metabolism
3. Alcoholism, which induces malnutrition
4. Hepatotoxins such as carbon tetrachloride, which injure liver tissue

Fat mobilization and oxidation. To prevent abnormal accumulation of fat in the liver, certain *lipotropic* factors are active in this organ. By a process of *transmethylation,* these lipotropic agents promote the production of lipoproteins, which transfer the fatty acids out of the liver.

A major example of such a lipotropic agent is choline, a component of the phospholipid, lecithin. Choline, sometimes classified as a B-complex vitamin, is synthesized from methionine, an essential amino acid. The therapeutic effect of protein in early liver disease may derive in some measure from its lipotropic constituent amino acid, methionine.

A summary of fat metabolism is shown in Fig. 3-7 (see also Fig. 7-2, p. 108).

The oxidation of fatty acids proceeds first through a gradual breakdown by 2-carbon fragments from the original carbon chain to form active acetate (acetyl CoA) and shorter chain fatty acids. The active acetate then enters the Krebs cycle (see pp. 23 and 24), and is oxidized to form carbon dioxide and water.

The role of the liver in fat metabolism may be summarized as the synthesis of fatty acids from carbohydrate, the synthesis of cholesterol from 2-carbon acetate fragments, the synthesis of bile acids (the liver is the sole source of bile acids), and the synthesis of phospholipids and lipoproteins from protein sources. The liver also removes phospholipids, cholesterol, lipopro-

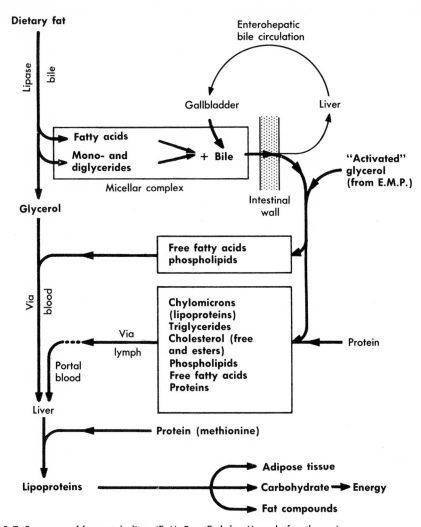

Fig. 3-7. Summary of fat metabolism. (E. M. P. = Embden-Meyerhof pathway.)

tein from plasma, and removes fatty acids from diet or deposit origin by degrading and oxidizing them when the body must call on fat as a major energy source. If oxidation is too rapid excess ketones are formed.

Hormonal influences on fat metabolism

Since fat and carbohydrate metabolism are so closely interrelated, the same hormones that affect carbohydrate metabolism also affect fat metabolism.

1. Growth hormone (GH), adrenocorticotrophic hormone (ACTH), and thyroid-stimulating hormone (TSH),

which are all secreted by the pituitary gland, increase the release of free fatty acids from adipose tissue by imposing energy demands upon the body.

2. Cortisone and hydrocortisone, which are secreted by the adrenal gland, cause the release of free fatty acids. Epinephrine and norepinephrine stimulate lipolysis, the breakdown of triglycerides.

3. The important lipogenic activity of insulin, which is secreted by the pancreas, has been described (pp. 20 and 21). Glucagon has an opposite effect

Table 3-3. Summary of factors affecting release of free fatty acids from adipose tissue

Increase release	Decrease release
Hormones	Insulin + glucose
Diabetes	(lipogenesis)
Starvation (fasting)	Feeding
Cold	

by increasing the release of free fatty acids from adipose tissue.

4. Thyroxin, which is secreted by the thyroid gland, affects fat metabolism by stimulating adipose tissue release of free fatty acids. It also lowers blood cholesterol.

Effect of body temperature on fat metabolism

Lowering of body temperature stimulates the release of unesterified fatty acids. These fatty acids supply fuel to return the body temperature toward normal. Table 3-3 summarizes the factors that affect the rate of mobilization of free fatty acids from adipose tissue.

Metabolism of cholesterol

Before the intestinal absorption of cholesterol can occur, bile and the pancreatic enzyme, cholesterol esterase, must be present. Cholesterol esterase catalyzes the esterification of cholesterol by fatty acids. By far the largest amount of cholesterol—80 to 90%—is absorbed in ester form.

The cholesterol esters and the small remaining amount of free cholesterol are then incorporated into the chylomicrons formed in the intestine wall, and are transported by way of the lymph to the portal blood. The blood level of cholesterol is normally maintained at 150 to 300 mg./100 ml.

Cholesterol may be synthesized by the liver as well as other tissues. Alteration of dietary cholesterol does not particularly affect serum cholesterol, and a low cholesterol diet probably has little therapeutic validity.

Cholesterol is excreted by the liver in bile. The liver, therefore, has a major cholesterol-regulating role, since it adds and removes cholesterol from the blood as needed.

GLOSSARY

cholecystokinin (Gr. *chole*, bile or gall; *kystis*, bladder; *kinein*, to move) a hormone that is secreted by the mucosa of the duodenum in response to the presence of fat. The cholecystokinin causes the gallbladder to contract. This contraction propels bile into the duodenum, where it is needed to emulsify the fat. The fat is thus prepared for digestion and absorption.

cholesterol a fat-related compound, a sterol ($C_{27}H_{45}OH$). It is a normal constituent of bile, and a principal constituent of gallstones. In body metabolism cholesterol is important as a precursor of various steroid hormones such as sex hormones, and adrenal corticoids. It has been associated with atherosclerosis, a disease of blood vessels characterized by the formation of localized plaques within or beneath the intimal surface of the vessel wall. Cholesterol is one of the major components of these fatty plaques. Cholesterol can be synthesized by the liver. It is widely distributed in nature, especially in animal tissue such as glandular meats and egg yolk.

chyle the milklike contents of the lacteals and lymphatic vessels of the intestine. It consists principally of absorbed fats. Chyle is carried from the intestine by the lymphatic vessels to the cisterna chyli. The cisterna chyli (the cistern or receptacle of the chyle) is a dilated sac at the origin of the thoracic duct, which is the common trunk that receives all the lymphatic vessels. The cisterna chyli lies in the abdomen between the second lumbar vertebra and the aorta. It receives the lymph from the intestinal trunk, the right and left lumber lymphatic trunks, and two descending lymphatic trunks. The chyle, after passing through the cisterna chyli, is carried upward into the chest through the thoracic duct and empties into the venous blood at the point where the left subclavian vein joins the left internal jugular vein.

chylomicrons (Gr. *chylos*, chyle; *mikros*, small) particles of fat appearing in the lymph and blood after a meal rich in fat. These particles are composed largely of triglycerides with lesser amounts of phospholipids, cholesterol, cholesterol esters, and protein. About two to three hours after a fat meal, the chylomicrons cause lactescence (milkiness) in the blood plasma; this is termed *alimentary lipemia*.

emulsifier an agent that breaks down large fat globules to smaller, uniformly distributed particles. This action is accomplished in the intestine chiefly by the bile acids, which lower surface tension of the fat particles. Emulsification greatly increases the surface area of fat, facilitating contact with fat-digesting enzymes.

enterohepatic circulation (Gr. *enteron,* intestine; *hepar,* liver) the circulation of bile from the liver to the gallbladder, then into the intestine, from which it is absorbed and carried by the blood back to the liver to be returned to the circulation. This continual circulation efficiently conserves the bile. Of the 20 to 30 gm. of bile used daily by the body, only about 0.8 gm. is eliminated in the feces and must be replenished by the liver.

essential fatty acid (EFA) a fatty acid which is (1) necessary for body metabolism or function, and (2) cannot be manufactured by the body and must therefore be supplied in the diet. The major essential fatty acid is linoleic acid ($C_{17}H_{31}COOH$). It is found principally in vegetable oils. Two other fatty acids usually classified as essential are linolenic acid and arachidonic acid.

ester a compound produced by the reaction between an acid and an alcohol with the elimination of a molecule of water. Esters are commonly liquids with characteristic fruity or flowery odors. Cholesterol esters are formed in the mucosal cells by combination with fatty acids, largely linoleic acid.

fatty acid the structural components of fats. See *glycerides.*

glycerides group name for fats, any of a group of esters obtained from glycerol by the replacement of one, two, or three hydroxyl (OH) groups with a fatty acid. Monoglycerides contain one fatty acid; diglycerides contain two fatty acids; triglycerides contain three fatty acids. These glycerides are the principal constituent of adipose tissue, and are found in animal and vegetable fats and oils.

glycerol a colorless, odorless, syrupy, sweet liquid; a constituent of fats usually obtained by the hydrolysis of fats. Chemically, glycerol is an alcohol; it is esterified with fatty acids to produce fats.

hydrogenation the process of adding hydrogen to unsaturated fats to produce a solid, saturated fat. This process is used to produce vegetable shortenings from vegetable oils.

hydrolysis the process by which a chemical compound is split into other compounds by taking up the elements of water. Common examples of hydrolysis are the reactions of digestion, in which the nutrients are split into simpler compounds by the digestive enzymes; that is, the conversion of starch to maltose, of fat to fatty acids and glycerol, and so on.

hyperlipemia excess quantity of fats and fatty substances in the blood.

lecithin (Gr. *lekithos,* egg yolk) a yellow-brown fatty substance, of the group called phospholipids. It occurs in animal and plant tissues and egg yolk. It is composed of units of choline, phosphoric acid, fatty acids, and glycerol. Commercial forms of lecithin, obtained chiefly from soybeans, corn, and egg yolk, are used in candies, foods, cosmetics, and inks. In the metabolism of fat in the liver, lecithin plays an important role. It provides an effective lipotropic factor, choline, which prevents the accumulation of abnormal quantities of fat.

linoleic acid the major essential fatty acid. It is unsaturated.

lipase (Gr. *lipos,* fat; *-ase,* the suffix for enzyme) any of a class of enzymes that break down fats. A small quantity of gastric lipase (lipase secreted by the gastric mucosa) acts on emulsified fats of cream and egg yolk. The major digestive lipase is pancreatic lipase, which acts upon fats in the small intestine. Pancreatic lipase was formely called *steapsin.* Enteric lipase acts within the mucosal cells.

lipids the group name for organic substances of fatty nature. The lipids include fats, oils, waxes, and related compounds.

lipogenesis the formation of fat.

lipolysis the breakdown of fat into its component fatty acids and glycerol.

lipoproteins compounds of fat with protein. The lipoproteins probably function as major carriers of lipids in the plasma, since most of the plasma fat is associated with them. Such a combination makes possible the transport of fatty substances in a predominantly aqueous medium such as plasma.

lipotropic factor (Gr. *lipos,* fat; *trope,* turning) an agent which has an affinity for lipids. It prevents or corrects an excess accumulation of fat in the liver. Choline is probably the most important of the lipotropic factors. Protein helps to prevent a fatty liver because it provides amino acids, such as methionine, that contribute to the synthesis of choline.

micellar bile-fat complex (L., *mica,* crumb, grain; *-ella,* diminutive suffix) a micelle is a particle formed by an aggregate of molecules; a microscopic unit of protoplasm. In micellar bile-fat complex, the particle is formed by the combination of bile salts with fat substances (fatty acids and glycerides) to achieve the absorption of fat across the intestinal mucosa.

phospholipids any of a class of fat-related substances which contain phosphorus, fatty acids, and a nitrogenous base. The phospholipids are essential elements in every cell, but seem to play a special role in the metabolism of fat within the liver.

saponification (L. *sapo,* soap; *facere,* to make) a characteristic reaction of fats and alkalis which produces soaps.

saturation (L. *saturare,* to fill) to cause to unite with the greatest possible amount of another substance, through solution, chemical combination, or the like. A saturated fat, for example, is one in which the component fatty acids are filled with hydrogen atoms. A fatty acid is said to be saturated if all available chemical bonds of its carbon chain are filled with hydrogen. If one bond remains unfilled, it is a monounsaturated fatty acid. If two or more bonds remain unfilled, it is a polyunsaturated fatty acid. Fats of animal sources are more saturated. Fats of plant sources are more unsaturated.

steroids Any of a large group of fat-related organic compounds, including sterols, bile acids, sex hormones, hormones of the adrenal cortex, and D vitamins.

References
Specific

1. Alfin-Slater, R. B.: The absorption, digestion, and metabolism of fats and of related lipids. In Wohl, M. G., and Goodhart, R. S., editors: Modern nutrition in health and disease, Philadelphia, 1964, Lea & Febiger.
2. Deuel, H. J., Jr.: The lipids: their chemistry and biochemistry, Vol. 1: chemistry, New York, 1951, Interscience Publishers.
3. Mead, J. F.: The metabolism of the polyunsaturated fatty acids, Amer. J. Clin. Nutr. 8:55, 1960.
4. Inglefinger, F. J.: Gastrointestinal absorption, Nutrition Today 2(1):2, 1967.
5. Phelps, C. P., Rubin, C. E., and Luft, J. H.: Electron microscope techniques for studying absorption of fat in man, Gastroent. 46:134, 1964.
6. Porte, D., Jr., and Entenman, C.: Fatty acid metabolism in segments of rat intestine, Amer. J. Physiol. 208:607, 1965.
7. Guyton, A. C.: Textbook of medical physiology, Philadelphia, 1966, W. B. Saunders Company, p. 908.

General

Barboriak, J. J., and others: Breakfast menu and blood lipids, J. Amer. Diet. Ass. 49:204, 1966.
Bierenbaum, M. L., and others: Fats and fatty acids in excess, J. Amer. Diet. Ass. 50:368, 1967.
Cantarow, A., and Trumper, M.: Clinical biochemistry, ed. 6, Philadelphia, 1962, W. B. Saunders Co.
Coons, C. M.: Fatty acids in foods, J. Amer. Diet. Ass. 34:242, 1958.
Council on Foods and Nutrition, American Medi-cal Association: Food fats, J.A.M.A. **179**:719, 1962.
Council on Foods and Nutrition, American Medical Association: Special shortenings, J.A.M.A. **187**:766, 1964.
Council on Foods and Nutrition, American Medical Association: The regulation of dietary fat, J.A.M.A. **181**:411, 1962.
Fatty acids in food fats, Home Economics Research Report No. 7, Agricultural Research Service, Washington, D. C., U. S. Department of Agriculture, 1959.
Feeley, R. M., and others: Fat metabolism in pre-adolescent children on all-vegetable diets, J. Amer. Diet. Ass. **47**:396, 1965.
Food and Nutrition Board: Dietary fat and human health, Publication No. 1147, National Academy of Sciences, National Research Council, Washington, D. C., 1966.
Gorman, J. C., and Moore, M. E.: Fatty acids in vegetarian diets, J. Amer. Diet. Ass. **50**:372, 1967.
Hansen, A. E., and others: Role of linoleic acid in infant nutrition, Pediatrics **31**:171, 1962.
Hardinge, M. G., and Crooks, H.: Fatty acid composition of food fats, J. Amer. Diet. Ass. **34**:1065, 1958.
Harper, H. A.: Review of physiological chemistry, ed. 11, Los Altos, Calif., 1967, Lange Medical Publications.
Hayes, O. B., and Rose, G.: Supplementary food composition table, J. Amer. Diet. Ass. **33**:26, 1957.
Kinsell, L. W., and others: Dietary considerations with regard to type of fat, Amer. J. Clin. Nutr. **15**:198, 1964.
Macdonald, I.: Interrelationship between the influences of dietary carbohydrates and fats on fasting serum lipids, Amer. J. Clin. Nutr. **20**:345, 1967.
Morse, E. H., and others: Lipid metabolism and the sulphur-containing amino acids, J. Amer. Diet. Ass. **48**:496, 1966.
Reviews: Body fat and adipose tissue, Nutr. Rev. **22**:99, 1964; Council report on dietary fat regulation, Nutr. Rev. **21**:36, 1963; Fat and cholesterol in the diet, Nutr. Rev. **23**:3, 1965.
Rice, E. E.: Composition of modern margarines, J. Amer. Diet. Ass. **41**:319, 1962.
Stefferud, A.: Food: the yearbook of Agriculture, 1959, Washington, D. C., 1959, U. S. Department of Agriculture.
Underwood, B. A., and others: Fatty acid absorption and metabolism in protein-calorie malnutrition, Amer. J. Clin. Nutr. **20**:226, 1967.
White, A., and others: Principles of biochemistry, ed. 3, New York, 1964, McGraw-Hill Book Company.
Wohl, M., and Goodhart, R.: Modern nutrition in health and disease, ed. 4, Philadelphia, 1968, Lea & Febiger.

CHAPTER 4

Proteins

The Dutch chemist, Mulder, first proposed the name *protein* in 1840, before much was known about these substances. The word *protein* comes from the Greek word *proteios,* meaning "primary, holding first place." Mulder applied the name well. Proteins make up the basic structure of all living cells and are an essential life-forming and life-sustaining ingredient of the diet of all animal organisms. The amount of protein in the diets of different cultures varies. In countries with adequate nutrition, it contributes from 10 to 15% of the total calories. In the average American diet, protein contributes approximately 14% of the total calories.

GENERAL AND CHEMICAL DEFINITIONS OF PROTEINS

General definition. Proteins may be defined as organic substances which upon hydrolysis or digestion yield their constituent unit building blocks—*amino acids.* Proteins are found in animal foods such as meat, milk, cheese, and egg, and to a lesser extent in plant foods such as grains and legumes. Entirely free protein, such as albumin in egg white, is rare in nature. Usually protein is found in connection with fats and carbohydrates. For example, in the animal food sources protein is usually associated with fat (meat, milk, cheese, egg yolk). In plants proteins are usually associated with carbohydrate (grains, legumes).

Chemical definition. A protein may be defined according to its basic elements. Like carbohydrate and fat, protein contains carbon, hydrogen, and oxygen. But protein

is unique in that it also contains nitrogen (16% of its total composition) and often other elements such as sulfur.

The structure of protein is also different from that of either carbohydrate or fat. The proteins are much more complex compounds with high molecular weights, which range from a few thousand to a million or more. A given protein contains a specific number of specific amino acids linked in a sequence that is specific for that protein. It is this very specificity of protein structure in a definite amino acid sequence that gives various tissues their unique form, function, and character.

CLASSIFICATION OF PROTEINS
Chemical structure

More is yet to be learned about the composition of specific proteins, but their general structure and chemical nature provide a basis for the rather loose classifications of simple proteins, compound proteins, and derived proteins.

Simple proteins. Simple proteins contain only amino acids or their derivatives. A few common examples of simple proteins are:
1. Albumin—lactalbumin in milk, serum albumin in blood
2. Globulin—ovoglobulin in egg, serum globulin in blood
3. Glutelins—glutens in wheat
4. Prolamines—zein in corn, gliadin in wheat
5. Albuminoids—collagen in supportive tissue, keratin in hair and skin, gelatin

Compound (conjugated) proteins. Compound proteins are compounds of simple proteins and some other nonprotein group.

Examples include:

1. Nucleoproteins (compounds of one or more proteins and nucleic acid)—purines, which are found in large amounts in glandular tissue
2. Glycoproteins and mucoproteins (compounds of a protein and carbohydrate)—mucin found in secretions from mucous membranes
3. Phosphoproteins (compounds of a protein and a phosphorus-containing radical other than phospholipid or nucleic acid)—casein, found in milk
4. Chromoproteins (compounds of a protein and a chromophoric, or pigmented group)—hemoglobin
5. Lipoproteins (compounds of a protein and a triglyceride or other lipid)—phospholipid or cholesterol
6. Metalloproteins (compounds of a protein and a metal such as copper or iron)—heme, the iron-binding portion of hemoglobin

Derived proteins. Derived proteins are fragments of various sizes. They are produced as large protein molecules initially and are progressively broken down during digestion. In order of size, from largest to smallest fragments of peptide chains, these derived proteins are proteoses, peptones, polypeptides, and peptides.

Function

Proteins may also be classified into seven broad categories according to their function in the body:

1. Structural proteins—collagen
2. Contractile proteins—muscle
3. Antibodies—gamma globulin
4. Blood proteins—albumin, fibrinogen, and hemoglobin
5. Hormones
6. Enzymes
7. Nutrient proteins—food sources of essential amino acids

AMINO ACIDS

Newer concepts of protein interpret them in terms of their constituent amino acids. A nursing student will need to rec-ognize the names of these amino acids and know something of their nature, for they will be encountered in clinical practice. For example, in pediatric nursing one learns of *phenylketonuria*, a disease in children caused by the body's inability to properly handle the essential amino acid *phenylalanine*. Proteins also have such an excellent buffering effect for peptic ulcer patients, because of the interesting *amphoteric* nature of amino acids.

Proteins should be viewed, then, in terms of their building blocks, amino acids. This chapter will look at the background of their discovery, and their unique dual structure.

History. Early in the 1800's, scientists recognized that proteins could be broken down (hydrolyzed) into a number of smaller structural units. Because these substances seemed to behave chemically with a dual nature—both acid and base—they were given the seemingly contradictory name *amino* (base) *acids*.

Glycine, the simplest amino acid, was identified in 1820; threonine was not identified until 1935. Since then, still other amino acids have been identified as metabolic products in the body. Much of the early work was contributed by Carl von Voit and his pupil, Max Rubner, in the late 19th century and by R. H. Chittenden in the early 20th century. These basic studies were expanded and developed by Thomas B. Osborne and L. B. Mendel at Yale, W. C. Rose at the University of Illinois, and many others.

Classification of amino acids

Essential and nonessential amino acids. It was largely the brilliant work of Dr. Rose[1] that established an important differentiation among the amino acids. He termed amino acids "essential" or "nonessential." This grouping is based on two factors: (1) whether the body can manufacture the particular amino acid, and (2) whether the amino acid is essential for normal growth and development.

In his experiments, Rose used young rats. He first fed the rats on a known mixture of purified amino acids. Then, one at a time, he removed an amino acid from the mixture. If the rat continued to grow normally, he classified that amino acid as nonessential. If the rat ceased to grow normally, or lost weight and died, he classified the amino acid as essential. It soon became apparent that in man, also, the protein requirement must be considered on the basis of the quality, and not merely the quantity of the protein. It was obviously not just a matter of the total amount of protein needed, but of the specific amino acids needed. For example, gelatin alone is a rather worthless protein, for it lacks three essential amino acids—tryptophan, valine, and isoleucine—and has only small amounts of leucine.

On the basis of these distinctions in body dependence, eight amino acids have been demonstrated to be essential for adults. The approximately twelve remaining amino acids are nonessential or dispensable. The body can manufacture them and they are not as necessary for normal growth and development. The following is a listing of the essential and nonessential proteins.

Essential	Nonessential*
Threonine	Glycine
Leucine	Alanine
Isoleucine	Aspartic acid
Valine	Glutamic acid
Lysine	Proline
Methionine	Hydroxyproline
Phenylalanine	Cystine
Tryptophan	Tyrosine
	Serine
	Arginine†
	Histidine†

Complete and incomplete proteins. According to the amount of essential amino acids that given proteins in foods possess, they have been broadly classified as complete or incomplete proteins. Complete pro-

*Three other amino acids, cysteine, citrulline, and hydroxylysine, may be added to the nonessential list. Although not naturally occurring, they are nonetheless metabolically active in the body.
†Arginine and histidine are necessary during growth, but not during adulthood; they may be called "semiessential."

teins are those that contain all the essential amino acids in sufficient quantity and ratio to supply the body's needs. These proteins are of animal origin: meat, milk (cheese), and egg. Incomplete proteins are those deficient in one or more of the essential amino acids. They are of plant origin: grains, legumes, and nuts. In a mixed diet, animal and plant proteins supplement one another. Even a mixture of plant proteins may provide an adequate, balanced ratio of amino acids. The value of variety in the diet is therefore self-evident. The comparative nutritive quality of protein foods is discussed later in this chapter as the question of protein requirement is considered (pp. 56-59).

Basic structure of amino acids

Amphoteric nature. As indicated by its name, an amino acid has a chemical structure which combines both acid and base (amino) factors. This important chemical structure gives to amino acids a unique amphoteric nature (Gr. *amphoteros,* both). This dual nature can be seen in the fundamental pattern of an amino acid as shown in the diagrams on p. 46. The acid factor is the carboxyl group (COOH) and the base factor is the amino group (NH_2). A radical which is specific for the individual amino acid is grouped around a central carbon atom.

As a result of its dual nature, an amino acid in solution can *ionize* (dissociate or separate into its constituent ions) to behave either as an acid or as a base, depending upon the pH of the solution. This means that amino acids have a great *buffer* capacity, which is an important clinical characteristic. The interesting term commonly used for this unique phenomenon is zwitterion. The term is taken from the German word *Zwitter,* meaning "hybrid" and the Greek word *ion,* meaning "wanderer." Amino acids behave like "hybrid wanderers," either acid or base, depending upon the buffering need presented by the particular solution they are in.

Peptide linkage. This acid-base chemical

$$\text{Base (amino group)} \longrightarrow \left(H-N \Big\backslash^H \right) \begin{pmatrix} O \\ \| \\ C-OH \end{pmatrix} \leftarrow \text{Acid (carboxyl group)}$$

$$H-N \text{—} C-H$$

$$(R) \leftarrow \text{Varying attached radical}$$

Fundamental amino acid pattern

$$\begin{array}{c} COOH \\ | \\ NH_2\text{—}C\text{—}H \\ | \\ CH_3 \end{array}$$

Alanine (attached radical a methyl group)

$$\begin{array}{c} COOH \\ | \\ NH_2\text{—}C\text{—}H \\ | \\ H \end{array}$$

Glycine (attached radical a single hydrogen atom)

$$\begin{array}{c} COOH \\ | \\ NH_2\text{—}C\text{—}H \\ | \\ CH_2 \end{array}$$

Phenylalanine (attached radical a complex carbon ring structure)

nature of amino acids also enables them to join in the characteristic chain structure of proteins. The amino group of one amino acid joins the carboxyl group of another. This characteristic chain structure of amino acids is called a peptide linkage. Long chains of amino acids which are linked in this manner are called *polypeptides* (Fig. 4-1).

Arrangement of peptide chains. Long polypeptide chains may be coiled or folded back upon themselves in a spiral shape called a *helix.* They are held together in some instances by additional cross-links of bonds involving sulfur and hydrogen. The helical shapes of these coils may be of two types: (1) *fibrous*—a protein which coils and unfolds upon contraction and relaxation, such as myosin in muscle fiber, and

(2) *globular*—a protein forming a dense compact coil, such as serum (albumin and globulin) and insulin.

The various component structures within the total structure of the protein molecule have been grouped according to increased complexity of arrangement. The *primary structure* is the basic polypeptide chain. The *secondary structure* is the helix with its coils linked to one another by cross-bonds usually of hydrogen or sulfur. The *tertiary structure* is the characteristic arrangements of helices which form specific layers on fibers of specific proteins.

FUNCTIONS OF PROTEIN

Growth and tissue maintenance. The primary function of dietary protein is the growth and maintenance of tissue. It does

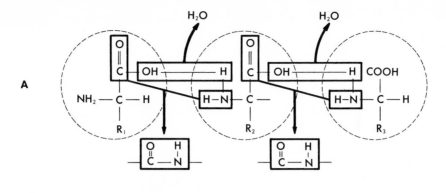

Fig. 4-1. Two stages in formation of peptide linkage by which amino acids are formed. **A,** Basic joining of the two amino acids, producing peptide bond and water. **B,** Polypeptide chain formed from numbers of specific amino acids linked in specific sequence. The different attached radicals (R_1, R_2 . . . R_{n-1}, R_n) determine the specific amino acids.

this by furnishing amino acids (of appropriate numbers and types) for efficient synthesis of specific cellular tissue proteins. In addition, protein supplies amino acids for other essential nitrogen-containing substances such as enzymes and hormones.

Specific physiological roles of amino acids. All amino acids supplied by protein participate in growth and tissue maintenance, but some also perform other important physiologic and metabolic roles.

Methionine is a methylating agent which participates in the formation of such nonprotein cellular constituents as choline. Methionine is also the precursor of the nonessential amino acid *cystine.*

Tryptophan is the precursor of the vitamin nicotinamide (niacin) and the precursor of the vasoconstrictor serotonin.

Phenylalanine is the precursor of the nonessential amino acid tyrosine. Together with tyrosine phenylalanine leads to formation of the hormones thyroxine and epinephrine.

Energy. Protein also contributes to the body's overall energy metabolism. After removal of the nitrogenous portion of the constituent amino acid, the amino acid residue may be either glycogenic (capable of being converted to carbohydrate) or ketogenic (capable of being converted to fatty acids). Only leucine, phenylalanine, and tyrosine are fully ketogenic, and isoleucine is weakly so. The remaining amino acids are glycogenic. It has been estimated that on an average, 58% of the total dietary protein becomes available as glucose and is oxidized as such to yield energy.

DIGESTION OF PROTEIN
Mechanical digestion

Mouth. Only mechanical breaking up of protein foods by mastication occurs in the mouth. Here the food particles are mixed with salivary secretions and pass as a semisolid mass into the stomach where the main chemical digestion of protein begins.

Chemical digestion

Stomach. Chemical digestion of protein begins in the stomach. In fact, the stomach's chief digestive function in relation to all foods is the partial enzymatic breakdown of protein. Three agents contained in the gastric secretions participate in different ways in this beginning hydrolysis. These agents are pepsin, hydrochloric acid, and rennin.

Pepsin, the main gastric enzyme specific for proteins, is first produced as an inactive substance, *pepsinogen,* by a single layer of cells (the chief cells) in the mucosa of the stomach wall. Pepsinogen requires hydrochloric acid for activation to the enzyme pepsin. This active pepsin then begins breaking the peptide linkages of protein to produce *proteoses* and *peptones.* These are shorter chain polypeptides which are still rather large protein derivatives. If the protein were held in the stomach longer, pepsin could continue this breakdown until individual amino acids resulted. However, with normal gastric emptying time, only the beginning stage is completed by the action of pepsin.

Hydrochloric acid (HCl) is necessary to convert inactive pepsinogen to the active enzyme pepsin. Gastric hydrochloric acid is an important catalyst in gastric protein digestion. Clinical problems can be anticipated for patients who lack proper hydrochloric acid secretion.

Rennin is a gastric enzyme important in the infant's digestion of milk. Rennin and calcium act on the casein of milk to produce a curd. By coagulating milk, rennin prevents too rapid a passage from the stomach. In adults, however, rennin is apparently absent from the gastric secretions.

Small intestine. Protein digestion begins in the acid medium of the stomach and continues in the alkaline medium of the small intestine. A number of enzymes from both pancreatic and intestinal secretions take part.

Pancreatic secretions. The protein-splitting enzyme *trypsin* is secreted first by the pancreas as an inactive substance called *trypsinogen.* Trypsinogen is activated to trypsin by the hormone *enterokinase,* which is produced by glands in the duodenal wall. This active enzyme trypsin acts on protein, and proteoses and peptones carried over from the stomach to produce shorter chain polypeptides and dipeptides.

The pancreas also produces another protein-specific enzyme, *chymotrypsin,* preceded by its inactive precursor, *chymotrypsinogen.* Chymotrypsin is activated by the activated trypsin present. Chymotrypsin has the same protein-splitting action as trypsin, and produces polypeptides and dipeptides. It also has more milk coagulating ability than trypsin.

Carboxypeptidase is one of a group of enzymes called peptidases. It is called *carboxypeptidase* because it attacks the end of the peptide chain where there is a free carboxyl (acid) group (COOH). It produces still simpler peptides and some free amino acids.

Intestinal secretions. Glands in the intestinal wall produce aminopeptidase and dipeptidase. These are two additional protein-splitting enzymes in the peptidase group.

Aminopeptidase attacks the amino (NH_2) linkages of the peptide chain. Through this cleavage action, aminopeptidase produces simpler short chain peptides and free amino acids.

Dipeptidase is the final enzyme of the protein-splitting system. It acts on the remaining dipeptides to produce free amino acids.

By this system, the pancreatic and intestinal secretions break down the large complex proteins into progressively smaller peptide chains, and amino acids are split off from the ends of these chains. The end products of protein digestion (amino acids) are then ready for absorption by the intestinal mucosa.

A summary of protein digestion is outlined for review in Table 4-1.

ABSORPTION OF PROTEIN INTO THE BLOODSTREAM

The end products of protein digestion are water-soluble amino acids. These amino acids are absorbed rapidly from the small

Table 4-1. Summary of protein digestion

Organ	Enzyme			Digestive action
	Inactive precursor	**Activator**	**Active enzyme**	
Mouth			None	Mechanical only
Stomach (acid)	Pepsinogen	Hydrochloric acid	Pepsin	Protein → proteoses and peptones
			Rennin (infants) (Ca necessary for activity)	Casein → coagulated curd
Intestine (alkaline)				
Pancreatic juice	Trypsinogen	Enterokinase	Trypsin	Protein, proteoses, peptones → polypeptides, dipeptides
	Chymotrypsinogen	Active trypsin	Chymotrypsin	Proteoses, peptones → polypeptides, dipeptides Also coagulates milk
			Carboxypeptidase	Polypeptides → simpler peptides, dipeptides, amino acids
Intestinal juice			Aminopeptidase	Polypeptides → peptides, depeptides, amino acids
			Dipeptidase	Dipeptides → amino acids

intestine directly into the portal blood system through the fine network of villous capillaries. Most of this amino acid absorption probably takes place in the proximal portion of the small intestine.

The mechanism of this absorptive transport is not completely known. Originally it was assumed that since amino acids are water soluble, all forms were absorbed through the intestinal wall by simple passive diffusion. However, more recent studies[2] indicate that far more activity is involved. This process is currently believed to include several aspects.

Active transport system. An active and selective transport system is present which is energy-dependent. The amino acids in their natural forms are transported by this active system; their isomers may be absorbed by free diffusion.

Vitamin B$_6$ cofactor. Vitamin B$_6$ (pyridoxine) in the form of pyridoxal phosphate appears to be intimately involved in the active transport of amino acids from the intestinal mucosa to the serosa. This vitamin also seems to play a role in the transport of amino acids into the cells for eventual metabolism. This relationship provides still another example of the concept of intimate interrelationships among the many nutrients and their metabolites in human nutrition.

Competition for absorption. Competition for absorption of the amino acids seems to exist. When a mixture of amino acids is fed to an organism, the quantitatively predominant amino acid may retard the absorption of the others. In the plasma, also, competition apparently exists among the circulating amino acids for entry into the cell.

Absorption of whole proteins. A few larger fragments of short-chain peptides may remain after digestion and be absorbed as such. Even whole proteins are sometimes absorbed intact. These larger molecules apparently cannot be used in protein synthesis as can free amino acids, but they may play a part in the development of immunity and sensitivity. For example, antibodies in the mother's colostrum (the pre-milk breast secretion) are passed on to her nursing infant.

METABOLISM OF PROTEIN

In human nutrition, the amino acids are the metabolic currency of protein. It is with the fate of these vital compounds that the metabolism of protein is ultimately concerned. The many metabolic processes involved in protein metabolism form a fascinating array of complex and intricately interwoven chemical activities. The metabolic activities of protein can be summarized under the three broad categories of *balance*, *building* tissue, (anabolism), and *breakdown* of tissue (catabolism). These activities may be remembered as the "three B's" of protein metabolism.

Balance

Throughout the body, many interdependent checks and balances exist. There is a constant ebb and flow of materials, a building up and breaking down of parts, and a depositing and mobilizing of constituents. Many body mechanisms maintain internal physiologic stability (equilibrium). The body has built-in controls which operate as coordinated responses of its parts to any situation that tends to disturb its normal condition or function. The resultant state of equilibrium is called *homeostasis,* and the various mechanisms designed to preserve it are called *homeostatic mechanisms.* This balance between body parts and functions is life-sustaining.

Increasingly, therefore, as more and more is being learned about human nutrition and physiology, older ideas of a rigid body structure are giving way to a concept of dynamic equilibrium. All body constituents are in a constant state of flux, although some tissues are more actively engaged

than others. This concept of dynamic equilibrium can be seen in carbohydrate and fat metabolism; however, it is especially striking in protein metabolism.

Protein turnover. Classic studies[3] with radioactive isotopes have clearly demonstrated that the body's protein tissues are continuously being broken down into amino acids and resynthesized. In such studies, when "labeled" amino acids are fed, they are rapidly incorporated into various body tissue proteins.

The rate of protein turnover varies in different tissues. It is highest in the intestinal mucosa, liver, pancreas, kidney, and plasma and lowest in muscle, brain, and skin tissue; there is almost no protein turnover in collagen tissue.

Endogenous body protein exists in a balance between two compartments—the tissue protein compartment and the plasma protein compartment. These endogenous stores are further balanced with exogenous dietary protein intake. Protein from one compartment may be drawn upon to supply a need in the other. For example, during fasting, resources from the body protein stores may be used for tissue synthesis. But the interesting fact is that even when the intake of protein and other nutrients is adequate, the tissue proteins are still being constantly broken down and reformed.

The adult body's state of stability, then, is the result of a balance between the rates of protein breakdown and resynthesis. In periods of growth, however, the synthesis rate is higher so that new tissue can be formed. In conditions of starvation and wasting diseases (and, more gradually, as the aging process in the elderly), the rate of breakdown exceeds that of synthesis and the body deteriorates.

Metabolic amino acid pool. Amino acids derived from endogenous tissue breakdown and amino acids from dietary protein both enter a common metabolic pool of amino acids. Thus, a balance of amino acids is maintained to supply the body's total needs. Shifts and balances between tissue breakdown and dietary protein ensure the con-

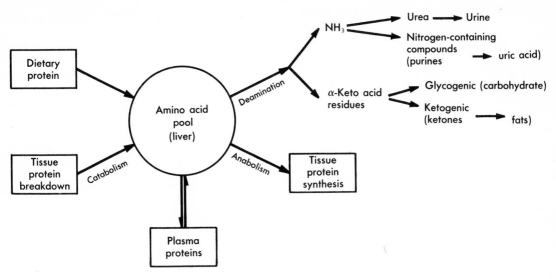

Fig. 4-2. Balance between protein compartments and amino acid pool.

stant availability of a balanced mixture of amino acids. From this amino acid pool, specific amino acids are supplied as needed for specific tissue protein synthesis and to make up body losses (Fig. 4-2).

Nitrogen balance. Nitrogen is also found in compounds other than amino acids. Nonprotein nitrogen is present in urea, uric acid, ammonia, creatine, creatinine, and other body tissues and fluids. *Total nitrogen balance* involves all these sources. The word balance refers to the balance between intake and output of a particular substance. The term *negative balance* is used to indicate that the output of the substance exceeds its intake. *Positive balance* is that state in which the intake of a given substance exceeds its output. *Total nitrogen balance* is the net result of all nitrogen gains and losses in all protein compartments, although it gives no picture of the shifts in distribution of nitrogen. For example, a tissue involved in a malignant neoplastic process may be robbing other tissues of nitrogen; yet this loss would not be reflected in total nitrogen balance. Nevertheless, the total nitrogen balance is a useful general measure of body equilibrium.

Nonprotein nitrogen plays a role in pro-

tein synthesis through its sparing effect on some amino acid requirements. By providing the amino group for transamination, it relieves the need for amino acid food sources to supply the nitrogen radical.

Building tissue (anabolism)

To maintain the vital balance in protein metabolism, amino acids have one of two possible fates in the body after absorption. They may be incorporated into tissue protein synthesis (*anabolism*), or they may be degraded or broken down into their constituent parts (*catabolism*). The products of protein catabolism are oxidized or excreted.

The building or synthesis of tissue protein is governed by a unique specificity with respect to the amino acid constituents that are required to produce a specific protein. This has been called the law of "all or none." All the necessary amino acids for a given protein must be present at the same time or the protein will not be formed. Specific selection and supply of amino acids are mandatory.

Since the advent of the electron microscope, scientists have been able to study the intricate workings of cell metabolism and develop hypotheses concerning the process by which protein is synthesized by the living organism. To understand the process of protein synthesis one must consider both the basic substances governing the process and the basic steps or stages necessary to build the specific peptide chains. The following brief explanation of some of these processes is highly oversimplified from the point of view of the physical chemist, but it may be found convenient as a basis for conceptualization.

Substances which govern protein synthesis

DNA (deoxyribonucleic acid). DNA has been identified as the controlling mechanism by which genetic design is passed from generation to generation. It is the key material in the chromosomes of the cell nucleus. Each gene is probably composed of a complex nucleic acid molecule. DNA is a large double-chain *polymer* (a compound of high molecular weight made up of many parts). It is composed of nitrogenous bases called nucleotides (purines, pyrimidines), a sugar (deoxyribose), and a phosphate group. DNA forms the basic pattern of the message code in each cell. This code or pattern determines what specific protein will be synthesized.

Messenger RNA (ribonucleic acid). RNA is formed by DNA in the cell nucleus and receives its own specific pattern imprint. (This relationship is similar to the way in which the waffle batter receives the imprint of the waffle iron pressed against it.) RNA differs from DNA, however, in that it is only a single strand structure, it has a different sugar (ribose), and one of its nitrogen bases is a different compound. Once it is formed in the cell nucleus by the DNA, it carries the message pattern transferred to it by DNA to the cell cytoplasm. This type of RNA has been designated "messenger RNA." (Another type of RNA, "transfer RNA," is described below.) Out in the cell, messenger RNA uses one of the membranous tubules of the endoplasmic reticulum as its working site. Here it attaches itself to the row of reticular granules (ribosomes) as an anchor point for its operations.

Ribosomes. Ribosomes are the small granules on the cell's network of endoplasmic reticulum. They are called *ribosomes* because they are minute bodies (Gr. *soma,* body) or spheres containing RNA (ribonucleic acid). The messenger RNA strand from the nucleus attaches itself to the ribosome and forms a template or mold to direct the lining up of amino acids in the exact sequence necessary to fit the master pattern for the desired protein. This is part of the marvelous *specificity* of protein synthesis at work.

Stages in the process of protein synthesis

Activated amino acids. For amino acids to be used in protein synthesis, they must first be activated. This means they must be energized in order to be capable of combining chemically with other substances. This is done in the cell's cytoplasm by an activating enzyme which is specific for each amino acid, plus an energizing phosphate compound—ATP (adenosine triphosphate) or AMP (adenosine monophosphate). The complex formed (enzyme + AMP + amino acid) produces an activated amino acid which is ready to go into its position in the protein molecule.

Transfer RNA. Many short chain RNA molecules (transfer RNA) occur free in the cell's cytoplasmic fluid. There appears to be specific transfer RNA molecules for each amino acid used. Each transfer RNA molecule attaches itself to its specific amino acid partner and carries it to the strand of messenger RNA which is anchored on the ribosome. The amino acid slips perfectly into its correct slot. One beside another, the amino acids line up at their specific fitting sites along the grid of the ribosomal template as the messenger RNA is guided into place by the transfer RNA.

Peptide linkage. The activated amino acids, which have been lined up side by side in a precise sequence, are joined to each other by peptide linkages to form long polypeptide chains. This is the specific

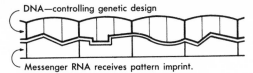

Stage 1: Preparation in cell nucleus: DNA transfers specific
protein pattern to messenger RNA

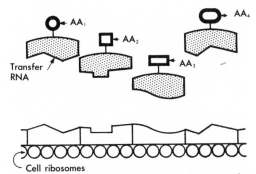

Stage 2: Activated amino acids in cell cytoplasm attach to
transfer RNA partner

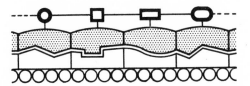

Stage 3: Transfer RNA carries the active amino acids into
position, and peptide linkage forms

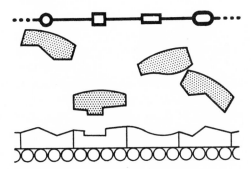

Stage 4: Newly formed polypeptide chain breaks free;
transfer RNA is released to repeat process

Fig. 4-3. Stages in protein synthesis.

polypeptide chain of the protein originally designated by the pattern coded on the DNA in the cell nucleus. The newly formed polypeptide chain breaks free from the ribosome, and the transfer RNA molecules are freed from the messenger RNA template. The transfer RNA molecules are now available to perform the process all over again. These three successive stages in protein synthesis are illustrated in Fig. 4-3.

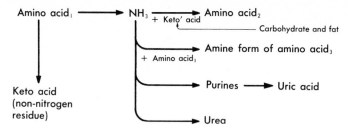

Fig. 4-4. Ways in which ammonia, derived from amino acid deamination, is disposed of by the body.

Breaking down tissue (catabolism)

If a given amino acid is not used in tissue protein synthesis, it may be degraded or oxidized to yield energy. A nitrogenous group and a non-nitrogen residue result from catabolism of amino acids.

Nitrogenous group (NH$_2$). The first step in the metabolic breakdown of amino acids is the splitting off of the nitrogenous portion (the amino group, NH$_2$) by hydrolysis. This process, which takes place chiefly in the liver, is called *deamination*. The ammonia (NH$_3$) which is formed may be handled in several ways (Fig. 4-4).

1. Ammonia may be converted in the liver to urea and excreted by the kidney in the urine. The conversion is completed by a special urea cycle in the liver.
2. The ammonia may also be used in production of purines and other nitrogen-containing compounds.
3. The ammonia may be combined with various carbohydrate derivatives of amino acid residues to form other amino acids. (Such amino acids would be nonessential because the body can manufacture them.) The process of transferring the amino group from an amino acid to a carbohydrate derivative or an amino acid residue is called *transamination*. The process is catalyzed by specific enzymes called *transaminases*. A vitamin B$_6$ derivative (pyridoxal phosphate) acts as a coenzyme. When tissue is damaged, transaminases are released and their level in plasma rises.

4. Ammonia may be taken up by an amino acid to produce still another form of that acid, the *amine* form. This process is called *amination*. For example, a glutamic acid molecule may take up an NH$_3$ radical to form glutamine. The NH$_3$ radical may then be liberated from the glutamine molecule in distal tubules of kidney and excreted. This process of amination and deamination provides an efficient way of removing a toxic substance (NH$_3$) from the body.

These four ways of processing ammonia furnish further illustrations of the body's constant metabolic interconversions between carbohydrate, protein, and fat.

Non-nitrogen residue. The non-nitrogen residue is called a *keto-acid*. The residue of a given amino acid is either *glycogenic* (leading to the formation of carbohydrate), or *ketogenic* (leading to the formation of fat). The ketogenic amino acids are phenylalanine, tyrosine, and leucine; isoleucine residue is also weakly ketogenic. The majority of the amino acids are glycogenic. Glycine, alanine, serine, threonine, valine, glutamic acid, aspartic acid, histidine, arginine, lysine, cystine, methionine, proline, and isoproline are all glycogenic. The glycogenic amino acid residues enter the Embden-Meyerhof glycolytic pathway at pyruvate (see Chapter 2), and the Krebs cycle at oxaloacetate and ketoglutarate. The ketogenic amino acid residues enter the same final oxidation pathways at active acetate (Fig. 4-5).

The intermediate metabolites from pro-

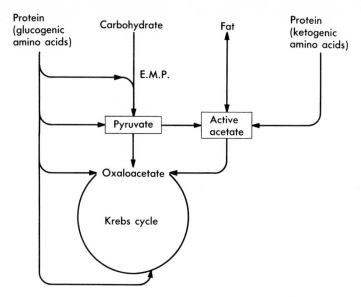

Fig. 4-5. Converging of glucogenic and ketogenic amino acids with carbohydrate and fat in the Embden-Meyerhof glycolytic pathway and the final common Krebs cycle for energy production.

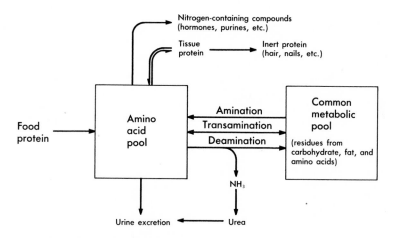

Fig. 4-6. Interrelationships between the amino acid pool and the common metabolic pool of residues from carbohydrates, fats, and amino acids.

tein, carbohydrate, and fat enter a common metabolic pool. There is constant interplay between this pool and the amino acid pool (Fig. 4-6). Finally, metabolites from all three basic nutrients enter the Krebs cycle and produce the end products CO_2 and H_2O.

During a fasting period, glycogen stores are rapidly depleted; fat stores are then reduced more slowly. Only after the fat stores are depleted does the body, in its attempt to maintain itself, begin to break down tissue protein. It is for this reason that a diet sufficient in carbohydrate calories has a protein-sparing effect.

Hormonal influences on protein metabolism

The anabolism and catabolism of protein are regulated by certain hormones.

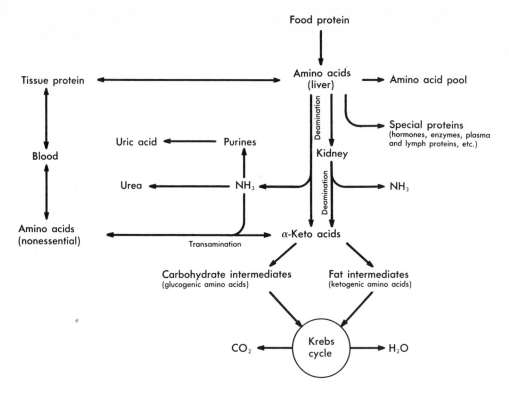

Fig. 4-7. Metabolic interrelationships between protein, carbohydrate, and fat.

Pituitary growth hormone (GH), androgens, insulin, and normal amounts of thyroid hormone all have an anabolic effect.

Growth hormone stimulates body cells to retain protein and to maintain a positive nitrogen balance. It also allows greater protein tissue synthesis during growth periods. *Androgens* (gonadotrophins), especially testosterone, stimulate tissue growth during puberty, chiefly in target reproductive organ tissue. *Insulin* is necessary for the protein synthesis effect of growth hormone and acts as an antagonist to the gluconeogenic effect of adrenocortical hormones. In normal amounts *thyroid hormone* works with growth hormone to stimulate protein synthesis.

Adrenal steroids and large amounts of thyroid hormone have a catabolic effect on protein metabolism. *Adrenal steroids* such as the glucocorticoids (cortisone, hydrocortisone) stimulate gluconeogenesis, deamination of amino acids, and conversion of the residue to glucose or glycogen. In this way, they act indirectly as protein catabolic agents.

Large doses of *thyroid hormone* stimulate excessive catabolism of muscle tissue. This effect is opposite to the anabolic action of the amounts normally secreted by the thyroid gland.

The summary of metabolic interrelationships among protein, carbohydrate, and fat given in Fig. 4-7 may be used for review.

PROTEIN REQUIREMENTS IN HUMAN NUTRITION
Factors which influence determination of protein requirements

Since protein is an essential nutrient, much study has been given to the question of how much protein the body actually requires. General requirements or recommendations for dietary protein intake have been developed on the basis of research pertaining to all age groups. A number of basic concepts influence (and confuse) one's understanding of the requirements of the various age groups.

Function of dietary protein. Because the primary purpose of furnishing protein in the diet is to supply amino acids in the quantity and kind necessary for growth and maintenance of tissue, the age and physical status of the individual should be taken into consideration when determining the amount required. Further, these amino acids must be supplied in an appropriate pattern for efficient synthesis of tissue protein and other nitrogen-containing substances. The nutritive value of a dietary protein is a measure of its ability to supply these needs. It can supply these needs, however, only if calorie needs are also met. Because protein's function is life-sustaining, a deficiency in this dietary factor has a profound effect on various organs of the body.

Metabolism of protein and amino acids. Knowing basic metabolic concepts is necessary to understand the body's protein requirement. The dynamic concept of protein compartments with an ebb and flow of nitrogen between tissue protein, dietary protein, and a common amino acid pool plays a role. Knowing the amount of protein reserves in the body is also necessary. Also, the concept of essential and nonessential amino acids aids in determining which specific amino acids the diet must supply. Moreover, the concept of the all or none law in protein synthesis aids in knowing which specific amino acids must be supplied at one time to produce a given tissue.

Nitrogen balance. The measure of net gain and loss of total nitrogen in all parts of the body gives a base for study of protein nutrition, although it gives no indication of internal shifts in distribution of nitrogen. An added difficulty is that this level is adaptive, and after a time, the body adapts to a lower or higher level of nitrogen. Nitrogen balance alone is not enough to determine protein requirement.

In reference to nitrogen balance, the nutritionist uses the term *biological value* of a food source. This measure of the nutri-

tive value of a given dietary protein refers to the percent of absorbed nitrogen that is retained by the body. However, some of the studies in this area are faulty. In some short-term observations, insufficient time is allowed for the organism to adapt to the diet change. In others, only a single tissue function is evaluated.

Digestibility factor. The degree to which a given protein is digested and absorbed will also influence the requirement for it. Absorption (digestibility) is affected by preparation and cooking and by the rate and completeness with which enzymes hydrolyze that specific protein.

Other factors affecting requirement. Other factors include the rate at which protein tissue is synthesized in the body at a given time, and the nature and caloric value of the diet as a whole. The nature of the diet influences the quantitative protein requirement because of the protein-sparing effect of the carbohydrate and fat contained in the diet. The timing of meals, interestingly enough, plays a role also. Allowing time intervals between ingestion of protein foods apparently lowers the competition for absorption sites and enzymes. Other obvious factors affecting the body's need for protein are fever, disease processes, traumatic injury to tissues, and the postsurgical state.

Measure of protein requirements

A source of confusion in the determination of requirements is the unclear terminology applied to standards. General terms such as minimum, average, adequate, and optimum are ambiguous. Does minimum mean the lowest adequate amount on record, the minimum requirement for the majority of the groups studied, or the minimum amount required to support growth? And how does one define optimum? Is it in terms of needed body reserves, or of stress? How much is optimum? Actually the desirable size of body reserves has not been established, for it depends on a variety of circumstances.

An attempt to overcome this difficulty in

terminology has brought into use the phrase "recommended allowances." But this phrase also poses some problems. It is based on an excess margin of safety. However, the question of the rational size of such a margin must still be answered. One investigator, W. C. Rose,[1] has defined the optimum (safe) level as twice the minimal requirement.

Basic measures. Two basic measures of protein requirement must be considered: *quantity* and *quality*.

Protein quantity would establish the total protein requirement. The United States standard has generally been set for adults at 0.9 gm. per kg. (2.2 lbs.) of body weight. This amounts to about 65 gm. (slightly more than 2 oz.) daily for a person weighing 70 kg. (143 lbs.). A total of 65 to 75 gm. daily are needed during pregnancy and lactation. The requirements for infants and children vary according to growth patterns (see Appendix L).

Since the value of a protein is dependent upon its content of essential amino acids, in the final analysis the measure of protein requirement must be based on *quality*, that is, on the essential amino acid content.

Guidelines for protein needs, based upon nitrogen balance studies determining specific amino acid requirements, have been developed. One widely used guideline is the provisional amino acid pattern outlined by the Food and Agriculture Organization, a division of the World Health Organization under the United Nations. This pattern is constructed according to the formula shown in Table 4-2. The amino acid that is required by the body in the smallest quantity is tryptophan. Tryptophan is therefore assigned the value of 1. Values for the other amino acids express the ratio between the body's tryptophan requirement and its need for each other amino acid. On the basis of the provisional amino acid pattern, an ideal proportionality pattern of amino acids is constructed, against which the amino acid ratios in different foods may be measured. According to this method of study, egg and milk ranked highest as reference proteins against which to measure other foods (Fig. 4-8).

Protein quality in terms of essential amino acid content is of great practical significance in world health problems. In countries where the diet is limited to a few foods and protein is available in only one main plant food source, the protein intake

Table 4-2. Food and Agriculture Organization* amino acid proportionality pattern for the adult based on essential amino acid requirements

Amino acid	Requirement (mg.)	Proportionality pattern	Pattern simplified in common use†
Tryptophan	250	1.0	1.0
Threonine	500	2.0	2.0
Isoleucine	700	2.8	3.0
Lysine	800	3.2	3.0
Valine	900	3.6	3.0
Total sulfur amino acid	950	3.8	3.0
(Methionine minimum)	(325)	(1.3)	
Leucine	1050	4.2	3.4
Total aromatic amino acid	1550	6.2	
(Phenylalanine minimum)	(325)	(1.3)	2.0

*Food and Agriculture Organization, Protein requirements, FAO Nutritional Studies, No. 16, Rome, 1957 (adapted).

†Leverton, R. M.: Amino acids. In Stefferud, A., editor: Food, the yearbook of agriculture, 1959, Washington, D. C. 1959, U. S. Department of Agriculture.

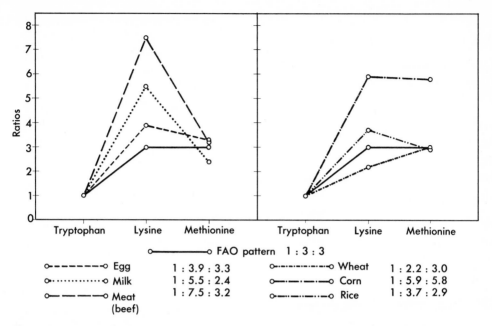

Fig. 4-8. Amino acid proportionality patterns of some animal and plant protein foods. Compare these with the amino acid pattern calculated by the Food and Agriculture Organization (FAO) to provide the daily adult requirements.

could be made adequate by introducing other complementary plant proteins to make up the lacking amino acids.

Summary

This discussion of requirements is intended to help the nursing student gain a sounder basis for teaching health to patients. The so-called protein requirements are not as rigid as they may appear when listed in National Research Council tables[4] (see Appendix L). Even the term "requirement" connotes an inflexible mandate, which simply is not the case.

The National Research Council's published standards for protein are intended to serve only as recommendations. They are designed to cover a wide range of need, and in order to provide a margin of safety to cover stress situations, they are approximately double the minimum allowances. They are not absolute, rigid requirements, but flexible *recommendations*. As such, they can serve only as rough guides, and should be adapted as needed to the individual patient.

There is a need for further research on proteins and amino acids. Better means of food analysis are needed to make food value tables more accurate and consistent. Further studies with animals are needed, as are studies with human subjects. Further research on protein deficiency diseases and field studies in areas of the world where protein malnutrition is prevalent are also needed.

Several general problems requiring further investigation have been identified by the National Research Council's Committee on Amino Acids:[5]

1. What are the role, desirable level, and means of maintenance of the so-called protein reserves?
2. What is the specific role of protein in the development of resistance to and recovery from various stresses?
3. What is the effect of protein on longevity and the so-called degenerative diseases?
4. What are the possible effects of excessive protein and amino acids?

In applying her knowledge of protein requirements to the individual patient, the nurse should always bear in mind that research along these and related lines is constantly modifying diet therapy. In order to cooperate intelligently with the physician and other members of the health team, she should maintain an open and inquiring mind toward news of these developments.

GLOSSARY

amino acid these compounds are the structural units of protein. Out of a total of twenty or more, ten are considered *essential*, or indispensable to life. (See *essential amino acid.*) The term "amino" represents the presence of the NH_2 group—a *base*. The unique chemical feature of the amino acids is that they contain *both* a base (NH_2, the amino group) and an acid (COOH, carboxyl group). Therefore, they are capable of both acid and base reactions (amphoteric chemical nature). The various food proteins, when digested, yield their specific constituent amino acids. These amino acids are then available for use by the cells as the cells synthesize specific tissue proteins.

amination the taking up of an amino group (NH_2) by an amino acid to produce the *amine* form of that acid. This process is one means by which toxic nitrogenous products such as ammonia (NH_3) are removed from the system and made ready for excretion.

amphoteric (Gr. *amphoteros,* both) having properties of both an acid and a base, and therefore able to function as either. Amino acids have this dual chemical nature because of their structure—they contain both an acid (carboxyl, COOH) and a base (amino, NH_2) group.

anabolism (Gr. *anabolē,* a building up) constructive metabolic processes that build up the body substances; the synthesis in living organisms of more complex substances from simpler ones. Anabolism *uses* energy; available energy generated by catabolic processes is taken up in forming the chemical bonds that unite the components of the increasingly complex molecules as they are developed in the anabolic processes. Anabolism is the opposite of catabolism.

catabolism (Gr. *katabolē,* a throwing down) the destructive phase of metabolism, the opposite of anabolism. Catabolism includes all the processes in which complex substances are progressively broken down into simpler ones. Catabolism usually involves the release of energy. Together, anabolism and catabolism constitute metabolism, which is the coordinated operation of anabolic and catabolic processes into a dynamic balance of energy and substance.

chymotrypsin a protein-splitting (proteolytic) enzyme produced by the pancreas that acts in the intestine. Together with trypsin, it reduces proteins to shorter chain polypeptides and dipeptides.

complete protein a protein that contains the essential amino acids in quantities sufficient for maintenance of the body and for a normal rate of growth. Such proteins are said to have a high biologic value. Egg, milk, cheese, and meat are complete protein foods.

deamination an initial step in the metabolic breakdown (catabolism) of amino acids, in which the amino group (NH_2) is split off. Deamination takes place chiefly in the liver. The nitrogenous group thus formed (NH_3, ammonia) may be: (1) converted to urea and excreted, (2) used in production of nitrogen-containing compounds such as purines, or (3) combined with carbohydrate derivatives or amino acid residues to form the amine form of that acid.

deoxyribonucleic acid (DNA) a complex, double chain protein of high molecular weight, which is the nucleic acid found in the chromosomes of the cell nucleus. It is believed to be the chemical basis of heredity and the carrier of genetic information for specific protein synthesis. DNA is composed of four nitrogenous bases (two purines, adenine and guanine; and two pyrimidines, thymine and cytosine), a sugar (deoxyribose), and phosphoric acid. A similar single chain nucleic acid, ribonucleic acid (RNA, in which the sugar is ribose), also functions with DNA in protein synthesis in the cell.

essential amino acid an amino acid that is indispensable to life and growth, and that the body cannot manufacture; it must be supplied in the diet. Eight amino acids are essential: threonine, leucine, isoleucine, valine, lysine, methionine, phenylalanine, and tryptophan.

homeostasis (Gr. *homoio,* similar; *stasis,* a standing) a state of equilibrium of the body's internal environment.

keto-acid the amino acid residue after deamination. The glycogenic keto-acids are used to form carbohydrates. The ketogenic keto-acids are used to form fats.

nitrogen balance the difference between intake and output of nitrogen in the body. If intake is greater, a positive nitrogen balance exists. If output is greater, a negative nitrogen balance exists. For example, during growth when new tissue protein is being formed, nitrogen is retained for protein synthesis, and a state of positive nitrogen balance prevails.

nucleoprotein a conjugated protein found in cell nuclei, that is formed from the combination of a protein with nucleic acid. Nucleoproteins are essential for cell division and reproduction. A common example of nucleoproteins are purines. Purines are found principally in meats, especially organ meats such as liver and heart.

pepsin the main gastric enzyme specific for proteins. Pepsin begins breaking large protein molecules into shorter chain polypeptides, proteoses, and peptones. Gastric hydrochloric acid is necessary to activate pepsin.

peptide linkage the characteristic joining of amino acids to form proteins. Such a chain of amino acids is termed a peptide. Depending upon its size, it may be a dipeptide fragment of protein digestion or a large polypeptide.

transamination the transfer of the amino group (NH_2) from an amino acid to a carbon residue to form another amino acid. The newly formed compound is classed a nonessential amino acid, since the body can synthesize it and is not dependent upon the diet to supply it.

trypsin a protein-splitting (proteolytic) enzyme secreted by the pancreas, that acts in the small intestine to reduce proteins to shorter chain polypeptides and dipeptides.

zwitterion (Ger. *Zwitter*, hybrid; Gr. *ion*, wandering) the term given to amino acids to describe their capacity, when ionized in a solution, to behave as either an acid or a base depending on the need of the solution in which they are present. This dual nature makes amino acids good buffer substances.

References

Specific

1. Rose, W. C., and others: The amino acid requirements of man, J. Biol. Chem. **217**:987, 1955.
2. Christensen, H. N., and Oxender, D. L.: Transport of amino acids into and across cells, Amer. J. Clin. Nutr. **8**:131, 1960.
3. Harper, H. A.: Review of physiological chemistry, ed. 11, Los Altos, California, 1967, Lange Medical Publications, p. 258.
4. Food and Nutrition Board: Recommended dietary allowances, 1968, ed. 6, Pub. 1694, Washington, D. C., 1968, National Academy of Sciences, National Research Council.
5. Food and Nutrition Board, Committee on Amino Acids: Evaluation of protein nutrition, Pub. 711, Washington, D. C., 1960, National Academy of Sciences, National Research Council.

General

Allison, J. B.: Nitrogen balance and the nutritive value of proteins, J.A.M.A. **164**:283, 1957.

Allison, J. B., and Wannemacher, R. W., Jr.: The concept and significance of labile and over-all protein reserves of the body, Amer. J. Clin. Nutr. **16**:445, 1965.

Burton, B. T., editor: The Heinz handbook of nutrition, New York, 1966, McGraw-Hill Book Co.

Cantarow, A., and Trumper, M.: Clinical biochemistry, ed. 6. Philadelphia, 1962, W. B. Saunders Co.

Council on Foods and Nutrition, American Medical Association: Protein and amino acid requirements of infants, J.A.M.A. **175**:100, 1961.

Hardinge, M. G., and others: Nutritional studies of vegetarians. J. Amer. Diet. Ass. **48**:25, 1966.

Harper, H. A.: Review of physiological chemistry, ed. 11, Los Altos, Calif., 1967, Lange Medical Publication.

Hartman, R. H., and Rice, E. E.: Supplementary relationships of proteins, J. Amer. Diet. Ass. **35**:34, 1958.

Holt, L. E., and others: The concept of protein stores and its implication in diet, J.A.M.A. **181**:699, 1962.

Howe, E. E., and others: Amino acid supplementation of cereal grains as related to the world food supply, Amer. J. Clin. Nutr. **16**:315, 1965.

Howe, E. E., and others: Amino acid supplementation of protein concentrates as related to the world protein supply, Amer. J. Clin. Nutr. **16**:321, 1965.

Joint FAO/WHO Expert Committee on Protein Requirements, FAO Nutr. Meet. Rep. Ser. No. 37; WHO Tech. Rep. Ser. No. 301, Rome, 1965.

Leverton, R. M.: Proteins; amino acids. In Food, the yearbook of agriculture, Washington, D. C., 1959, U. S. Department of Agriculture.

Leverton, R. M., and others: The quantitative amino acid requirements of young women, J. Nutr. **58**:59, 1956.

McCollum, E. V.: A history of nutrition, Boston, 1957, Houghton Mifflin Company.

Milner, M.: Protein food problems in developing countries, Food Technology **16**:51, 1962.

Mitchell, H. S.: Protein limitation and human growth, J. Amer. Diet. Ass. **44**:165, 1964.

Orr, M. L., and Watt, B. K.: Amino acid content of foods, Home Economics Research Report, No. 4, Washington, D. C., 1957, U. S. Department of Agriculture.

Reviews: Protein Digestion and Metabolism, Nutr. Rev. **20**:67, 1962; Protein and amino acid requirements, Nutr. Rev. **20**:235, 1962.

Standal, B. R.: Amino acids in oriental soybean foods, J. Amer. Diet. Ass. **50**:397, 1967.

Stare, F. J., editor: Protein nutrition, a monograph, Ann. N. Y. Acad. Sci. **69**:855, 1958.

Swendseid, M. E., and others: Plasma amino acid response to glucose administration, Amer. J. Clin. Nutr. **20**:243, 1967.

Todhunter, E. N.: Some classics in nutrition and dietetics, J. Amer. Diet. Ass. **44**:100, 1964.

Watts, J. H., and others: An evaluation of the FAO amino acid reference pattern in human nutrition, J. Nutr. **75**:295, 1961.

White, H., and others: Principles of biochemistry, ed. 3, New York, 1964, McGraw-Hill Book Co.

Wohl, M., and Goodhart, R., editors: Modern nutrition in health and disease, ed. 3, Philadelphia, 1964, Lea & Febiger.

CHAPTER 5

Energy metabolism

Energy is the basis of ongoing life. It is the power of an organism to do its work. Fundamental laws of physical existence ultimately revolve around the production of energy. The study of nutrition is concerned with the basic question of how the human body transforms the elements in its food into energy.

Several important interrelated concepts are involved in the study of energy metabolism. These deal with such basic questions as:

1. What are energy and metabolism?
2. How is energy measured?
3. How does the human body get its energy?
4. How is energy controlled in human metabolism?
5. How are basal and total energy needs determined?

DEFINITIONS OF ENERGY AND METABOLISM

The word *energy* comes from two Greek roots, *en* meaning "in" and *ergon* meaning "work." The Greeks put the two roots together to form *energon*, meaning "active." Hence, energy is that force or power that enables the body to carry on life-sustaining activities. Death is the cessation of this activity. The word *metabolism* also comes from two roots, *meta* meaning "beyond" and *ballein* meaning "to throw." The Greeks put these two roots together to form the noun *metabolē*, meaning "change." Metabolism is the total of all those chemical processes in the body by which substances initially in food are "thrown beyond themselves" to be changed into other substances. This very phrase gives the feel of the power involved in the processes that nurture and sustain life. *Energy metabolism* deals with the very real and dynamic concept underlying all life—*change.* It is these constant, multiple changes in the forms of physiologic constituents that produce energy.

MEASUREMENT OF ENERGY (Calories)

Since the body can perform work only as energy is released, and since all work takes the form of heat production, energy may be measured in terms of heat equivalents. Such a heat measure is the *calorie.* In nutritional and physiologic studies, the unit of measure is the large calorie or kilocalorie, which is equal to 1,000 small calories. A kilocalorie is the amount of heat required to raise 1 kg. of water 1° C.

The caloric values of various foods have been determined by the use of a metal instrument, which is called a bomb calorimeter because its shape resembles that of a bomb. A weighed amount of a food is placed into the core of the calorimeter, and the instrument is immersed in water. The food is then ignited by an electric spark in the presence of oxygen and burned. The increase in temperature of the surrounding water indicates the number of calories given off by the oxidation of the food.

The average caloric value of each of the three major nutrients is known as its respective *fuel factor.* One gm. of carbohydrate yields 4 calories, 1 gm. of fat yields 9 calories, and 1 gm. of protein yields 4 calories.

These figures should be remembered because they are constantly used in computing diets.

ENERGY IN THE HUMAN BODY

Energy cycle. It is clear that energy is not created. It exists in many forms and is constantly being transformed. In the human body, energy is available in four basic forms for life processes: *chemical, electrical, mechanical,* and *thermal.* It is constantly being cycled through these forms. In this perpetual cycle of energy, the ultimate source of power is the sun with its vast reservoir of nuclear reactions. Through the process of photosynthesis, with water and carbon dioxide as raw materials, plants transform the sun's energy into food storage forms. In the body, these food sources are converted to the basic energy unit of glucose, which is burned to release energy.

Water and carbon dioxide are the end products of this process of oxidation.

Transformation of energy—free and potential (Fig. 5-1). Metabolism is the process of converting chemical energy to other forms of energy for the body's work. This chemical energy is changed to *electrical energy* as in brain and nerve activity, *mechanical energy* as in muscle contraction, *thermal energy* as in regulation of body temperature, and to other types of *chemical energy* as in the synthesis of new compounds. In all these work activities of the body heat is given off.

In human metabolism, as in any energy system, energy is always present as either *free* or *potential* energy. Free energy is the energy involved at any given moment in the performance of a task. It is unbound and in motion. Potential energy is the energy that is stored, or bound, in various chemi-

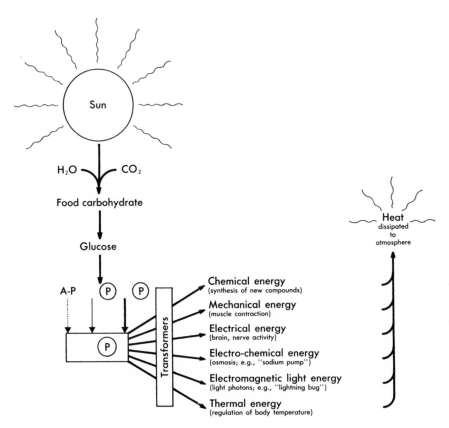

Fig. 5-1. Transformation of energy from its primary source (the sun) to various forms for biological work, by means of metabolic processes ("transformers").

cal compounds, and is available for conversion to free energy as needed. Energy stored in the sugar molecule is potential energy. When it is burned, free energy is released and work results. As work is done, energy in the form of heat is given off.

Whether the energy system is electrical, mechanical, thermal, or chemical, in the course of the many reactions that comprise its operation, free energy is decreased and the reservoir of potential energy is secondarily diminished. Therefore, the system must be constantly refueled from some outside source. In the human energy system, this source is food.

CONTROL OF ENERGY IN HUMAN METABOLISM

Controlled energy system — chemical bonding. The energy in any system may be uncontrolled and destructive, as in an atomic bomb used for warfare; or it may be controlled and constructive, as in an atomic reactor used for research and industry. In the human body also, the energy produced in its many chemical reactions, if "exploded" all at once, could be destructive. The mechanism by which energy is controlled in the human system is *chemical bonding.* The chemical bonds that hold the elements of the compounds together consist of energy. As long as that compound remains constant, energy is being exerted to maintain the atomic constellation that is characteristic for that molecule. It is in this sense that potential energy is stored in the compound. When the compound is broken into its parts, energy is released, and it becomes free energy. It is a characteristic of free energy that it immediately involves itself in the bonding of other atoms, which results either in a rearrangement of the atoms within the same compound or in new compounds.

The three types of chemical bonds by which energy is transferred in the body are *covalent bonds, hydrogen bonds,* and *phosphate bonds.*

Covalent bond. Valence refers to the chemical combining power of an element.

A common example of covalent bonds are those shared between neighbor carbon atoms in the core of an organic compound:

-C-C-C-

Hydrogen bond. Hydrogen bonds are weaker bonds which attach hydrogen to various compounds. They are less rich in energy than covalent bonds. The very fact that they can be broken easily gives them physiologic importance. They can alter molecular shapes, as in protein molecules, and they can be transferred or passed readily from one substance to another.

High-energy phosphate bond. Phosphate (PO_4) bonds (the bonds that attach the phosphate radical to a compound) play an important role in energy metabolism. Since the phosphate radical is highly labile, more energy is required to bind it than to bind carbon or most other radicals, and more free energy is released when the phosphate bond is broken. Many phosphate bonds are referred to as high-energy bonds. The sign $\sim$ is used to indicate them. An example of such a high energy compound is adenosine triphosphate, commonly called ATP: $A - PO_4 \sim PO_4 \sim PO_4$.

Dr. Harold Harper[1] has called ATP the "currency of the cell," which may be "cashed in" by the body for energy as needed to perform its work. Like storage batteries, these PO_4 bonds become the controlling force of any further energy needs.

Although more energy is required to bind the phosphate radical to any compound than is required to bind, for example, a carbon radical, there are some compounds in which the amount of energy required to bind the phosphate radical is relatively low. In such compounds, the phosphate bond is called a low-energy phosphate bond.

Examples of low-energy phosphate bonds include those formed by the phosphorylation of glucose (glucose-6-phosphate, glucose-1-phosphate), which activates glucose for participation in cell metabolism. Later in the total process of oxidating glucose, high-energy phosphate bonds are formed.

Controlled reaction rates—enzymes, co-enzymes, and hormones. The many chemical reactions that make up the finely developed energy systems in cell metabolism must also have controls. Some of the chemical reactions that break down proteins, for example, if left to themselves (as in sterile decomposition), would span several years. Such reactions must be accelerated, or else it might take years to get the needed energy from a meal. At the same time, they must be regulated so that too fast a reaction will not produce energy in a single explosion. Enzymes and coenzymes control biologic oxidation of the cells. The enzymes and coenzymes control numerous other biologic processes as well. The hormones also play a regulatory role in cell oxidation.

Enzymes. Dr. David Green,[2] a noted enzymologist, once called enzymes "chemical keys of breath-taking eloquence." They are indeed just that! Life simply cannot go on without them.

The word "enzyme" comes from a Greek word meaning "in yeast." It was originally used because the first observations were of something in yeast which caused the fermentation of glucose to produce alcohol. All enzymes that have been isolated thus far are protein substances. They are produced in the cells, apparently under the control of specific genes. One specific gene is believed to control the making of one specific enzyme, and there are thousands of enzymes in each cell.

The substance upon which a particular enzyme works is called its *substrate.* Enzymes possess a remarkable and highly significant degree of specificity for their special substrates; that is, a particular enzyme usually will act only on its own particular substrate. Like the interlocking pieces of a jigsaw puzzle, the specific shapes of enzyme and substrate must fit together perfectly or the reaction will not take place. In this vital lock and key mode of action, the enzyme and substrate first combine in a complex, then break apart and produce the new reaction products and the original unchanged enzyme.

Enzyme + substrate → Enzyme-substrate complex
Activated enzyme-substrate complex →
Reaction products + enzyme

While the substrate is locked in place with the enzyme, the enzyme places specific stress upon it to break certain bonds and rearrange certain molecules. When unlocking occurs, different reaction products are released and the enzyme breaks away unchanged, ready to perform its remarkable feat over and over again. (Compare this action with that shown in Fig. 5-3.)

Coenzymes. The completion of reactions such as those involved in cellular oxidation to yield energy requires coenzymes. In respiratory chains for oxidation in the cells oxygen was originally thought to enter into the process and to take part in the reactions. It is now known that energy is generated by a system of hydrogen ion transfer from product to product, with formation of high energy phosphate compounds (ATP) along the way. The coenzymes act as a series of acceptors of the bouncing hydrogen ion, until the hydrogen finally combines with oxygen to form water (Fig. 5-2).

Three such systems play a part in this hydrogen ion transfer to yield energy:

1. The *dehydrogenases,* with niacin as part of the coenzyme (nicotinamide-adenine dinucleotide → reduced nicotinamide-adenine dinucleotide [NAD → NADH]; nicotinamide-adenine dinucleotide phosphate → reduced nicotinamide-adenine dinucleotide phosphate [NADP → NADAH])

2. The *flavoprotein system,* containing riboflavin coenzymes

3. The *cytochrome system* (a "cousin" of hemoglobin), containing iron

An example of a dehydrogenase of clinical significance is *lactic dehydrogenase* (LDH), which catalyzes the change of lactic acid to pyruvic acid in muscle. When heart muscle is damaged, as in a myocardial infarction, the enzyme is released from the cells and accumulates in the blood. Hence, a rise in the blood level of this enzyme is used as a diagnostic measure.

It may be helpful to think of the coen-

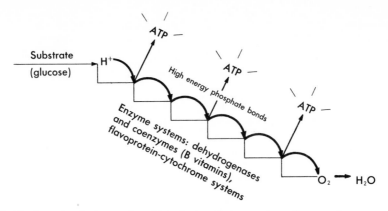

Fig. 5-2. The bouncing hydrogen ion—biological oxidation in the cell to produce energy. Energy in the form of ATP (high-energy phosphate bonds) is produced through transfer of H⁺ and electrons by means of enzyme systems (dehydrogenases and coenzymes, the B vitamins, and the flavoprotein-cytochrome systems). These enzyme chains are coupled with the glycolytic pathway and the Krebs cycle.

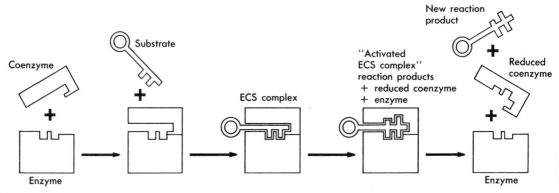

Fig. 5-3. Lock and key concept of the action of enzyme, coenzyme, and substrate to produce new reaction products.

zyme as another substrate, for in receiving the material transferred the coenzyme is changed or reduced (Fig. 5-3).

Enzyme + coenzyme + substrate →
    Enzyme-coenzyme-substrate complex
Activated enzyme-coenzyme-substrate complex →
    Reaction products + reduced coenzyme + enzyme

Hormones. The word "hormone" comes from the Greek word *hormaein* meaning "set in motion" or "to spur on." Hormones are secretions of the endocrine glands, and they perform many regulatory functions in the body. In energy metabolism they act as chemical messengers to trigger or control enzyme action. For example, the rate of ox-

idative reactions in the tissues (the body's metabolic rate) is controlled by thyroxine from the thyroid gland, which in turn is controlled by thyrotropic hormone from the anterior pituitary gland. Another familiar example is the controlling action of insulin from the pancreas upon the rate of glucose utilization in the tissues. Steriod hormones also have the capacity to regulate the cell's ability to synthesize enzymes.

Types of metabolic reaction. The two types of reaction constantly going on in energy metabolism are anabolism and catabolism. Each requires energy; therefore, each causes a decrease in free energy.

Anabolism is the synthesis of a more complex substance. Energy is required to generate this synthesis. The more complex the substance the greater is its potential or bound energy.

Catabolism is the breakdown to simpler substances. This process releases free energy, but it also uses up some free energy for the breakdown. Therefore, there is a constant energy deficit which must be supplied by food. When food is not available, as in periods of fasting or starvation, the body draws for energy on its own stores:

1. Only a 12 to 48 hour reserve of glycogen exists in liver and muscle; this amount is quickly depleted.
2. Storage of energy (as protein) exists in limited amounts in the muscle mass, but in greater volume than glycogen stores.
3. The capacity for storage in the adipose tissue is virtually unlimited. This stored fat provides needed energy, but the supply varies from person to person and from circumstance to circumstance.

ENERGY METABOLISM—
CALORIE REQUIREMENTS
Basal metabolism

Basal metabolism is a measure of the energy produced in the maintenance of the body at rest after a twelve hour fast. The basal metabolic rate (BMR) is the rate of internal chemical activity of resting tissue.

It is interesting to compare the contribution of various body tissues to the rate of basal metabolism. Certain small but vitally active tissues—brain, liver, gastrointestinal tract, heart, kidney—together make up less than 5% of the total body weight, yet they contribute about 60% of the total basal metabolic processes. Although resting muscle and adipose fat tissue are far larger in mass, they contribute much less to the body's BMR.

Methods of measuring the BMR. Both direct and indirect methods of calorimetry have been used to measure the BMR. In direct methods, a chamber large enough for a person to enter is used and his body's heat production is measured. Obviously, such an instrument is large and costly, and is therefore limited to research studies.

For clinical purposes, the far more simple indirect calorimetry is sufficiently accurate. This method measures the exchange of gases in respiration while the subject is at rest. Usually, the calories are computed according to an average of the amount of oxygen consumed during two six-minute periods. In indirect calorimetry, metabolic rates are based on the *respiratory quotient* (RQ). This is the ratio between the volume of carbon dioxide given off and the volume of oxygen consumed:

$$\frac{\text{Volume } CO_2 \text{ produced}}{\text{Volume } O_2 \text{ consumed}} = RQ$$

It has been found that energy calculated in this manner is equivalent to the heat given off by the body. The BMR is calculated for a given person in terms of the number of calories given off per hour per square meter of body surface area, with corrections for age, sex, height, and weight. The results are then expressed in percent of variation above or below the normal number of calories per square meter of body surface area for a person of like height, weight, age, and sex. The ranges usually given as normal are −10 to +10 percent, which includes about 75% of normal people, and −15 to +15 percent, which includes about 95% of normal people.

Conditions necessary for accuracy. When the BMR test is administered, certain conditions are necessary for accuracy. It is the nurse's responsibility to check the following:

1. The patient must have been in a fasting state (nothing by mouth; NPO) for the previous twelve hours. This assures that no digestive or absorptive activities are going on.
2. The patient must be in a relaxed state, both mental and physical. There should be a quiet atmosphere, with at least a half hour of bed rest preceding the test.

3. The patient should be recumbent during the test.
4. The patient should be fully awake.
5. The room temperature should be 20° to 25° C. (68° to 77° F.).

Factors that influence BMR. A number of factors influence the BMR and should be considered when interpreting results of tests.

1. Rates tend to be higher during growth periods. Generally, the BMR slowly rises during the first five years of life, levels off, rises again just before and during puberty, and then declines into old age.
2. Surface area influence is relatively constant. Smaller persons of each sex tend to have a higher rate of metabolism per unit of surface area than larger persons.
3. Because of relative sex differences in body mass, women usually have a lower BMR than men.
4. The BMR rises during pregnancy, because of increases in muscle mass of the uterus, size of mammary glands, fetal mass and placenta, cardiac work, and respiratory rate. This totals a 20 to 25% increase over the nonpregnant state, or about 300 calories.
5. The BMR also rises during the lactation period, because milk production utilizes energy. This is a large increase (about 60% or 1,000 calories) because breast milk has a value of 30 calories per ounce, and the average daily production is about 30 ounces.
6. Fever increases the BMR about 7% for each 1° C. rise.
7. Although the effect of climate has been debated, most investigators indicate that the BMR rises in response to lower temperatures as a compensatory mechanism to maintain body temperature.
8. Small BMR differences have been recorded among people of different races. For example, the BMR of some Oriental individuals is lower than the rates of their Caucasian counterparts, and higher rates were noted in some Eskimos.
9. Diseases involving increased cellular activity (cancer, leukemia, polycythemia, certain anemias, cardiac failure, hypertension, dyspnea, emphysema) usually increase the BMR.
10. In starvation and malnutrition the BMR is usually lowered.
11. Thyroxin stimulates the BMR. The principal use of BMR testing in clinical practice is in the diagnosis of thyroid disease.
12. Obesity seems to have little effect on the BMR, although it may lower the rate somewhat.

Other influences on calorie requirements

Muscular work. Exercise is the other large factor which accounts for individual calorie requirements. The effects of various activities on energy metabolism have been

Table 5-1. Energy expenditure per hour during different activities for a man weighing 70 kg.*

Activity	Calories per hour
Sleeping	65
Awake, lying still	77
Sitting at rest	100
Standing relaxed	105
Dressing and undressing	118
Sewing (tailoring)	135
Typewriting rapidly	140
Light exercise	170
Walking slowly (2.6 mph)	200
Active exercise	290
Severe exercise	450
Swimming	500
Running (5.3 mph)	570
Very severe exercise	600
Walking very fast (5.3 mph)	650
Walking upstairs	1,110

*From Guyton, A. C.: Textbook of medical physiology, ed. 3, Philadelphia, 1966, W. B. Saunders Co., p. 980.

measured by the oxygen consumption method (indirect calorimetry). Some representative calorie expenditures are given in Table 5-1.

Mental effort. Mental effort as in studying demands few if any calories. Feelings of fatigue following periods of study, for example, are due not to vast cerebral activity, but to various amounts of muscle tension involved.

Emotional state. Calories are expended during heightened emotional states because metabolic activity rises as muscle tension, restlessness, and agitated movements increase.

Diet. Food intake increases the expenditure of calories for digestion and absorption. Protein especially has a high specific dynamic action.

Total energy requirements

The total daily energy requirement of an individual is the number of calories necessary to replace daily basal metabolic loss, plus loss from exercise and other activities.

These general calorie needs for various ages as indicated in the 1968 revisions of recommendations by the National Research Council are listed in Table 5-2.

GLOSSARY

adenosine triphosphate (ATP) a compound of adenosine (a nucleotide containing adenine

Table 5-2. Recommended daily calorie allowances*

	Age (yrs.)	Weight (lbs.)	Height (in.)	Calories
Men	18 to 35	154	69	2,800
	35 to 55	154	68	2,600
	55 to 75+	154	67	2,400
Women	18 to 35	128	64	2,000
	35 to 55	128	63	1,850
	55 to 75+	128	62	1,700
	(Pregnant)			(+ 200)
	(Lactating)			(+1,000)
Infants	0 to ⅙	9 (4 kg.)	22	Kg × 120
	⅙ to ½	15 (7 kg.)	25	Kg × 110
	½ to 1	20 (9 kg.)	28	Kg × 100
Children	1 to 2	26	32	1,100
	2 to 3	31	36	1,250
	3 to 4	35	39	1,400
	4 to 6	42	43	1,600
	6 to 8	51	48	2,000
	8 to 10	62	52	2,200
Boys	9 to 12	77	55	2,500
	12 to 15	95	59	2,700
	15 to 18	130	67	3,000
Girls	10 to 12	77	56	2,250
	12 to 14	97	61	2,300
	14 to 16	114	62	2,400
	16 to 18	119	63	2,300

*Food and Nutrition Board, Recommended dietary allowances, ed. 7, Washington, D. C., 1968, National Academy of Science, National Research Council.

and ribose) which has three phosphoric acid groups. ATP is a high-energy phosphate compound important in energy exchange for cellular activity. The splitting off of the terminal phosphate bond ($\sim PO_4$) of ATP to produce ADP (adenosine diphosphate) releases bound energy and transfers it to free energy, available for body work. The re-forming of ATP in cell oxidation again stores energy in the high-energy phosphate bonds for use as needed. They may be considered to act as biological storage batteries which can be charged and discharged according to conditions in the cell.

basal metabolism (Gr. *basis,* base; *metabolē,* change) the amount of energy needed by the body for maintenance of life when the person is at digestive, physical, and emotional rest. The amount of oxygen consumed at rest is used as a measure of the basal energy requirements, and is expressed as calories per square meter of body surface per hour. This basal metabolic rate (BMR) is reported as the percent of variation in the person above or below the normal number of calories required for a person of like height, weight, age, and sex.

calorie (L. *calor,* heat) a measure of heat. The *energy* required to do the work of the body is measured as the amount of *heat* produced by the body's work. The energy value of a food is expressed as the number of calories a specified portion of that food will yield when oxidized, either in the body or on being burned. Physicists use several different standard calories in investigative work. The calorie commonly used in metabolic and dietetic studies is the large calorie or kilocalorie, which is the amount of heat required to raise 1 kg. of water 1° C.

calorimetry (L. *calor,* heat; Gr. *metron,* measure) the measurement of heat loss. An instrument for measuring heat output of the body or the energy value of foods is called a calorimeter.

chemical bonding the mutual attachment of various chemical elements to form chemical compounds. The chemical bonds that hold the elements of a compound together consist of stored potential energy. When the compound is broken up into its parts, free energy is released to do the body's work.

coenzyme (L. *co,* together; Gr. *en,* in; *zymē,* leaven) enzyme-activators required by some enzymes to produce their reactions. Coenzymes are diffusible, heat-stable substances of low molecular weight which combine with inactive proteins called *apoenzymes.* Each such combination of apoenzyme and coenzyme forms an active compound or a complete enzyme called a *holoenzyme.* A number of the B vitamins function as coenzymes in the energy-producing pathways in cell metabolism.

energy (Gr. *en,* in or with; *ergon,* work) the ca-

pacity of a system for doing work; available power. Energy is manifest in various forms—motion, position, light, heat, and sound. Energy is interchangeable among these various forms, and is constantly being transformed and transferred among them.

enzyme a complex organic substance originating in living cells and capable of producing certain chemical changes in other organic substances by catalytic action. An enzyme is usually named for the substance on which it acts (its substrate) with the addition of the suffix -ase. For example, an enzyme that splits a protein may be called by the general name of proteinase. Enzymes are specific in their action; they will act only on a certain substance and no other. Some enzymes require coenzymes to make them active.

fuel factor the calorie value (energy potential) of food nutrients; that is, the number of calories 1 gram of the nutrient yields when oxidized. The fuel factor for carbohydrate is 4; for protein, 4; and for fat, 9. These basic figures are used in computing diets and calorie values of foods.

hormone (Gr. *hormaein,* to spur on or to set in motion) a compound, produced in an endocrine organ (an organ of internal secretion; a ductless gland), secreted by the endocrine organ into the bloodstream, and transported by body fluids to a specific receptor or target organ, whose function the hormone controls. Most hormones are complex proteins. They are usually active in minute quantities. In energy metabolism, a hormone does not supply energy, but acts as a chemical messenger, which triggers or controls enzyme action or synthesis.

respiratory chain the series of chemical reactions in the cell's oxidation systems which transfer hydrogen ions or electrons to produce ATP (high-energy phosphate compounds). For example, the *riboflavin-cytochrome systems* couple with the glucose oxidation pathways and Krebs cycle to produce such forms of energy.

respiratory quotient the ratio between the volume of CO_2 produced and the volume of O_2 consumed: $\dfrac{CO_2}{O_2} = RQ$. This ratio is used in indirect calorimetry as a basis for determining metabolic rates.

substrate the specific organic substance on which a particular enzyme acts.

References
Specific
1. Harper, H. A.: Review of physiological chemistry, ed. 11, Los Altos, California, 1967, Lange Medical Publications, p. 480.
2. Cooley, D. J.: Enzymes: chemical keys to health and disease, Today's Health **39:**42, 1961.

General

Bogert, L. J., Briggs, G., and Calloway, D.: Nutrition and physical fitness, ed. 8, Philadelphia, 1966, W. B. Saunders Co.

Burton, B. T., editor: The Heinz handbook of nutrition, New York, 1966, McGraw-Hill Book Co.

Cantarow, A., and Trumper, M.: Clinical biochemistry, ed. 6, Philadelphia, 1962, W. B. Saunders Co.

Consolazio, C. F., and others: Physiological measurements of metabolic functions in man, New York, 1963, McGraw-Hill Book Co.

Food and Agriculture Organization of the United Nations: Calorie requirements, FAO Nutritional Studies, No. 15, Rome, 1957.

Food and Agriculture Organization of the United Nations: Energy yielding components of food and computation of calorie values, Comm. on Calories Conversion Factors and Food Composition Tables, Washington, D. C., 1947.

Food and Agriculture Organization of the United Nations: Nutrition and working efficiency, Basic Study No. 5, Rome, 1962.

Food and Nutrition Board: Recommended dietary allowances, (1968 review), National Academy of Science, National Research Council, Washington, D. C., 1968.

Guyton, A. C.: Textbook of medical physiology, ed. 3, Philadelphia, 1966, W. B. Saunders Co.

Harper, H. A.: Review of physiological chemistry, ed. 11, Los Altos, Calif., 1967, Lange Medical Publications.

Keys, A.: Energy requirements of adults, J.A.M.A. **142**:33, 1950.

Konishi, F.: Food energy equivalents of various activities, J. Amer. Diet. Ass. **46**:186, 1965.

Moore, M., and others: Energy expenditure of preadolescent girls, J. Amer. Diet. Ass. **49**:409, 1966.

Richardson, M., and McCracken, E.: Energy expenditures of women performing selected activities, Home Economics Research Report, No. 11, U. S. Department of Agriculture, Washington, D. C., 1960.

Sargent, D.: An evaluation of basal metabolic data, Home Economics Research Report, No. 14, U. S. Department of Agriculture, Washington, D. C., 1961.

Stefferud, A., editor: Food: the yearbook of agriculture, 1959, Washington, D.C., 1959, U.S. Department of Agriculture.

Watt, B. K.: Revising the tables in "Agriculture Handbook No. 8," J. Amer. Diet. Ass. **44**:261, 1964.

Watt, B. K., and Merrill, A. L.: Composition of foods—raw, processed, prepared, Handbook No. 8, rev., U. S. Department of Agriculture, 1963.

Whedon, G.: New research in human energy metabolism, J. Amer. Diet. Ass. **35**:682, 1959.

Widdowson, E. M.: Development of British food composition tables, J. Amer. Diet. Ass. **50**:363, 1967.

Wilder, R.: Calorimetry: the basis of the science of nutrition, Arch. Int. Med. **103**:146, 1959.

Wohl, M. G., and Goodhart, R. S., editors: Modern nutrition in health and disease, ed. 4, Philadelphia, 1968, Lea & Febiger.

Wu Leng, W. T.: Problems in compiling food composition data, J. Amer. Diet. Ass. **40**:19, 1962.

CHAPTER 6

Vitamins: fat-soluble vitamins

INTRODUCTION

Probably no other group of nutritional elements has so captured interest and stimulated concern among biochemists, members of the health professions, and the general public as has the vitamin group. Over the past six decades the discoveries of the vitamins have formed a fascinating chapter in nutrition history. Numerous scientists have contributed to this unfolding story. Casimir Funk, a Polish chemist working at the Lister Institute in London in the early 1900's, with little financial means to carry on his experimental work, ordinarily fed his pigeons rice polishings which he swept up from the floor of a granary. That source of food supply was eventually closed to him, and he began to purchase rice which was whole-grain but polished. The pigeons soon developed a paralytic disease. Funk wondered whether the change of diet was related to the onset of the paralysis, and again fed the birds the waste polishings and they recovered. Funk then sought some substance in the grain hulls that would account for the different response in the birds. In 1911 he discovered a nitrogen-containing material which he thought was an amine. Because it was apparently vital to life, he called it *vitamine* ("vital-amine"). The final "e" was dropped later, when other similarly vital substances turned out to be a variety of organic compounds. The name "vitamin" has been retained to designate compounds of this class.

One by one the list of vitamins has grown. Two characteristics mark a compound for assignment to the vitamin (or accessory factor) group: (1) it must be a vital organic dietary substance, which is neither a carbohydrate, fat, mineral, nor protein, but is necessary in very small quantities to the performance of particular metabolic functions or to the prevention of an associated deficiency disease, and (2) it cannot be manufactured by the body, and, therefore, must be supplied in food.

Because of the intricacies of the human body, many such substances probably exist in addition to those already discovered. Those that have been discovered have probably been recognized because they exist in relatively small quantities in foods. Deficiencies are, therefore, more likely to occur, to be observed, and to be questioned.

The study of vitamins

Vitamins are usually grouped according to solubility. Although this distinction is sometimes an arbitrary one, it is still used for want of a better basis. The fat-soluble group includes vitamins A, D, E, and K. The water-soluble group includes vitamin C and the B-complex vitamins. This chapter will be concerned only with the fat-soluble group. The water-soluble vitamins will be considered in Chapter 7.

To clarify the current concepts concerning each known vitamin, this Chapter and Chapter 7 will consider the answers to the following questions:

1. What is the nature of each vitamin?

2. How does the body handle each vitamin and how is it absorbed into the bloodstream?
3. What is each vitamin's role in body functions?
4. What are the body's requirements for each vitamin?
5. What are the food sources for each vitamin?

THE FAT-SOLUBLE VITAMINS
Vitamin A (retinol)
Chemical and physical nature of vitamin A

In 1917, E. V. McCollum and his coworkers at Johns Hopkins University in Baltimore demonstrated that an eye disease, xerophthalmia, was caused specifically by a lack of a fat-soluble substance. McCollum called this substance vitamin A.[1,2]

Chemically, vitamin A is a primary alcohol of high molecular weight ($CO_{20}H_{29}OH$). Because it has a specific function in the retina of the eye, and because it is an alcohol, it has been given the name retinol. However, it is still commonly referred to by its letter name.

Vitamin A is soluble in fat and in ordinary fat solvents. Because it is insoluble in water, it is fairly stable in general cooking. It oxidizes readily, however, upon prolonged exposure to temperatures higher than those ordinarily used in cooking. Antioxidants, such as vitamin E, have been used with vitamin A to preserve it.

In its natural form, vitamin A is found only in animal sources, and is usually associated with lipids. As an ester with fatty acids, it is deposited in such tissues as kidney, lung, fat depots, and especially liver. Since so limited an amount of vitamin A existed as such in these animal sources, investigators looked for a precursor in plants which the animals consumed. They believed that the animals must convert such a precursor in their bodies to vitamin A and this proved to be the case.

Provitamin A (carotene). The ultimate source of all vitamin A is plants. The precursor of vitamin A (provitamin A) is a substance called carotene ($C_{40}H_{56}$) which is found in certain plant pigments. It is called carotene because it was first identified in the yellow pigment of carrots.

During the early study of these substances and their relation to vitamin A, confusion arose from the fact that the carotenes have such a deep, intense color, while pure vitamin A is colorless.

Several forms, α-, β-, and γ-carotene, have been found in deep yellow and green plants. Another form with similar properties, crytoxanthin, has been found in yellow corn. Of these, β-carotene is the most significant to human nutrition, and is the most common precursor of vitamin A. About two-thirds of the vitamin A necessary in human nutrition is supplied by β-carotene.

Carotene occurs as crystals in plant cells. Cooking, by weakening the cell wall, helps to release these crystals, thus aiding their absorption in the intestine.

Vitamin A absorption

Substances that aid absorption. Vitamin A enters the body in two forms: as the preformed vitamin from animal sources, and as carotene. Bile salts, pancreatic lipase, and fat aid in the absorption of vitamin A and carotene by the body.

Bile salts. Since oxygen easily destroys vitamin A, the natural antioxidant bile salts help to stabilize the vitamin. Therefore, clinical conditions affecting the biliary system, such as obstruction of the bile ducts, infectious hepatitis, and cirrhosis of the liver, hinder vitamin A absorption. This is caused more by the rapid oxidation of the unprotected vitamin than by any primary defect in the absorptive process itself. Bile also aids in the absorption of vitamin A, as it does of other fat-related substances, since it serves as a vehicle of transport through the intestinal wall.

Pancreatic lipase. The fat-splitting enzyme lipase is necessary for initial saponification or hydrolysis in the upper intestine of fat emulsions or oil solutions of the vitamin. This enzyme is not required for absorption of an aqueous dispersion form of the vitamin. Therefore, in conditions where secretion of pancreatic lipase is curtailed, such as in cystic fibrosis, the aqueous dispersion form would be preferred.

Fat. The presence of some fat in the intestine, simultaneously absorbed, is apparently required for effective absorption of the vitamin. This seems to be more true of carotene than of vitamin A.

A warning must be given here about the nonfood fat, mineral oil. This oil is not digested by the body, but goes through the gastrointestinal tract intact. If it is present in the intestine along with fat-soluble vitamins, such as vitamin A or carotene, it absorbs them and carries them out also. Therefore, mineral oil should never be used with meals; nor should it be taken immediately before or after eating.

Carotene conversion and absorption. In the intestinal wall, during absorption, some of the carotene is converted to vitamin A. Animals vary greatly in their ability to make this conversion. The efficiency with which it is accomplished in man is not known, but it probably varies in different conditions. Thyroid hormone appears to stimulate this conversion. Some studies seem to indicate that conversion is impaired in uncontrolled severe diabetes and in lipoid nephrosis, and that it is also affected by the amount and quality of protein in the diet. Normal whole blood levels of carotene range from 80 to 120 μg. per 100 ml. (about 100 to 300 I.U. per 100 ml.). Serum levels are lower (40 to 100 I.U. per 100 ml., or about 40 to 60 μg. per 100 ml.). When carotene levels exceed 250 μg. per 100 ml., as occasionally occurs with a large dietary intake, an interesting condition called xanthosis cutis develops. The skin takes on a deep yellow color that is particularly noticeable in the palms, ear lobes, and soles of the feet. It can be distinguished from jaundice because the sclerae or mucous membranes are not affected. It is harmless, and fades in a few days after the quantity of ingested carotene is reduced.

Route of absorption and storage. The route of absorption of vitamin A and caro-

tene is the same as that of fat. They enter the lymphatic system and are carried through the thoracic duct into the portal vein and then to the liver for storage and distribution. The liver is by far the most efficient storage organ. It contains about 90% of the total vitamin A in the body. This amount is sufficient to supply the body's needs for three to twelve months. Liver stores, as well as plasma levels, are reduced, however, during periods of infectious disease such as pneumonia and rheumatic fever. At such times supplements of vitamin A may be indicated. Vitamin E may be given with the supplement to help prevent the rapid oxidation of vitamin A.

Influence of disease and age. Other conditions diminishing vitamin A absorption and utilization are intestinal diseases such as celiac, sprue, and colitis, which cause changes in the absorptive surface tissue of the mucosa. Age is also a factor in vitamin A absorption. In the newborn infant, especially the premature infant, absorption is poor. With advancing age, the elderly person may experience increasing difficulties with absorption also.

Physiologic functions of vitamin A

Vitamin A has important functions in a number of human tissues. Its role in visual adaptation to light and dark has been well established, and studies indicate that it has a number of more generalized functions that influence epithelial tissue, growth, development of teeth and endocrine function.

Vision. The ability of the eye to adapt to changes in light is dependent upon the presence of a light sensitive pigment, *rhodopsin* (commonly known as visual purple) in the rods of the retina. Rhodopsin is a conjugated protein, that is, it is made up of a protein attached to a nonprotein substance. The protein is *opsin;* the nonprotein part is a vitamin A compound called *retinene.*

When light hits the retina, rhodopsin is split into its two parts, opsin and retinene. In the dark the two components recombine to form visual purple again. Normally, there is more than enough vitamin A in

$$\text{Rhodopsin (visual purple)} \underset{\text{Dark}}{\overset{\text{Light}}{\rightleftharpoons}} \text{opsin} + \text{retinene} \rightleftharpoons \text{vitamin A}$$

$$\text{(light-sensitive pigment)} \qquad\qquad\qquad\qquad\qquad \text{(retinol)}$$

the pigment layer behind the rods and cones to ensure constant adjustments to variances in light. When the body is deficient in vitamin A, less retinene is available for formation of visual purple; the rods and cones become increasingly sensitive to light changes, which causes night blindness. This condition can usually be cured in a half hour or so by an injection of vitamin A, which is readily converted into retinene and then into visual purple.

The cones of the retina contain another pigment, visual violet, which influences color vision and the ability to see in bright light. Vitamin A is required as a component of this pigment also, but there is no evidence that vitamin A can cure color blindness.

Epithelial tissue. Vitamin A has a vital role in the formation and maintenance of healthy, functioning epithelial tissue, which forms the body's primary barrier to infections. The epithelium includes not only the skin but also the mucous membranes lining the ocular and oral cavities, and the gastrointestinal, respiratory, and genitourinary tracts.

Without vitamin A, the epithelial cells become dry and flat, and gradually harden to form scales that slough off. This process is called *keratinization*. Keratin is a protein that forms dry, scalelike tissue such as nails and hair. When the body is deficient in vitamin A, many epithelial tissues may undergo keratinization.

1. In the eye, the cornea dries and hardens. This condition, called *xerophthalmia*, may progress to blindness in extreme deficiency of vitamin A. The tear ducts dry, which robs the eye of its cleansing and lubricating means, and infection follows easily.

2. In the respiratory tract ciliated epithelium in the nasal passages dries, and the cilia are lost. A barrier to entry of infection is, therefore, removed. The

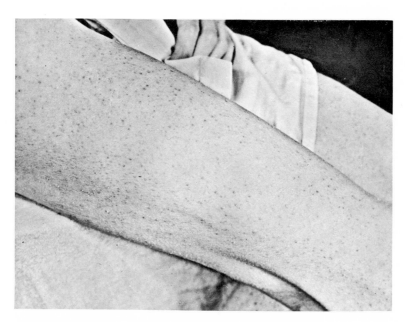

Fig. 6-1. Follicular hyperkeratosis caused by vitamin A deficiency. (From files of Therapeutic Notes, Parke, Davis & Co., Detroit, Michigan; courtesy Dr. Orson D. Bird.)

salivary glands dry, and the mouth becomes dry and cracked, open to invading organisms.

3. In the gastrointestinal tract the secretory function of mucous membranes is diminished, so that tissue sloughs off, which affects digestion and absorption.

4. In the genitourinary tract, as epithelial tissue breaks down, problems such as urinary tract infections, renal calculi, and vaginal infections become more common.

5. As the skin becomes dry and scaly, small pustules or a hardened, pigmented, papular eruption may appear around the hair follicles. This condition resulting from vitamin A deficiency is called *follicular hyperkeratosis* (Fig. 6-1).

Growth. It has been observed for some time that vitamin A deficiency is associated with retarded growth, but the mechanism is unknown. In man, nutritional deficiency usually involves multiple factors that make it difficult to isolate specific nutrient influences. For this reason, most studies of the effect of vitamin A on growth have been made in animals, where environment and variables can be controlled. Apparently, vitamin A contributes in some essential way to the growth of skeletal and soft tissues, perhaps through an effect upon protein synthesis, mitosis, or stability of cell membranes.

Teeth. Certain epithelial cells surrounding tooth buds in fetal gum tissue become specialized cup-shaped organs *(ameloblasts)* for forming the enamel structure of the developing tooth. Each cell carries out the fascinating task of producing and depositing minute prisms of enamel substance that eventually form the erupted tooth. Inadequate vitamin A produces faulty enamel-forming epithelial cells, which impairs the soundness of the tooth structure.

Endocrines. Studies with radioactive iodine have indicated that vitamin A defi-

---

TO PROBE FURTHER
Clues to the growth puzzle

As is so often the case when there are no pat answers to puzzles in the functioning of the human body, clues may be found that point to possible solutions. Animal experiments in controlled laboratory situations have frequently provided the keys. Such is true concerning vitamin A's relation to growth.

Nitrogen uptake (necessary to protein synthesis) was found to be decreased in vitamin A deficiency in young, growing rats, but not in fully grown ones. This may suggest that vitamin A is required for growth of tissue but not for maintenance.[*]

In young animals deprived of vitamin A, bone growth slows, especially in the cranium and spine, while nerve tissue continues to grow. The result is overcrowding of the skull and spine, and mechanical compression damage to nerve tissue with paralysis and degeneration.

Mucopolysaccharides, the ground substance of collagenous tissue, are especially affected by vitamin A deficiency.

Protein synthesis is adversely affected by vitamin A deficiency.[†]

[*]Brown, E. F., and Morgan, A. F.: The effect of vitamin A deficiency upon the metabolism of the rat, J. Nutr. **35:**425, 1948.
[†]Roels, O. A.: Present knowledge of vitamin A, Nutr. Rev. **24:**129, 1966.

Table 6-1. National Research Council recommended daily vitamin A allowances

	Age (yrs.)	Recommended I.U.
Men	(All)	5,000
Women	(All)	5,000
Pregnancy		+1,000
Lactation		+3,000
Infants	Up to 1 year	1,500
Children	1 to 3	2,000
	3 to 6	2,500
	6 to 9	3,500
Boys	9 to 12	4,500
	12 to 18	5,000
Girls	9 to 12	4,500
	12 to 18	5,000

ciency reduces the rate of thyroxin formation. Also, goiter has been shown to occur more frequently in persons whose diet is deficient in vitamin A than in the general population.

Vitamin A requirement

The requirement for vitamin A is difficult to establish precisely because of the number of variables that modify the vitamin A requirement. The amount stored in the liver, the form in which it is taken (as carotene or vitamin A), the medium in which taken (oil or aqueous dispersion), illness, and gastrointestinal defect all would have a bearing on the requirement.

National Research Council recommendations. To cover such variables, the recommendations of the National Research Council allow a margin of safety above minimal needs (Table 6-1).

Vitamin A is commonly measured in International Units (I.U.). One I.U. is equivalent to the biological activity* of 0.6 μg. (0.006 mg.) of pure β-carotene or 0.3 μg. of retinol.

---

*The "biological activity" of a vitamin is measured in rats according to its ability to forestall the development of a disease that is associated with deficiency of that specific vitamin.

Hypervitaminosis A. In this vitamin-conscious, health-obsessed age, where the vitamin bottle is a common addition to the dining table and foods, it is clearly possible to take potentially toxic amounts of vitamins A and D. Vitamins are substances that are required in *small* amounts. These small amounts are vital, but too much of some vitamins can be dangerous.

Hypervitaminosis A is manifested by joint pain, thickening of long bones, loss of hair, and jaundice. Such a case has been reported in an infant whose mother mistakenly gave vitamin A concentrate (dosage in *drops*) in amounts required for liver oil (dosage in *teaspoons*).[3]

Food sources of vitamin A

There are few animal sources of preformed vitamin A. These include liver, kidney, cream, butter, and egg yolk. The major contributors are the yellow and green vegetable and fruit sources of carotene (carrots, sweet potatoes, squash, apricots, spinach, collards, broccoli, and cabbage). A number of commercial products may be fortified with vitamin A. Margarine, for example, is fortified with 15,000 I.U. of vitamin A per pound.

In summary, vitamin A deficiency may occur for three basic reasons:

1. Inadequate dietary intake
2. Poor absorption (lack of bile or defective absorbing surface)
3. Inadequate conversion of carotene (liver or intestinal disease).

Vitamin D
Chemical and physical nature of vitamin D

A chemical characteristic of vitamin D, its resistance to oxidation, led to its discovery in 1922 by McCullom's group[1] at Johns Hopkins University. He eliminated vitamin A from a sample of cod liver oil by oxidation, and named the undestroyed factor vitamin D. Vitamin D has since been identified as a group of sterols varying in potency. The crystalline form is white and odorless. All forms are soluble in fat and in organic solvents, but not in water. They are heat stable, and are not easily oxidized.

The two D vitamins most important in nutrition are D_2 and D_3. D_2 is formed by irradiating the provitamin D_2 (ergosterol) that is found in ergot and in yeast. The irradiated product is known as calciferol or viosterol.

Vitamin D_3 occurs in fish liver oils (and also in human skin). Provitamin D_3 (7-dehydrocholesterol) is converted to the active form by sunlight.

Vitamin D is unique among the vitamins in two respects. It occurs naturally in only a few common foods (mainly in fish oils and a little in egg and milk), and it can be formed in the body by exposure of the skin to ultraviolet rays either from the sun or from a lamp.

Vitamin D absorption

Absorption of vitamin D accompanies that of calcium and phosphorus in the small intestine. Since vitamin D is fat-soluble, this absorption requires the presence of bile salts. Vitamin D, like vitamin A, is absorbed by mineral oil so if mineral oil is taken, it should be ingested separately from food. Moreover, as with vitamin A, diseases such as celiac syndrome, sprue, and colitis hinder its absorption.

Synthesis of vitamin D in the skin. Synthesis in the skin upon exposure to sunlight is unique to vitamin D. Recent studies[4] have shown, however, that synthesis occurs *on,* rather than *in,* the skin. After exposure to ultraviolet light, each subject's skin was washed, and the washings were found to have antirachitic properties. The skin washings from a control group not exposed to ultraviolet light had little potency. (Moral: Don't go swimming *after* a sunbath, but before!)

After being produced on or in the skin, vitamin D is absorbed through the skin and carried to the liver and other organs for use. A relatively small amount is stored in the liver, compared with the liver's much larger capacity for vitamin A storage. Vita-

min D is excreted from the circulating blood by way of the bile.

Physiologic functions of vitamin D

Vitamin D in the body is predominantly associated with calcium and phosphorus. It influences the absorption of these minerals and their deposit in bone tissue. Here again is demonstrated a vital interdependency among the nutrients in the body's overall functioning.

Absorption of calcium and phosphorus. The primary action of vitamin D is to facilitate the absorption of calcium from the small intestine. This absorption appears to take place by active transport in the proximal segment of the small intestine, and throughout the remainder of the intestine by passive diffusion. The absorption of phosphorus is apparently secondary. Within the lumen of the intestine, calcium is bound to phosphorus as calcium phosphate. As calcium is removed from the intestine, uncombined phosphorus remains. Its absorption through the intestinal wall follows that of calcium. Vitamin D probably is responsible for the more rapid absorption of calcium; it makes the cell membranes more permeable to calcium, but not to phosphorus.

Calcification. After the absorption of calcium and phosphorus through the intestinal wall, vitamin D continues to work in partnership with calcium and phosphorus in the calcification aspect of bone formation. Tracer studies with radioactive isotopes have shown that vitamin D directly increases the rate of mineral accretion and resorption in bone, by which the tissue is built and maintained.

Renal phosphate clearance. Vitamin D also has an important effect on the kidney's handling of phosphates. When the body is deficient in vitamin D, as in rickets (a disease of bone formation, Fig. 6-2), the renal threshold for phosphate excretion is lowered, and the kidney excretes more phosphate than normal. Therapeutic doses of vitamin D raise the renal threshold by causing more tubular reabsorption, which

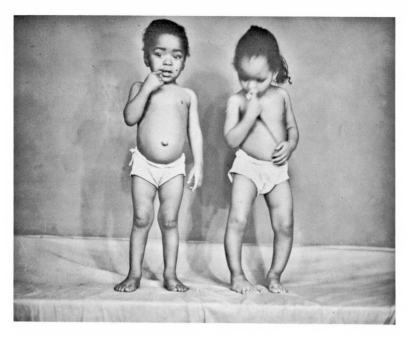

Fig. 6-2. Rachitic children. Note the knock-knees on the child on the left and the bowlegs on the child on the right. (From files of Therapeutic Notes, Parke, Davis & Co., Detroit, Michigan; courtesy Dr. Tom Spies and Dr. Orson D. Bird.)

conserves the plasma phosphate level. This renal mechanism gives another interesting example of the body's tenacious effort to adapt to the presence of disease and to maintain the integrity of the blood even at the expense of the tissue. The initial problem in rickets is lack of calcium due to absence of vitamin D. In order to preserve the vital balance between calcium and phosphorus in the blood, the kidney lowers its threshold point for phosphate and excretes more of it. If this adjustment were not made, the ratio of calcium to phosphorus would not be corrected, and tetany would result.

Citrate metabolism. Vitamin D also seems to play a role in citrate metabolism. Citrate is an important organic acid involved in many metabolic functions, including mobilization of minerals from bone tissue and removal of calcium from the blood. The removal of calcium results in an anticoagulant effect. This anticoagulant effect gives vitamin D a useful role in producing blood plasma and serum for medi-

cal use. In animal experiments, doses of vitamin D have produced increases in the citrate levels in many tissues such as bone, blood, kidney, heart, and the small intestine. Moreover, some investigators have even cured human rickets with citrate therapy alone. Orange juice given at the rate of 600 to 700 ml. daily also proved effective therapy for rickets.

Knowledge about the physiologic role of vitamin D has been gained mainly through studies of its relation to rickets. More recent studies,[5] however, have indicated that this vitamin functions throughout the body in the movement of various divalent cations (for example, Mg^{++}). This is suggested by the wide dispersion of the vitamin in many systems and tissues.

Vitamin D requirement

Difficulties in establishing requirements for vitamin D arise from the limited number of food sources available and lack of knowledge of precise body needs. Also the degree to which the body is able to produce vitamin D in response to irradiation is not precisely known. Thus, one's way of living determines the degree of exposure to sunlight, and would therefore influence one's individual need for additional vitamin D. A city dweller living in a high-rise apartment or in a tenement, and working indoors, needs more than a farmer who works out-of-doors all day. Elderly people or invalids who do not go out-of-doors have need for supplementary vitamin D. Growth demands in childhood, and in pregnancy and lactation, necessitate increased intake.

National Research Council recommendations. The National Research Council recommends 400 I.U. daily for children and for women during pregnancy and lactation. No statement is made concerning adult need, which indicates that in most instances general exposure to sunlight is sufficient. One I.U. of vitamin D is equivalent to the biological activity of 0.025 μg of pure crystalline vitamin D_3.

Hypervitaminosis D. As with vitamin A, it is possible to ingest excess quantities of vitamin D, and so to produce toxicity. This is a special danger in infant feeding practices where fortified milk, fortified cereal, plus variable vitamin supplements are used. The infant needs only 400 I.U. daily; whereas the amount in all of the above items can easily total 4,000 I.U. or more. As vitamin D is now commonly added to many infant foods, it seems wise to reconsider the need for supplementation with vitamin D preparations.

Symptoms of vitamin D toxicity are calcification of soft tissue such as lungs and kidney, and bone fragility. Renal tissue is particularly prone to calcify; glomerular filtration is affected and overall function is impaired.

Food sources of vitamin D

Few natural food sources of vitamin D exist. The two basic vitamins D_2 and D_3 occur only in yeast and fish liver oils. The main food sources are those to which crystalline vitamin D has been added, or in which vitamin D has been produced by irradiation. Milk, because it is so commonly used, has proved to be the most practical carrier, and it is now a widespread commercial practice to standardize the added vitamin D content at 400 I.U. per quart. Milk is also a good companion for the vitamin because it provides calcium and phosphorus as well. Butter substitutes are also fortified.

Vitamin E
Chemical and physical nature of vitamin E

Early vitamin research in animals led to observations that a certain factor was necessary for their reproduction. Between 1922 and 1924, the identification of this factor as an alcohol was reported.[6] Because of its function and chemical nature, it was named *tocopherol* (Gr. *tokos,* childbirth; *phero,* to bring; suffix-*ol,* alcohol). Tocopherol has come to be known as the antisterility vitamin, but it has been demonstrated to have this effect only in the rat and not in man— all specious advertising claims for its contribution to potency, virility, and the like notwithstanding! Pure vitamin E was finally isolated in 1936 from wheat germ oil. Its chemical structure was defined, and its synthesis achieved in 1938.

A number of related compounds have since been discovered. In reality, vitamin E is a group of vitamins. Three of these, designated α-, β-, and γ-tocopherol, display the greatest biologic activity. Of these three, α-tocopherol is the most significant.

Vitamin E is a pale yellow oil, stable to acids but not to alkalis, and it is insoluble in water. It is also stable to heat. It oxidizes very slowly, which is one of its most important chemical characteristics.

Vitamin E absorption

Vitamin E is believed to be absorbed like the other fat-soluble vitamins through bile salts and fats. Storage takes place in different body tissues, but especially in adipose tissue.

Maternal transfer of vitamin E to the infant. The amount of vitamin E that crosses the placenta is apparently limited to immediate fetal needs. The amount transferred to the infant through mother's milk is apparently greater. Therefore, vitamin E levels in breast-fed infants rise more rapidly than in bottle-fed infants. Vitamin E values in human colostrum range from 0.13 to 3.6 mg. per 100 ml., and in human milk from 0.10 to 0.48 mg. per 100 ml., with a mean of 0.24 mg. per 100 ml. This is about twice the value found in an infant feeding formula made of evaporated cow's milk diluted with an equal quantity of water.[6]

Physiologic functions of vitamin E in animals

The functions of vitamin E that have been determined up to this time are mainly those that have been demonstrated in laboratory animals and in animals important to commerce and industry. Even its role in animals gives it an important, though indirect, value to man. Such animals are of tremendous worth in research, and in everyday life to supply food, clothing, and other human needs. A summary of these findings in animals may give some clues to the possible role of vitamin E in human nutrition.

Reproduction. Classic studies have established the role of vitamin E in the reproductive function of the rat (an animal widely used in nutrition research, from which some of the most important discoveries have come). In the female rat, a deficiency of vitamin E causes poor placental implantation with consequent fetal resorption. In the male rat, a deficiency of vitamin E causes testicular degeneration, with atrophy of spermatogenic tissue and consequent permanent sterility.

Muscle integrity. Vitamin E seems to be necessary, for both the structure and function of smooth muscle, skeletal muscle, cardiac muscle and vascular tissue. There is evidence that in a large number of animal species vitamin E deficiency causes muscular dystrophy. Affected muscles display various stages and forms of degenera-tion such as pallor, fragmentation of fibers, edema, nuclear breakdown, necrosis, calcification, fibrosis, and pigmentation. In some animals, cardiac muscle fibrosis leads to failure and death. Accelerated respiration with increased oxygen uptake is observed.

Liver integrity. Of interest are studies relating vitamin E to integrity of liver tissue. Massive liver necrosis in rats, was made worse by vitamin E deficiency and improved by vitamin E treatment. The condition had been induced by a low-protein diet which was especially low in cystine, an amino acid that contains sulfur. If the diet was supplemented with cystine, vitamin E, and a newly discovered "factor 3" (a selenium compound) liver necrosis was prevented; if it had already occurred, it was reversed.[7]

Red blood cell integrity. Vitamin E is an effective antioxidant. Tests with strong oxidating agents such as hydrogen peroxide have indicated that the presence of vitamin E protects red blood cells against hemolysis. Vitamin E may preserve the integrity of the erythrocyte by inhibiting the action of the oxidase in hemoglobin on the unsaturated fatty acids of the cell membrane, and may protect cellular unsaturated lipids from oxidative breakdown.

Coenzyme factor in tissue respiration. There is some evidence that vitamin E may function as a cofactor in various enzyme systems involved in cell respiration or in biosynthesis of cellular substances such as DNA. It is suggested that vitamin E may serve as an electron transfer agent in the cell's energy metabolism system (see p. 65).

Role of vitamin E in human nutrition

The preceding studies have been summarized to show how much must be learned about vitamin E in relation to its possible clinical applications. These studies suggest exciting directions for future research. Do these findings relate to human nutrition, and if so, in what ways? Although no specific role of vitamin E in human metabolism has been clearly established, there are several possibilities.

Antioxidant agent. Already the antioxidant property of vitamin E is being made use of in commercial products to retard spoilage. Vitamin E is also added to therapeutic forms of vitamin A to protect the vitamin A from oxidizing before it is absorbed.

Anemias. The evidence concerning the role of vitamin E in erythrocyte protection has excited inquiry into possible relationships between this vitamin and blood dyscrasias. Several investigators have reported that plasma vitamin E levels are low in newborn infants, and that erythrocytes tested in dilute hydrogen peroxide showed increased hemolysis. Malnourished infants with macrocytic anemia have responded to vitamin E therapy with a favorable hematologic response.[8]

Malabsorption and muscle defects. Cystic fibrosis of the pancreas causes steatorrhea. Patients with this disease have demonstrated low plasma vitamin E levels and increased erythrocyte hemolysis in the peroxide test. Muscle lesions similar to those seen in animal studies have been found postmortem in patients with cystic fibrosis.[9] Low plasma vitamin E levels and skeletal muscle lesions have also been reported in patients with kwashiorkor.[9]

Relation to unsaturated fatty acid metabolism. Vitamin E may prove to have a definite correlation with protection of unsaturated fatty acids, especially linoleic acid, in the body. One study in a group of adults seems to indicate that the vitamin E requirement can be directly correlated with the amount of polyunsaturated fatty acids in the diet.[10]

Vitamin E requirement

Although the exact biochemical mechanism by which vitamin E functions in the body is still unknown, it is clearly an essential nutrient. In the revised dietary allowances recommended by the National Research Council in 1968, a statement is made concerning vitamin E requirement for the first time. The recommended allowance as I. U. is 1.25 times the body weight in kilo-

Table 6-2. Vitamin E requirements

	Age	Vitamin E (I. U.)
Infants	0 to 1	5
Children	1 to 6	10
	6 to 10	15
Boys	10 to 14	20
	14 to 18	25
Girls	10 to 14	20
	14 to 18	25
Men	(all ages)	30
Women	(all ages)	25
Pregnancy		30
Lactation		30

grams.[3] This calculation gives the recommended values in Table 6-2.

Food sources of vitamin E

The richest sources of vitamin E are the vegetable oils. Curiously enough, these are also the richest sources of polyunsaturated fatty acids. Other food sources include milk, eggs, muscle meats, fish, cereals, and leafy vegetables.

Vitamin K
Chemical and physical nature of vitamin K

In 1929, Professor Henrik Dam, biochemist at the University of Copenhagen, discovered a hemorrhagic disease in chicks fed a fat-free diet. Later he determined that the absent factor responsible was a blood-clotting vitamin which he called "Koagulationsvitamin," or vitamin K. In 1939, he succeeded in isolating and identifying the vitamin from alfalfa. In 1943, he was a recipient of the Nobel Prize for physiology and medicine in recognition of this brilliant work.

As with most of the vitamins, not one but several forms of vitamin K comprise a group of substances with similar biologic activity. There are three main K vitamins. Two occur in nature, and are fat soluble: K_1 (phylloquinone or phytonadione), which was isolated from alfalfa by Dam;

and K_2 (farnoquinone), which was isolated from putrefied sardine meal by other
investigators.[1] Vitamin K_3 has been made
synthetically and has wide clinical use. It
is *menadione,* one of several so-called vitamins that are synthetic products with
similar structures and properties. A water-
soluble form of menadione (its diphosphate
ester) is available for clinical use in patients in whom a fat-soluble form would be
less readily metabolized. Because vitamin
K is sensitive to light and irradiation, it
should be kept in dark bottles.

Vitamin K is synthesized by the normal
intestinal bacteria so an adequate supply is
generally present. Since the intestine of a
newborn infant is sterile at birth, however,
the supply of vitamin K is inadequate until
normal bacterial flora of the intestine develop about the third or fourth day of life.

Absorption of vitamin K

The natural fat-soluble vitamins K_1 and
K_2 require bile salts for absorption, and
therefore enter the metabolic system by
way of the upper segment of the small intestine. They are absorbed with other fat-
related products by the way of the abdominal lacteals into the lymphatic system,
and then into portal blood and the liver.
Vitamin K is apparently stored in small
amounts, as considerable quantities are excreted after administration of therapeutic
doses.

Physiologic functions of vitamin K

Blood clotting. The major function of
vitamin K is to catalyze the synthesis of
prothrombin by the liver (Fig. 6-3). Without vitamin K the whole vital process of
blood clotting cannot be initiated. It acts
as a catalyst, either as an enzyme or coenzyme. The mechanism for the production of prothrombin in the liver is not
known, but in the absence of functioning
liver tissue, vitamin K cannot act. When
liver damage has caused hypoprothrom-
binemia, and this in turn has led to hemor-

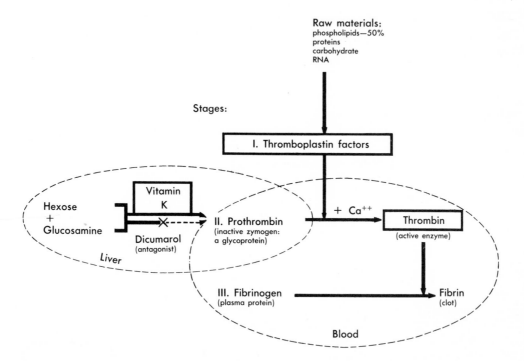

Fig. 6-3. The three stages of blood clotting. Note the role played by vitamin K in the production
of prothrombin. Dicumarol, an anticlotting drug, acts as an antagonist (antimetabolite) to vitamin
K and therefore inhibits the clotting mechanism at the start.

rhage, vitamin K is an ineffective therapeutic agent.

Clinical applications. A number of clinical situations, therefore, have important relationships with vitamin K.

Obstetrics. Since the intestinal tract of the newborn is sterile, the infant has no vitamin K during the first few days of life until normal bacterial flora develops. During this immediate postnatal period, hemorrhage may, therefore, occur. This condition is called hemorrhagic disease of the newborn. Vitamin K therapy may be given to the mother before delivery, but the effectiveness of placental transfer is debatable. Therefore, a prophylactic dose of vitamin K is usually given to the infant soon after delivery.

Biliary disease and surgery. Any condition of the biliary tract affecting the flow of bile will prevent the proper absorption of vitamin K. Since vitamin K is a fat-soluble material, bile is necessary for its absorption. Bleeding tendencies would be enhanced in obstruction of the bile ducts, jaundice, gallbladder disease, hepatic injury, or liver disease. Water-soluble forms of vitamin K are available for therapeutic use. Parenteral use of menadione or oral administration of bile salts together with vitamin K may be indicated to counteract the delayed clotting.

Surgical procedures involving the biliary tract, such as operations on the common bile duct or removal of the gallbladder, usually necessitate vitamin K therapy to prevent excessive hemorrhage.

Intestinal disease. Vitamin K deficiency is common in diseases such as celiac disease and sprue, which affect the absorbing mucosa of the small intestine, or other diarrheal diseases, such as ulcerative colitis, that cause rapid loss of intestinal contents. Intravenous administration of vitamin K may be indicated.

Antibiotic therapy. Prolonged use of antibiotics may adversely affect the normal bacterial flora of the intestine, so that vitamin K deficiency occurs.

Anticoagulant therapy. Use of heparin or bishydroxycoumarin (Dicumarol) in anticoagulant therapy for coronary thrombosis or thrombophlebitis may counteract vitamin K. The molecular structure of Dicumarol is similar to that of vitamin K, and it acts as an antimetabolite or antagonist to vitamin K because of the lock-and-key concept of enzyme action (see Fig. 5-3, p. 66). Dicumarol almost fits into vitamin K's spot in the enzyme-substrate complex. It therefore gets in the way, and prevents the normal reaction of vitamin K and prothrombin. This accounts for its anticoagulant action. In case of an overdose of the anticoagulants, vitamin K may be used as an antidote.

Coenzyme role. Recent studies suggest that vitamin K may have an additional metabolic function as an essential factor in oxidative phosphorylation (see p. 22).

Vitamin K requirement

No requirement for vitamin K is stated, since a deficiency of vitamin K is unlikely except in the clinical situations indicated. An adequate amount is usually ensured because (1) the intestinal bacteria constantly synthesize a supply, and (2) the amount the body needs is apparently small. The liver, however, must produce prothrombin if vitamin K is to be effective.

Food sources of vitamin K

The items from which the natural vitamins K_1 and K_2 were originally extracted by Dam and others—alfalfa and putrefied sardine meal—are hardly human foods. However, vitamin K is also found in green leafy vegetables, such as cabbage, spinach, kale, and cauliflower. Lesser amounts are found in tomatoes, cheese, egg yolk, and liver.

A summary of the fat-soluble vitamins is presented in Table 6-3 for review.

GLOSSARY

ameloblasts (Old Fr. *amel*, enamel; Gr. *blastos*, germ) special epithelial cells surrounding tooth buds in gum tissue, which form cup-shaped organs for producing the enamel structure of the

Table 6-3. Summary of fat-soluble vitamins

Vitamin	Physiological functions	Results of deficiency	Requirement	Food sources
A (retinol)	Production of rhodopsin (visual purple)	Xerophthalmia	Adult: 5,000 I.U.	Liver
Provitamin A (carotene)	Formation and maintenance of epithelial tissue Toxic in large amounts	Night blindness Keratinization of epithelium Follicular hyperkeratosis Skin and mucous membrane infections Faulty tooth formation	Pregnancy: 6,000 I.U. Lactation: 8,000 I.U. Children: 1,500 to 5,000 I.U. depending on age	Cream, butter, whole milk Egg yolk Green and yellow vegetables Yellow fruits Fortified margerine
D (calciferol)	Absorption of calcium and phosphorus Calcification of bones Renal phosphate clearance Toxic in large amounts	Rickets Faulty bone growth Osteomalacia in adults	400 I.U. (children; pregnant or lactating women)	Fish oils Fortified or irradiated milk
E (tocopherol)	Related to action of selenium Antioxidant with vitamin A and unsaturated fatty acids Hemopoiesis Reproduction (in animals)	Hemolysis of red blood cells; anemia Possible protection of unsaturated fatty acids Sterility (in rats)	Adult: 25 to 30 mg.	Vegetable oils
K (menadione)	Blood clotting, necessary for synthesis of prothrombin Possible coenzyme in oxidation phosphorylation Toxic in large amounts	Hemorrhagic disease of the newborn Bleeding tendencies in biliary disease or surgical procedures Deficiency in intestinal malabsorption (sprue, celiac disease, colitis) Prolonged antibiotic therapy Anticoagulant therapy (Dicumarol counteracts)	Unknown	Green leafy vegetables Cheese Egg yolk Liver

developing teeth. Insufficient vitamin A causes faulty production of ameloblasts, and therefore impairs the soundness of tooth structure.

antioxidant any substance that inhibits oxidation. Oxidation is a catabolic chemical process, that breaks down or changes a substance by the introduction of oxygen. An antioxidant inhibits or slows such a deteriorating change. Vitamin E acts as an antioxidant in commercial products to retard spoilage.

carotene provitamin A. Carotene, which occurs in certain plant pigments, is the natural precursor that the animal body converts to vitamin A.

follicular hyperkeratosis a vitamin A deficiency condition in which the skin becomes dry and scaly, and small pustules or hardened, pigmented, papular eruptions form around the hair follicles.

hypervitaminosis a toxic condition that results from intake of excess quantity of certain vitamins. The fat-soluble vitamins, especially A and D, have this distinct potential because they are stored by the body. The danger of toxicity does not hold for water-soluble vitamins, as the body eliminates any excess in the urine.

international units the measure commonly used for vitamins A and D. The amount of the vitamin comprising a unit is determined by its biological activity in rats; that is, the amount of the vitamin required to cure or prevent a disease that is associated with a deficiency of that specific vitamin.

keratinization (Gr. *keras, kerat,* horn) a process occurring in vitamin A deficiency states, in which the epithelial cells either slough off or become dry and flattened, then gradually harden, and forming rough horny scales. This process may occur in the cornea, the respiratory tract, the gastrointestinal tract, the genitourinary tract, or the skin.

precursor (L. *praecursor,* forerunner) a substance that precedes and is converted into a second substance. For example, carotene is a natural substance in plant pigments which the body converts to vitamin A. Thus, carotene is the precursor of vitamin A.

prothrombin (Gr. *pro,* before; *thrombos,* a clot) a protein (globulin) circulating in the plasma, essential to the clotting of blood. Prothrombin is produced by the liver. The process requires the presence of vitamin K.

retinol vitamin A; so named because of its chemical nature (an alcohol) and its function in the eye in the production of retinene, a necessary component of rhodopsin (visual purple).

rickets a childhood disease that results from deficient deposition of calcium and phosphorus in developing cartilage and newly forming bone, producing abnormal bone shape and structure.

Rickets is due primarily to vitamin D deficiency, which affects the absorption of calcium and phosphorus from the intestine, their deposition in bone tissue, and the reabsorption of phosphorus by the renal tubules.

tocopherol (Gr. *tokos,* childbirth; *pherein,* to bring) vitamin E; so named because of its association with reproduction in rats.

vitamin (L. *vita,* life; *amine*) any of a group of organic substances essential in small quantities to normal metabolism, found in minute amounts in natural foodstuffs; sometimes produced synthetically. Deficiencies of vitamins cause specific diseases and disorders.

References
Specific

1. Kagan, B. M., and Goodhart, R. S.: The vitamins. In Wohl, M. G., and Goodhart, R. S., editors: Modern nutrition in health and disease, Philadelphia, 1964, Lea & Febiger.
2. McCollum, E. V.: Early experiences with vitamin A—a restrospect, Nutr. Rev. **10**:161, 1952.
3. Breslau, R. C.: Hypervitaminosis A. Acute vitamin A toxicity, Arch. Pediat. **74**:178, 1957.
4. Kleiner, I. S., and Orten, J. M.: Biochemistry, ed. 7, St. Louis, 1966, The C. V. Mosby Co., p. 347.
5. Harper, H. A.: Physiological chemistry, ed. 10, Los Altos, California, 1967, Lange Medical Publications, pp. 67-68.
6. Gordon, H. H., and Nitowsky, J. M.: Vitamin E. In Wohl, M. G., and Goodhart, R. S., editors: Modern nutrition in health and disease, Philadelphia, 1964, Lea & Febiger, pp. 378-379.
7. Schwarz, K.: Factor 3, selenium, and vitamin E, Nutr. Rev. **18**:193, 1960.
8. Oski, F. A., and Barnes, L. A.: Vitamin E deficiency: a previously unrecognized cause of hemolytic anemia in the premature infant, J. Pediat. **70**:211, 1967.
9. Blanc, W. A., Reid, J. D., and Andersen, D. H.: Avitaminosis E in cystic fibrosis of the pancreas, Pediatrics **22**:494, 1958.
10. Horwitt, M. K.: Vitamin E and lipid metabolism in man, Amer. J. Clin. Nutr. **8**:451, 1961.

General

Bergen, S. S., Jr., and Roels, O. A.: Hypervitaminosis A.: report of a case, Amer. J. Clin. Nutr. **16**:265, 1965.
Burton, B. T., editor: Heinz handbook of nutrition, New York, 1966, McGraw-Hill Book Co.
Campbell, J. A., and Morrison, A. B.: Some factors affecting the absorption of vitamins, Amer. J. Clin. Nutr. **12**:162, 1963.

Cheldelin, V. H.: Nomenclature of the vitamins, Nutr. Rev. **9**:289, 1951.

Committee on Nutrition, American Academy of Pediatrics: The prophylactic requirement of toxicity of vitamin D. Pediatrics **35**:1022, 1965.

Cooley, D. G.: What is a vitamin? Today's Health **41**:20, 1963.

Council on Foods and Nutrition, American Medical Association: Fortification of nonfat milk solids with vitamins A and D, J.A.M.A. **197**:1107, 1966.

Council on Foods and Nutrition, American Medical Association: Importance of vitamin D milk, J.A.M.A. **159**:1018, 1955.

Council on Foods and Nutrition, American Medical Association: Vitamin preparations as dietary supplements and as therapeutic agents, J.A.M.A. **169**:41, 1959.

Dicks-Bushnell, M. W., and Davis, K. C.: Vitamin E content of infant formulas and cereals, Amer. J. Clin. Nutr. **20**:262, 1967.

Dinning, J. S.: Vitamin E responsive anemia in monkeys and man, Nutr. Rev. **21**:289, 1963.

Elliott, R. A., and Dryer, R. L.: Hypervitaminosis A: report of a case in an adult, J.A.M.A. **161**:1157, 1956.

Food and Nutrition Board, National Academy of Science, National Research Council: Recommended dietary allowances, 1968, Rev., ed. 7, Publication No. 1694, Washington, D. C., 1968.

Harris, R. S., and Thimann, K. V., editors: Vitamins and hormones: advances in research and application, New York, Academic Press (an annual publication).

Horwitt, M. K.: Vitamin E in human nutrition—an interpretive review, Borden's Review **22**:1, 1961.

Horwitt, M. K., and others: Polyunsaturated lipids and tocopherol requirements, J. Amer. Diet. Ass. **38**:231, 1961.

Jeghers, H., and Marraro, H.: Hypervitaminosis A: its broadening spectrum, Amer. J. Clin. Nutr. **6**:335, 1958.

Johnson, B. C.: Dietary factors and vitamin K, Nutr. Rev. **22**:225, 1964.

Joliffe, N., editor: Clinical nutrition, ed. 2, New York, 1962, Harper and Row.

McCollum, E. V.: Early experiences with vitamin A—a retrospect, Nutr. Rev. **10**:161, 1952.

McLaren, D. S.: Xerophthalmia: a neglected problem. Nutr. Rev. **22**:289, 1964.

McLaren, D. S., and others: Xerophthalmia in Jordan, Amer. J. Clin: Nutr. **17**:117, 1965.

Oski, F. A., and Barnes, L. A.: Vitamin E deficiency: a previously unrecognized cause of hemolytic anemia in the premature infant, J. Pediat. **70**:211, 1967.

Pereira, S. M., and others: Vitamin A therapy in children with kwashiorkor, Amer. J. Clin. Nutr. **20**:297, 1967.

Review: Availability of vitamins and minerals in tablet form, Nutr. Rev. **24**:101, 1966.

Review: Interrelationships between vitamins A and E, Nutr. Rev. **23**:82, 1965.

Review: Intestinal absorption of vitamin A, Nutr. Rev. **22**:86, 1964.

Review: The metabolic role of vitamin E, Nutr. Rev. **23**:90, 1965.

Review: Toxic reactions of vitamin A, Nutr. Rev. **22**:109, 1964.

Review: Vitamin A intoxication in infancy, Nutr. Rev. **23**:263, 1965.

Roels, O. A.: Present knowledge of vitamin A, Nutr. Rev. **24**:129, 1966.

Roels, O. A.: Present knowledge of vitamin E, Nutr. Rev. **25**:33, 1967.

Rosenberg, H. R.: The fiftieth anniversary of Casimir Funk's "Vitamines," Nutr. Rev. **20**:353, 1962.

Sebrell, W. H., Jr., and Harris, R. S., editors: The vitamins: chemistry, physiology, and pathology, (3 vols.) New York, 1954, Academic Press, Inc.

Stefferud, A., editor: Food, the yearbook of agriculture, 1959, Washington, D. C., 1959, U. S. Department of Agriculture.

Udall, J. A.: Human sources and absorption of vitamin K in relation to anticoagulation stability, J.A.M.A. **194**:127, 1965.

Verner, J. V., Jr., and others: Vitamin D intoxication: report of two cases treated with cortisone, Ann. Int. Med. **48**:765, 1958.

Vietti, T. J., and others: Observations on the prophylactic use of vitamin K in the newborn infant, J. Pediat. **56**:343, 1960.

Vietti, T. J., and others: Vitamin K, prophylaxis in the newborn, J.A.M.A. **176**:791, 1961.

Vitamin Manual, Kalamazoo, Mich., 1963, The Upjohn Co.

Wohl, M. G., and Goodhart, R. S., editors: Modern nutrition in health and disease, ed. 3, Philadelphia, 1964, Lea & Febiger.

Wolf, G.: Some thoughts on the metabolic role of vitamin A, Nutr. Rev. **20**:161, 1962.

CHAPTER 7

Vitamins: water-soluble vitamins

B-COMPLEX VITAMINS

The story of the B vitamins is a compelling one because it is the story of many people dying of a puzzling, age-old disease which other people observed and sought to cure. It was eventually learned that common, everyday food held the answer. The paralyzing disease beriberi had plagued the Orient for centuries and caused many men in many places to search for its solution. As early as 1882, a Japanese Naval medical officer, Takaki, reported that he had cured beriberi in sailors of the Japanese Navy by giving them less rice and more vegetables, barley, meat, and canned milk.

A few years later Christian Eijkman, a Dutch doctor at a prison in the Netherlands East Indies, observed the same type of paralysis in prison inmates and began to seek the answer through experiments with pigeons. Since he had little money for his research he fed the pigeons scraps of the prison food, which was mostly polished rice. The same type of paralysis developed in the pigeons. When the unsympathetic prison director refused Eijkman permission to use the prison scraps, he was forced to buy some cheap natural (unmilled) rice to feed the birds. The dying birds revived and were soon well again. Eijkman experimented with numerous birds and the same results followed. He could produce the disease and cure it simply by changing the diet! He reported his findings in 1897.

Eijkman's first theory was that the disease resulted from a poison in polished rice that was neutralized by an antidote in the hulls. Although this theory was wrong, his observation was an important clue. An associate of Eijkman, Dr. Grijns, offered another clue in 1901 with the idea that the disease was caused by something vital that was present in the polishings but was absent in the polished rice. In 1911, Casimir Funk, isolated the vital nitrogen compound in the hulls which he called a "vitamine" (see p. 72).

The international search gained momentum in the field and in the laboratory. A dedicated American, R. R. Williams, in the foreign service as chief chemist at the Philippine Bureau of Science from 1909 to 1916, applied these new findings and made tremendous strides in control and eradication of infantile beriberi by using extracts of rice polishings. In 1916, another American scientist then at the University of Wisconsin, E. V. McCollum, named the food factor "water-soluble B," because it was thought to be a single vitamin.

The widening search, however, proved that vitamin B was not a single substance, but about a dozen vitamin and vitamin-related factors. The B-complex family of vitamins is now recognized.

The B vitamins, originally believed to be important only in preventing the deficiency diseases that led to their discovery, have now been identified with many important metabolic functions. They serve as vital partners in many reactions as coenzymes in energy metabolism. Grouping them according to their function is therefore a useful step before the significance of each in relation to human nutrition is discussed.

Group I: Classic disease factors

1. Thiamine (vitamin B_1)—antiberiberi factor or antineuritic vitamin, called "aneurin" in Europe and some other areas; essential in carbohydrate metabolism
2. Riboflavin (vitamin B_2, formerly known as G)—essential in tissue respiration, hence in growth; and to the prevention of various skin disorders such as cheilosis (cracking at the corners of the mouth)
3. Niacin—nicotinic acid, originally called P-P factor (pellagra-preventing factor); a coenzyme essential to tissue oxidation and cell metabolism

Group II: More recently discovered coenzyme factors

1. Pyridoxine (vitamin B_6)—essential coenzyme with amino acids; need for pyridoxine is increased in high protein diets
2. Pantothenic acid—essential part of coenzyme A or active acetate (Reread p. 22 to identify this pivotal key in the metabolism of carbohydrate, fat, and protein.)
3. Lipoic acid—coenzyme associated with thiamine in carbohydrate metabolism; a fatty acid, not a true vitamin
4. Biotin (formerly vitamin B_7 or H)—coenzyme in carbon dioxide fixation reactions in energy metabolism

Group III: Cell growth and blood-forming factors

1. Folic acid (formerly vitamin B_9 or B_{10})—a group of factors essential to the growth and reproduction of cells; associated with anemias because of their vital role in formation of red blood cells.
2. Para-aminobenzoic acid (PABA)—part of folic acid molecule; sulfonamide antagonist; not a true vitamin
3. Cobalamin (vitamin B_{12})—red, cobalt-containing vitamin group; the antipernicious anemia factor; extrinsic factor (Castle)

Group IV: Other related nutrition factors (pseudo-vitamins)

1. Inositol—lipotropic agent in animal nutrition
2. Choline—essential metabolite, nerve mediator, lipotropic agent

CLASSIC DISEASE FACTORS
Thiamine (B_1)

The search of many persons for the antiberiberi factor led eventually to a successful conclusion. In 1924, two Dutch workers in Java, Jansen and Donath, isolated and identified thiamine hydrochloride from rice polishings as the beriberi-preventive ma-

terial. Subsequently, in 1935, the American workers, Williams and his associates,[1,2] finally synthesized thiamine, and the answer to the puzzle of beriberi was found. Its basic metabolic functions were essentially clarified during the 1930's.

Nature of thiamine

Thiamine hydrochloride is a white crystalline material, sometimes described as having a nutlike and yeasty odor. It is water-soluble and stable when dry, but is destroyed by alkalis. It is absorbed more readily in the acid medium of the proximal duodenum than in the lower duodenum, where the acidity of the chyme is counteracted by alkaline intestinal secretions. Thiamine is not stored in large quantities in the tissues. The tissue content is highly relative to heightened metabolic demand (fever, increased muscular activity, pregnancy, and lactation) or to composition of the diet. Carbohydrate increases the need for thiamine, while fat and protein spare thiamine. In addition, thiamine is constantly excreted in the urine.

Physiologic functions of thiamine

Coenzyme in carbohydrate metabolism. The manifestations of beriberi—polyneuritis, muscle weakness, and gastrointestinal disturbances—can be traced to physiologic problems related to the basic metabolic function of thiamine. When actively combined with phosphorus as thiamine pyrophosphate (TPP), thiamine plays a key role as a coenzyme in carbohydrate metabolism.

As stated in Chapter 5 on Energy Metabolism, enzymes act as *catalysts*. They not only speed up reactions that would otherwise be too slow, but also make possible the dynamic turnover of compounds without which life could not exist. The active partners in these processes are the coenzymes.

For glucose oxidation thiamine is such a coenzyme during decarboxylation and transketolation. *Decarboxylation* is the reaction in which pyruvate is converted to active acetate and carbon dioxide is removed. The enzyme is called a *decarboxylase;* thiamine pyrophosphate acts as a *cocarboxylase.* This enables pyruvate to enter the Krebs cycle to produce vital energy. If there were no thiamine there could be no energy (see p. 23).

In the hexose monophosphate shunt pathway for glucose oxidation, thiamine diphosphate (TDP) acts as a coenzyme in the important reaction which provides active glyceraldehyde. This is a key link providing activated glycerol for lipogenesis for the conversion of glucose to fat (see pp. 24 and 25). The process is called *transketolation* (keto-carrying), and the enzyme is a *transketolase.* Thiamine diphosphate is the key activator which provides the high energy phosphate bond. Ionized magnesium (Mg^{++}) is another cofactor present.

Clinical effects of thiamine deficiency

If thiamine is not present in sufficient amounts to provide the key energizing coenzyme factor in the cells, clinical effects will be reflected in the gastrointestinal system, the nervous system, and the cardiovascular system.

Gastrointestinal system. Various manifestations such as anorexia, indigestion, severe constipation, gastric atony, and deficient hydrochloric acid secretion may occur as a result of thiamine deficiency. As the cells of the smooth muscles and secretory glands are not able to receive sufficient energy from glucose, they cannot do their proper work in digestion to provide still more glucose, and a vicious cycle ensues as deficiency continues.

Nervous system. The central nervous system is extremely dependent upon glucose

Table 7–1. National Research Council allowances for thiamine in relation to calories

	Age (yrs.)	Calories	Thiamine (mg.)
Adult			
Men	18 to 35	2,800	1.4
	35 to 55	2,600	1.3
	55 to 75+	2,400	1.2
Women	18 to 35	2,000	1.0
	35 to 55	1,850	1.0
	55 to 75+	1,700	1.0
Pregnaoncy		+200	(+0.2) 1.2
Lactatin		+1,000	(+0.5) 1.5
Infants	0 to 1/6	480	0.2
	1/6 to 1/2	770	0.4
	1/2 to 1	900	0.5
Children	1 to 2	1,100	0.6
	2 to 3	1,250	0.6
	3 to 4	1,400	0.7
	4 to 6	1,600	0.8
	6 to 8	2,000	1.0
	8 to 10	2,200	1.1
Boys	10 to 12	2,500	1.3
	12 to 14	2,700	1.4
	14 to 18	3,000	1.5
Girls	10 to 12	2,250	1.1
	12 to 14	2,300	1.2
	14 to 16	2,400	1.2
	14 to 18	2,300	1.2

for energy to do its work. Without sufficient thiamine to help provide this need, neuronal activity is impaired, alertness and reflex responses are diminished, and general apathy and fatigue result. If thiamine deficiency continues, damage or degeneration of myelin sheaths of nerve fibers causes increasing nerve irritation, which produces pain and prickly or deadening sensations. Paralysis may gradually result if the process continues unchecked in a severe deficiency state.

Cardiovascular system. If the thiamine deficiency persists, the heart muscle weakens and cardiac failure may result. Also, smooth muscle of the vascular system may be involved causing peripheral vasodilation. As a result of the cardiac failure, peripheral edema may be observed in the extremities.

Thiamine requirement

The requirements for thiamine in human nutrition are usually stated in terms of the direct relation of thiamine to carbohydrate and energy metabolism, expressed as caloric intake. The studies of various investigators have indicated that the daily adult thiamine requirements are from 0.23 to 0.5 mg. per 1,000 calories. The National Research Council allowances recommend, therefore, 0.5 mg. per 1,000 calories, with a minimum of 1.0 mg. for any intake between 1,000 and 2,000 calories. The correlations of thiamine with calories are shown in Table 7-1.

Clinical applications. Several important factors influence thiamine requirements and should be recognized in care of patients:

1. During growth periods of infancy, childhood, and especially adolescence, thiamine needs are increased.
2. Increased needs accompany gestation because of the increased metabolic rate characteristic of pregnancy and production of milk.
3. The larger the body and its tissue volume, the greater its cellular energy requirements.
4. Fevers and infections increase cellular energy requirements, which also increase thiamine needs. Geriatric patients and those with chronic illness require particular attention to avoid deficiencies.

Food sources of thiamine

Good sources are lean pork, beef, liver, whole or enriched grains, and legumes. Eggs, fish, and a few vegetables are fair sources. Thiamine is less widely distributed in food than some of the other vitamins, such as A and C, and the quantities of thiamine in these foods are less than the naturally available quantities of vitamins A and C. Therefore, a deficiency of thiamine is a distinct possibility in the average diet, especially when calories are markedly curtailed, and in some highly inadequate special therapeutic diets.

Riboflavin (B₂)

Although as early as 1897 a London chemist named Blythe had observed a water-soluble pigment with peculiar yellow-green fluorescence in milk whey, it was not until 1932 that riboflavin was actually discovered by workers in Germany.[3,4] The chemical group name, flavins (L. *flavus*, yellow), was given to the related compounds. Later, because the vitamin also contained the pentose sugar d-ribose the term *riboflavin* was officially adopted.

Nature of riboflavin

Riboflavin is a yellow-green fluorescent pigment which forms yellowish brown needlelike crystals. It is water soluble and relatively stable to heat, but is easily destroyed by light and irradiation. It is stable in acid media and is not easily oxidized. However, it is sensitive to strong alkalis. Absorption seems to occur readily in the upper section of the small intestine and to be facilitated by combining with phosphorus in intestinal mucosa. Storage is relatively limited, although some amounts are found in liver and kidney. Day-to-day tissue turnover needs must be supplied by the diet.

Urinary excretion varies according to intake and state of tissue depletion.

Physiologic functions of riboflavin

Coenzyme in protein metabolism. Just as thiamine is a partner in carbohydrate metabolism, riboflavin is a vital factor in protein metabolism. It, too, combines with phosphorus to form essential coenzymes in tissue respiration systems. The enzymes of which riboflavin is an important constituent are called *flavoproteins.* Two such riboflavin enzymes, flavin mononucleotide and flavin adenine dinucleotide, operate at vital reaction points in the respiratory chains of cellular metabolism.

Flavin mononucleotide (FMN) is riboflavin phosphate activated with a high energy phosphate bond. It is part of the enzyme systems which remove the amino group (NH_2) from certain amino acids. This process is called *deamination* (see Chapter 4 on Protein Metabolism).

Flavin adenine dinucleotide (FAD) is a riboflavin enzyme that contains two high energy phosphate bonds. It is a highly active form which operates in many reactions affecting amino acids, fatty acids, and carbohydrate. It helps in the deamination of glycine, an essential amino acid, and in the oxidizing of some of the lower fatty acids, such as butyric acid. It also acts in one of the systems of H^+ transfer in cellular oxidation (see Chapter 5). One such system is located in the Krebs cycle between succinic acid and fumaric acid (see Figs. 2-6, p. 23 and 5-2, p. 66).

Clinical effects of riboflavin deficiency

Manifestations of riboflavin deficiency center around tissue inflammation and breakdown.

1. Wound aggravation—even minor tissue injuries easily become aggravated and do not heal easily
2. Mouth—cheilosis develops and the

Table 7-2. National Research Council allowances for riboflavin in relation to protein (1968 revision)

	Age (yrs.)	Protein (gm.)	Riboflavin (mg.)
Men	18 to 22	60	1.6
	22 to 75+	65	1.7
Women	18 to 75+	55	1.5
Pregnancy		65	1.8
Lactation		75	2.0
Infants	0 to ⅙	10	0.4
	⅙ to ½	14	0.5
	½ to 1	16	0.6
Children	1 to 2	25	0.6
	2 to 3	25	0.7
	3 to 4	30	0.8
	4 to 6	30	0.9
	6 to 8	35	1.1
	8 to 10	40	1.2
Boys	10 to 12	45	1.3
	12 to 14	50	1.4
	14 to 18	60	1.5
Girls	10 to 12	50	1.3
	12 to 14	50	1.4
	14 to 18	55	1.5

lips become swollen, crack easily, and characteristic cracks develop at the corners of the mouth

3. Nose—cracks and irritation develop at nasal angles
4. Tongue—the tongue becomes swollen and reddened (glossitis)
5. Eyes—extra blood vessels develop in the cornea (corneal vascularization), and the eyes burn, itch, and tear
6. Skin—a scaly, greasy eruption may develop, especially in skin folds (seborrheic dermatitis)

Since nutritional deficiencies are usually multiple rather than single, riboflavin deficiencies seldom occur alone; they are especially likely to occur in conjunction with deficiencies of other B vitamins and protein.

Riboflavin requirement

The body's requirement for riboflavin is related not so much to total caloric intake, as it is to body size, metabolic rate, and rate of growth, all of which are related to protein intake. The lower the protein intake the more riboflavin is excreted and lost. Studies indicate that tissue stores of riboflavin are not maintained when the dietary intake of this vitamin is less than 1.0 mg. daily and that 1.3 mg. or more daily is necessary to maintain tissue reserves.

For practical purposes, the general National Research Council allowances for riboflavin have been stated in terms of metabolic body size: 0.7 mg. per kilogram of body size. The relation to protein intake is shown in Table 7-2.

Clinical applications

Attention should be given to certain risk groups or clinical situations in which riboflavin needs may be increased or where deficiencies are more likely to occur.

1. Cheap high-starch diets which are limited in protein foods such as milk, meat, and vegetables may be deficient in riboflavin.
2. Gastrointestinal disorders or chronic illness may result in a riboflavin deficiency because food intake is affected by such disorders as anorexia, by poor tolerance, or by prolonged use of a too limited special diet. Disorders that affect absorption of nutrients can also cause riboflavin deficiency.
3. Wound healing, as in surgical procedures, trauma, and burns, increases the need for riboflavin because of the increased need for protein.
4. Periods of normal body stress such as growth periods, pregnancy, and lactation increase the need for riboflavin.

Food sources of riboflavin

The most important food source of riboflavin is milk. One of the pigments in milk, *lactoflavin*, is the milk form of riboflavin. Each quart of milk contains 2 mg. of riboflavin, which is more than the daily requirement. Other good sources are the active organ meats (liver, kidney, and heart), and some vegetables contribute additional amounts. Cereals are poor sources unless they are enriched by commercial processing, which is now a common practice.

Since riboflavin is water-soluble and destroyed by light, considerable loss can occur in open, excess-water cooking. Therefore, covered containers and limited water are indicated.

Niacin (nicotinic acid, B₅)

Discovery of niacin. The discovery of niacin was the result of man's age-old struggle with disease. The disease associated with niacin deficiency is pellagra, which is characterized by a typical dermatitis and often has fatal effects on the nervous system. The unraveling of the mystery of pellagra forms a classic example of the interworking of talents and techniques from medicine, public health, epidemiology, nutrition, and nursing.

Observations of pellagra were first recorded in 18th century Spain and Italy, where it was endemic in populations subsisting largely on corn. In the early 1900's Joseph Goldberger, a United States Public

Health Service physician studying the problem of pellagra, worked in an orphanage in the rural southern United States. He noticed that although the majority of the children in the orphanage had pellagra in some degree, a few did not. He traced the absence of pellagra in the few to their pilfering of milk and meat from the orphanage's limited supply. His investigations established the relation of the disease to a certain food factor, which he called the P-P (pellagra preventive) factor or vitamin G. Casimir Funk, in London, isolated nicotinic acid from rice polishings in 1911, but did not recognize its disease-preventive significance. It was not until 1937 that Conrad Elvehjem,[5,6] a scientist at the University of Wisconsin, definitely associated the vitamin

with pellagra by using it to cure the related disease, black tongue, in dogs.

Relation of niacin to tryptophan. As further study of the vitamin and pellagra continued, a new mystery developed concerning the relation of niacin to the essential amino acid, tryptophan. Again, curious observations were made. Why was pellagra rare in some population groups whose diets were actually low in niacin, whereas it was common in other groups whose diets were higher in niacin? And why did milk, which is low in niacin, have the ability to cure or prevent pellagra? Why was pellagra so common in groups subsisting on high-corn diets?

At the University of Wisconsin, in 1945, Willard Krehl and his associates finally dis-

TO PROBE FURTHER
Niacin coenzymes and the "bouncing H^+"

In the chain of agents that pass ionized hydrogen (H^+) and electrons along the distributing line to the waiting consumer, oxygen, two niacin compounds play key roles. This intricate network of systems within the cell provides energy precisely in the amounts necessary and at the time of need, which prevents waste and maintains orderly control (see Fig. 5-2, p. 66).

These two niacin compounds are:
1. NAD (nicotinamide adenine dinucleotide) Coenzyme I; formerly called DPN (diphosphate nucleotide); the new term, expresses the structure of the compound, and is based on recognition of the important presence of the vitamin
2. NADP (nicotinamide adenine dinucleotide phosphate) Coenzyme II; formerly called TPN (triphosphate nucleotide)

In this oxidation system (the so-called respiratory chain) the niacin coenzymes often operate in partnership with thiamine and riboflavin coenzymes. For example, in the pivotal entry reaction of pyruvate into the Krebs final energy cycle, both niacin and thiamine coenzymes (NAD and TPP) are necessary. In the Krebs cycle itself, both niacin coenzymes (NAD and NADP) and riboflavin coenzymes (the flavoprotein system) operate together with cytochromes to generate bursts of energy (high energy phosphate bonds at several different raction points).

The total effect is similar to that of a generator. Energy is constantly produced and stored in "batteries" from which the body's cells may derive "current" when energy is needed. The carbon dioxide and water that are left at the end of these reactions are really by-products, but the controlling purpose of the entire series of reactions is to produce *energy*.

covered that *tryptophan is a precursor of niacin.*[7,8] Here again was a vital link of a B vitamin with protein. Milk prevents pellagra because it is high in tryptophan. Almost exclusive use of corn contributes to pellagra because corn is low in tryptophan. Populations subsisting on diets low in niacin may never have pellagra because they happen to be also consuming adequate amounts of tryptophan. Gelatin is so poor a source of protein because it lacks tryptophan, whereas meat combines tryptophan and niacin.

This tryptophan-niacin relation led to the development of a unit of measure called *niacin equivalent.* It was calculated that in a person with average physiologic needs, approximately 60 mg. of tryptophan pro-

duces 1 mg. of niacin. This amount of tryptophan was designated as a niacin equivalent. Dietary requirements are now usually given in terms of total milligrams of niacin and niacin equivalents.

Chemical nature of niacin. Two forms of niacin exist. Niacin (nicotinic acid) is easily converted to its amide form, *nicotinamide,* which is water-soluble, stable to acid and heat, and forms a white powder when crystallized.

Physiologic functions of niacin

Coenzyme in tissue oxidation. Niacin is a partner with riboflavin in the cellular coenzyme systems that convert proteins and fats to glucose, and that oxidize glucose to release controlled energy. In these systems,

Table 7-3. National Research Council niacin equivalent allowances in relation to calories and protein (1968 revision)

	Age (yrs.)	Calories	Protein (gm.)	Niacin (mg. equiv.)
Men	18 to 22	2,800	60	18
	22 to 35	2,800	65	18
	35 to 55	2,600	65	17
	55 to 75+	2,400	65	14
Women	18 to 35	2,000	55	13
	35 to 55	1,850	55	13
	55 to 75+	1,700	55	13
Pregnancy		2,200	65	15
Lactation		3,000	75	20
Infants	0 to 1/6	480	10	5
	1/6 to 1/2	770	14	7
	1/2 to 1	900	16	8
Children	1 to 2	1,100	25	8
	2 to 3	1,250	25	8
	3 to 4	1,400	30	9
	4 to 6	1,600	30	11
	6 to 8	2,000	35	13
	8 to 10	2,200	40	15
Boys	10 to 12	2,500	45	17
	12 to 14	2,700	50	18
	14 to 18	3,000	60	20
Girls	10 to 12	2,250	50	15
	12 to 14	2,300	50	15
	14 to 16	2,400	55	16
	16 to 18	2,300	55	15

the oxidation of glucose often takes place in the absence of free oxygen simply by the removal of hydrogen ions. These ions are passed down the line between the successively simpler compounds that comprise these systems to the eventual receiver oxygen, and the end product is water. (See Chapter 5 on Energy Metabolism.)

Clinical effects of niacin deficiency

Since riboflavin and niacin have close interrelationships in cell metabolism, clinical manifestations of their deficiency closely parallel. Furthermore, if one of these two components is deficient, the other is usually deficient as well. General niacin deficiency is manifest as weakness, lassitude, anorexia, indigestion, and various skin eruptions. More specific manifestations involve the skin and nervous system. Skin areas exposed to sunlight are especially affected, and they develop a dark, scaly dermatitis. If deficiency continues, the central nervous system becomes involved, and confusion, apathy, disorientation, and neuritis develop.

Niacin requirement

Studies with human requirements for niacin have indicated that the minimum for necessary tissue stores is about 9 mg. per 1,000 calories. Many factors affect requirement such as age and growth periods, pregnancy and lactation, illness, tissue trauma, body size, and physical activity. The National Research Council recommendations (6.6 mg. per 1,000 calories and not less than 13 niacin equivalents at intakes of less than 2,000 calories) are about 50% higher than minimum requirements, to provide a safety margin to cover variances in individual need. These recommendations also allow for the contribution of tryptophan (in terms of niacin equivalents) from the dietary protein sources (Table 7-3).

Food sources of niacin

Meat is a major source of niacin. Peanuts, beans, peas, are also good sources. Enrichment makes good sources of all the grains; otherwise corn and rice are poor, because they are low in tryptophan. Oats are also low in niacin. Fruits and vegetables generally are poor sources.

MORE RECENTLY DISCOVERED COENZYME FACTORS
Pyridoxine (B$_6$)

Discovery.[9,10] It was Joseph Goldberger, continuing his work with B vitamins, who suggested in 1926 that the group contained a factor that cured a particular dermatitis in rats. Because of this property, the factor was at first called *adermin* (or the rat-anti-dermatitis factor). In 1939, Harris synthesized the factor, and noted that its chemical structure was distinguished by having a pyridine ring and so named it pyridoxine. In 1942, Snell's group isolated in animal tissue and synthesized the two companion products, pyridoxal and pyridoxamine. Umbreit and his group followed in 1945 with their report of coenzyme functions of the vitamin in its phosphate forms. The activity of another B vitamin in metabolic coenzyme reactions throughout the body was being clearly and systematically brought into view.

Chemical nature of pyridoxine

Three forms of vitamin B$_6$ occur in nature—pyridoxine, pyridoxal, and pyridoxamine. In the body, all three forms undergo conversion to pyridoxal phosphate. By far the most potent and active forms in body metabolism are the phosphate derivatives of pyridoxal and pyridoxamine. The term *pyridoxine* or simply vitamin B$_6$ is used to designate the entire group, as well as one of its components.

Pyridoxine is a water-soluble, heat-stable vitamin that is sensitive to light and alkalis. It is absorbed in the upper portion of the small intestine, and is found throughout the body tissues, which is evidence of its many essential metabolic activities. There is evidence that intestinal bacteria also produce this vitamin, but the full extent of this source and the degree to which it is utilized by the body are as yet undetermined.

Physiologic functions of pyridoxine

Coenzyme in protein metabolism. In its active phosphate forms (B_6-PO_4), pyridoxine is an active coenzyme factor in many types of reaction in amino acid in metabolism:

1. Pyridoxine is active in decarboxylation. An example is the reaction that converts glutamic acid to γ-aminobutyric acid, a substance found in gray matter in the brain. Since aminobutyric acid affects central synaptic activity, it is a regulatory factor for the neurons. Also important to brain function is another such B_6-PO_4-dependent reaction involved in the conversion of tryptophan to serotonin. Serotonin, a potent vasoconstrictor, stimulates cerebral activity and brain metabolism.

2. Pyridoxine also aids in deamination. By removing the amino groups from amino acids, such as serine and threonine, B_6-PO_4 helps to render carbon residues availables for energy.

3. In transmination reactions (transfer of amino groups), B_6-PO_4 acts as a coenzyme which splits off NH_2 and transfers it to a new carbon skeleton, which forms a new amino acid or other compound. This passage of the amino group from compound to compound is much like the hydrogen ion transfer systems in which thiamine, niacin, and riboflavin operate.

4. In transsulfuration (transfer of sulfur) B_6-PO_4 aids reactions of the sulfur-containing amino acids, as in the transfer of sulfur from methionine to another amino acid (serine) to form the derivative cysteine.

5. Pyridoxide is involved in nicotinic acid formation from tryptophan. Through its involvement in this reaction, B_6-PO_4 plays a role in niacin supply.

6. There is evidence that B_6-PO_4 is necessary for the incorporation of the amino acid glycine and succinate (a glucose metabolite in the Krebs cycle) into *heme*, the essential protein core of hemoglobin.

7. In amino acid absorption, B_6-PO_4 appears also to operate as part of an active transport system in the intestinal wall which aids in the absorption of amino acids and their entry into cells.

Coenzyme in carbohydrate and fat metabolism. To a lesser extent, B_6-PO_4 also plays a role in carbohydrate metabolism. By way of the transfer systems such as decarboxylation and transamination, metabolites are provided for energy-producing fuel in the Krebs cycle. B_6-PO_4 also participates in the conversion of the essential fatty acid, linoleic acid, to another fatty acid, arachidonic acid.

Clinical effects of pyridoxine deficiency

It is evident from such an impressive list of metabolic activities that pyridoxine may hold a key to a number of clinical problems.

Anemia. A hypochromic, microcytic anemia has been observed in several patients even in the presence of a high serum iron level. A deficiency of B_6-PO_4 was demonstrated by a tryptophan load test, and the anemia was subsequently cured by supplying the deficient vitamin.

Central nervous system disturbances. By virtue of its role in the formation of the two regulatory compounds in brain activity, serotonin and γ-aminobutyric acid, $B_6 PO_4$ may have a place in control of related neurological conditions. In infants deprived of the vitamin, there is increased hyperirritability that progresses to convulsive seizures. A classic object lesson occurred in the early 1950's when infants fed a commercial milk formula in which most of the pyridoxine content had inadvertently been destroyed by high-temperature autoclaving, subsequently had convulsions. The seizures ceased soon after a B_6-supplemented formula was instituted.

Tuberculosis. Experience with isoniazid (isonicotinic acid hydrazide; INH) used as a chemotherapeutic agent for tuberculosis has shown it to be an antagonist for pyridoxine. By inhibiting the conversion of glutamic acid (the only amino acid the brain metabolizes), isoniazid has caused a side effect of neuritis in some patients. Treatment with large doses (50 to 100 mg. daily) of pyridoxine prevents this effect.

Physiologic demands in pregnancy. Pyridoxine deficiencies during pregnancy have been demonstrated by tryptophan load tests and subsequently alleviated by supplementation with vitamin B_6. Fetal growth, in addition to creating greater maternal metabolic demands, increases the pyridoxine requirement. For some years, vitamin B_6 has been used to treat the hyperemesis of pregnancy, but there is no real evidence to substantiate this practice.

Pyridoxine requirement

For the first time in its 1968 recommendations, the National Research Council has made a statement concerning vitamin B_6 needs. Although exogenous vitamin B_6 is mandatory, the amount required is very small so that a deficiency is unlikely. Some of the vitamin is provided by bacterial synthesis in the intestine, but just how much is available from this source is not known. Since vitamin B_6 is involved in amino acid metabolism, the need for vitamin B_6 varies with dietary protein intake. It seems that for adults approximately 1 mg. daily is minimal. However, the Council has set a recommended allowance of 2 mg. per day for adults to assure a safety margin for variances in individual need.

Food sources of pyridoxine

Pyridoxine is fairly widespread in foods, but many sources provide only very small amounts. Good sources include yeast, wheat and corn, liver and kidney, and other meats. There are limited amounts in milk, eggs, and vegetables.

Pantothenic acid
Nature of pantothenic acid

The presence of pantothenic acid in all forms of living things, and the amount of it throughout body tissues accounts for the name given it by its discoverers. Pantothenic comes from the Greek word *pantothen* which means "in every corner" or "from all sides." It is a white crystalline compound. Pantothenic acid was isolated and synthesized by R. J. Williams between 1938 and 1940.[11]

Intestinal bacteria synthesize considerable amounts of pantothenic acid. This, together with its widespread natural occurrence, makes deficiency unlikely. Deficiency states have been studied for the most part by inducing them in animals. Manifestations of deficiency are similar to those of other B vitamins. An additional manifestation, adrenal necrosis, has been observed in the deficient animals. This condition is related to the role of pantothenic acid in steroid synthesis.

Physiologic functions of pantothenic acid

Coenzyme role in metabolism. The coenzyme role of pantothenic acid is vital to overall body metabolism. In the metabolism of carbohydrate, active acetate (p. 23) is the point at which important reactions in a number of directions can involve carbohydrates, fats, and proteins. Pantothenic acid is an essential constituent of the enzyme CoA, which forms this key compound, and as such has extensive metabolic responsibility as an activating agent. The process of *acetylation* by the enzyme CoA is one of the prime chemical reactions of the body. Activation by pantothenic acid is necessary in the following reactions.

1. Activation of acetic acid to form active acetate enables the acetic acid derived from carbohydrate, fat, and amino acids to enter the Krebs cycle.
2. Activation of fatty acids provides for lipogenesis for oxidation of fat for energy, or for production of intermediate products such as ketones.
3. Activation of amino acids allows them to combine in a number of synthesis reactions such as the formation of fat products (ketogenic reactions) or the formation of carbohydrate products (glycogenic reactions).
4. Radioactive isotope studies have

shown that active acetate is a direct precursor of cholesterol.

5. Steroid hormones formed by the adrenal and sex glands are closely related to cholesterol, and, therefore, to active acetate.
6. Activation of succinic acid from the Krebs cycle and glycine are necessary constituents of the first step in the formation of heme for hemoglobin synthesis.
7. Active acetate may combine with the sulfonamide drugs to facilitate their excretion.

Pantothenic acid requirement

The quantitative requirement for pantothenic acid in man has not been established since deficiency is not likely. Studies with adults have shown that daily excretion rates range from 2.5 to 9.5 mg. The daily intake of pantothenic acid in an average American diet of from 2,500 to 3,000 calories is about 10 to 20 mg. Therefore, a deficiency is not probable except perhaps under extreme metabolic stress.

Food sources of pantothenic acid

Sources of pantothenic acid are widespread. Yeast and metabolically active tissues such as liver and kidney are rich sources. Egg, especially the yolk, and skimmed milk contribute more. Fair additional sources include lean beef, milk, cheese, legumes, broccoli, kale, sweet potatoes, and yellow corn.

Lipoic acid

Nature of lipoic acid

The continuing study of thiamine as a coenzyme in carbohydrate metabolism revealed that this metabolic system required other coenzyme factors in addition to thiamine. One of these additional coenzymes, reported by Reed in 1951,[12] was discovered in work with lactic acid bacteria. On analysis, this new factor proved to be a fat-soluble acid, and was named *lipoic acid* (Gr. *lipos,* fat). Subsequent study of its structure in natural sources proved it to be a *sulfur*-containing fatty acid ($LipS_2$; LSS). Although lipoic acid is not a true

vitamin, because its coenzyme function is closely related to thiamine, it is classified here with the B-vitamin group.

Physiologic function of lipoic acid

Coenzyme role in metabolism. Lipoic acid is an essential coenzyme that functions with thiamine in the initial decarboxylation step of pyruvate (p. 23). Pyruvate, a key product in carbohydrate metabolism, is formed in the beginning pathway of glucose oxidation (Embden-Meyerhof glycolytic pathway, p. 22). This key reaction, oxidative decarboxylation, enables pyruvate ultimately to enter the Krebs cycle to produce energy. Lipoic acid, because it has two sulfur bonds of high energy potential (LSS), combines with the active thiamine coenzyme with two high-energy phosphate bonds (thiamine pyrophosphate, TPP) to reduce pyruvate to active acetate, thereby sending it into the final energy cycle.

A review of Chapter 7 up to this point reveals not one, but *five* B vitamins are involved, together with ionized magnesium (Mg^{++}), in this one key reaction in energy metabolism—oxidative decarboxylation (Fig. 7-1).

This same type of team reaction occurs at a later point in the Krebs cycle. It is a striking illustration of that important general concept of the interdependent relationships among the various nutrients giving life to the organism. "No man is an island," said the poet John Donne. Indeed, it seems that no nutrient is an island—even when it occurs in microorganisms!

Lipoic acid requirement

A quantitative requirement for lipoic acid in human nutrition has not been established. Only a minute amount appears to be needed for oxidative decarboxylation in microorganisms, and lipoic acid is widespread in active tissues. Further study may prove that this coenzyme is of even greater significance than is now known.

Food sources of lipoic acid

Lipoic acid is found in many biological materials, including yeast and liver.

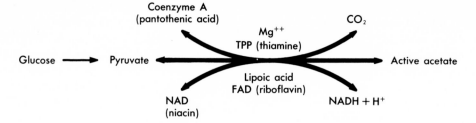

Fig. 7-1. Conversion of pyruvate to active acetate (acetyl CoA), illustrating the team action of five B vitamins and one mineral (magnesium).

Biotin

Biotin, a member of the B-complex group of vitamins, has been called a "micro-micronutrient" because such minute traces of it perform its metabolic task. Its potency is great. A natural deficiency is unknown.

Nature of biotin

Biotin is a water-soluble vitamin factor, and was first identified and synthesized from egg yolk in 1936 by German workers.[13,14] Previously, a curious syndrome characterized by eczema and paralysis had been observed in rats fed large amounts of raw egg white. This condition was counteracted by a factor in other foods such as egg yolk. The corrective factor was subsequently identified as biotin, and the vitamin has been called the "anti-egg white injury" factor. Further study showed that the injurious substance in egg white, *avidin*, was a carbohydrate-containing protein, which apparently combines with biotin in the intestine and prevents its absorption. Biotin deficiency in human beings from such a cause is unlikely, unless one had an unusual taste for large amounts of raw eggs, but it has been known to occur.

Physiologic functions of biotin

Coenzyme role in metabolism. Biotin, even in very small amounts appears to function as a coenzyme mainly in carboxylation and deamination.

Carboxylation (carbon dioxide fixation, or carbon dioxide addition). Biotin serves as a coenzyme with active acetate in reactions that transfer carbon dioxide from one compound and fix it onto another. Examples of this combination of cofactors at work are:

1. Initial steps in synthesis of some fatty acids
2. Conversion reactions involved in synthesis of some amino acids
3. Carbon dioxide fixation in forming purines

Deamination. Biotin serves as a coenzyme with deaminases in splitting off the amino group from certain amino acids (aspartic acid, serine, threonine).

Biotin requirement

The human requirement for biotin has not been established in quantitative terms, since the amount needed for metabolism is so small. This coenzyme occurs in many natural foods, and is apparently synthesized by intestinal bacteria.

Food sources of biotin

Examples of excellent food sources of biotin include egg yolk, liver, kidney, tomatoes, and yeast.

CELL GROWTH AND BLOOD-FORMING FACTORS
Folic acid (B$_9$)

The isolation and identification of folic acid are associated with laboratory studies of anemias and growth factors in animals. In 1938, Stokstad and Manning[15] described a growth factor for chicks which they named vitamin U. Later, in 1945, folic acid was obtained from liver and synthesized by Angier and Stokstad and their associates.[16] The vitamin was given the name *folic acid*

(L. *folium,* leaf) or *folicin,* because a major source of its extraction was dark green leafy vegetables such as spinach. The reduced form of folic acid has since been discovered. It is *folinic acid,* first called *citrovorum factor* (CF) because it supplies an essential growth factor of a lactobacillus, *L. citrovorum.*

Nature of folic acid

Folic acid is a conjugated substance made up of three acids, one of which is the amino acid glutamic acid. It is water-soluble and forms yellow crystals. As with many of the B vitamins, folic acid is a group of related compounds which have similar actions in the body. It is absorbed throughout the small intestine. Apparently some amount is synthesized by intestinal bacteria.

Physiologic functions of folic acid

Coenzyme for single carbon transfer. The basic metabolic role of folic acid is to act as a necessary coenzyme in the important task of transferring single carbon (C_1) units for attachment in many interconversions. A number of key compounds are formed by these conversions.

1. *Purines* are part of a group of materials called *nucleoproteins,* which are essential constituents of all living cells. Because nucleoproteins are intimately related to the nuclear substance of the cells, they are involved in cell division and in the transmission of inherited traits. It is clear, then, that any factor involved in the formation of nucleoproteins, such as folic acid, would play a vital role in cell growth and reproduction. Purines are therefore found in large quantity in tissues with very active cellular growth and reproduction, such as glandular tissue.

2. *Thymine* is an essential nucleoprotein material which forms a key part of DNA (deoxyribonucleic acid), the all-important material in the cell nucleus that is responsible for transmitting genetic characteristics (see p.

52). Folic acid participates in the reactions that synthesize thymine.

3. Folic acid performs its basic C_1-carrier role in the formation of heme, the iron-containing protein in *hemoglobin.* It is therefore not surprising that folic acid deficiencies would greatly affect blood cell formation.

Clinical applications

Anemias. Through continued study of *pernicious anemia* it has been determined that other factors, not folic acid, are necessary to prevent this deficiency disease. Although the administration of folic acid results in blood cell regeneration in patients with pernicious anemia, its effect is not permanent; nor does it control the degenerative neurological problems associated with the disease. Vitamin B_{12}, which was discovered after folic acid, proved to be the fully effective agent, both for blood regeneration and for the neurological defect. The American Medical Association and the Food and Drug Administration have therefore recommended that no more than 0.4 mg. of folic acid be included in nonprescription multivitamin preparations, as this would suffice for common needs while at the same time it would not mask the development of pernicious anemia and prevent its diagnosis. A *nutritional megaloblastic anemia* due to simple folic acid deficiency has been clearly described, however. A report of seven cases[17] indicated low serum folic acid in the face of normal serum B_{12} levels, and a rapid hematological response to treatment with folic acid alone.

Some cases of *macrocytic anemia of pregnancy,* and *megaloblastic anemia of infancy* have been attributed to dietary folic acid deficiency. In one reported instance[18,19] a mother with macrocytic anemia and her three-month-old nursing infant with megaloblastic anemia both responded to folic acid given to the mother alone.

Sprue. Folic acid has also been demonstrated to be effective in the treatment of sprue, a gastrointestinal disease characterized by intestinal lesions, malabsorption defects, diarrhea, macrocytic anemia, and general malnutrition. Response to folic acid has been excellent; both the blood-forming and gastrointestinal defects have been corrected.

Leukemia. A potent folic acid antagonist, *aminopterin,* has been used in the treatment of malignant neoplastic disease such as leukemia. An *antagonist* is a compound whose molecular configuration is almost, but not precisely, like that of a compound that is involved in a normal or abnormal metabolic process. An enzyme and its substrate combine by a lock-and-key interaction (see p. 65), in which a molecule of the substrate (the "key") fits into particular sites on a molecule of the enzyme (the "lock"). An antagonist is so similar in molecular structure to a specific enzyme that its molecule can compete with the molecule of that particular enzyme or coenzyme for the position of forming the lock. Once an antagonist molecule has got into the lock position, however, the slight dissimilarity between its configuration and that of the enzyme molecule prevents the key from fitting into it exactly, and the reaction will not proceed (see Fig. 5-3, p. 66).

Folic acid is intimately involved in the normal synthesis of substances such as nucleic acid within the cell nucleus, which are responsible for cellular growth. Aminopterin, because it is an antagonist of folic acid, is able to block the rapid development of cells that is characteristic of malignant neoplastic disease. Unfortunately, although temporary remissions have been achieved with aminopterin, the leukemic cells seem to develop a resistance to the antagonist with continued use and its effectiveness is overcome.

Folic acid requirement

Folic acid requirements have been set for the first time by the National Research Council in its 1968 recommendations. The average American diet contains about 0.6 mg. of total folic acid activity (as measured by *L. casei* assay). To cover variances in need and in the amount of available folic

acid in foods, the recommendation for adults is set at 4 mg. daily. During pregnancy 8 mg. daily is recommended; for lactation, 5 mg. Stress such as disease and growth may increase the requirement.

Food sources of folic acid

Liver, kidney, fresh green leafy vegetables, and asparagus are rich sources of folic acid. Fruit, milk, poultry and eggs are relatively poor sources.

Para-aminobenzoic acid (PABA)
Nature of para-aminobenzoic acid

Para-aminobenzoic acid is a structural unit of folic acid. Although it is not a true vitamin, PABA is sometimes listed as a separate factor because it is essential to the growth of certain microorganisms. However, its main role in human nutrition is secondary to that of folic acid; it is an essential component in folic acid formation.

Clinical application

In pharmaceutical levels, not as a vitamin, PABA has been reported to be effective in the treatment of some rickettsial diseases. The rickettsial diseases are disorders in man and animals caused by microscopically small parasites of the genus *Rickettsia.* They were named for their discoverer, H. T. Ricketts, who was a pathologist at the American University of Chicago in the late 1800's and early 1900's. These minute organisms, which resemble small rod-shaped bacterial cells, live in the intestinal tract of arthropods (mites, ticks, fleas, lice). When the arthropod bites a human being, the rickettsial parasite may be transmitted to the person's blood. It is capable of causing serious disease such as typhus or Rocky Mountain spotted fever.

The clinical use of PABA in attempts to combat rickettsial diseases is based on the concept of metabolic antagonism. PABA acts as an antagonist to a recently discovered material essential to these organisms, para-oxybenzoic acid. The rickettsial organisms are killed because PABA blocks their essential metabolite.

Cobalamin (Vitamin B_{12})

When folic acid was found to be lacking in full effectiveness as a specific agent in the control of pernicious anemia, the search continued for the remaining piece in the disease puzzle. In 1948 two groups of workers—one in America[20,21] and one in England[22]—crystallized a red compound from liver which they numbered vitamin B_{12}. In the same year, it was clearly shown that this new vitamin could control both the blood-forming defect and the neurological involvement in pernicious anemia.

Soon afterward a method of producing the vitamin through a process of fermentation with microorganisms was developed. This remains the main source of commercial supply.

Nature of vitamin B_{12}

Continued study of the vitamin's chemistry revealed its unique structure. B_{12} is the only vitamin that contains cobalt. It is a complex red crystalline compound of high molecular weight, with a single cobalt atom at its core ($C_{63}H_{90}O_{14}N_{14}PCo$). It has been given the generic name of *cobalamin*. It occurs as a protein complex in foods, so that its food sources are mostly of animal origin. The ultimate source, however, might be designated as microorganisms in the gastrointestinal tract of herbivorous animals. Such microorganisms are found in large amounts in the rumen (first stomach, containing cud) of cows. Apparently some synthesis occurs in the intestinal bacterial of man also, although the amount supplied from this source is not known.

Absorption of vitamin B_{12}

Absorption of vitamin B_{12} appears to take place in the ileum. It must be prepared for absorption, however, by two gastric secretions. It is the only human nutrient known to require exposure to stomach secretions before it can be absorbed. Hydrochloric acid in the stomach begins to split the B_{12} from its peptide bonds, and this splitting is continued by a group of enzymes in the intestine. The free B_{12} combines with *intrin-sic factor*—a mucoprotein enzyme that is secreted by glands in the fundus and cardia of the stomach (though not in the pylorus). The combined material is conveyed to the ileum. In the presence of calcium, it remains for several hours attached to ileal receptors and is then carried by the blood to various organs where it is utilized or stored.

Storage of vitamin B_{12}

Vitamin B_{12} is stored in active body tissues. Organs holding the greatest amounts are the liver, kidney, heart, muscle, pancreas, testes, brain, blood, spleen, and bone marrow. Even these amounts are very minute, but because they are so vital the body apparently holds tenaciously to its small supply. The stores are very slowly depleted. For example, a characteristic type of anemia, caused by loss of gastric secretions necessary for absorption of vitamin B_{12}, develops after surgical removal of the stomach. But this anemia does not become apparent until three to five years after the gastrectomy.

Physiologic function of vitamin B_{12}

Methylation in general metabolism. Vitamin B_{12} appears to have many metabolic interrelationships with the basic nutrients. It seems to be tied to protein metabolism, since the requirement for B_{12} increases as protein intake increases. Also, there is evidence that vitamin B_{12} is related to the utilization of fat and carbohydrate. The role of B_{12} in these various aspects of general metabolism seems to be associated with *methylation*, a process of forming or transferring key methyl groups (CH_3). In this role, B_{12} has been viewed as participating in the synthesis of nucleic acid and vital proteins in the cell. Coenzyme forms of B_{12} called *cobamides* have been found in tissue.

Hematopoiesis. A well-established role of vitamin B_{12} is its participation in the formation of red blood cells, and, therefore, in the control of pernicious anemia. It has been postulated that B_{12} has an indirect effect upon blood cell formation through activa-

TO PROBE FURTHER
B_{12} absorption defect in pernicious anemia*

Tracer studies with radioactive cobalt (Co_{60}) have given valuable additional information concerning the B_{12} absorption defect in pernicious anemia. Since a single cobalt atom is the core structure of vitamin B_{12}, radioactive cobalt may be incorporated into the B_{12} complex. The routing and activity of the vitamin can then be followed by various devices that detect the precise location of radioactivity in the body. The amount of radioactive substance necessary to label a compound so that it can be traced as it travels through the body is called a tracer dose.

A tracer dose of the vitamin is given by mouth, and the amount absorbed is determined by subtracting the quantity of radioactive substance that is excreted from the total amount of the tracer dose. After an interval, a second dose of radioactive B_{12} is given, but on this occasion a dose of intrinsic factor is given at the same time. The amount absorbed is again calculated and compared with the amount that was absorbed when no intrinsic factor is given. Without intrinsic factor, only from 10 to 20% of the vitamin is absorbed.

The amount taken up by the liver after absorption has also been checked by counting radioactivity with instruments applied to the surface of the body over the liver.

---

*Shilling, R. F.: A new test for intrinsic factor activity, J. Lab. Clin. Med. **42**:946, 1953; Glass, G. B. J., and others: Assay of intrinsic factor preparations: comparsion of hepatic uptake of radioactive Co_{60} -B_{12} with the hematopoietic response in pernicious anemia, J. Lab. Clin. Med. **46**:60, 1955.

---

tion of folic acid coenzymes. Within the developing red blood cell, activities that are dependent upon folic acid are indirectly controlled by vitamin B_{12}. Perhaps this link with folic acid explains why folic acid may alleviate pernicious anemia only temporarily, and why the folic acid must be supplemented by vitamin B_{12} if the pernicious anemia is to be corrected over a long period.

Clinical applications

Pernicious anemia. The discovery of B_{12} as a specific controlling factor in pernicious anemia was a great clinical breakthrough. Now a patient with this defect can be given from 15 to 30 μg. of B_{12} daily in intramuscular injections during a relapse, and can be maintained afterward by an injection of about 30 μg. every thirty days. This con-

trols both the hematopoietic disorder and the degenerative effects on the nervous system.

Sprue. Like folic acid, vitamin B_{12} has been effective in the treatment of the intestinal syndrome of sprue. However, it seems most effective when used in conjunction with folic acid. Therefore, its role may be indirect in that it may facilitate the action of folic acid.

Vitamin B_{12} requirement

The amount of exogenous vitamin B_{12} needed for normal human metabolism appears to be very small. Reported minimum requirements have been from 0.6 to 1.2 μg. per day, with a range upward to approximately 2.8 μg. to allow adequately for individual variance. The ordinary diet easily provides this much and more. For example, one cup of milk, one egg, and four ounces of meat provide 2.4 µg.

In its 1968 revisions, the National Research Council recommends a daily intake of 5 µg for adults. This amount allows a margin of safety to cover variance in individual need, absorption, and body stores.

Food sources of vitamin B$_{12}$

Vitamin B$_{12}$ is supplied almost entirely by animal foods. The richest sources are liver and kidney, and lean meat, milk, egg, and cheese supply additional amounts.

Natural dietary deficiency is rare. The only reported manifestations of deficiency (general nervous symptoms, sore mouth and tongue, paresthesia, amenorrhea) have come from a group of true vegetarians, "Vegands," who live in Great Britain, and from other vegetarian groups in India.

PSEUDOVITAMINS

Certain substances, although they are not true vitamins, are nonetheless related to vitamins in their activity and are usually classified with the B complex. These additional essential nutritional factors include inositol and choline. Lipoic acid and PABA, as indicated previously, may also be considered pseudovitamins.

Inositol
Nature of inositol

Inositol is a chemical compound found in meat extractives, and is closely related in composition to glucose. It was first commonly called "muscle sugar" and given the name inositol from two Greek roots: *inos,* meaning sinews; and *-ose,* the suffix for sugars. It appeared to be an intermediary between aromatic substances and glucose.

Some years ago it was observed that certain patients' clinical records indicated a relationship between inositol and diabetes. Diabetic patients excreted larger amounts of inositol in the urine than did nondiabetics. It was not until much later, during the vitamin research of the 1940's, that the substance was used in animal experiments and a true deficiency state identified. In rats, early work showed that alopecia (baldness) of a particular type was found to be directly associated with inositol deficiency. A denuded area around the eyes gave the animals a curious speckled eye appearance. Although this relationship between inositol and alopecia in animals has been proved untrue, the initial belief that inositol was an essential nutritional factor led investigators to group it with the vitamins.

Phytic acid, found in grains, is a hexaphosphate ester of inositol. Phytic acid binds calcium in the intestine to form calcium phytate. It may therefore prove to be a cause of rickets.*

Inositol is stored largely in muscle tissue, particularly heart muscle and skeletal muscle. It is also stored in brain and eye tissue and in red blood cells. Apparently some is synthesized by intestinal bacteria.

Physiologic functions of inositol

No specific role of inositol in human nutrition has been established. Some evidence of a lipotropic effect (an affinity for fat, which enables some substances to decrease fat deposits in the liver) in animals led to its use in patients with cirrhosis. However, it failed to prove effective in reducing hepatic fat in such patients.

Requirement of inositol

The requirement is unknown since the role of inositol in human nutrition is undetermined.

Food sources of inositol

Inositol is abundantly distributed in nature. It occurs in fruits, especially citrus fruits, in grains, nuts, and legumes. Animal sources include meat and milk.

---

*Notice the difference between the two words, "rickettsial" and "rickets." As explained in the section on PABA (p. 102), the term rickettsial diseases is based on the name of the discoverer of a group of microorganisms, Dr. Howard T. Ricketts. The term *rickets* is thought to have developed from an old English misspelling of the Greek word *rachitis.* The word rachitis is still a correct name for the group of diseases more familiarly known as rickets.

Table 7-4. Summary of B complex vitamins

Vitamin	Physiological functions	Clinical applications	Requirement	Food sources
Thiamine (B₁)	Coenzyme in carbohydrate metabolism: TPP—decarboxylation TDP—transketolation	Beriberi (deficiency) GI*: anorexia, gastric atony, indigestion, deficient hydrochloric acid CNS*: fatigue, apathy, neuritis, paralysis CV*: cardiac failure, peripheral vasodilation and edema of extremities	0.4 mg. per 1,000 calories	Pork, beef, liver, whole or enriched grains, legumes
Riboflavin (B₂)	Coenzyme in protein of energy metabolism (flavoproteins) FMN (flavin mononucleotide) FAD (flavin adenine dinucleotide)	Wound aggravation Cheilosis (cracks at corners of mouth) Glossitis Eye irritation; photophobia Seborrheic dermatitis	0.6 mg. per 1,000 calories	Milk, liver, enriched cereals
Niacin (nicotinic acid) (precursor—tryptophan)	Coenzyme in tissue oxidation to produce energy (ATP) NAD (nicotinamide adenine dinucleotide) NADP (nicotinamide adenine dinucleotide phosphate)	Pellagra (deficiency) Weakness, lassitude, anorexia Skin: scaly dermatitis CNS: neuritis, confusion	14-19 mg. (niacin equivalent)	Meat, peanuts, enriched grains
Pyridoxine (B₆)	Coenzyme in amino acid metabolism Decarboxylation Deamination Transamination Transsulfuration Niacin formation from tryptophan Heme formation Amino acid absorption	Anemia (hypochromic microcytic) CNS: hyperirritability, convulsions, neuritis Isoniazid is an antagonist for pyridoxine Pregnancy: anemia	0.2 mg.	Wheat, corn, meat, liver
Pantothenic acid	Coenzyme in formation of active acetate (CoA)—acetylation	Contributes to: Lipogenesis Amino acid activation Formation of cholesterol Formation of steroid hormones Formation of heme Excretion of drugs		Liver, egg, skimmed milk

Vitamin	Physiologic function	Clinical applications	Requirement	Food sources
Lipoic acid (sulfur-containing fatty acid)	Coenzyme (with thiamine) in carbohydrate metabolism to reduce pyruvate to active acetate Oxidative decarboxylation	Undetermined (see Thiamine)		Liver, yeast
Biotin	Coenzyme in decarboxylation (synthesis of fatty acids, amino acids, purines); deamination	Undetermined		Egg yolk, liver
Folic acid	Coenzyme for single carbon transfer—purines, thymine, hemoglobin Transmethylation	Blood cell regeneration in pernicious anemia but not control of its neurological problems Megaloblastic anemia Macrocytic anemia of pregnancy Sprue treatment Aminopterin is folic acid antagonist	0.4 mg. Pregnancy: 0.8 mg. Lactation: 0.5 mg.	Liver, green leafy vegetables, asparagus
PABA (part of folic acid)		Treatment of rickettsial diseases Anemias (see Folic acid)		Same as folic acid
Cobalamin (B_{12})	Coenzyme in protein synthesis Formation of nucleic acid and cell proteins—red blood cells Transmethylation	Extrinsic factor in pernicious anemia—combines with intrinsic factor of gastric secretions for absorption; forms red blood cells (with folic acid) Sprue treatment (with folic acid)	5 µg.	Liver, meats, milk, egg, cheese
Inositol	Lipotropic agent (?)	Undetermined		Citrus fruit, grains, meat, milk
Choline	Lipotropic agent Forms nerve mediator—acetylcholine	Fatty liver—hepatitis, cirrhosis (undetermined in human nutrition)		Meat, cereals, egg yolk

*GI = gastrointestinal; CNS = central nervous system; CV = cardiovascular.

Choline
Nature of choline

Choline is a second essential nutritional factor with vitaminlike activity and has long been known as a chemical compound. It was isolated from bile in 1862. It probably cannot be classified as a vitamin as the body can manufacture choline, and uses it in quantities larger than the small amounts that form part of the definition of the true vitamins (see p. 72). This biosynthesis of choline is established in animal experiments; it is not yet proved for man.

Choline deficiency states produced in animals include fatty liver and hemorrhagic kidney disease, but choline deficiency states have not been observed in man.

Choline is closely related to protein metabolism. Two essential amino acids are used by the animal body in the synthesis of choline. Serine serves as a base, and methionine donates three methyl groups to complete it. Transferring these key single carbon groups to form vital products of metabolism is the important process of *transmethylation,* in which folic acid and vitamin B_{12} are coenzyme factors. Adequate dietary protein is therefore essential to supply building materials.

Choline is also a key component of two fat-related products. *Lecithin* is a phospholipid important in the metabolism of fat by the liver. *Sphingomyelin* is a phospholipid in brain and nerve tissue.

Physiologic functions of choline

Lipotropic agent. Choline seems to be an important lipotropic agent in hepatic fat metabolism. Lipotropic means "having an affinity for fat" (Gr. *lipos,* fat; *tropein,* to turn).

To prevent the accumulation of damaging amounts of fat in the liver, fat must be changed within the liver from storage forms to vehicular or transportation forms. Any substance that has an affinity for fat, and therefore attaches itself to fat in such a way that it changes the fat from a storage form into a transportation form, is called a lipotropic substance. The way in which choline acts in relation to hepatic fat has not been fully elucidated, but it is known that choline participates in phospholipid turnover. This turnover is the conversion of fatty acids to lipoproteins, the form in which they may be carried to the fat depots. This lipotropic role of choline may assume vital importance in liver disease such as hepatitis

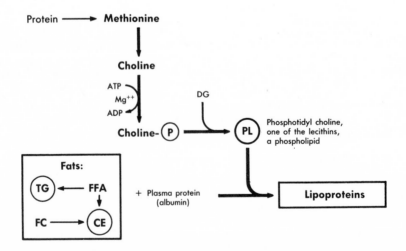

Fig. 7-2. Role of choline as a lipotropic agent in converging of fats to lipoproteins (transport form) for removal from the liver to adipose depots. Note that choline is produced from the essential amino acid methionine. (DG = diglyceride, TG = triglyceride, FFA = free fatty acid, FC = free cholesterol, CE = cholesterol ester, PL = phospholipid.)

or cirrhosis. This important lipotropic role of choline is shown in Fig. 7-2.

Acetylcholine. Choline combines with active acetate to form acetylcholine, which reportedly functions as a mediator in nerve activity. There is some evidence that acetylcholine may have an influence on cell permeability.

Choline requirement

Dietary requirement for choline has not been stated. Materials required for its synthesis are choline precursors such as methionine.

Food sources of choline

Choline is widely distributed in foods, usually in association with proteins. Good sources include egg yolk, meat, cereals, and legumes. There is very little choline in fruits and vegetables.

A summary of the B vitamins and their roles in the body is given in Table 7-4.

VITAMIN C (ASCORBIC ACID)

Discovery. The fact that discovery is often the result of keen observation and asking why is illustrated in the history of the recognition of vitamin C and its association with the hemorrhagic disease scurvy. Documents describing the typical manifestations are as ancient as an Egyptian papyrus which dates from about 1500 B.C. The Greek "father of medicine," Hippocrates, was concerned about scurvy. Crusaders of the 13th century observed the toll of the disease in their ranks. Jacques Cartier, exploring America in 1536, provided a clue to the cause of the disease when he wrote in his log that he cured his dying men "almost overnight," simply by giving them a brew made from pine needles and bark. Officers of sailing vessels contributed further bits of information. In 1600, Captain Lancaster of the East India Company stated that he kept his crew hearty merely by the addition of a mandatory "three spoonfuls of lemon juice every morning." In 1753, the English naval surgeon, James Lind, concluded that the key must lie in a food factor in citrus fruit.

The result was the official order for one ounce of lemon or lime juice daily in every British sailor's food ration, and a name that stuck—"limies."

Thus the ground was laid for the research of the Norwegian scientists, Holst and Fröhlich, who in 1907 reproduced the disease in animals by feeding them a diet deficient in foods containing *ascorbic acid* (*a*, without; L. *scorbutus*, scurvy). In 1928 Szent-Györgyi, while working on cell oxidation in adrenal tissue, isolated a substance from the adrenals, and later from cabbage and from orange juice, which he believed to be a hexuronic acid derivative; he did not test it for antiscorbutic effect. In 1932, Charles Glen King[23] and W. A. Waugh, at the University of Pittsburgh, isolated and identified a hexuronic acid in lemon juice, and demonstrated that it prevented or cured scurvy. The name ascorbic acid was given to this substance because of its antiscorbutic properties. The centuries-old scourge of scurvy had been defeated.[24]

Nature of vitamin C

Vitamin C is an odorless, white crystalline powder, that is soluble in water but not in fat. It is an unstable, easily oxidized acid, and it can be destroyed by oxygen, alkalis, and high temperatures. It also reacts with the metallic ions of iron and copper.

A comparison of the chemical structure of vitamin C with glucose (Fig. 7-3) shows some striking similarities. Glucose is the natural precursor of vitamin C. Plants make the conversion from glucose to produce the vitamin. Almost every animal species can also make ascorbic acid and, therefore, do not require a food source for this vitamin. The exceptions includes man, monkeys, guinea pigs, a rare Indian fruit bat, and the red-vented bulbul (a bird). These species lack the enzyme necessary to make the conversion from l-gulonic acid to ascorbic acid, and the material is diverted into other metabolites. Scurvy, then, in the final analysis can really be called a disease of genetic origin, an inherited metabolic error. A defect in carbohydrate metabolism results

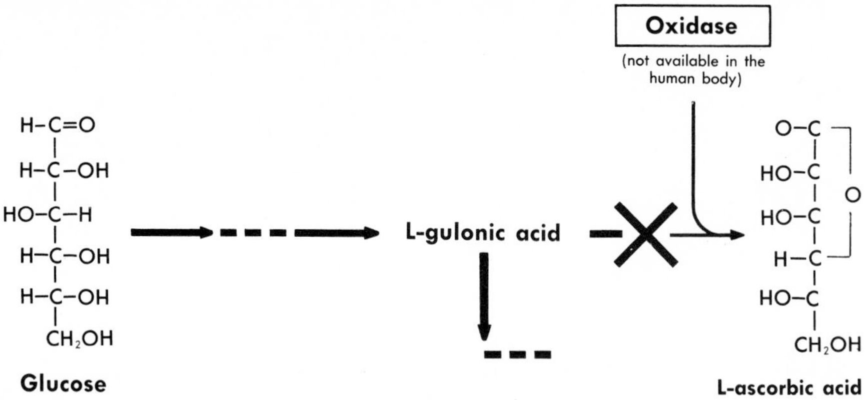

Oxidase
(not available in the human body)

H–C=O				O–C
H–C–OH				HO–C
HO–C–H				HO–C
H–C–OH				H–C
H–C–OH				HO–C
CH₂OH				CH₂OH

Glucose   → → → → L-gulonic acid → ✕ →   L-ascorbic acid

Fig. 7-3. Metabolic relation of glucose to ascorbic acid. In man, the absence of oxidase prevents this reaction, making the intake of preformed ascorbic acid in food necessary.

from the lack of an enzyme, which in turn results from the lack of a specific gene.

Metabolism of vitamin C

Vitamin C is easily absorbed from the small intestine. Absorption is hindered by a lack of hydrochloric acid or by bleeding from the gastrointestinal tract. Vitamin C is not stored in single tissue depots, but is more generally distributed throughout body tissues. The amount of vitamin C in white blood cells is used as a general indicator of the degree of body tissue saturation. A small amount (from 1.0 to 1.2 mg. per 100 ml.) circulates in blood plasma, and any excess is readily excreted. Excretion depends upon the quantity ingested and the state of tissue stores. Sufficient vitamin C for needs in early infancy is present in breast milk. Cow's milk does not contain an adequate supply for the requirements of the human infant, so formulas must be supplemented with ascorbic acid.

Physiologic functions of vitamin C

Intercellular cement substance. The well established role of vitamin C in human nutrition concerns the provision of an intercellular cementing substance which is necessary to build supportive tissue. The presence of vitamin C is required to build and maintain bone matrix, cartilage, dentine, collagen, and connective tissue. Just

how vitamin C functions in this process is not known, but when vitamin C is absent the important ground substance does not develop into collagen. When vitamin C is given, formation of cartilagenous tissue follows quickly. *Collagen* is a protein substance that exists in many tissues of the body, such as the white fibers of connective tissue. The term is derived from two Greek words: *kolla*, glue; and *gennan*, to produce. Evidently vitamin C must help provide the glue.

Vascular tissue particularly is weakened without the cementing substance of vitamin C to provide firm capillary walls. Therefore, vitamin C deficiency states are characterized by fragile, easily ruptured capillaries with consequent diffuse tissue bleeding. Clinical conditions include easy bruising, pinpoint peripheral hemorrhages (Fig. 7-4), bone and joint hemorrhages, easy bone fracture, poor wound healing, and friable bleeding gums with loosened teeth (gingivitis).

General body metabolism. Continuing research is bringing to light facts that raise interesting questions and may indicate an even broader role of vitamin C in general body metabolism. The fact that there is a greater concentration of vitamin C in the more metabolically active tissues such as adrenal, brain, kidney, liver, pancreas, thymus, and spleen, than in less active tissues,

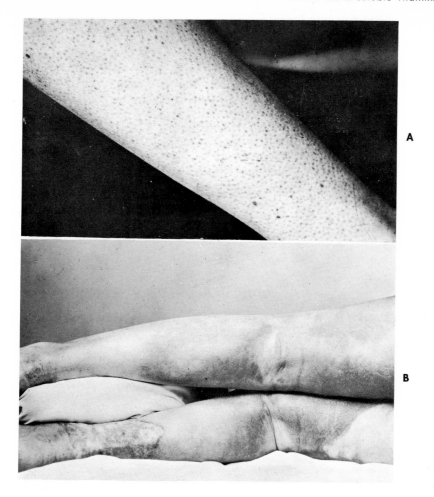

Fig. 7-4. **A,** Perifollicular hemorrhages of early scurvy. **B,** Ecchymosis of scurvy. (From Merck Report, May 1956, Merck and Co., Inc., Rahway, N. J.)

and that there is more vitamin C in a child's actively multiplying tissue than in adult tissue must mean there are vital interrelationships among vitamin C, protein, and cell metabolism processes.

In the formation of hemoglobin and maturation of red blood cells vitamin C influences the removal of iron from ferritin (the protein-iron-phosphorus complex in which iron is stored), particularly in reticuloendothelial cells of the liver, spleen, and bone marrow. Because of this reaction more iron is made available in the body fluids. Vitamin C also influences the conversion in the liver of folic acid to a related compound, folinic acid. This is the citrovorum factor

(p. 101) which has been used in the treatment of megaloblastic anemia.

A relationship of vitamin C to several amino acids may be indicated by certain observations made in the search for protein links:

1. Metabolism of phenylalanine and tyrosine is defective in premature infants who lack adequate vitamin C. In several reactions, tyrosine is not converted properly without vitamin C.

2. Vitamin C seems to participate in the synthesis of hydroxyproline from proline. This may be related to its role in collagen formation.

Large amounts of vitamin C are present in adrenal tissue; a dose of ACTH depletes the adrenal tissue of this substance.

Clinical applications

Wound healing. The significant role of vitamin C in cementing the ground substance of supportive tissue makes it an important agent in wound healing. This has evident implications for vitamin C therapy in surgery, especially where extensive tissue regeneration is involved. For example, during the acute stage, a patient who has undergone mastectomy or a severe burn may need from 1 to 2 gm. daily of vitamin C, which is ten times or more the usual daily allowance.

Fevers and infections. Infectious processes deplete tissue stores of vitamin C and necessitate additional intake. Apparently this is especially true of infection with bacteria. Optimum tissue stores of vitamin C help maintain resistance to infection.

Reaction to stress. Any body stress—injury, fracture, general illness, shock—calls on vitamin C tissue stores. This seems indicated by the large concentration of the vitamin in adrenal tissue.

Growth periods. Additional vitamin C is needed during growth periods (infancy and childhood) and during pregnancy to supply demands for fetal growth and maternal tissues.

Vitamin C requirement

Difficulties in establishing requirements for vitamin C involve questions concerning individual tissue need, and whether minimum or optimum intakes are desired. Although studies indicate that a lower intake (from 20 to 30 mg. daily) may suffice for the average adult, the National Research Council's revised allowances recommend 60 mg. daily for optimum margins to cover variances in tissue demand (Table 7-5).

In considering vitamin C requirements, it seems wise to follow such logical recommendations as those of the National Research Council to provide safety ranges for optimum need. At the same time, it seems

Table 7-5. National Research Council daily allowances for vitamin C (1968 revision)

	Age (yrs.)	Vitamin C (mg.)
Men		60
Women		55
Pregnancy		60
Lactation		60
Infants	0 to 1	35
Children	1 to 10	40
Boys	10 to 12	40
	12 to 14	45
	14 to 18	55
Girls	10 to 12	40
	12 to 14	45
	14 to 18	50

wise to avoid extravagant and wasteful excesses in the name of good health when the situation does not demand therapeutic measures.

Food sources of vitamin C

Because of the ease with which vitamin C can be oxidized, the handling, preparation, cooking, and processing of any food source should be considered in evaluating its contribution of the vitamin. Well-known sources include citrus fruit and tomatoes. Less regarded, but good additional sources, include cabbage, sweet potatoes, white potatoes, and green and yellow vegetables. Other sources are seasonal, local, or regional foods such as berries, melons, chili peppers, green peppers, guavas, pineapple, chard, kale, turnip green, broccoli, and asparagus.

A summary of vitamin C and its role in the body is given in Table 7-6.

BIOFLAVONOIDS
Nature of bioflavonoids

In the mid 1930's, Szent-Györgyi and his coworkers[25] isolated a material from citrus rind that they called *citrin*. Their initial tests of it with scorbutic guinea pigs, re-

Table 7-6. Summary of vitamin C (ascorbic acid)

Physiological functions	Clinical applications	Requirement	Food sources
Intercellular cement substance: 1. collagen formation 2. firm capillary walls General metabolism: 1. makes iron available for hemoglobin and maturation of red blood cells 2. influences conversion of folic acid to "citrovorum factor" (folinic acid)	Scurvy (deficiency) Megaloblastic anemia Wound healing; tissue formation Fevers and infections Stress reactions Growth periods	60 mg. daily (adults)	Citrus fruits Tomatoes Cabbage Potatoes Strawberries Melon Chili peppers

ported in 1936, seemed to indicate that this new substance was effective, together with ascorbic acid, in decreasing capillary permeability and in curing scurvy. Therefore, they named the substance "Permeabilitäts-Vitamin," or vitamin P.

Continued study proved that citrin was the flavanone hesperidin, which is one of a widely occurring group of natural pigments in flowers, fruits, grains, and vegetables. These substances were called *flavonoids* because of their basic yellow coloring (L., *flavus*, yellow). Some of these materials are naturally occurring yellow dyes.

Nutritional significance of bioflavonoids

The early high hopes held for the flavonoids, however, did not materialize. Szent-Györgyi reported in 1938[25] that subsequent tests did not confirm the results of his earlier experiments, and similar work in other laboratories verified his conclusions. As a result, in 1950 the Joint Committee on Biochemical Nomenclature of the American Society of the American Society of Biological Chemists and the American Institute of Nutrition recommended that the term "vitamin P" be discontinued. Since then the term "bioflavonoid" has been used instead, although the term "vitamin P" may still appear occasionally in the literature.

In the two decades since Szent Györgyi's original work, numerous workers have studied the effects of the flavonoids (*citrin* from citrus rind and *rutin* from buckwheat) on capillary fragility, infections, the common cold, hypertension, and various hemorrhagic disorders. As yet, no therapeutic value has been demonstrated. Though the bioflavonoids may possess mild pharmacological properties under certain conditions, they have no known nutritional functions, and they cannot be considered essential nutrients.

GLOSSARY

antagonist a substance that counteracts the action of another substance. The antagonist prevents the normal action because its molecular structure is so like that of the first substance that it *almost* fits into the first substance's position in a metabolic process. It gets in the way and prevents the reaction from taking place.

beriberi (Sinhalese *beri*, weakness) a disease of the peripheral nerves caused by a deficiency of thiamine (vitamin B_1). It is characterized by pain (neuritis) and paralysis of the extremities, cardiovascular changes, and edema. Beriberi is common in the Orient where diets consist largely of milled rice with little protein.

bioflavonoids compounds that are widely distributed in nature as pigments in flowers, fruits, tree barks, vegetables, and grains. In the late 1930's, a bioflavonoid material found in the peel of citrus fruit (citrin) was thought to have antiscorbutic properties (decreasing capillary fragility), and was termed "Permeabilitäts-Vitamin," or "vitamin P." However, these results were refuted by later tests, and in 1950 the term "vitamin P" was officially dropped. Since then, the term "bioflavonoid" has replaced it. Continuing attempts to determine its role, if any, in capillary fragility, treatment of the common cold, and so on, have yielded no data that support any valid clinical role for the flavonoids.

biotin a B vitamin, sometimes called the "anti-egg white injury" factor because it was discovered as the preventive substance for a curious eczema and paralysis observed in rats fed large amounts of raw egg white. In very small amounts, biotin appears to function as a coenzyme in metabolism during carboxylation and deamination reactions. It is found mainly in egg yolk.

cheilosis (Gr. *cheilos,* lips) a riboflavin deficiency condition in which the lips become swollen, crack easily, and characteristic cracks form at the corners of the mouth.

choline though not a true vitamin, choline is sometimes grouped with the B complex because it has vitamin-like activity related to animal growth. Choline has a vital role in nutrition as a lipotropic agent in the liver, by preventing fat accumulation there. Choline is synthesized from the essential amino acid, methionine, and is a key component of the phospholipid lecithin. Choline also combines with active acetate to form the important compound acetylcholine, which mediates nerve activity.

citrovorum factor folinic acid, a derivative of folic acid, which has been used in the treatment of megaloblastic anemia. Vitamin C influences this conversion of folic acid to folinic acid in the liver.

cobalamin (B$_{12}$) the B vitamin that controls pernicious anemia. B$_{12}$ is the extrinsic factor, which combines with the intrinsic factor (a mucoprotein enzyme of the gastric secretions) to be absorbed and carried to various organs for use or storage. Many of its functions seem to be linked to those of folic acid, perhaps indicating that B$_{12}$ may activate folic acid. B$_{12}$ is a distinctive B vitamin. It is a large, complex compound of high molecular weight with a single red cobalt atom at its core. Its dietary sources are almost entirely animal foods—liver, lean meat, milk, egg, cheese. The only known natural dietary deficiency has been observed in true vegetarians.

collagen (Gr. *kolla,* glue; *gennan,* to produce) the protein in connective tissue and bones which helps give support, structure, and cohesiveness to the whole body. Collagen has a gelatin-like quality.

decarboxylation removal of the carboxyl group from certain chemical compounds to form other compounds. In the important decarboxylation of pyruvate to form active acetate (and hence its entrance into the Krebs cycle to produce energy) thiamine is part of the necessary coenzyme TPP. Thiamine is a vital key that unlocks and releases energy for action of muscles and nerves.

ferritin the protein-iron-phosphorus complex in which iron is stored, particularly in reticuloendothelial cells of the liver, spleen, and bone marrow. Vitamin C helps to make iron available for use by influencing its removal from the ferritin complex.

flavin adenine dinucleotide (FAD) a riboflavin enzyme containing two high-energy phosphate bonds. It is a highly active coenzyme that operates in many reactions that affects amino acids, glucose, and fatty acids.

flavin mononucleotide (FMN) a riboflavin phosphate compound which acts as a coenzyme in the deamination of certain amino acids.

flavoproteins the enzymes of which riboflavin is an important constituent (FMN and FAD).

folic acid the B vitamin (B$_9$) discovered as a factor in the control of pernicious anemia. Folic acid only temporarily aids in regenerating the red blood cells in pernicious anemia and does not control the associated degenerative neurological problems. Vitamin B$_{12}$ has since been found to be the fully effective agent. A nutritional megaloblastic anemia due to folic acid deficiency has been clearly described, however, as well as a macrocytic anemia of pregnancy. Folic acid functions in metabolism as a coenzyme for transferring single carbon (C$_1$) units for attachment in many reactions. In this role, folic acid is a key substance in cell growth and reproduction through aiding in the formation of nucleoproteins and hemoglobin.

hematopoiesis (Gr. *haima,* blood; *poiein,* to form) the formation of blood.

inositol an intermediary compound between aromatic substances and glucose, classed in the B complex because it has vitamin-like activity. It seems to possess some lipotropic ability, but as yet its precise role in human nutrition is undetermined. Inositol occurs in grains, especially wheat, as an ester with phosphoric acid (phytin).

lactoflavin the form in which riboflavin occurs in milk.

lipoic acid a sulfur-containing fatty acid. Although it is not a true vitamin, lipoic acid is classed with the B vitamins, because its coenzyme function is closely related to thiamine.

NAD (nicotinamide adenine dinucleotide) a niacin compound with two high-energy phosphate bonds, which functions as an important coenzyme in tissue oxidation to release controlled energy.

NADP (nicotinamide adenine dinucleotide phosphate) a niacin compound with three high-energy phosphate bonds, which acts as a vital coenzyme in the "respiratory chains" of tissue oxidation within the cell; controlled energy is made available by this reaction.

niacin a B vitamin, nicotinic acid, the lack of which produces pellagra. Important niacin compounds (NAD and NADP) function as key coenzymes in glucose oxidation. Niacin's relation to pellagra was discovered by Joseph Goldberger. Meat is a major source of niacin; also peanuts, enriched grains, and legumes. The essential amino acid, tryptophan, is a precursor of niacin.

niacin equivalent a unit of measure used for the amount of tryptophan (60 mg.) which produces 1 mg. of niacin in the body. Because tryptophan is a precursor of niacin and thus an additional source, dietary requirements for niacin are usually given in terms of total niacin and niacin equivalents.

PABA (para-aminobenzoic acid) though not a true vitamin, PABA is a structural component of folic acid. Its action as an essential cell growth factor is secondary to that of folic acid. Clinically, PABA has been used to treat some rickettsial diseases. It is effective because it acts as an antagonist to a material essential to the growth of the rickettsiae.

pantothenic acid (Gr. *pantothen,* from every side) a B vitamin found widely distributed in nature and occurring throughout body tissues. Pantothenic acid is an essential constituent of the enzyme CoA, which has extensive metabolic responsibility as an activating agent of a number of compounds in many tissues.

pellagra (L. *pelle,* skin; Gr. *agra,* seizure) a deficiency disease caused by a lack of niacin in the diet and an inadequate amount of protein containing the amino acid, tryptophan, a precursor of niacin. Pellagra is characterized by skin lesions which are aggravated by exposure to sunlight, and by gastrointestinal, mucosal, neurological, and mental symptoms. Four "D's" often associated with pellagra are dermatitis, diarrhea, dementia, and death.

pernicious anemia a chronic, macrocytic anemia occurring most commonly in Caucasians after age 40. It is caused by the absence of the intrinsic factor normally present in gastric juice. The intrinsic factor is necessary for the absorption of vitamin B_{12}, the extrinsic factor required for proper formation of red blood cells. Pernicious anemia is controlled by intramuscular injections of vitamin B_{12}.

pyridoxine (vitamin B_6) In its active phosphate forms (B_6-PO_4), pyridoxine functions as an important coenzyme in many reactions in the metabolism of amino acids, and to a lesser extent in the metabolism of glucose and fatty acids. Clinically, pyridoxine deficiency produces a hypochromic, microcytic anemia and disturbances of the central nervous system. Isoniazid (INH), used to treat tuberculosis, is a pyridoxine antagonist and produces side effects of pyridoxine deficiency. Large doses of pyridoxine prevent these side effects of neuritis.

riboflavin a B vitamin (B_2); a yellow-green pigment that contains ribose. B_2 is found mainly in milk as lactoflavin, and also in leafy green vegetables and organ meats. Riboflavin forms coenzymes (FMN and FAD) important in the metabolism of amino acids, glucose, and fatty acids.

rickettsial diseases diseases in man and in animals caused by microscopic parasites of the genus *Rickettsia.* These are minute pathogenic organisms about midway in size between bacteria and viruses. They live in the intestinal tract of arthropods such as mites, ticks, fleas, and lice and are transmitted to humans by these biting insects. They cause such diseases as typhus and Rocky Mountain spotted fever.

scurvy a hemorrhagic disease caused by lack of vitamin C. Without vitamin C, the intercellular cement substance provided by this vitamin is missing; therefore, capillary walls, bone matrix, cartilage, collagen, and connective tissue are not properly formed. As a result, diffuse tissue bleeding occurs, limbs and joints are painful and swollen, bones thicken due to subperiosteal hemorrhage, ecchymoses (large irregular discolored skin areas due to tissue hemorrhages) form, bones fracture easily, wounds do not heal well, gums are swollen and bleeding, and with teeth loosen.

TDP (thiamine diphosphate) the activating coenzyme (acting with the enzyme *transketolase*) necessary for the transketolation reaction in the hexose monophosphate shunt (glucose oxidation) by which active glyceraldehyde is formed for lipogenesis (synthesis of fats).

thiamine a major B vitamin (B_1); essential for the normal metabolism of carbohydrates and fats. It acts as a coenzyme (TPP and TDP) in two key reactions: (1) decarboxylation by which active acetate is formed from pyruvate, and (2) transketolation by which intermediate products are formed between carbohydrate and fat. A deficiency of thiamine hinders energy production and proper functioning of muscles and nerves. Muscle weakness and nerve irritation result, involving the gastrointestinal tract, the cardiovascular system, and the central nervous system. Extreme continued deficiency produces beriberi, paralysis, edema, and death. Thiamine is found in whole or enriched grains, meats, and legumes.

transketolation transfer of the first 2-carbon group (CH_2OH—$\overset{O}{\overset{\|}{C}}$—) from one sugar to another in the hexose monophosphate shunt (glucose oxidation pathway). This transfer produces active glyceraldehyde, a necessary component for synthesizing fats (triglycerides). The reaction requires thiamine diphosphate (TDP) as an activating coenzyme.

References
Specific
1. Williams R. R.: Toward the conquest of beriberi, Cambridge, Massachusetts, 1961, Harvard University Press.

2. Williams, R. R.: Recollections of the "beri-beri-preventing substance," Nutr. Rev. **11:** 257, 1953.
3. Horwitt, M. K.: Thiamine, riboflavin, and niacin. In Wohl, M. G., and Goodhart, R. S., editors: Modern nutrition in health and disease, Philadelphia, 1964, Lea & Febiger, p. 385.
4. György, P.: Early experiences with riboflavin—a retrospect, Nutr. Rev. **12:**97, 1954.
5. Elvehjem, C. A.: Early experiences with niacin—a retrospect, Nutr. Rev. **11:**289, 1953.
6. Todhunter, E. N.: The story of nutrition. In Stefferud, A., editor: Food, the yearbook of agriculture, 1959, Washington, D. C., 1959, U. S. Department of Agriculture, p. 7.
7. Goldsmith, G. A.: Niacin-tryptophan relationships in man and niacin requirements, Amer. J. Clin. Nutr. **6:**479, 1958.
8. Goldsmith, G. A., and others: Efficiency of tryptophan as a niacin precursor in man, J. Nutr. **73:**172, 1961.
9. György, P.: The history of vitamin B_6, Amer. J. Clin. Nutr. **4:**313, 1956.
10. Lepkovsky, S.: Early experiences of pyridoxine—a retrospect, Nutr. Rev. **12:**257, 1954.
11. Williams, R. J.: Early experiences with pantothenic acid—a retrospect, Nutr. Rev. **12:** 65, 1954.
12. Reed, L. J., and others: Crystalline α-lipoic acid: a catalytic agent associated with pyruvate dehydrogenase, Science **114:**93, 1951.
13. Harper, H. A.: A review of physiological chemistry, ed. 10, Los Altos, California, 1965, Lange Medical Publications, p. 86.
14. Sydenstricker, V. P.: "Egg-white injury" in man and its cure with a biotin concentrate, J.A.M.A. **118:**1199, 1942.
15. Viltner, R. W.: Folic acid. In Wohl, M. G., and Goodhart, R. S., editors: Modern nutrition in health and disease, Philadelphia, 1964, Lea & Febiger, p. 410.
16. Angier, R. B., Stokstad, E. L. R., and others: The structure and synthesis of the liver L. casei factor, Science **103:**667, 1946.
17. Unglaub, W. G., and Goldsmith, G. A.: Folic acid and vitamin B_{12} in medical practice, J.A.M.A. **161:**623, 1956.
18. Streiff, R. R., and Little, A. B.: Folic acid deficiency in pregnancy, New Eng. J. Med. **276:**776, 1967.
19. Giles, C., and Shuttleworth, E.: Megaloblastic anemia of pregnancy and the puerperium, Lancet **7061:**1341, 1958.
20. Rickes, E. L., and others: Crystalline vitamin B_{12}, Science **107:**396, 1948.
21. West, R.: Activity of vitamin B_{12} in Addisonian pernicious anemia, Science **107:**398, 1948.
22. Smith, E. L.: Purification of anti-pernicious anemia factors from liver, Nature **161:**638, 1948.
23. King, C. G.: Early experiences with ascorbic acid—a retrospect, Nutr. Rev. **12:**1, 1954.
24. Lorenz, A. J.: The conquest of scurvy, J. Amer. Diet. Ass. **30:**665, 1954.
25. Pearson, W. N.: Flavonoids in human nutrition and medicine, J.A.M.A. **164:**1675, 1957.

General

Abt, A. F., and others: Vitamin C requirements of man re-examined, Amer. J. Clin. Nutr. **12:**21, 1963.
Baker, E. M., and others: Vitamin B_6 requirement for adult man, Amer. J. Clin. Nutr. **15:**59, 1964.
Best, C. H., and Taylor, N. B., editors: The physiological basis of medical practice, ed. 8, Baltimore, 1966, The Williams and Wilkins Co.
Bridgers, W. F.: Present knowledge of biotin, Nutr. Rev. **25:**65, 1967.
Bring, S. V., and Raab, F. P.: Total ascorbic acid in potatoes, J. Amer. Diet. Ass. **45:**149, 1964.
Council on Foods and Nutrition, American Medical Association: Importance of vitamin C in the diet, J.A.M.A. **160:**1470, 1956.
Coursin, D. B.: Present status of vitamin B_6 metabolism, Amer. J. Clin. Nutr. **9:**306, 1961.
Drapanas, T., and others: Role of the ileum in the absorption of vitamin B_{12} and intrinsic factor, J.A.M.A. **184:**337, 1963.
FAO/WHO of the United Nations, Requirements of vitamin A, thiamine, riboflavin, and niacin, FAO Nutr. Meet. Rep. Ser. No. 41; WHO Tech. Rep. Ser. No. 362, Rome, 1967.
Food and Nutrition Board, National Research Council, National Academy of Sciences: Recommended dietary allowances, Rev. 1968, Publ. 1694, Washington, D. C., 1968.
György, P.: Reminiscences on the discovery and significance of some of the B vitamins, J. Nutr. **91:**5, 1967.
Harper, H. A.: Review of physiological chemistry, ed. 11, Los Altos, Calif., 1967, Lange Medical Publications.
Heyssell, R. M., and others: Vitamin B_{12} turnover in man, Amer. J. Clin. Nutr. **18:**176, 1966.
Horwitt, M. K.: Nutritional requirements of man, with special reference to riboflavin, Amer. J. Clin. Nutr. **18:**458, 1966.
Hsu, J. M.: Effect of deficiencies of certain B vitamins and ascorbic acid on absorption of vitamin B_{12}, Amer. J. Clin. Nutr. **12:**170, 1963.
Joliffe, N.: Clinical nutrition, ed. 2, New York, 1962, Harper and Row.
King, C. G.: Early experiences with ascorbic acid—a retrospect, Nutr. Rev. **12:**1, 1954.
Lopez, A., and other: Influence of time and temperature on ascorbic acid stability, J. Amer. Diet. Ass. **50:**308, 1967.

Lorenz, A. J.: The conquest of scurvy, J. Amer. Diet. Ass. **30**:665, 1954.

Mangay Chung, A. S., and others: Folic acid, vitamin B_6, pantothenic acid, and vitamin B_{12} in human dietaries, Amer. J. Clin. Nutr. **9**:573, 1961.

McCollum, E. V.: The paths to the discovery of vitamins A and D, J. Nutr. **91**:11, 1967.

Noble, I.: Ascorbic acid and color of vegetables, J. Amer. Diet. Ass. **50**:304, 1967.

Pearson, W. N.: Flavonoids in human nutrition and medicine, J.A.M.A. **164**:1675, 1957.

Reviews: The citrovorum factor, Nutr. Rev. **9**:24, 1951; Nutrition and metabolic bone disease in the elderly, Nutr. Rev. **25**:71, 1967; Riboflavin deficiency and anemia in man, Nutr. Rev. **23**:197, 1965; Vitamin B_6 components in various foods, Nutr. Rev. **23**:78, 1965.

Rivers, J. M.: Ascorbic acid in metabolism of connective tissue, N. Y. State J. Med. **65**:1235, 1965.

Santini, R., and others: The distribution of folic acid active compounds in individual foods, Amer. J. Clin. Nutr. **14**:205, 1964.

Sherlock, P., and Rothschild, E. O.: Scurvy produced by a Zen macrobiotic diet, J.A.M.A. **199**:794, 1967.

Stefferud, A., editor: Food: the yearbook of agriculture, 1959, Washington, D. C., 1959, U. S. Department of Agriculture.

Streiff, R. R., and Little, A. B.: Folic acid deficiency in pregnancy, New Eng. J. Med. **276**:776, 1967.

Sydenstricker, V. P.: History of pellagra, its recognition as a disorder of nutrition and its conquest, Amer. J. Clin. Nutr. **6**:409, 1958.

Unglaub, W. B., and Goldsmith, G. A.: Folic acid and vitamin B_{12} in medical practice, J.A.M.A. **161**:623, 1956.

Viltner, R. W.: Vitamin B_6 in medical practice, J.A.M.A. **159**:1210, 1955.

Vitale, J. J.: Present knowledge of folacin, Nutr. Rev. **24**:289, 1966.

Wachstein, M.: Evidence of abnormal vitamin B_6 metabolism in pregnancy and various disease states, Amer. J. Clin. Nutr. **4**:369, 1956.

Wilson, T. H.: Intrinsic factor and B_{12} absorption —a problem in cell physiology, Nutr. Rev. **23**:33, 1965.

Wohl, M. G., and Goodhart, R. S., editors: Modern nutrition in health and disease, ed. 4, Philadelphia, 1967, Lea & Febiger.

CHAPTER 8

The minerals

One remaining group of nutrients is essential to man—the minerals. Minerals are inorganic elements widely distributed in nature, and many of them have vital roles in metabolism. Their metabolic roles are as varied as the minerals are themselves. These substances, which appear so inert in comparison with the complex, organic, vitamin compounds, fulfill an impressive variety of metabolic functions. They are builders, activators, regulators, transmitters, and controllers. For example, ionized sodium and potassium exercise all-important control over shifts in the locale of body fluids; dynamic calcium and phosphorus provide structural body framework; oxygen-hungry iron gives a core to heme in hemoglobin; brilliant red cobalt is the atom at the core of vitamin B_{12}; and iodine is a necessary constituent of thyroxine. Far from being static, inert body materials, the minerals are active participants in the overall metabolic process.

The minerals found in the human body may be grouped according to whether they are present in large amounts (major minerals), are present in small amounts and have a known function (trace minerals), or are present in small amounts but their function is not understood. There are seven minerals in each of these three groups. The major minerals contribute from 60 to 80% of all the inorganic material in the body.

Group I: Major minerals

Calcium (Ca)	Phosphorus (P)
Magnesium (Mg)	Sulfur (S)
Sodium (Na)	Chlorine (Cl)
Potassium (K)	

Group II: Trace minerals

Iron (Fe)	Cobalt (Co)
Copper (Cu)	Zinc (Zn)
Iodine (I)	Molybdenum (Mo)
Manganese (Mn)	

Group III: Function unknown

Fluorine (Fl)	Cadmium (Cd)
Aluminum (Al)	Chromium (Cr)
Boron (Br)	Vanadium (V)
Selenium (Se)	

Each of the minerals in Groups I and II is known to act dynamically in human physiology. Each mineral will be considered separately. In order to trace the metabolic activity of each mineral, the answers to the following four questions will be considered:

1. How much of each mineral normally occurs in the body and in what chemical form is it found?
2. What does each mineral do in the body, where and how does it act?
3. What is the clinical significance of each mineral, and what are some of its relationships to health and disease?
4. How much of each mineral is required in food and what are the food sources of each mineral?

MAJOR MINERALS
Calcium
Occurrence in the body

Of all the minerals in the human body, calcium is present in by far the largest amounts. It comprises about 1.5 to 2.0% of the total body weight. A person weighing 120 pounds has about two pounds of calcium in his body. Ninety-nine percent of this mineral is in skeletal tissue (bones and teeth) as deposits of the calcium salts dahllite or apatite.

The remaining 1% of the total body calcium performs highly important metabolic tasks. This 1% occurs in the plasma and other body fluids.

The approximate distribution of calcium in plasma and interstitial fluids is indicated in Fig. 8-1 (p. 122). The normal serum calcium level is about 10 mg. per 100 ml. of serum or 5 mEq. per liter. The narrow normal range of 9 to 11 mg. per 100 ml. indicates how strictly this level must be guarded and maintained. The main guardian of the serum calcium level is the parathyroid hormone, which will be discussed later in this chapter.

The 1% of total body calcium that appears in the body fluids occurs in three forms (1) nondiffusible, (2) diffusible, and (3) diffusible but a constituent of an organic complex. These three fractions are normally in equilibrium.

1. About half of the calcium in the plasma and other body fluids is bound with the plasma proteins, albumin and globulin. This is the nondiffusible fraction. Since the levels of plasma proteins vary, the size of this fraction also varies.
2. Diffusible calcium is ionized free calcium (Ca^{++}) and makes up the other half of the calcium in the plasma. It has the greatest physiologic effect of the three fractions. It exerts a profound influence on metabolism and function of bone, the nervous system, and the heart.
3. About 5% of the plasma calcium is diffusible, but occurs as part of organic complexes such as citrate and other substances.

Metabolism of calcium

The metabolism of calcium, like that of any substance, may be considered in two broad aspects: (1) as a substance in its own right, and (2) according to the physiologic function it performs in the body. It is taken for granted that calcium is important to the body, and inquiry is made into the ways in which the body maintains its calcium level. This leads directly to the concept of *homeostasis* (Gr. *homois,* unchanging; *stasis,* standing), which means to maintain a state of balance. Modern physiologists emphasize that every state of balance is maintained *dynamically* by constant interaction of the components that make up the whole. Calcium may also be looked at as a functioning component of the total body. Calcium is not only maintained by metabolic functions of the body; it contributes *to* the total metabolic interactions of the body, and therefore has its own physiologic functions.

Homeostasis. Balance mechanisms are constantly at work to maintain the level of calcium in the circulating plasma within its narrow normal range. The concepts that have emerged from physiologists' study of these mechanisms are basic to the understanding of the metabolism of many substances and are highly significant. As they apply to calcium, these homeostatic mechanisms involve four interrelated metabolic activities:

General metabolic concept	Application to calcium homeostasis
1. Maintenance of intestinal absorption-excretion balance	1. Intestinal adjustment of calcium absorption and excretion
2. Renal adjustment of excretion (the kidney threshold)	2. Renal adjustment of calcium excretion in the urine
3. Maintenance of a storage compartment	3. Maintenance of calcium stores in bone
4. Hormonal regulation	4. Parathyroid hormone control of calcium homeostasis

These mechanisms may be organized around two basic pairs of balances: (1) absorption-excretion balance and (2) deposition-mobilization balance.

Absorption-excretion balance

Absorption. From 10 to 30% of the calcium in an average diet is absorbed through the intestine. Absorption apparently takes place chiefly in the proximal intestinal tract (the duodenal area), where the pH tends to be lower than in the distal portion of the intestine because the acidity of the gastric juices has not yet been reduced. Calcium salts are relatively insoluble in a less acid medium. Vitamin D is necessary for the absorption of calcium through the intestinal mucosa. It appears to have some direct effect upon the mucosa, which increases its active transport of calcium across the membrane.

Calcium absorption is increased by greater body need, calcium ion concentration, carbohydrate and protein intake, and the acidity of the intestinal medium.

BODY NEED. During periods of greater body demand, such as growth or depletion states, more calcium is absorbed. For example, utilization of calcium is much more efficient in children of countries where the diet is low in calcium than in children studied in the United States, whose diets are high in calcium.

CALCIUM ION CONCENTRATION IN EXTRA-CELLULAR FLUID. Even a small change in the concentration of ionized calcium in the extracellular fluid is reflected in a several-fold rise in the rate of calcium absorption. The maintenance of ionized calcium concentration within this narrow range is controlled by the parathyroid hormone (see p. 121).

PROTEIN INTAKE. A greater percentage of calcium is absorbed when the diet is high in protein than when it is low in protein. This is probably due to the influence of the amino acids lysine, arginine, and serine upon intestinal pH and upon the formation of soluble calcium–amino acid complexes.

CARBOHYDRATE INTAKE. Lactose especially seems to enhance the absorption of calcium in the ileum, perhaps through action of the lactobacilli to produce lactic acid, which lowers the pH. It is interesting that the only source of lactose is milk, which also contributes the major amount of calcium—a fortunate combination.

ACIDITY. Generally, lower pH favors solubility of calcium and consequently its absorption.

Factors that decrease calcium absorption include vitamin D deficiency, excess fat, the calcium to phosphorus ratio, the presence of oxalic or phytic acids, and the alkalinity of the intestinal medium.

VITAMIN D DEFICIENCY. If there is a deficiency in vitamin D, calcium cannot be absorbed into the bloodstream.

FATS. Excess fat in the diet, or poor absorption of fats, results in an excess of free fatty acids in the intestine. The fatty acids combine with free calcium to form insoluble calcium soaps—a process called *saponification*. These insoluble soaps are excreted, with consequent loss of the incorporated calcium.

CALCIUM TO PHOSPHORUS RATIO. The optimal *dietary ratio* of calcium to phosphorus is 1 : 1 in the diet of children, and of women during the latter half of pregnancy and during lactation. Other adults require phosphorus in an amount one to one-half times the intake of calcium. If either mineral is taken in excess of this ratio, absorption of both is hindered and excretion of the lesser mineral is increased. For example, excess phosphorus in relation to the amount of calcium in the intestine will result in the formation of more calcium phosphate, which binds the calcium and makes it unavailable for absorption.

The amounts of calcium and phosphorus in the serum are normally maintained in a definite relationship called the *serum calcium to phosphorus ratio*. This ratio is the product (solubility product) of calcium × phosphorus, expressed in milligrams of each mineral per 100 ml. of serum. Since the serum level of calcium is normally 10 mg. per 100 ml., and that of phosphorus is normally 4 mg. per 100 ml. in adults (5 mg. per 100 ml. in children), the normal calcium to phosphorus ratios are $10 \times 4 = 40$ for adults and $10 \times 5 = 50$ for children. Briefly expressed, the ratios are Ca : P = 40 (adult) and Ca : P = 50 (child).

OXALIC ACID. Oxalic acid, a constituent of some foods, combines with calcium to produce calcium oxalate, a relatively insoluble compound, and thus prevents calcium absorption. The classic example is the unavailability of the calcium in spinach because of the oxalic acid also present in this leaf.

PHYTIC ACID. Phytic acid, found in the outer hulls of many cereal grains, especially wheat, also forms an insoluble compound with calcium—calcium phytate—which prevents the absorption of calcium.

ALKALINITY. Calcium is insoluble in an alkaline medium, and therefore is poorly absorbed.

Excretion. The quantity of calcium excreted tends to balance the quantity absorbed. Amounts ingested in excess of need, and amounts remaining unabsorbed, are excreted in the feces. From an average American diet, which contains ample amounts of this mineral, 70 to 90% of the total calcium ingested is so excreted. When calcium from food is plentiful, the body absorbs it less efficiently than when it is scarce.

When the calcium level in serum is high as a result of excess bone destruction or mobilization of calcium from any storage site, the excess calcium is excreted primarily in the urine. Ordinarily, however, about 99% of the ionized calcium filtered by the renal glomeruli is reabsorbed in the renal tubules.

Calcium is also excreted through the intestinal digestive secretions, especially the bile. The intestinal juices contain about 500 mg. of calcium.

Deposition-mobilization balance

The second large homeostatic balance mechanism involves bone as a major site of calcium storage—the bone compartment of the total metabolic pool of calcium.* Formerly, bone tissue was thought of as an

---

*A metabolic pool is not to be thought of as a collection of a certain substance in any one place. When a physiologist talks about a metabolic pool, he is speaking of the total available reserves of a specific substance in the storage sites of the body. There may be one, or several, such sites. He frequently speaks of the "compartments" of this pool. The substances that are ascribed to pools are not necessarily liquids. For example, one speaks of a metabolic pool of calcium, 99% of which is in the bone compartment.

inert site of static deposit of calcium for storage. It has been demonstrated that this is not true. Bone is a dynamic tissue, characterized by a constant turnover of calcium; balance results from an ongoing process of accretion and resorption. Circulating ionized calcium is constantly being deposited in bone, while the calcium stored in bone is perpetually mobilized and withdrawn. The calcium in the bone compartment appears to be divided into two portions. This division is not a spatial separation; rather, there are two forms of calcium in bone which participates in this dynamic exchange at two different levels of activity. There is a more actively exchangeable reservoir of about 4 gm. in equilibrium with the free plasma ionized calcium, and there is a much larger, more stable calcium bone reserve which exchanges slowly. Parathyroid hormone and vitamin D influence this exchange of calcium.

Parathyroid hormone (PH). The parathyroid gland is particularly sensitive to changes in the circulating plasma level of free ionized calcium. When this level drops, the parathyroid releases its hormone, which acts in three ways to restore the normal calcium level: (1) it stimulates the intestinal mucosa to increase the absorption of calcium; (2) it mobilizes calcium rapidly from the bone compartment; and (3) it causes renal excretion of phosphate. These combined activities restore calcium and phosphorus to their correctly balanced ratio in the blood. Tetany* results from a decrease in the free ionized serum calcium; the action of parathyroid hormone prevents tetany (see also Clinical Application, p. 123).

VITAMIN D. Vitamin D seems to play a role in the deposition of calcium in the bone matrix. Studies have shown that vitamin D has a direct effect upon the calcification of bone tissue; however, its effect on calcium absorption from the intestine is much

---

*Do not confuse *tetany* with *tetanus*. Although they come from the same Greek word *teinein* meaning "to stretch," they refer to very different syndromes. *Tetany* is due to abnormal calcium metabolism; *tetanus* is an acute infectious disease.

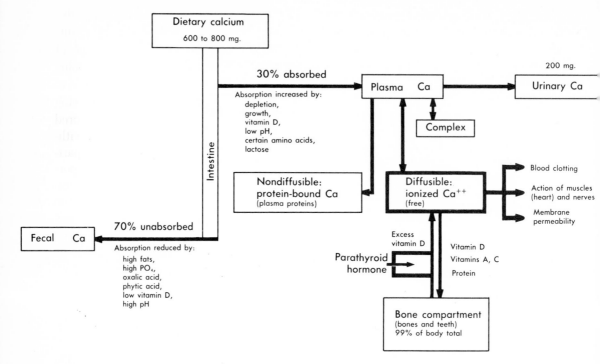

Fig. 8-1. Calcium metabolism. Note the relative distribution of calcium in the body.

greater. The effect of parathyroid hormone is greater at the point of bone calcium mobilization. The cooperative action of these two factors is a good example of synergistic* behavior of metabolic controls.

The overall relationship of the various factors involved in calcium absorption and metabolism may be visualized in Fig. 8-1.

Physiologic function of calcium

Bone and teeth formation. The physiologic function of 99% of the calcium in the body is to build and maintain skeletal tissue. This intricate and delicately balanced process is carried on by two types of cells. *Osteoblasts* continually form new bone matrix, in which calcium phosphate is deposited, and bone crystals develop. *Osteoclasts* continually balance this activity by absorbing bone tissue; they engulf

---

*Synergism is the cooperative action of two or more factors, which in acting together produce a total effect greater than the sum of their separate effects. Many biological and physiological interactions provide examples of synergism.

(phagocytize) and digest minute bone crystals.

Calcium phosphate deposits are important to *tooth formation*. As the teeth develop, tooth-forming organs (ameloblasts) deposit calcium and other constituents; then mineral exchange continues, as in bone. This exchange occurs mainly in the dentine and cementum; very little occurs in the enamel.

Blood clotting. The remaining 1% of the body's calcium performs several vital physiologic functions. In blood clotting, calcium ions enhance bonding between fibrin molecules and give stability to the fibrin threads required for conversion of prothrombin to thrombin (see Fig. 6-3, p. 83).

Muscle contraction and relaxation. Ionized serum calcium plays an important role in the initiation of muscle contraction. Each muscle fiber contains hundreds of small contractile units called *myofibrils*, which are composed of the muscle protein filaments, *myosin* and *actin*. Alongside each myofibril is a fine system of tubes—the *tubu-*

lar reticulum. Calcium is firmly bound to this reticulum. When the signal for contraction comes, the calcium is suddenly released, ionized, and mobilized. The free calcium ions activate the chemical reaction between myosin and actin filaments that releases a large amount of energy from ATP and brings about contraction. The calcium ions are then immediately bound back on the reticulum, causing relaxation. Other elements, such as magnesium and potassium, are also involved in this process. The catalyzing action of calcium ions upon the muscle protein filaments myosin and actin, which allows the sliding contraction between them to occur, is particularly vital in the contraction-relaxation cycle of the *heart muscle.*

Nerve transmission. Calcium is required for normal transmission of nerve impulses. Calcium ions in the extracellular fluid at the neuromuscular junction apparently cause the excitatory transmitting substance *acetylcholine* (see p. 109) to rupture through the separating membranes at the tips of the many nerve branches and excite the muscle fiber.

Cell wall permeability. Ionized calcium controls the passage of fluid through cell walls by affecting cell wall permeability. This is apparently the result of calcium's influence upon the integrity of the intercellular cement substance.

Enzyme activation. Calcium ions are important activators of certain enzymes, such as adenosine triphosphatase (ATPase), in the energy release for muscle contraction. They play a similar role with other enzymes, including lipase and some members of the protein-splitting enzyme system.

Clinical application

Tetany. A decrease in ionized serum calcium causes tetany, a state marked by severe, intermittent spastic contractions of the muscle and by muscular pain. It is manifested by a characteristic carpopedal spasm of the muscles in the upper extremity which causes flexion of wrist and thumb with extension of the fingers *(Trousseau's sign).*

Tetany-like responses may be caused by an increase in serum phosphorus fraction in the calcium to phosphorus ratio (p. 120), which causes a decrease in calcium level to maintain the solubility product of calcium × phosphorus. For example, a so-called milk tetany has been reported in newborn infants fed undiluted cow's milk. The ratio of phosphorus to calcium in cow's milk is greater than in human milk, and the kidneys of these infants could not clear this phosphate load. Phosphorus therefore accumulated in the serum. The rise in serum phosphorus caused a compensatory decrease in serum calcium; this in turn caused typical tetanic muscular spasms.

Occasional leg cramps of pregnancy have been attributed by some observers to a similar rise in phosphorus intake, if the gravid woman drinks an excess of the recommended amount of milk.

Rickets. As indicated in the discussion of vitamin D's relation to calcium and phosphorus in producing rickets (p. 78), when adequate calcium and phosphorus are not absorbed, proper bone formation cannot take place.

Renal calculi. The majority of renal stones are composed of calcium. A predisposing factor to the formation of renal calculi may be an increase in the amount of calcium that must be excreted in the urine as calcium is mobilized or withdrawn from the bone compartment. Immobilization of the body is one state which causes such resorption of calcium from bone stores into the blood. This has definite clinical implications. When a full body cast or some other orthopedic device immobilizes the body for a long period, dietary calcium intake should be adequate but should not exceed the usual daily allowance; if renal stones have already occurred, the amount of calcium in the diet should be somewhat reduced.

Hyperparathyroidism and hypoparathyroidism. Because calcium and phosphorus metabolism are so directly controlled by parathyroid hormone, conditions of the parathyroid gland that increase or decrease the secretion of its hormone will immediately be reflected in abnormal metabolism of these two minerals.

Dietary requirements of calcium

The National Research Council recommended allowances (1968 revision) for calcium are 800 mg. daily for men or women, increased to 1.3 gm. during pregnancy and lactation. Infants younger than one year should have 400 to 600 mg., and children should have from 0.7 to 1.4 gm. daily.

Food sources of calcium

Dairy products supply the bulk of dietary calcium. One quart of milk contains about 1 gm. of calcium, and cheese contains a comparable amount. Secondary sources contribute much smaller quantities. These include egg yolk, green leafy vegetables, legumes, nuts, and whole grains. If the average American diet contained no dairy products, one would be hard pressed to account for more than about 300 mg. of calcium.

Phosphorus

Phosphorus is closely associated with calcium in human nutrition. Both minerals occur in the same major food source—milk. Both function in the major task of bone building. Both are related to vitamin D in the absorption process. Both are regulated metabolically by parathyroid hormone. The two exist in the blood serum in definite ratio to one another.

Although phosphorus has been called the "metabolic twin" of calcium, it has some unique characteristics and functions. As the role of phosphorus in metabolism is considered here and the expected similarities to calcium are found, characteristics that distinguish it from calcium should also be looked for.

Occurrence in the body

Phosphorus comprises from 0.8 to 1.1% of the total body weight. The body of a person weighing 120 pounds would contain about 1.2 pounds of phosphorus. From 80 to 90% of this phosphorus is in the skeleton (including the teeth) compounded with calcium. The remaining 20% is, unlike calcium, uniquely distributed in every living cell, where it participates as an essential component in interrelationships with proteins, lipids, and carbohydrates to produce energy, to build and repair tissues, and to act as a buffer.

The serum phosphorus level normally ranges from 3 to 4.5 mg. per 100 ml. in adults and is somewhat higher, 4 to 7 mg. per 100 ml., in children. The higher range during growth years is a significant clue to its role in cell metabolism.

The total inorganic serum phosphorus exists in the form of the two balancing buffer anions: $HPO_4^=$ (phosphate), 2.1 mEq. per liter; and $H_2PO_4^-$ (phosphoric acid), 0.26 mEq. per liter. Other phosphorus in the body occurs as a constituent of organic compounds.

Absorption-excretion

The absorption of phosphorus is closely related to that of calcium. Equal amounts of the two minerals in the diet is an optimal ratio; excess of either causes increased fecal excretion of the other. Apparently phosphorus is more efficiently absorbed than calcium, as only 30% of the ingested phosphorus (bound to calcium) is excreted in the feces and about 70% is absorbed, compared with only 10 to 30% of dietary calcium that is absorbed.

The absorption of phosphorus is apparently secondary to that of calcium. Vitamin D enhances, but is not required for, the absorption of phosphorus. The direct action of vitamin D is on the absorption of calcium, and the absorption of phosphorus follows.

Since phosphorus occurs in food as a phosphate compound, mainly with calcium, the first step is the splitting off of phosphorus for absorption as the free mineral. Factors similar to those that influence calcium absorption also affect phosphorus absorption. For example, an excess of calcium or other material that may bind phosphorus in insoluble salts (such as aluminum or iron) will inhibit its absorption.

The kidneys provide the main excretory mechanism for regulation of the serum phosphorus level. The *renal threshold for phosphate* means that the amount of phosphate excreted by the kidney is relative to the serum phosphorus level. If the serum phosphorus level falls, the renal tubules return more phosphorus to the blood; if the serum phosphorus level rises, the renal tubules excrete more. When the diet lacks sufficient phosphorus, the renal tubules conserve phosphorus by returning it to the blood. By this means, normal serum phosphorus levels are maintained through the work of the kidney. The amount of phosphorus excreted in the urine of a person ingesting an average diet is from 0.6 to 1.0 gm. every twenty-four hours.

Metabolism of phosphate

Role of parathyroid hormone. The homeostatic mechanism by which the kidneys maintain the serum phosphorus level is controlled by the parathyroid hormone. This action is usually interdependent with calcium balance. When the serum phosphate level rises, the parathyroid hormone blocks renal tubular resorption of phosphorus, so that more phosphorus is excreted in the urine. The serum phosphorus level and the calcium to phosphorus ratio are returned to normal.

The balance concept is also applicable to the equilibrium existing between the phosphorus in the bone compartment and in the circulating serum. These various balance relationships may be visualized in Fig. 8-2.

Physiologic functions of phosphorus

Eighty percent of body phosphorus contributes to mineralization of bones and teeth. As a component of calcium phosphate, it is constantly being deposited and reabsorbed in the dynamic process of bone formation.

Far out of proportion to the relatively small amount of the remainder, 20% of body phosphorus is intimately involved in overall human metabolism. Its vital role is indicated by its presence in every living cell. The various metabolic functions of phosphorus illustrate again the over-arching

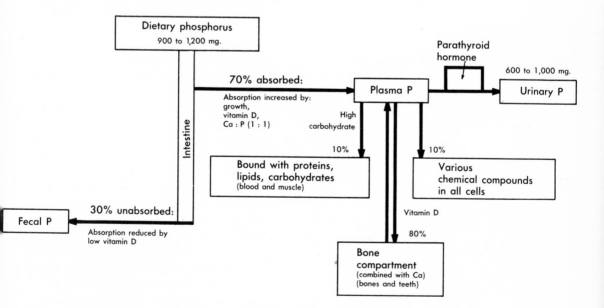

Fig. 8-2. Relative distribution and interchange of phosphorus in the body.

concept of interrelatedness of the nutrients.

Absorption of glucose and glycerol. By the process of *phosphorylation*, phosphorus combines with glucose and glycerol (from fat) to promote the absorption of these substances from the intestine. Phosphorylation also promotes the renal tubular reabsorption of glucose, by which this sugar is conserved and returned to the blood.

Transport of fatty acids. By combination with fat as phospholipids, phosphorus helps to provide a vehicular form for fat.

Energy metabolism. Phosphorus is an essential part of such key cellular nucleoprotein substances as DNA and phosphatides, which also participate in the formation of numerous enzymes in the pathways for glucose oxidation and final energy production. These nucleoprotein substances are a key power source in the high-energy phosphate bonds of such compounds as ATP.

Buffer system. The phosphate buffer system of phosphoric acid and phosphate contributes additional control of acidotic and alkalotic states in the blood.

Clinical application

Situations involving physiologic changes in serum phosphorus level include growth and recovery from diabetic acidosis.

Growth. Growing children usually have high serum phosphate levels, probably resulting from high levels of growth hormone.

State of recovery from diabetic acidosis. Active carbohydrate absorption and metabolism use much phosphorus, depositing it with glycogen, thus causing temporary hypophosphatemia.

Situations involving pathologic changes in serum phosphorus level include hypophosphatemia and hyperphosphatemia.

Hypophosphatemia. Intestinal diseases such as sprue and celiac disease in which phosphorus absorption is hindered, or bone diseases such as rickets or osteomalacia in which the calcium to phosphorus balance is upset, are characterized by low serum phosphorus levels. The serum phosphorus level is also low in primary hyperparathyroidism,

because the excess quantity of parathyroid hormone secreted results in excessive renal tubular excretion of phosphorus. Symptoms of hypophosphatemia include muscle weakness, because the muscle cells are deprived of phosphorus essential for energy metabolism.

Hyperphosphatemia. Renal insufficiency or hypoparathyroidism causes excess accumulation of serum phosphate. As a result, the calcium side of the calcium to phosphorus ratio is low, which causes tetany.

Dietary requirement of phosphorus

During growth, pregnancy, and lactation, the ratio of phosphorus to calcium in the diet is ideally 1 : 1. In ordinary adult life, the intake of phosphorus is about one to one-half times that of calcium. In general, since these two minerals are found in the same food sources, if calcium needs are met adequate phosphorus will be assured.

The National Research Council (1968 revision) recommends a phosphorus allowance equal to that for calcium for all ages except the young infant. For the infant the proportion of phosphorus is lower than calcium.

Food sources of phosphorus

Milk and milk products are the most significant sources of phosphorus, as they are for calcium. Because the role of phosphorus in cell metabolism assures the presence of phosphorus in muscle cells, lean meats are also a good source.

Magnesium
Occurrence in the body

Magnesium, an essential nutrient, occurs in the body in appreciable quantities. There are about 25 gm. in an adult, and 70% of this is combined with calcium and phosphorus in the bone salts complex. The remaining 30% is distributed in various soft tissues and body fluids.

Plasma magnesium values range from 1.4 to 2.5 mg. per 100 ml. Unlike calcium, magnesium occurs predominantly in the red blood cells and there is relatively little in the serum. About 80% of the blood magnesium is ionized and diffusible. The remainder is probably bound with serum protein, as is the nondiffusible calcium. Muscle tissue contains more magnesium than calcium; blood contains more calcium than magnesium.

Absorption-excretion

On an average diet about 45% of ingested magnesium is absorbed, and 55% is excreted in the feces. Absorption apparently occurs in the upper small intestine; none appears to be absorbed in the colon. Urinary excretion is relatively low, as the kidney conserves magnesium efficiently. Aldosterone increases the renal clearance of magnesium, as it does that of potassium.

Factors that inhibit calcium absorption also hinder magnesium absorption. These include the presence of excess fat, phosphate, calcium, or alkalis. As with calcium, parathyroid hormone also increases magnesium absorption from the intestine. Vitamin D, however, apparently does not affect magnesium absorption.

Metabolic functions of magnesium

Ionized magnesium is essential to cellular metabolism of both carbohydrate and protein because it is a significant cation of the intracellular fluid. The following are the metabolic functions of magnesium.

1. In carbohydrate metabolism ionized magnesium (Mg^{++}) serves as an activator of many enzymes in the reactions of the initial Embden-Meyerhof glycolytic pathway for glucose oxidation (oxidative phosphorylation).
2. In protein metabolism ionized magnesium is a coenzyme in protein synthesis in the cell ribosomes.
3. Magnesium is a constituent of molecules formed in the processes of growth and maintenance of tissues.
4. Magnesium is related to cortisone in the regulation of the blood phosphorus level.
5. Decreased ionized magnesium con-

centration causes vasodilatation and inhibits smooth muscle action. Normally ionized magnesium, like potassium, is concentrated in the intracellular fluid. Any changes in this concentration produce neuromuscular irritability. A tetany-like syndrome has been observed in animals fed a low magnesium diet.

Clinical application

Gastrointestinal disorders. In prolonged diarrhea or vomiting, or in diseases characterized by intestinal malabsorption, excessive amounts of magnesium may be lost. Fundamental to the treatment of such states is the restoration of the lost water by mouth or intravenously. This is called rehydration. Rehydration must be accompanied by adequate magnesium replacement; if it is not, the resulting low serum magnesium level may give rise to general neuromuscular irritability, manifested by tremor, spasm, and increased startle response to sound and touch.

Alcoholism. A tetany-like syndrome has been studied in persons with chronic alcoholism in whom magnesium deficiency has developed.

Serum cholesterol levels. Some recent study indicates a possible correlation of the serum magnesium level with the serum cholesterol level. As yet, this relationship is unclear.

Dietary requirement of magnesium

A natural magnesium deficiency in man is unlikely. Balance studies indicate that the average adult needs from 250 to 300 mg. per day. The National Research Council (1968 revision) has set adult recommendations at 350 mg. daily for men and 300 mg. for women. Any deficiency would probably be long-term and cumulative, and may have a role in chronic cardiovascular, neuromuscular, and renal diseases.

Food sources of magnesium

Magnesium is relatively widespread in nature. Its main sources include nuts, soybeans, cocoa, seafood, whole grains, dried beans, and peas.

Sodium

Occurrence in the body

Sodium, crucially important to many metabolic activities, is one of the more plentiful of the minerals in the body. Of the 4 oz. or so in the body of a person weighing 154 lbs., about one-third is present in the skeleton as inorganic bound material. The remaining two-thirds are in the extracellular fluids. This extracellular ionized sodium (Na^+) is largely distributed in plasma, and in nerve and muscle tissue. Normal blood serum values range from 136 to 145 mEq. per liter or from 310 to 340 mg. per 100 ml.

Absorption-excretion

Sodium is readily absorbed from the intestine, and normally only about 5% of all excreted sodium is lost in the feces. Larger amounts are passed by this route in such abnormal states as diarrhea. Ninety-five percent of the sodium that leaves the body is excreted in the urine. The renal control of sodium excretion is regulated largely by hormones of the adrenal gland, especially the powerful mineralocorticoid *aldosterone*. The aldosterone mechanism for sodium conservation is one of the major homeostatic controls of body sodium, and hence of body water.

Metabolic function of sodium

Fluid balance. Ionized sodium is the major cation of the extracellular fluid. Variations in the concentration of ionized sodium largely determine the shift of water by osmosis from one body area to another. These shifts of water from one part of the body to another are the means whereby substances in solution in the body water can circulate between the cells and the fluid that surround them. Such shifts also protect the body against large fluid losses. The role of sodium in the maintenance of fluid balance is discussed in Chapter 9 on Water and Electrolytes.

Acid-base balance. Through its associa-

tion with chloride and bicarbonate ions, ionized sodium is an important factor in the regulation of the acid-base balance in the body.

Cell permeability. Cell permeability is affected by the sodium pump associated with glucose metabolism and cellular exchange of ionized sodium (see p. 18). By an active mode of transport of this type, sodium appears to be essential to the passage of such materials through cell walls.

Normal muscle irritability. Sodium ions play a large part in transmitting electro-chemical impulses along nerve and muscle membranes and, therefore, maintain normal muscle irritability or excitability. Potassium and sodium ions balance the response of nerves to stimulation, the travel of nerve impulses to muscles, and the resulting contraction of the muscle fibers.

Clinical application

Fluid-electrolyte and acid-base balance. Many clinical applications of these balance mechanisms, which are essential to health and to life itself, will be discussed in the next chapter. Suffice it to say here that perhaps no other physiologic activity is so broad in scope or so profound in its effect on body systems (especially the cardiovascular, renal, and gastrointestinal systems) as the mechanisms by which the fluid-electrolyte and acid-base balances are maintained.

Muscle action. Abnormal serum levels of sodium may adversely affect the function of muscles, for example, the heart muscle. The consequences of serum sodium abnormalities on muscular function are, however, less profound than those of serum potassium abnormalities.

Dietary requirement of sodium

The specific dietary requirement for sodium is not stated. Apparently the body can function on a rather wide range of exogenous sodium through the operation of mechanisms designed to conserve or excrete this mineral. The amount of sodium in the average American diet (4 gm. of sodium, in the average 10 gm. of table salt consumed daily) is about ten times the quantity that the body requires for the maintenance of an adequate balance. An intake of about 5 gm. of table salt, or 2 gm. sodium, (NaCl) has been recommended for adults. For those with a family history of hypertension, the recommended quantity in food is even less—from 1 to 2 gm. salt daily.

Food sources of sodium

Common salt, used in cooking and for seasoning, is the main dietary source of sodium. Other food sources include milk, meat, egg, and certain vegetables such as carrots, beets, spinach and other leafy greens, celery, artichokes, and asparagus.

Potassium
Occurrence in the body

Like sodium, potassium is a vital mineral element associated with physiologic fluid balance. This role will be discussed in greater detail in the next chapter.

Potassium is about twice as plentiful as sodium in the body. The body of an average man weighing 154 pounds contains about 9 oz. (4,000 mEq.) of potassium. By far the larger portion is found inside the cells; potassium is the major cation (K^+) of the intracellular fluid (see p. 160). However, the relatively small amount in extracellular fluid has a significant effect on muscle activity, especially heart muscle. The normal blood serum values for potassium range from 3.5 to 5.0 mEq. per liter, or 14 to 20 mg. per 100 ml. In comparison, the cell concentration is about 115 mEq. per liter of cell water.

Absorption-excretion

Potassium ingested in food is easily absorbed from the small intestine. A considerable amount of potassium is also secreted into the intestine as a component of the digestive juices, but is later reabsorbed during the continuous cycle of gastrointestinal circulation of water and electrolytes. Very little potassium is lost in the feces.

Urinary excretion is the principal route of loss. Since maintenance of serum potassium within the narrow normal range is vital to heart muscle action and is an indicator of electrolyte balance, the kidney guards potassium carefully. The ability of the renal glomeruli and tubules to filter, reabsorb, secrete, and excrete potassium is so remarkable that the well-functioning kidney can maintain normal serum levels even in the face of relatively large injections of potassium. Changes in acid-base balance are reflected in compensatory changes in the amount of potassium excreted in the urine.

Hormones of the adrenal cortex, especially aldosterone, also influence potassium excretion. As a part of the aldosterone mechanism that conserves sodium, ionized potassium is excreted instead of ionized sodium, the two ions being exchanged for one another in the renal tubule (see p. 169).

Metabolic functions of potassium

Fluid-electrolyte balance. As the major cation of the intracellular fluid, ionized potassium functions in balance with the extracellular ionized sodium to maintain the normal osmotic pressures and water balance that maintain the integrity of the cellular fluid.

Acid-base balance. Ionized potassium also exerts an influence upon acid-base balance through its operation with ionized sodium and ionized hydrogen.

Muscle activity. Ionized potassium plays a significant role in the activity of striated (skeletal and cardiac) muscle. As indicated, ionized potassium functions with ionized sodium and calcium to regulate neuromuscular excitability and stimulation, transmission of electrochemical impulses, and contraction of muscle fibers. This effect of ionized potassium is particularly notable in the action of heart muscle. Even small variations in serum potassium concentration are reflected in electrocardiographic changes. *Excess* serum potassium (hyperkalemia), a common and life-threatening complication of renal failure, severe dehydration, or shock, causes the heart to dilate and become flaccid, which slows its rate. Eventually, transmission of the electrochemical impulse that mediates the flow of the beat through the heart may be blocked between the atrium and the ventricles (atrioventricular block). An increase in serum potassium concentration to only two to three times the normal level may weaken cardiac contractions sufficiently to cause death.

Low serum potassium concentrations (hypokalemia) may cause muscle irritability and paralysis. The heart may develop gallop rhythm, tachycardia, and finally cardiac arrest.

Carbohydrate metabolism. When blood glucose is converted to glycogen for storage, potassium is stored with the glycogen. It has been calculated that for every 1 gm. of glycogen stored, 0.36 mM. of potassium is also retained. When a patient in diabetic acidosis is treated by the administration of insulin and glucose, glycogen is rapidly produced and stored. The potassium that is to be stored with the glycogen is quickly withdrawn from the serum. The resulting hypokalemia may be fatal. For this reason, the treatment of diabetic acidosis usually includes replacement of serum potassium.

Protein synthesis. Potassium is required for the storage of nitrogen as muscle protein. When muscle tissue is broken down, potassium is lost together with the nitrogen in muscle protein. Replacement therapy—the administration of amino acids to provide for resynthesis of muscle protein—should therefore also include potassium to ensure nitrogen retention.

Clinical application

As with sodium, variances in potassium levels have far-reaching clinical implications in fluid-electrolyte and acid-base balances. These are discussed in greater detail in Chapter 9. Other clinical situations related to potassium may be grouped under *elevated* or *decreased* serum potassium states.

Hyperkalemia (elevated serum potassium). Any condition that results in renal failure precludes the normal adjustment and clearance of ionized potassium. Serum potassium then rises to toxic levels. The too-rapid intravenous administration of potassium may also cause hyperkalemia. Hyperkalemia from either cause results in characteristic weakening of heart action, mental confusion, poor respiration (caused by weakening of the respiratory muscles), and numbness of extremities.

Hypokalemia (low serum potassium). Hypokalemia of dangerous degrees may be caused by a prolonged wasting disease with tissue destruction and malnutrition, or by prolonged gastrointestinal loss of potassium as in diarrhea, vomiting, or gastric suction. The continuous use of certain diuretic drugs, such as chlorothiazide (Diuril) or acetazolamide (Diamox), increases ionized potassium excretion, and may leave the serum potassium level abnormally low. It is therefore recommended that the administration of such drugs be interrupted at intervals, and that patients taking such agents receive potassium for replacement.

Heart failure and subsequent depletion of ionized potassium in heart muscle makes the myocardial tissue more sensitive to digitalis toxicity and arrhythmia (irregular contractions). To prevent these complications of cardiac failure, potassium should be given, especially when potassium-depleting diuretics are also used.

Diabetic acidosis, as indicated, requires replacement of potassium when insulin and glucose are given, to offset the rapid withdrawal of potassium for incorporation with glycogen storage.

Dietary requirement of potassium

No dietary requirement is specified for potassium. The usual diet contains from 2 to 4 gm. daily, which seems ample for common need. No deficiency is likely, except in the clinical situations described in the preceding sections.

Food sources of potassium

Potassium is widely distributed in natural foods. Legumes, whole grains, certain fruits, leafy vegetables, and meats supply considerable amounts. Many other foods are supplementary sources.

Chlorine
Occurrence in the body

Chlorine occurs in the body as the chloride ion (Cl^-). It accounts for about 3% of the body's total mineral content. Ionized chlorine is the major anion of the extracellular fluid. The cerebrospinal fluid has the highest concentration of chloride (124 mEq. per liter, or 440 mg. per 100 ml.). The normal range for plasma level is from 95 to 105 mEq. per liter or 340 to 370 mg. per 100 ml. A relatively large amount of ionized chlorine is found in the gastrointestinal secretions, especially as a component of gastric hydrochloric acid.

Absorption-excretion

Chloride is almost completely absorbed in the intestine with only a functional fecal loss. Excretion is accomplished chiefly through the kidney. Like sodium, chloride is a threshold substance. It is largely conserved by reabsorption in the renal tubules, where it is returned to the circulating plasma. This reabsorption is enhanced by the adrenal hormone aldosterone. The reabsorption of chlorine is secondary to aldosterone's control over the renal reabsorption of sodium.

Since ionized chlorine is a major component of the gastrointestinal circulation, relatively large losses may occur in prolonged vomiting or diarrhea.

Metabolic functions of chlorine

Fluid-electrolyte balance. Together with ionized sodium, ionized chlorine in the extracellular fluid helps to maintain water balance and to regulate osmotic pressure.

Acid-base balance. By participating in the chloride-bicarbonate shift mechanism, which operates between the plasma and the red blood cells, ionized chlorine plays a special role in maintaining a constant pH in the blood. In response to changes in carbon dioxide tension in erythrocytes, ionized chlorine goes into the red blood cell in exchange for HCO_3 (the chloride-bicarbon-

ate shift). This provides constant bicarbonate buffering for the rapidly formed carbonic acid (H_2CO_3) from water and CO_3. These reactions are then reversed in the lungs as carbon dioxide is expired.

Gastric acidity. Chloride, secreted by the mucosa of the stomach as gastric hydrochloric acid, provides the necessary acid medium for digestion in the stomach, and for the activation of enzymes (such as conversion of the pepsinogen to active pepsin for initial protein splitting).

Clinical application

Gastrointestinal disorders. As is true of sodium and potassium, large amounts of chlorine may be lost during continued vomiting, diarrhea, or tube drainage, which would contribute the complications of hypochloremic alkalosis to the clinical state produced by dehydration. Prompt replacement of chloride is essential.

Alkalosis. Gastric secretions such as hydrochloric acid are low in sodium but high in chloride. When such secretions are lost, bicarbonate replaces the depleted chloride ions. A type of metabolic alkalosis called hypochloremic alkalosis results. Potassium deficiency is a frequent accompaniment.

Endocrine disorders. Cushing's disease, which is caused by hyperactivity of the adrenal cortex, or excessive quantities of ACTH or cortisone given as therapy may produce hypokalemia and hypochloremic alkalosis may result.

Requirement and sources of chlorine

No quantitative statement of human requirement for chloride has been established. Almost the sole dietary source is as a partner to sodium in table salt ($NaCl$). When sodium intake is adequate, chloride will be amply supplied.

Sulfur
Occurrence in the body

Sulfur, an essential element, occurs in the body in a number of organic and inorganic forms. The inorganic forms of sulfur are the sulfates of sodium, potassium, and magnesium. Organic sulfur is divided into non-protein sulfur and protein sulfur. Nonprotein organic sulfur includes sulfalipids and sulfatides. The following is a list of protein sulfurs.

1. Sulfur-containing amino acids—methionine and cystine
2. Glycoproteins—conjugates of sulfate and sulfuric acid with carbohydrate derivatives, such as chondroitin-sulfuric acid in cartilage, tendon and bone matrix
3. Detoxification products—conjugates such as phenol and cresol sulfuric acids, and indoxyl sulfate; some of these products are formed in part from bacterial putrefactive activity in the intestine
4. Other organic compounds such as heparin, insulin, thiamine, biotin, lipoic acid, and coenzyme A
5. Keratin—the protein of hair and skin

Sulfur occurs in some form throughout the body, and is present in all cells, usually as an essential constituent of cell protein. The plasma sulfur level ranges from 0.7 to 1.5 mEq. per liter.

Absorption-excretion

Inorganic sulfate is absorbed in the intestine as such, and goes directly into the portal blood circulation. The sulfur-containing amino acids, methionine and cystine, are split off from protein during digestion, and are also absorbed into the portal circulation. These two amino acids are the most important sources of sulfur in the body.

Sulfur is excreted by the urine. Since sulfur enters the body chiefly with protein, the amount excreted varies directly with the amount of protein ingested and with the extent of tissue protein breakdown.

Metabolic functions of sulfur

Maintenance of protein structure. Disulfide linkages (-S-S-) form an important secondary structure between parallel peptide chains to maintain the stability of proteins.

Activation of enzymes. Many enzymes depend upon a free sulfhydryl group (-SH)

to maintain their activity. Therefore, sulfur participates in tissue respiration or biologic oxidation.

Energy metabolism. The sulfhydryl group also forms a high-energy sulfur bond similar to the high-energy phosphate bond (see pp. 64, 99). This is an important aspect of the metabolic activity of acetyl coenzyme A(CoA.SH) or active acetate.

Detoxification. Sulfur participates in several important detoxification reactions, by which toxic materials are conjugated with active sulfate and converted to a nontoxic form and excreted in the urine.

Clinical application

Cystine renal calculi. A relatively rare hereditary defect in renal tubular reabsorption of the amino acid cystine causes excessive urinary excretion of cystine (cystinuria) and repeated production of kidney stones formed of cystine crystals. They are yellowish in color because of the high sulfur content. A low-methionine diet is given to reduce the intake and synthesis of these sulfur-containing amino acids.

Requirement and sources of sulfur

No quantitative dietary requirement has been specified for sulfur. The major food sources are proteins containing methionine and cystine. Cystine may be synthesized in the body from its precursor methionine.

The major minerals are summarized in Table 8-1.

TRACE MINERALS

Seven essential minerals have been grouped as *trace elements* because they occur in the body in relatively small amounts—even minute amounts in most cases. Each, however, performs some vital function in human nutrition. These seven minerals are iron (Fe), copper (Cu), iodine (I), manganese (Mn), cobalt (Co), zinc (Zn), and molybdenum (Mo).

Iron
Occurrence in the body

The body contains about 45 mg. of iron per kilogram of body weight. To calculate the amount of iron in the body the formula 2.2 lb. = 1 kg. is used. A person weighing 55 kg. (121 lb.) would have about 2.5 gm. of iron.

This iron is distributed in the body in four main forms which point to its basic metabolic functions.

Transport iron. A very small amount of iron (from 0.05 to 0.18 mg. per 100 ml.) is found in the plasma. This iron is being transferred from one point of use to another. While it is transferred, it is bound with one of the plasma β-globulins. The plasma protein that binds iron in this compound form and transports it is called *transferrin.*

Hemoglobin. About 75% of the body's iron is in hemoglobin. The greatest amount of the body's iron, about 70%, is found in red blood cells as a constituent of hemoglobin. Another 5% of the total body iron is a part of muscle hemoglobin—myoglobin.

Storage iron. About 20% of the total body iron is in various organs in storage form as the protein-iron compound *ferritin.* The main storage organs are the liver, spleen, and bone marrow.

Cellular tissue iron. The remaining 5% of total body iron is distributed throughout all cells as a major component of oxidative enzyme systems for production of energy.

Absorption, transport, storage, excretion

In the body, iron follows a unique system of interrelated absorption-transportation-storage-excretion. The system is unique in that the optimal levels of body iron are not maintained by urinary excretion, as is the case with most plasma constituents. Rather, the mechanisms of control lie in an absorption-transportation-storage complex.

Absorption. Iron enters the body usually as ferric iron (Fe^{+++}) in food. It is reduced in the acid medium of the stomach to ferrous iron (Fe^{++}), the form necessary for absorption. Only about 10 to 30% of the ingested iron is absorbed, and this occurs mostly in the stomach and duodenum. The remaining 70 to 90% is eliminated in the feces.

Probably in a complex with amino acids, iron is carried into the mucosal cells of the intestine, where it combines with a protein, *apoferritin,* to form ferritin. The factor that chiefly controls the absorption or rejection of ingested iron is the amount of ferritin already present in the intestinal mucosa. When all available apoferritin has been bound to iron to form ferritin, any additional iron that arrives at the binding site is rejected, returned to the lumen of the intestine, and passed on for excretion in the feces.

A number of factors influence the absorption of iron. Those which favor or facilitate absorption include:

1. The amount of reserve ferritin present in mucosal cells correlates with the body's need for iron. In deficiency states, or in periods of extra demand as in growth or pregnancy, mucosal ferritin is lower, and more iron is absorbed. When tissue reserves are ample or saturated, iron is rejected and excreted.

2. Ascorbic acid (vitamin C) aids in absorption of iron by its reducing action and effect on acidity, changing dietary iron to the ferrous form in which it can be absorbed. Other metabolic reducing agents have similar effects.

3. The hydrochloric acid that is a normal constituent of gastric secretions provides the optimum acid medium for the preparation of iron for utilization.

4. An adequate amount of calcium helps to bind and remove agents such as phosphate and phytate, which if not removed would combine with iron and inhibit its absorption.

The following are factors that hinder iron absorption:

1. Phosphate, phytate, and oxalate are binding agents that remove iron from the body. Therefore, a diet high in phosphate, phytate, or oxalate leads to a decrease in iron absorption.

2. Surgical removal of stomach tissue (gastrectomy) reduces the number of cells

Table 8-1. Summary of major minerals

Mineral	Metabolism	Physiologic functions	Clinical application	Requirement	Food sources
Calcium (Ca)	Absorption according to body need, aided by vitamin D; favored by protein, lactose, acidity; hindered by excess fats and binding agents (phosphates, oxalates, phytate) Excretion chiefly in feces, 70 to 90% of amount ingested Deposition-mobilization in bone compartment constant; deposition aided by vitamin D Parathyroid hormone controls absorption and mobilization	Bone formation Teeth Blood clotting Muscle contraction and relaxation Heart action Nerve transmission Cell wall permeability Enzyme activation (ATPase)	Tetany—decrease in ionized serum calcium Rickets Renal calculi Hyperparathyroidism Hypoparathyroidism	Adults: .8 gm. Pregnancy and lactation: 1.3 gm. Infants: .7 gm. Children: 0.8 to 1.4 gm.	Milk Cheese Green leafy vegetables Whole grains Egg yolk Legumes, nuts
Phosphorus (P)	Absorption with calcium aided by vitamin D; hindered by excess binding agents (calcium, aluminum and iron) Excretion chiefly by kidney according to renal threshold blood level Parathyroid hormone controls renal excretion balance with blood level Deposition-mobilization in bone compartment constant	Bone formation Overall metabolism: Absorption of glucose and glycerol (phosphorylation) Transport of fatty acids Energy metabolism (enzymes, ATP) Buffer system	Growth Hypophosphatemia: Recovery state from diabetic acidosis Sprue, celiac disease (malabsorption) Bone diseases (upset Ca : P balance) Hyperphosphatemia: Renal insufficiency Hypoparathyroidism Tetany	Adults: 1½ times calcium intake Pregnancy and lactation: 1.3 gm. Infants: 0.2 to 0.5 mg. Children: 0.8 to 1.4 gm.	Milk Cheese Meat Egg yolk Whole grains Legumes, nuts
Magnesium (Mg)	Absorption increased by parathyroid hormone; hindered by excess fat, phosphate, calcium Excretion regulated by kidney	Constituent of bones and teeth Activator and coenzyme in carbohydrate and protein metabolism Essential intracellular fluid (ICF) cation Muscle and nerve irritability	Tremor, spasm; low serum level following gastrointestinal losses	300 to 350 mg. Deficiency in man unlikely	Whole grains Nuts Meat Milk Legumes

Mineral	Metabolism	Physiological functions	Clinical applications	Requirement	Food sources
Sodium (Na)	Readily absorbed Excretion chiefly by kidney, controlled by aldosterone, acid-base balance	Major extracellular fluid (ECF) cation Water balance; osmotic pressure Acid-base balance Cell permeability; absorption of glucose Muscle irritability; transmission of electrochemical impulse and resulting contraction	Fluid shifts and control Buffer system Losses in gastrointestinal disorders	About 0.5 gm. Diet usually has more: 2 to 6 gm.	Table salt (NaCl) Milk Meat Egg Baking soda Baking powder Carrots, beets, spinach, celery
Potassium (K)	Secreted and reabsorbed in digestive juices Excretion guarded by kidney according to blood levels; increased by aldosterone	Major ICF cation Acid-base balance Regulates neuromuscular excitability and muscle contraction Glycogen formation Protein synthesis	Fluid shifts Losses in: Starvation Diabetic acidosis Adrenal tumors Heart action—low serum potassium (tachycardia, cardiac arrest) Treatment of diabetic acidosis (rapid glycogen production reduces serum potassium) Tissue catabolism—potassium loss	About 2 to 4 gm. Diet adequate in protein, calcium, and iron contains adequate potassium	Whole grains Meat Legumes Fruits Vegetables
Chlorine (Cl)	Absorbed readily Excretion controlled by kidney	Major ECF anion Acid-base balance—chloride-bicarbonate shift Water balance Gastric hydrochloric acid—digestion	Hypochloremic alkalosis in prolonged vomiting, diarrhea, tube drainage	About 0.5 gm. Diet usually has more: 2 to 6 gm.	Table salt
Sulfur (S)	Absorbed as such and as constituent of sulfur-containing amino acid, methionine Excreted by kidney in relation to protein intake and tissue catabolism	Essential constituent of cell protein Activates enzymes High-energy sulfur bonds in energy metabolism Detoxification reactions	Cystine renal calculi Cystinuria	Diet adequate in protein contains adequate sulfur	Meat Egg Cheese Milk Nuts, legumes

that secrete hydrochloric acid. The acid medium necessary for iron reduction is therefore not provided.

3. Severe infection hinders iron absorption.

4. Malabsorption syndromes or any disturbance that causes diarrhea or steatorrhea will hinder iron absorption.

Transport. Mucosal ferritin delivers ferrous iron to the portal blood system. The iron is converted back to the ferrous state by oxidation. As ferrous iron, it combines with a plasma β-globulin, *transferrin* (or siderophilin), to form a ferric-protein complex which is the plasma transport form of iron. Transferrin is about 30 to 40% saturated with iron, and the remaining 60 to 70% forms an unsaturated, unbound, latent reserve in the plasma for handling iron.

Storage. The plasma transferrin then conveys iron to the various body cells for storage and utilization. About 1 gm. is distributed throughout all the cells as an essential element in energy-producing enzyme systems. The main storage organs, however, are the liver, spleen, and bone marrow, which participate in the forming of red blood cells. In these sites, the iron is stored as ferritin and as hemosiderin. Hemosiderin is a secondary, less soluble compound. It is a protein-bound ferric oxide with 35% iron. Hemosiderin formation increases as excess iron accumulates, such as during rapid destruction of red blood cells in hemolytic anemia. From these storage compounds, iron is mobilized for hemoglobin synthesis as needed. In the average adult, from 20 to 25 mg. of iron is involved daily in hemoglobin synthesis. But the body avidly conserves the iron that it uses in the synthesis of hemoglobin. As red cells are destroyed after an average life span of about 120 days, approximately 90% of the iron that is released is conserved, and is used over and over and over again. These iron absorption-storage mechanisms are diagrammed in Fig. 8-3. These relationships should be carefully compared.

Excretion. As indicated, since the main regulatory mechanism for control of iron levels is at the point of absorption, only very minute amounts are lost by excretion—about 0.5 to 1.0 mg. daily. Average trace amounts excreted are 0.1 mg. in the urine; 0.2 to 0.5 mg. in feces; and 0.05 to 1.0 mg. in sweat. In girls and women, monthly menstrual losses are about 20 mg. About 400 to 900 mg. of iron is lost during a usual pregnancy and delivery.

Metabolic functions of iron

Essentially, iron serves two major purposes in human metabolism.

Hemoglobin formation. Iron is the core of the heme molecule, the fundamental protein of hemoglobin. Hemoglobin in the red blood cell is the oxygen transport unit of the blood that conveys oxygen to the cells for respiration and metabolism.

Cellular oxidation. Though in smaller amounts, iron also functions in the cells as a vital component of enzyme systems for oxidation of glucose to produce energy. In the Krebs cycle, for example, iron is a constituent of the *cytochrome* compounds which are used in the oxidative chains producing high-energy ATP bonds (see p. 65).

Clinical application

Normal life cycle. During growth, the demand for positive iron balance is imperative. The newborn infant has at birth about a three to six months' supply of iron which was stored in the liver during fetal development. Since milk does not supply iron, supplementary iron-rich foods must be added to prevent the classic milk anemia of young children. Iron is also needed during continued growth, and to build up reserves for the physiologic stress of adolescence, especially the onset of menses in girls.

The woman's need for iron is increased during pregnancy, to maintain the increased total number of red blood cells in an expanded circulating blood volume, and to supply the iron for storage in the developing fetal liver. Finally, normal blood loss during delivery reduces iron stores.

Abnormal clinical situations. Because of the unique physiologic controls of the

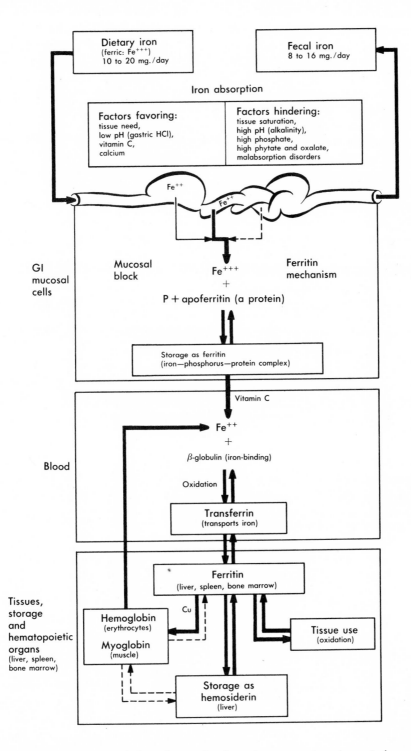

Fig. 8-3. Summary of iron metabolism, showing its absorption, transport, main use in hemoglobin formation, and its storage forms (ferritin and hemosiderin).

body's iron content, clinical abnormalities may result from either a deficiency or an excess of iron.

Deficiency of iron results in a hypochromic microcytic anemia. This lack of iron or inability to use it, may be due to one of several causes:

1. An inadequate supply of iron in the diet—nutritional anemia
2. Excessive blood iron loss—hemorrhagic anemia
3. Inability to form hemoglobin in the absence of other necessary factors such as vitamin B_{12}—pernicious anemia (p. 103)
4. Lack of gastric hydrochloric acid necessary to liberate iron for absorption—postgastrectomy anemia
5. The presence of iron inhibitors of absorption such as phosphate or phytate; or mucosal lesions which affect absorbing surface, leading to *malabsorption anemia*

Excessive amounts of iron may accumulate in the body because of the lack of an efficient excretory mechanism, and iron storage capacities may become saturated. This build-up of iron may be due to one of several causes:

1. Excess iron intake or excess red blood cell destruction, as in malaria or hemolytic anemias (which releases excess iron into the serum) produces a condition known as *hemosiderosis* (Gr., *hemo*, blood; *sidero*, iron). (An unusually high iron intake—about 200 mg. per day—and the resulting hemosiderosis has been reported among the Bantu natives of Africa. Their high corn diet is low in phosphates to bind iron, and they cook their food in heavy iron pots. It seems that the continuous high iron intake with little phosphate to hinder its absorption results in excessive liver storage and liver damage. This condition has been called Bantu siderosis.)
2. Excess intravenous iron or repeated transfusions may cause an accumulation of iron. This is associated with long-standing aplastic or hemolytic anemias with excess breakdown of red blood cells.
3. Hemochromatosis, a rare disease which occurs chiefly in males, is believed by some investigators to be genetically transmitted. Saturation of the body tissues with iron causes a bronze coloration, liver damage, and severe diabetes. Recently, a potent iron-chelating agent *desferrioxamine,* has been developed for use in treating such conditions. (The word *chelate* comes from the Greek word, *chele,* meaning claw.) A chelating agent is a substance that can grasp and incorporate a metallic ion in its molecular structure, which binds it and removes the ion from a tissue or from the circulating blood.

Dietary requirements of iron

The recommended allowances of the National Research Council (1968 revision) list a general daily adult dietary intake of 10 mg. of iron for men and 18 mg. for women during the childbearing years. This greater amount is needed to cover menstrual losses and the demands of pregnancy. It is doubtful that the woman's ordinary diet can supply this larger quantity of iron, and fortification with iron supplements is probably desirable. Infant allowances are 6 to 15 mg.; recommendations for children start at 15 mg. from ages one to three, and increase to 10 mg. for children ages three to twelve. The daily need is 18 mg. for boys twelve to eighteen and for girls from age ten on through the reproductive years.

Iron needs vary with age and situations, and these allowances are designed to provide margins for safety.

Food sources of iron

Organ meats, especially liver, are by far the best sources of iron. Other food sources include meats, egg yolk, whole wheat, seafood, green leafy vegetables, nuts, and legumes.

Copper
Occurrence in the body

Broadly speaking, copper seems to behave in the body as a companion to iron. The two are metabolized in much the same way, and share some functions.

The adult human body contains from 100 to 150 mg. of copper, distributed mainly in muscle, bone, the liver, heart, kidneys, and central nervous system. A small quantity is bound to plasma protein. The serum values are highly variable but range from 130 to 230 μg. per 100 ml. In the serum, about 5% of the copper is bound with albumin, and about 95% is bound with an α-globulin as the copper-binding protein *ceruloplasmin*.

Absorption-transport-storage-excretion

Absorption. Copper is known to be absorbed in the proximal portion of the small intestine, though the mechanism for its absorption is not well understood.

Transport and storage. The absorbed copper is first taken up by the plasma albumin and probably is initially transported in this bound form. Within twenty-four hours, however, the copper is bound by an α-globulin to form ceruloplasmin. From 50 to 75% of the total body copper is stored in muscle mass and bones, with high concentrations in the liver, heart, kidneys, and central nervous system.

The main route of excretion is the intestine. Some additional copper is lost in urine, sweat, and in menstrual flow.

Metabolic functions of copper

Copper is associated with iron in several important metabolic functions:

1. Copper, like iron, is involved in the cytochrome oxidation system of tissue cells for energy production, as well as being a constituent of several other oxidative enzymes for amino acids.
2. Copper is essential, together with iron, in the formation of hemoglobin. A copper-containing protein, *erythrocuprein*, is in red blood cells.
3. Copper seems to promote absorption of iron from the gastrointestinal tract.

Copper also appears to be involved in transporting iron from the tissues into the plasma.

In addition to these iron-related functions, copper is involved in two other areas of metabolism: (1) bone formation, and (2) brain tissue formation and maintenance of myelin in the nervous system.

Clinical application

Deficiency states in man are unknown. However, low plasma copper levels (*hypocupremia*), due to urinary loss of ceruloplasmin have been observed in nephrosis. Sprue, because of malabsorption of copper can also cause low plasma levels.

An excess accumulation of copper occurs in a rare inherited condition known as Wilson's disease, that is characterized by degenerative changes in brain tissue (basal ganglia) and in the liver. Large amounts of copper are absorbed and storage is increased in the liver, brain, kidneys, and cornea. A copper-chelate, penicillamine, is used to bind the excess copper and cause it to be excreted.

Requirement and food sources

Balance studies indicate that adults require about 2.5 mg. of copper daily. Infants and children require about 0.05 mg. per kilogram of body weight.

Copper is widely distributed in natural foods. The average daily diet contains from 2.5 to 5.0 mg. Therefore, given a sufficient caloric intake, copper will be amply supplied.

Iodine
Occurrence in the body

Iodine is a trace element associated mainly with the thyroid gland. The total iodine in the body is from 20 to 50 mg. Approximately 50% is in the muscles, 20% in the thyroid gland, 10% in the skin, 6% in the skeleton. The remaining 14% is scattered in other endocrine tissue, in the central nervous system, and in plasma transport. By far the greatest iodine tissue concentration, however, is in the thyroid.

TO PROBE FURTHER
The iodine pump and thyroxine formation

The cell membranes of the thyroid gland have a tremendous specific capacity to take up or trap iodides by an active transport mechanism. The concentration of iodides in these structures is normally about twenty-five times that of their concentration in the blood plasma. Highly active thyroid cells can accomplish an iodide concentration some 350 times that in blood.

Studies* with radioactive iodine (I^{131}) have traced the interesting interrelated role of iodine with protein in thyroxine formation. A neutral protein of large molecular weight, *thyroglobulin,* secreted into the thyroid follicle forms both the working base for synthesizing the hormone and the molecular storage complex for holding it until needed. This complex is called *colloid.* The amino acid tyrosine, a part of the thyroglobulin molecule, forms the base structure which, through successive stages of iodination, finally builds the hormone *thyroxine* (Fig. 8-4).

---

*Wolff, J.: Transport of iodide and other anions in the thyroid gland, Physiol. Rev. **44:**45, 1964.

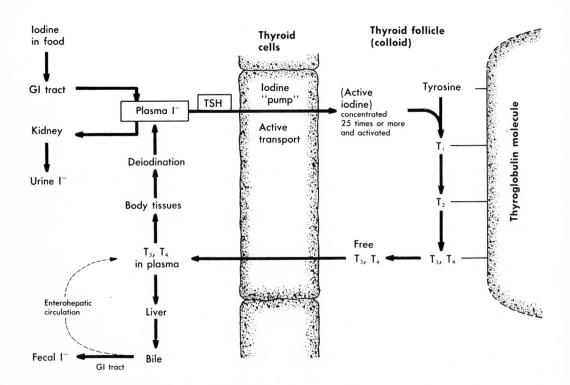

Fig. 8-4. Summary of iodine methabolism, showing active iodine pump in the thyroid cells and the synthesis of thyroxine in the colloid tissue of the thyroid follicles. (TSH = thyroid stimulating hormone; T_1 = monoiodotyronine; T_2 = diiodotyrosine; T_3 = triiodothyronine; T_4 = tetraiodothyronine

Absorption-excretion

Ingested iodine is absorbed in the small intestine as iodides. These are loosely bound with proteins and are conveyed by the blood to the thyroid gland. About one-third of it is selectively absorbed by the thyroid cells and removed from circulation. The remaining two-thirds is usually excreted in the urine within two to three days after ingestion. A pituitary hormone, TSH (thyroid stimulating hormone, or thyrotropic hormone) stimulates the uptake of iodine by the thyroid cells. The amount of TSH that is released by the pituitary is, in turn, governed by the level of thyroid hormone in the circulating blood. This circular or feedback mechanism normally maintains a healthy balance between supply and demand. Such a feedback mechanism is the characteristic pattern for governing all of the hormones from the several endocrine glands that are controlled by the pituitary (master) gland.

Metabolic function of iodine

Iodine participates in the synthesis of the thyroid hormone. This is the only known function of iodine in human metabolism. The thyroid hormone (thyroxine) in turn stimulates cell oxidation, apparently by increasing oxygen uptake and reaction rates of enzyme systems handling glucose. Therefore, iodine indirectly exerts tremendous influence upon overall body metabolism.

The free thyroxine with its associated iodine is secreted into the blood stream and bound to plasma protein for transport to body cells as needed. This transport form of iodine is called serum *protein-bound iodine* (PBI). The serum level of PBI normally ranges from 4 to 8 μg. per 100 ml. After being used to stimulate oxidation in the cell, thyroxine is degraded in the liver, and the iodine is excreted in bile as inorganic iodide.

Clinical application

Thyroid function. Both hyperthyroidism and hypothyroidism affect the rate of iodine uptake and utilization. Endemic colloid goiter is a classic condition characterized by great enlargement of the thyroid gland. Endemic colloid goiter occurs in residents of areas where the water and soil (and therefore locally grown foods) contain little iodine. The thyroid gland that is starved for iodine cannot produce a normal quantity of thyroxine. The amount of thyroxine that is secreted into the blood stream is therefore too low to shut off TSH secretion by the pituitary. The pituitary persists in putting out TSH, and these large quantities of TSH continue to stimulate the thyroid gland, calling upon it to produce the thyroxine that it cannot supply. The only response that the iodine-starved gland can make is to increase the amount of thyroglobulin (colloid), which then accumulates in the thyroid follicles. Such a gland becomes increasingly engorged, and may attain a tremendous size, weighing 500 to 700 gm. (1 to 1½ lb.) or more.

Tests for iodine metabolism

The PBI test measures the amount of iodine that is bound to thyroxine and in transit in the plasma. A small amount of free inorganic iodide may also be present. The normal range is from 4 to 8 μg. per 100 ml. of serum. Values below 4 indicate hypothyroidism; those above 8 indicate hyperthyroidism. Unfortunately, falsely high readings may result from the presence in the system of other iodine compounds, such as certain iodine-containing radiopaque substances that may have been administered in conjunction with x-ray studies, or iodine-containing therapeutic agents. Mercurial diuretics may cause falsely low readings.

Radioactive I[131] tests are tests that use radioactive iodine to measure the uptake and utilization of iodine by the thyroid gland.

The iodine cycle and dental caries. Prevention of dental caries has been attributed to the iodine cycle, which involves the salivary secretion of iodine. It is believed that increased saliva flow, by raising the concentration and secretion of iodine by the parotid and submaxillary glands, inhibits the formation of dental caries.

Requirement and food sources of iodine

Balance studies indicate that the human adult needs to ingest from 100 to 200 μg. of iodine daily, and that the basal requirement is about 25 μg. The National Research Council (1968 revision) has recommended daily adult allowances of 140 μg. for young men and 100 μg. for young women. These needs normally decrease with age. The demand is increased during periods of accelerated growth such as adolescence and pregnancy.

Seafood provides a considerable amount of iodine; however, the quantity in natural sources varies broadly, depending upon the iodine content of the soil. The average diet falls somewhat below the requirement. The commercial iodizing of table salt (1 mg. to every 10 grams of salt) provides the main dietary source of iodine.

Manganese
Occurrence in the body

In industry, manganese is a metallic element used chiefly as an alloy in steel to give it toughness. In nutrition, traces of manganese serve as essential activating agents that strengthen and stimulate a number of vital metabolic reactions. Only about 10 mg. of manganese is present in the adult body, chiefly in the liver and kidneys, with small amounts in other tissues such as the retina, bones, and salivary glands. Blood values are very low—4 to 20 μg. per 100 ml. have been reported.

Absorption-excretion

Manganese, like iron, is poorly absorbed by the intestine; much is rejected by the intestine, and that which is rejected is eliminated directly in the feces. The small quantity that is absorbed in the small intestine, however, enters the blood stream and is transported, loosely bound with protein, to the tissues for storage and utilization.

Excretion of manganese takes place almost entirely through the intestine. In addition to that which was rejected and eliminated directly, a small amount of the manganese that has been used by the tissues is ultimately carried to the bile, which returns it into the intestine, where this amount also is excreted with other body wastes. Little or no manganese is excreted in the urine.

Metabolic functions of manganese

Studies of animals have clearly demonstrated the essential nature of manganese to a number of their metabolic functions. Although the participation of manganese has not been clearly shown in all of the parallel functions in human nutrition, studies with radioactive manganese (Mn^{56}) have shown that its active uptake sites are the cell mitochondria, in which the cell enzyme systems operate. Therefore, it seems that the function of manganese in human nutrition may well be to participate in key coenzymes in these reactions.

Some of these reactions include:
1. *Urea formation*—activates an enzyme in the formation of urea; may help prevent ammonia toxicity
2. *Protein metabolism*—activates amino acid interconversions; activates peptidases for splitting specific amino acids such as leucine
3. *Carbohydrate metabolism*—activates several conversion reactions of the glycolytic pathway and Krebs cycle in glucose oxidation
4. *Fat metabolism*—activates the serum fat-clearing factor, lipoprotein lipase, and operates as a cofactor in the synthesis of long chain fatty acids

Clinical application

Though many clinical evidences of manganese deficiency have been established in animals, none have been observed in humans. However, an industrial disease syndrome, representing *inhalation toxicity* occurs in miners and other workers who undergo prolonged exposure to manganese dust. The excess manganese accumulates in the liver and central nervous system, and eventually produces severe neuromuscular manifestations that resemble those of Parkinson's disease.

Requirement and food sources of manganese

Whether there is a specific human requirement of manganese is unknown. The average diet provides from 3 to 9 μg. daily, which seems highly adequate.

The best food sources of manganese are of plant origin: cereal bran, soybeans, legumes, nuts, tea, and coffee. Animal foods are relatively poor sources.

Cobalt
Occurrence in the body

Cobalt occurs in only minute traces in the body tissues, and the main storage area is the liver. As an essential constituent of vitamin B_{12}, cobalt is largely associated with red blood cell formation. The normal blood level, representing the element in transit and in erythrocytes, is about 1 μg. per 100 ml.

Absorption-excretion

Variable amounts of cobalt are absorbed, and apparently quickly excreted in the urine. Unabsorbed cobalt is lost in feces. The main form in which it is absorbed and used is as a constituent of vitamin B_{12}.

Metabolic function of cobalt

The basic function of cobalt in human nutrition that has been demonstrated is that of a constituent of vitamin B_{12}, an essential factor in the formation of red blood cells. The widespread distribution of cobalt in nature, and its ready uptake by plants lead one to speculate about possible broader functions. As yet, however, such have not been established.

Clinical application

Deficiency of cobalt per se is well known to have deleterious effects in animals. In man, a deficiency of cobalt is associated only with a deficiency of vitamin B_{12} and the consequent development of pernicious anemia (see p. 103).

Excess of cobalt has led to polycythemia, a condition characterized by the formation of an excess number of red blood cells which contain a relatively high concentration of hemoglobin.

Requirement and food sources of cobalt

The quantitative human requirement of cobalt is unknown, but is evidently minute. For example, as small an amount as .045 to .09 μg. daily maintains bone marrow function in patients with pernicious anemia.

Cobalt is widely distributed in nature; however, for man's chief need—as a constituent of vitamin B_{12}—cobalt is best obtained in the preformed vitamin, that is synthesized in animals by gastrointestinal bacteria.

Zinc
Occurrence in the body

Zinc occurs in the human body in amounts larger than those of other trace elements except iron. The body's total zinc content, from 1.3 to 2.3 gm., is distributed in many tissues including the pancreas, liver, kidney, lung, muscles, bones, eye (cornea, iris, retina, and lens), endocrine glands, prostate secretions, and spermatozoa. The plasma zinc level is about 120 μg. per 100 ml.

Absorption-excretion

After zinc is absorbed in the small intestine, it combines with plasma proteins for transport to the tissues. Isotope studies indicate that it first concentrates in the liver, pancreas, kidneys, and pituitary; then predominantly in red blood cells and bone, after which it appears to remain in circulation and use as long as from 8 to 12 months.

Excretion of zinc is largely intestinal. Unabsorbed zinc is eliminated immediately. Zinc that has entered the blood and tissues is gradually excreted into the intestine in pancreatic and intestinal secretions, and a small amount is also excreted in the bile.

Except in disease states, zinc is rarely excreted in the urine.

Metabolic functions of zinc

Enzyme constituent. Zinc functions mainly as an essential constituent of carbonic anhydrase, carboxypeptidase, and lactic dehydrogenase.

Zinc is an integral part of *carbonic anhydrase,* which acts as a carbon dioxide carrier, especially in red blood cells. It takes up carbon dioxide from cells, combines it with water to form carbonic acid (H_2CO_3), and then releases carbon dioxide from the capillaries into the alveoli of the lung. This enzyme also functions in the renal tubule cells in the maintenance of acid-base balance, in mucosal cells, and in glands of the body.

Zinc is a cofactor of the protein-splitting enzyme, *carboxypeptidase,* which removes the carboxyl group (COOH) from peptides to produce amino acids. Zinc, therefore, has a key role in protein digestion.

Zinc is a part of *lactic dehydrogenase.* This enzyme is essential for the interconversion of pyruvic acid and lactic acid in the glycolytic pathway for glucose oxidation. Thus, zinc also plays a part in carbohydrate digestion.

Two additional roles of zinc in metabolism are important but their significance is less well understood:

Insulin. Zinc combines readily with insulin in the pancreas; zinc-insulin serves perhaps as the storage form of this hormone. The diabetic pancreas contains about half the normal amount of zinc.

Leukocytes. A considerable quantity of zinc bound to protein is present in leukocytes although its function in white cells is unknown. The leukocytes of patients with leukemia contain about 10% less zinc than normal.

Clinical application

A possible relation of zinc metabolism with liver disease has aroused the interest of investigators. In cirrhosis, serum zinc levels are low, urinary excretion is increased, and postmortem studies have revealed reduced zinc concentrations in the liver. It is speculated that the disease may increase the need for zinc, and therefore deficiency results from the usual intake.

Requirement and food sources of zinc

No specific quantitative requirement for zinc has been established in man. Balance studies indicate that a daily intake of 0.3 mg. per kilogram of body weight is adequate. Since the usual intake on an average diet is from 10 to 15 mg., deficiency is unlikely.

Zinc is easily obtained in widespread natural sources.

Molybdenum
Occurrence in the body and function of molybdenum

Amounts of molybdenum in the body are very minute. This trace mineral is present in bound form as an integral part of various enzyme molecules, and thus functions in facilitating the action of the specific enzyme involved. Examples of molybdenum-containing enzymes are xanthine oxidase and liver aldehyde oxidase.

In purine catabolism, xanthine oxidase catalyzes the oxidation of xanthine to uric acid. It has been isolated from milk and liver.

Liver aldehyde oxidase, a flavoprotein, catalyzes the oxidation of aldehydes to corresponding carboxylic acid.

Requirement and food sources of molybdenum

Food sources of molybdenum include legumes, whole grains, milk, leafy vegetables, and organ meats. There is no known requirement.

MINERALS WITH UNKNOWN FUNCTION

Several other minerals occur in trace amounts in the body, but their essential function is not clear. These include fluorine (Fl), selenium (Se), aluminum (Al), boron, (Bo), cadmium (Cd), and chromium (Cr).

Fluorine

The only relationship thus far established for fluorine in human metabolism is its association with dental health. Basic observations have centered around the results of an excess intake of fluorine, and of a small intake.

Excess intake

Endemic dental fluorosis has been observed in communities where the natural fluorine content of the water supply is high. The largest known such region in the United States is the West Texas Panhandle. Apparently fluorine excesses act upon teeth in the budding stage of formation, so that by the time they erupt their enamel is mottled, pitted, and discolored. Adults who habitually eat excessive quantities of fluoride may suffer from osteosclerosis. Osteosclerosis is abnormal density of the skeletal bone, which in some cases is so mild that it can barely be detected by x-ray, but in other instances it is so severe as to be called crippling fluorosis.

Small intake

Dental caries have been demonstrated to be largely preventable by the addition of a small amount of fluorine to fluorine-poor drinking water, or by the topical application of fluoride solutions to young developing teeth. Public health authorities advocate the fluoridation of public drinking water in the amount of 1 part per million in areas where the drinking water is low in fluoride content. The mechanism by which fluorine prevents dental caries is unknown.

Selenium

Interest in selenium has recently centered about the discovery of a potent, metabolically active, selenium-containing compound called "factor 3", which was observed to protect the liver against fatty infiltration and necrosis. This action of selenium may be related to that of vitamin E, as the two substances appeared to act synergistically in curing the hepatic disease and certain muscle disorders induced in animals.

The function of selenium involved is probably that of a cofactor for enzyme systems related to cell oxidation. Perhaps such a role may ultimately be proved for this trace element in human nutrition also.

Aluminum

The amount of aluminum ingested in the average human diet ranges widely from about 10 mg. to more than 100 mg. daily. This element is found in many plant and animal foods. Despite this wide intake and distribution, no clear function in human nutrition has been established. A clue may be present in model systems studies of certain transaminase reactions with amino acids. The mechanism and significance of these reactions are not clear, however.

The total aluminum content of the adult human body is from 50 to 150 mg.

Boron

Minute traces of boron are found in body tissues, but no clues to its purpose have been discovered. Boron has been found to be essential for plant nutrition and growth, but experiments in animals have not demonstrated any evidences of deficiency after boron deprivation.

Cadmium

That traces of cadmium are present in body tissues has been known for some time. Not until 1960, however, was cadmium isolated as a definite component of a metal-containing protein. This protein, metallothionein, found in the renal cortex of the horse, contains cadmium, zinc, and sulfur. The significance of this cadmium-containing protein is not yet clear, but it points to the possibility that the mineral functions in some basic biologic system.

Chromium

The minute traces of chromium present in the body were not recognized until two decades ago, when analytic methods were developed that were sufficiently sensitive to

Table 8-2. Summary of trace minerals

Mineral	Metabolism	Physiologic function	Clinical application	Requirement	Food source
Iron (Fe)	Absorption according to body need controlled by mucosal block—ferritin mechanism; aided by vitamin C, gastric hydrochloric acid Transport—transferrin Storage—ferritin, hemosiderin Excretion from tissue in minute quantities; body conserves and re-uses	Hemoglobin formation Cellular oxidation (cytochrome system producing ATP)	Growth (milk anemia) Pregnancy demands Deficiency—anemia Excess—hemosiderosis; hemochromatosis	Men: 10 mg. Women: 18 mg. Pregnancy: 18 mg. Lactation: 18 mg. Children: 10 to 18 mg.	Liver Meats Egg yolk Whole grains Enriched bread and cereal Dark green vegetables Legumes, nuts
Copper (Cu)	Transported bound to an α-globulin as ceruloplasmin Stored in muscle, bone, liver, heart, kidney and central nervous system	Associated with iron in: Enzyme systems Hemoglobin synthesis Absorption and transport of iron Involved in bone formation and maintenance of brain tissue and myelin sheath in nervous system	Hypocupremia: Nephrosis Malabsorption Wilson's disease—excess copper storage	2 to 2.5 mg. Diet provides 2 to 5 mg.	Liver Meat Seafood Whole grains Legumes, nuts
Iodine (I)	Absorbed as iodides, taken up by thyroid gland under control of thyroid-stimulating hormone (TSH) Excretion by kidney	Synthesis of thyroxine, the thyroid hormone, which regulates cell oxidation	Deficiency—endemic colloid goiter; cretinism	Men: 140 μg. Women: 100 μg. Infants: 25 to 45 μg. Children: 55 to 140 μg.	Iodized salt Seafoods
Manganese (Mn)	Absorption limited Excretion mainly by intestine	Activates reactions in: Urea formation Protein metabolism Glucose oxidation Lipoprotein clearance and synthesis of fatty acids	No clinical deficiency observed in humans Inhalation toxicity in miners	Unknown Diet provides 3 to 9 μg.	Cereals Soybeans Legumes, nuts Tea, coffee

Mineral	Metabolism	Physiologic functions	Clinical applications	Food sources
Cobalt (Co)	Absorbed chiefly as constituent of vitamin B$_{12}$	Constituent of vitamin B$_{12}$, essential factor in red blood cell formation	Deficiency associated with deficiency of vitamin B$_{12}$—pernicious anemia	Supplied by preformed vitamin B$_{12}$
Zinc (Zn)	Transported with plasma proteins. Excretion largely intestinal. Stored in liver, muscle, bone, and organs	Essential enzyme constituent: Carbonic anhydrase, Carboxypeptidase, Lactic dehydrogenase. Combines with insulin for storage of the hormone	Possible relation to liver disease	Unknown. Average diet supplies 10 to 15 mg. Widely distributed. Liver. Seafood
Molybdenum (Mo)	Minute traces in the body	Constituent of specific enzymes involved in: Purine conversion to uric acid, Aldehyde oxidation		Unknown. Organ meats, Milk, Whole grains, Leafy vegetables, Legumes
Fluorine (Fl)	Deposited in bones and teeth. Excreted in urine	Associated with dental health	Small amount prevents dental caries. Excess causes endemic dental fluorosis	Water (1 ppm. Fl)
Selenium (Se)		Associated with fat metabolism	Constituent of "factor 3" which acts with vitamin E to prevent fatty liver	
Chromium (Cr)		Associated with glucose metabolism	Infants unable to metabolize sugar and adult diabetics showed definite improvement when small amounts of chromium added to diet. Possible link with cardiovascular disorders and diabetes	

detect them. There are about twenty parts of chromium in one billion parts of blood; however, certain cell proteins can achieve concentrations of chromium much higher than this. The greater concentration in cells has led to studies of chromium which indicate a probable role in glucose metabolism. In animals made chromium-deficient by deprivation, fasting blood sugar levels were elevated and glycosuria followed. In man, recent studies showed the ability of chromium to raise abnormally low fasting blood-sugar levels and to improve faulty uptake of sugar by body tissues. Physicians working in Jerusalem with refugee infants suffering from severe malnutrition and an inability to use sugar found that when small amounts of chromium were added to their diet, the infants made rapid recovery.

The average daily human diet apparently contains from 80 to 100 μg. of chromium, of which only 2 to 5 μg. is absorbed. The absorbed chromium is stored in the tissues, from which it is released when glucose is ingested. It seems, however, that tissue levels are by no means consistent. Wide variances have been found in samples taken from different sites and at different times. Further study is needed to determine chromium's role in metabolism and its nutritional significance. In the meantime, it is interesting to speculate concerning its possible link with chronic disease processes such as cardiovascular disorders and diabetes.

The trace minerals are summarized in Table 8-2.

GLOSSARY

anemia blood condition characterized by decrease in number of circulating red blood cells, hemoglobin, or both. Anemias may be caused by lack of dietary iron intake, hemorrhage, lack of other substances necessary to form hemoglobin (vitamin B_{12}), lack of factors necessary for absorption of iron (hydrochloric acid), or to intestinal diseases affecting absorbing surface.

apoferritin (Gr. *apo*, from away, separation; L. *ferr*, iron) protein base in intestinal mucosa cells, which will bind with iron (from food) to form ferritin, the storage form of iron.

bone compartment the body's total content of skel-

etal tissue. The bone compartment contains 99% of the body's total metabolic calcium pool.

calcitonin a quick-acting hormone secreted by the parathyroids in response to hypercalcemia, which acts to induce hypocalcemia. A similar substance from the thyroid gland, thyrocalcitonin, also lowers calcium levels. These substances are believed to participate in the feedback mechanism that controls and maintains stable blood calcium levels.

calcium to phosphorus ratio (Ca:P ratio) since calcium and phosphorus are intimately related in metabolism, two ratios between them are significant. (1) The dietary calcium to phosphorus ratio affects absorption of these minerals; a 1:1 ratio is ideal for growth, pregnancy, and lactation periods. Otherwise, for adults a 1:1½ ratio of calcium to phosphorus is required. (2) The serum calcium to phosphorus ratio is the solubility product of the two minerals in the serum. An increase in one mineral causes a decrease in the other to maintain a constant product of the two. The normal serum level of calcium is 10 mg. per 100 ml.; of phosphorus, 4 mg. per 100 ml. in adults (5 in children). Thus, the normal serum calcium to phosphorus ratio for adults is 40 (10 × 4); and for children is 50 (10 × 5).

calculus (L. pebble) (pleural, *calculi*) any abnormal accretion within the body of material which forms a "stone." Calculi are usually composed of mineral salts. The most commonly formed renal calculi are composed of calcium salts.

chelate (Gr. *chele,* claw) a chemical compound capable of grasping and incorporating a metallic ion into its molecular structure. By binding the metal, the chelate removes it from a tissue or from the circulating blood. For example, *desferrioxamine* is a chelating agent developed by chemists for the treatment of hemochromatosis, a disease in which excess iron is stored in body tissue. The desferrioxamine removes iron from the tissues and transports it to excretion sites.

chloride-bicarbonate shift the exchange of bicarbonate for chloride in red blood cells. To provide constant bicarbonate buffering for the rapidly forming carbonic acid from water and carbon dioxide ($H_2O + CO_2$), chloride replaces bicarbonate in the cell, which allows bicarbonate to participate in the carbonic acid-base bicarbonate buffer system. In the lungs, as carbon dioxide is expired, the reaction forming carbonic acid is reversed, and bicarbonate is not needed, so the shift changes.

cystinuria a condition caused by a rare hereditary defect. It is characterized by excessive urinary excretion of cystine (a sulfur-containing amino acid). In this disease, cystine crystals often accumulate and form characteristic, small, smooth, yellow kidney stones—cystine renal calculi.

feedback mechanism the mechanism that regulates production and secretion, by an endocrine gland (A_g), of its hormone (A_h), which stimulates another endocrine gland (T_g; the *target gland*) to produce its hormone (T_h). As T_g produces sufficient T_h to supply the body's needs, the blood level of T_h rises. This rise in the blood level of T_h signals A_g to stop secreting A_h. The blood level of A_h then gradually falls. T_g is no longer stimulated to produce T_h. The blood level of T_h therefore declines. When it falls below the body's need, A_g recognizes this as its signal to produce more A_h. The rise in A_h tells T_g to increase its production of T_h. Example: The anterior pituitary-thyroid interaction. Here, A_g is the anterior pituitary gland; T_g is the thyroid gland. The anterior pituitary secretes thyroid-stimulating hormone (TSH). TSH stimulates the thyroid to secrete thyroxine. When the blood level of thyroxine reaches optimum, the anterior pituitary ceases to secrete TSH. The thyroid thereupon stops secreting thyroxine, and the blood level of thyroxine falls. When it falls below the level needed by the body, the anterior pituitary responds to this low blood level of thyroxine by again liberating TSH into the blood stream.

ferritin the protein-iron compounds in which iron is stored in the tissues—the storage form of iron in the body. The so-called ferritin mechanism in the mucosal cells of the stomach and small intestine regulates iron absorption. When the ferritin protein compound is saturated with iron, no more iron is absorbed.

fluoridation the process by which fluorine is added to a substance. Proper fluoridation of public water supplies in areas where the fluorine content is naturally low has been demonstrated to control the incidence of dental caries.

goiter (L. *guttur,* throat) endemic colloid goiter is an enlargement of the thyroid gland caused by lack of sufficient available iodine to produce the thyroid hormone, thyroxine.

hemochromatosis (Gr. *haima,* blood; *chroma,* color) a disturbance of iron metabolism in which excessive iron storage causes a bronze discoloration of skin and viscera, liver and pancreas damage, and diabetes (bronzed diabetes). The condition is believed to be genetically transmitted by a defect occurring chiefly in males.

hemoglobin (Gr. *haima,* blood; L. *globus,* globe) the protein which gives the color to red blood cells. Hemoglobin is a conjugated protein composed of an iron-containing pigment called heme and a simple protein, globin. Hemoglobin is the oxygen carrier of the blood, and combines with oxygen to form oxyhemoglobin.

hemosiderin (Gr. *haima,* blood; *sideros,* iron) an insoluble iron oxide-protein compound, in which iron is stored in the liver if the amount of iron in the blood exceeds the storage capacity of ferritin. Such accumulation of excess iron occurs in diseases that are accompanied by rapid destruction of red blood cells (malaria, hemolytic anemia).

hemosiderosis a condition in which large amounts of the iron storage compound hemosiderin are deposited, especially in the liver and spleen. Hemosiderosis may occur as the result of excessive breakdown of red blood cells in diseases such as malaria and hemolytic anemias, or after multiple blood transfusions.

hyperkalemia excessive amounts of potassium (K) in blood plasma. Hyperkalemia is a serious complication of renal failure, severe dehydration, or shock; it causes the heart to dilate, and the heart rate is slowed by weakened contractions. Potassium plays a vital role with ionized sodium and calcium (Na^+ and Ca^+) in regulating neuromuscular stimulation, transmission of electrochemical impulses (such as those that mediate the flow of the beat through the heart), and contraction of muscle fibers.

hyperphosphatemia high serum phosphorus. Hyperphosphatemia may be caused by renal insufficiency because the kidney cannot excrete phosphorus adequately, or by hypoparathyroidism which causes an insufficient secretion of parathyroid hormone, which regulates the renal excretion of phosphorus. When serum phosphorus rises, serum calcium falls, causing tetany.

hypochloremic alkalosis excessive loss of gastric secretions, (hydrochloric acid) results in loss of chlorides and bicarbonate replaces the depleted chloride ions. Hypochloremic alkalosis (a type of metabolic alkalosis) results. Such gastrointestinal disorders as excessive vomiting may lead to hypochloremic alkalosis. Therefore, prompt replacement of chloride is essential.

hypocupremia low serum copper level. Hypocupremia may be caused by urinary loss of *ceruloplasmin* (the copper-binding protein of the plasma) in nephrosis; or by malabsorption of copper in sprue.

hypokalemia low blood potassium. Hypokalemia is a serious complication of severe diarrhea, for example, in which large amounts of potassium are lost in intestintal secretions. Hypokalemia may also result from rapid glycogenesis during the recovery phase of diabetic acidosis. Replacement therapy in both instances should involve added potassium.

hypophosphatemia low serum phosphorus. Hypophosphatemia may be caused by decreased absorption of phosphorus as in intestinal diseases (sprue, celiac disease); or to an upset serum calcium to phosphorus ratio as in bone disease (rickets, osteomalacia); or to excess secretion of parathyroid hormone with resulting excessive renal excretion of phosphorus, as in primary hyperparathyroidism.

ionized calcium (Ca⁺⁺) free, diffusible form of calcium in the blood and other body fluids. Although free ionized calcium makes up a very small amount of the total body calcium (1%) it exerts a profound influence on the function of bone, the heart, and the nervous system. (The remaining 99% of the total body calcium is deposited as calcium salts in bone tissue.)

myofibrils (Gr. *myo,* muscle; L. *fibrilla,* small fiber) the contractile element in muscle tissue, a tiny fiber running parallel to the cellular long axis. Calcium ions activate the chemical reaction between the constituent muscle protein filaments, myosin and actin, which releases a burst of energy from ATP bonds and brings about contraction of the myofibril units in the muscle.

myoglobin muscle protein (globin) that contains iron (also called *myohemoglobin*).

osteoblasts (Gr. *osteo,* bone; *blastos,* germ) bone forming cells.

osteoclasts (Gr. *osteo,* bone; *klan,* to break) giant, multinuclear cells found in depressions on bone surfaces, which cause resorption of bone tissue and the formation of canals.

parathyroid hormone (PH) hormone of parathyroid gland, which controls calcium and phosphorus metabolism in three ways: (1) it stimulates the intestinal mucosa to increase calcium absorption, (2) it mobilizes calcium rapidly from bone, and (3) it causes renal excretion of phosphate. All of these responses act together as needed to regulate the circulating amounts of calcium and phosphorus to maintain them within normal levels.

PBI protein-bound iodine. The PBI test is used to measure thyroid activity by determining the amount of iodine that is bound to thyroxine and in transit in the plasma.

polycythemia a condition characterized by the presence of excess red blood cells that contain a high concentration of hemoglobin. There are several types of polycythemia. One type may be caused by an excess of cobalt. Cobalt is the core of vitamin B_{12}, which is an essential factor in red blood cell formation.

radioactive I¹³¹ tests tests of thyroid function using a radioactive isotope of iodine, I¹³¹. After the test dose is administered, the uptake and utilization of iodine by the thyroid gland is measured by tracing the I¹³¹.

sulfhydryl group the -SH radical which forms high-energy sulfur bonds in chemical compounds. These are similar to the high-energy bonds formed by phosphates in compounds such as ATP. In such compounds, sulfur participates in important tissue respiration (oxidation) reactions.

synergism (Gr. *syn,* with or together; *ergon,* work) the joint action of separate agents in which the total effect of their combined action is greater than the sum of their separate actions. Each agent potentiates the action of the other.

tetany a disorder caused by abnormal calcium metabolism. Severe, intermittent, tonic contractions of the extremities and muscular pain occur, which are usually caused by lowered blood calcium levels. A characteristic diagnostic sign is the inward muscular spasm of the wrist called Trousseau's sign.

thyroid-stimulating hormone (TSH) a hormone secreted by the anterior pituitary gland which regulates uptake of iodine and synthesis of thyroxine by the thyroid gland.

thyroxine the iodine-containing hormone produced by the thyroid gland.

transferrin an iron-binding protein complex, a serum β-globulin; the transport form of iron in the body.

Wilson's disease a rare hereditary disease of abnormal copper metabolism. Large amounts of copper are absorbed by, and accumulate in, the liver, brain, kidneys, and cornea. The disease produces degenerative changes in brain and liver tissue. A copper-chelate, *penicillamine,* is used to bind the excess copper and excrete it.

References

General

General mineral

Comar, C. L., and Bronner, F.: Mineral metabolism, New York, 1962, Academic Press, Inc.

Davis, G. K.: Excess minerals in the diet, J. Amer. Diet. Ass. **51:**46, 1967.

Food and Nutrition Board: Recommended dietary allowances, 1968 rev., ed. 7, Publ. No. 1694, National Academy of Science, National Research Council, Washington, D. C., 1968.

Schutte, K. H.: The biology of the trace elements: their role in nutrition, Philadelphia, 1964, J. B. Lippincott Co.

Underwood, E. J.: Trace elements in human and animal nutrition, New York, 1962, Academic Press, Inc.

Calcium and phosphorus

Chakmakjian, Z. H., and Bethune, J. E.: Sodium sulfate treatment of hypercalcemia. New Eng. J. Med. **275:**862, 1966.

Council on Food and Nutrition, American Medical Association: Symposium on human calcium requirements, J.A.M.A. **185:**588, 1963.

FAO/WHO Expert Committee: Calcium requirements, WHO Tech. Rep. Series No. 230, Rome, 1962.

Greenwald, E., and others: Effect of lactose on calcium metabolism in man, J. Nutr. **79:**531, 1963.

Hegsted, D. M.: Nutrition, bone, and calcified tissue, J. Amer. Diet. Ass. **50**:105, 1967.

Holemans, K. C., and Meyer, B. J.: A quantitative relationship between the absorption of calcium and phosphorus, Amer. J. Clin. Nutr. **12**:30, 1963.

Johansen, E.: Nutrition, diet, and calcium metabolism in dental health, Amer. J. Public Health **50**:1089, 1960.

Lutwak, L.: Osteoporosis—a mineral deficiency disease?, J. Amer. Diet. Ass. **44**:173, 1964.

Report: Kinetic response to dietary calcium changes, J.A.M.A. **199**:35, 1967.

Wenger, J., and others: The milk-alkali syndrome: hypercalcemia, alkalosis, and temporary renal insufficiency during milk-antacid therapy for peptic ulcer, Amer. J. Med. **24**:161, 1958.

Magnesium

Briscoe, A. M., and Ragan, C.: Effect of magnesium or calcium metabolism in man, Amer. J. Clin. Nutr. **19**:296, 1966.

Caddell, J. L.: Studies in protein-calorie malnutrition. II. A double-blind clinical trial to assess magnesium therapy, New Eng. J. Med. **276**:535, 1967.

Caddell, J. L., and Goddard, D. R.: Studies in protein-calorie malnutrition. I. Chemical evidence for magnesium deficiency, New Eng. J. Med. **276**:533, 1967.

Friedman, F., and others: Primary hypomagnesemia with secondary hypocalcemia in an infant, Lancet **1**:687, 1967.

Hathway, M. L.: Magnesium in human nutrition, Home Econ. Res. Rep. No. 19, U. S. Department of Agriculture, Washington, D. C., 1962.

Kahil, M. E., and others: Magnesium deficiency and carbohydrate metabolism, Diabetes **15**:734, 1966.

Review: Magnesium deficiency, Nutr. Rev. **20**:335, 1962.

Review: Magnesium Metabolism, Nutr Rev. **20**:250, 1962.

Seelig, M. S.: The requirement of magnesium by the normal adult, Amer. J. Clin. Nutr. **14**:342, 1964.

Smith, W. O., and others: The Clinical Expression of Magnesium Deficiency, J.A.M.A. **174**:77, 1960.

Vallee, B. L., and others: The magnesium tetany syndrome in man, New Eng. J. Med. **262**:155, 1960.

Wacker, W. E. C.: Magnesium metabolism, J. Amer. Diet. Ass. **44**:362, 1964.

Fluoride

Ast, D. B., and Schlesinger, E. R.: The conclusion of a ten-year study of water fluoridation, Amer. J. Public Health **46**:265, 1956.

Bernstein, D. S., and others: Prevalence of osteoporosis in high- and low-fluoride areas in North Dakota, J.A.M.A. **197**:499, 1966.

Knutson, J. W.: Fluoridation—where are we today? Amer. J. Nursing **60**:196, 1960.

Report: Fluoride protects against bone loss, J.A.M.A. **200**:31, 1967.

Waldbott, G. L.: Fluoride in food, Amer. J. Clin. Nutr. **12**:455, 1963.

Iron

Bothwell, T. H., and Clement, A. F.: Iron metabolism, Boston, 1962, Little, Brown and Company.

Brown, E. B.: The absorption of iron, Amer. J. Clin. Nutr. **12**:205, 1963.

Finch, C. A.: Iron balance in man, Nutr. Rev. **23**:129, 1965.

Mendel, G. A.: Iron metabolism and etiology of iron-storage diseases: an interpretative formulation. J.A.M.A. **189**:45, 1964.

Review: Iron deficiency anemia, Nutr. Rev. **20**:164, 1962.

Review: Iron storage in bone marrow, Nutr. Rev. **21**:99, 1963.

Scott, D. E., and Pritchard, J. A.: Iron deficiency in healthy young college women, J.A.M.A. **199**:897, 1967.

Copper

Cartwright, G. E.: The question of copper deficiency in man, Amer. J. Clin. Nutr. **15**:94, 1964.

Cartwright, G. E.: The relationship of copper, cobalt, and other trace elements to hemopoiesis, Amer. J. Clin. Nutr. **3**:11, 1955.

Cartwright, G. E., and Wintrobe, M. M.: Copper metabolism in normal subjects, Amer. J. Clin. Nutr. **14**:224, 1964.

Copper cooking utensils, J.A.M.A. **200**:426, 1967.

Cordano, A., and Graham, G. G.: Copper deficiency complicating chronic intestinal malabsorption, Pediatrics **38**:596, 1966.

Hook, L., and Brandt, I. K.: Copper content of some low-copper foods, J. Amer. Diet. Ass. **49**:202, 1966.

Report: Preventing Wilson's disease sequelae (abnormal copper metabolism), J.A.M.A. **200**:41, 1967.

Sodium and potassium

Cooper, G. R., and Heap, B.: Sodium ion in drinking water. II. Importance, problems, and potential applications of sodium-ion-restricted therapy, J. Amer. Diet. Ass. **50**:37, 1967.

Dahl, L. K.: Salt, fat, and hypertension, Nutr. Rev. **18**:97, 1960.

Krehl, W. A.: Sodium, a most extraordinary dietary essential, Nutrition Today, **1**:16, 1966.

Krehl, W. A.: The potassium depletion syndrome, Nutrition Today **1**:20, 1966.

Potassium imbalance: programmed instruction, Amer. J. Nurs. **67**:343, 1967.

Report: Sodium intake in pregnancy: two views, J.A.M.A. **200**:42, 1967.

Review: Salt in the infant's diet, Nutr. Rev. **25**:82, 1967.

Seftel, H. C., and M. C. Kew: Early and intensive potassium replacement in diabetic acidosis, Diabetes **15**:694, 1966.

White, J. M., and others: Sodium ion in drinking water. I. Properties, analysis, and occurrence, J. Amer. Diet. Ass. **50**:32, 1967.

Trace elements

Council on Foods and Nutrition, American Medical Association, The use of aluminum cooking utensils in the preparation of foods, J.A.M.A. **146**:477, 1951.

Glinsmann, W. H., and others: Plasma chromium after glucose administration, Science **152**:1243, 1966.

Lang, V. M., and others: Manganese metabolism in college men consuming vegetarian diets, J. Nutr. **85**:132, 1965.

Mertz, W.: Biological role of chromium, Fed. Proc. **26**:186, 1967.

Prasad, A. S.: Nutritional metabolic role of zinc, Fed. Proc. **26**:172, 1967.

Prasad, A. S.: Zinc metabolism, Springfield, Ill., 1966, Charles C Thomas, Publisher.

Vought, R. L., and Landon, W. T.: Dietary sources of iodine, Amer. J. Clin. Nutr. **14**:186, 1964.

Vought, R. L., and Landon, W. T.: Iodine intake and excretion in healthy nonhospitalized subjects, Amer. J. Clin. Nutr. **15**:124, 1964.

CHAPTER 9

Water and electrolytes

Water is the one nutrient most vital to man's existence. Man can survive far longer without food than without water. Only air is a more constant need. Fulfilling the body's need for a continuous supply of water and maintaining the body's water composition are major economic, nutritional, and physiologic tasks.

Several basic concepts are essential to understanding of the uses of water in the human body. First, there is the idea of a unified whole. Man is one continuous body of water. The "sea within" is held in shape by a protective envelope of skin. Water diffuses freely to all parts and is controlled only by the water's own chemical potential. In this warm, fluid, chemical environment, life processes are sustained. Second, there is the concept of compartments of water within the whole. These compartments are separated by membranes. The quantities of water contained in each compartment are balanced by forces that maintain an equilibrium among the parts. Third, basic to an understanding of these balancing forces, there is the concept of particles (charged electrolytes and other solutes) in the water solution. It is the concentration and distribution of these particles that determines internal shifts and balances in body water.

Involved throughout is the unifying concept of homeostasis. The body has a tremendous resilience through its capacity to employ numerous, finely-balanced homeostatic mechanisms which protect its vital fluid supply. To relate these various parts to the whole, the following questions should be considered carefully:

1. Where is the water in the body and how is it distributed?
2. What is the overall balance between intake and output of water?
3. What forces control the distribution of water?
4. What is the role of the gastrointestinal tract in water distribution and use?
5. What is the role of the kidney with respect to body water?
6. How do hormones influence water balance?

BODY WATER AND ITS DISTRIBUTION

The body of the adult human male has been found by various investigators to be from 55 to 65% water; that of a woman is from 50 to 55% water. The higher water content in men is generally because of the greater muscle mass. (Striated muscle contains more water than any body tissue other than blood.) The remaining 40% of a man's weight is about 18% protein and related substances, 15% fat, and 7% minerals.

The body water performs three functions that are essential to life: (1) it helps give structure and form to the body through the turgor it provides for tissue, (2) it gives the aqueous environment that is necessary for cell metabolism, and (3) it provides the means for maintaining a stable body temperature.

The body water may be thought of as the total water outside the cells plus the total water inside the cells. These two quantities of water have been called compartments of body water: (1) the *extracellular fluid compartment* (ECF) is made

153

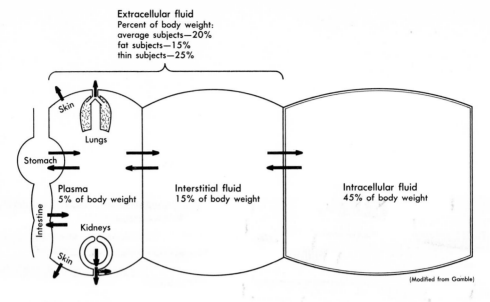

Fig. 9-1. Body fluid compartments. Note the relative total quantities of water in the intracellular compartment and in the extracellular compartment.

up of all the water outside the cells, and (2) the *intracellular fluid compartment* (ICF) is made up of all the water inside the cells.

Extracellular fluid compartment (ECF)

The collective water outside the cells makes up about 20% of the total body weight. Approximately one-fourth of this (5% of body weight) is contained in the blood plasma. The remaining three-fourths (15% of body weight) is made up of water surrounding the cells, water in dense tissue, and water in transit secretions. *Plasma* includes the total extracellular fluid within the heart and blood vessels. The *interstitial fluid and lymph* include the fluid environment in which the cells are bathed; it provides a transfer medium for materials entering and leaving the cells. *Fluid in dense tissue* includes water in dense connective tissue, cartilage, and bone. *Fluid in transit* includes transcellular water in cerebrospinal fluid and in secretions such as those of the salivary glands, thyroid gland, liver, pancreas, gallbladder, gastrointestinal tract, gonads, various mucous membranes, skin, kidneys, and eye spaces.

Intracellular fluid compartment (ICF)

The total water inside the body cells amounts to about twice that outside the cells. This is not surprising, since the cell is the basic unit of structure of the entire body, and the cells are the sites of the vast basic metabolic activity of the body. The intracellular fluid compartment makes up about 40% of the total body weight.

These relative total amounts of body water in the different compartments are compared in Fig. 9-1.

OVERALL WATER BALANCE: INTAKE AND OUTPUT

The average adult metabolizes from 2½ to 3 liters of water per day in a constant turnover balanced between intake and output. Normally, water enters and leaves the body by various routes, controlled by such basic mechanisms as *thirst* and *hormonal control of renal excretion.* Thirst is a distinct physical sensation and a conscious demand for water caused by (1) extracellular dehydration, (2) low cardiac output, or hemorrhage, (3) intracellular dehydration, and (4) dryness of the mouth. The hormonal regulation of renal excretion is under the control of the antidiuretic hormone (ADH; also called vasopressin) which is secreted by the pituitary gland. These mechanisms of dehydration and hormone control will be discussed later. First, the routes of water intake and water output will be compared.

Water intake

Water enters the body in three main forms: (1) as preformed water in liquids, (2) as preformed water in foods, and (3) as a product of oxidation.

Preformed water in liquids. Water and other beverages are the main source of ingested fluid. From 1,200 to 1,500 ml. of liquid is ingested daily in this form.

Preformed water in foods. Foods vary with respect to their water content from those with a large amount such as tomatoes, oranges, and watermelon to those that contain little water, such as dried fruit and legumes. The water ingested in foods that are eaten (rather than as liquid that is drunk) contributes from 700 to 1,000 ml. daily.

Water of oxidation. When nutrients are burned or oxidized in the body, one of the end products is water. The amount of metabolic water produced varies with different nutrients. For example, 100 grams of fat produces 107 grams of water; 100 grams of carbohydrate produces 55 grams of water; and 100 grams of protein produces 41 grams of water. On the whole, from 200 to 300 ml. of water is contributed daily from the body's metabolic activity. This brings the daily water intake from 2,100 to 2,800 ml.

Water output

Water leaves the body through the kidneys, the skin, the lungs, or the feces.

Kidneys. The kidneys of an adult normally excrete from 1 to 2 liters of urine daily. The water in this total amount is made up of two portions, the obligatory water excretion and the facultative water excretion. *Obligatory water excretion* is the amount of water that the kidney is "obligated" to excrete in order to rid the body of its daily load of urinary solutes. Since about 15 ml.

of water is required to dissolve 1 gm. of solute, the quantity of obligatory water excretion depends upon how large a load of metabolic end products (solutes such as urea and other metabolites) is seeking excretion, and also upon the concentrating power of the kidney. The average obligatory water excretion of an adult is approximately 900 ml. daily. *Facultative water excretion* occurs in addition to obligatory water loss. An additional 500 ml., more or less, may be excreted according to fluctuating body need and the renal tubular reabsorption rate.

Skin. About 350 ml. of water is lost daily through the skin by diffusion. Because man is unaware of this loss, it is called *insensible water loss.* An additional 100 ml. may be lost in normal perspiration. Heavier sweating, caused by heat and/or increased activity, may cause the loss of 250 ml. of water, more or less, according to body need. Therefore, under usual circumstances, from 450 to 700 ml. of water is lost daily through the skin. Excessive sweating, or loss of skin as in extensive burns, further increases the water output.

Lungs. An insensible water loss of about 350 ml. occurs daily through normal respiration vapor. This amount varies with climate, being least in hot, humid weather and greatest in very cold temperatures.

Feces. A small amount of water, from 150 to 200 ml., is usually lost daily through intestinal elimination. In abnormal conditions such as diarrhea or dysentery much greater losses will occur.

On the average, daily water output from the adult body totals about 2,600 ml. This comparative intake and output balance is summarized in Table 9-1.

FORCES INFLUENCING WATER DISTRIBUTION

Forces that influence and control the distribution of water in the body revolve around two factors: (1) the *solutes* (particles in solution in body water) and (2) the *membranes* that separate the water compartments.

Table 9-1. Approximate daily adult intake and output of water

Intake (replacement) ml. per day		Output (loss)		
			Obligatory (insensible) ml. per day	Additional (according to need) ml. per day
Preformed		Lungs	350	
Liquids	1,200 to 1,500	Skin		
In foods	700 to 1,000	Diffusion	350	
		Sweat	100	±250
Metabolism (oxidation		Kidneys	900	±500
of food)	200 to 300	Feces	150	
Total	2,100 to 2,800		1,850	750
	(approx. 2,600 ml. per day)		(approx. 2,600 ml. per day)	

Solutes

Three types of solutes influence internal shifts and balances of body water. These are electrolytes, plasma proteins, and organic compounds of small molecular size.

Electrolytes. Certain inorganic compounds (usually an acid, an alkali, or a salt) partly dissociate into their constituent ions when they are dissolved in water. An *ion* is an atom or a group of atoms that carries an electrical charge. This charge may be *positive*, because the atom has *lost* one of the negatively charged electrons that orbit around its nucleus, or *negative*, because the atom has *gained* a negatively charged orbiting electron. The word *ion*, which is derived from the Greek word meaning "wanderer," emphasizes that such an atom wanders freely in a solution, dissociated from the compound of which it was a part. A compound that dissociates into ions when in solution is called an *electrolyte* (Gr. *electron*, amber + *lytos*, a solution). This term refers to the fact that a solution containing one of these substances can transmit an electric current. If an electric current is passed through a volume of water in which an electrolyte is dissolved, the ions that dissociate themselves from the electrolyte migrate toward the pole that carries the electric charge opposite to the electric

charge of that particular ion; the positively charged ions cluster around the negative pole, and the negatively charged ions migrate to the positive pole. The two forms of ions are cations and anions. A *cation* is an ion that carries a positive charge (Na^+, K^+, Ca^{++}, Mg^{++}); an *anion* is an ion that carries a negative charge (Cl^-, HCO_3^-, $HPO_4^=$, $SO_4^=$). Electrolytes constitute a major force controlling fluid balances within the body (see also pp. 158 and 159).

Plasma proteins. Plasma proteins are organic substances of large molecular size, mainly albumin and globulin, which influence the shift of water from one compartment to another. They are called colloids (Gr. *kolla*, glue) and form *colloidal solutions.* Such a solution is a mixture of large, gelatinous particles or molecules which do not readily pass through separating membranes. Therefore, they normally remain in the blood vessels, where they exert a *colloidal osmotic pressure* (COP), which maintains the integrity of the blood volume in the vascular compartment.

Organic compounds of small molecular size. Organic compounds of small molecular size include such substances as glucose, urea, and amino acids. Because of their small size, they diffuse freely and therefore affect water balances only if they occur in unusually large amounts. For example, the large amount of glucose in the urine of a patient with uncontrolled diabetes causes an abnormal osmotic diuresis or excess water output.

Separating membranes

Two basic types of separating membranes are involved in the movements of water and solutes within the body. These are the capillary wall and the cell wall. The capillary wall is a relatively free or rapid membrane, across which electrolytes pass readily. The cell wall is a slow membrane, and is more difficult to penetrate. It is composed essentially of a lipid matrix, covered on either surface by a layer of protein. The metabolic processes within the cell usually govern the passage of electrolytes (and therefore water) across this barrier.

Mechanisms for movement of water and solutes across membranes

According to the type of membrane and the number of particles in the involved solution, water and solutes move across membranes by one or more of five mechanisms: osmosis, diffusion, active transport, filtration, or pinocytosis.

Osmosis. The word, osmosis comes from the Greek word *osmos* meaning "to push" or "to thrust." Osmosis is the process by which water molecules pass through a semi-permeable membrane separating two solutions. The molecules pass from the more dilute solution (water concentration is *higher*, the solute concentration is *lower*) to the more dense solution (water concentration is *lower*, the solute concentration is *higher*). Osmotic pressure is created by the difference in molecular pressure on either side of the membrane. The process may be thought of as a thrusting force in which water molecules, relatively unimpeded by the presence of many solute particles, push through the membrane more freely than the molecules that are laden with solute. It may also be thought of as a pulling force exerted by the denser solution, in which the burden of solute particles hinders the movement of the water molecules. As a consequence, the solution that is laden with solutes draws to itself a greater number of water molecules to enhance its mobility. Whether osmosis is thought of as a pushing or a pulling force, it tends to equalize the concentration of solutes and the fluid pressure on each side of a membrane. As it does so, it effectively controls the movement of water from place to place in the body.

Diffusion. The word diffusion comes from the Latin word *diffundere,* meaning "to spread" or "pour forth." It is the process by which particles in solution spread throughout the solution and across separating membranes, from the place of highest solute

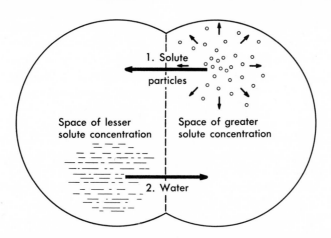

Fig. 9-2. Movement of molecules, water, and solutes by osmosis and diffusion.

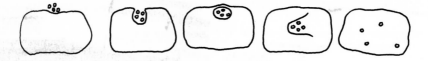

Fig. 9-3. Pinocytosis—engulfing of large molecules by the cell.

concentration to all spaces of lesser solute concentration. The movements of molecules in osmosis and diffusion are compared in Fig. 9-2.

Active transport. Many times a significant movement of substances across a membrane is accomplished even against the usual pressure gradient. This may be compared to a person swimming upstream or walking uphill against gravity's pull. Obviously such movement against pressure requires energy. In the case of substances moving across membranes in the body, the requisite energy comes from metabolism in the cells. Usually some vehicle or mechanism of transport is needed in addition. An example of such active transport is the operation of the sodium pump by which glucose is absorbed from the intestinal lumen and into individual cells (see Fig. 2-3, p. 18). Other molecules such as amino acids and fatty acids enter and leave cells by a similar means of active transport.

Filtration. Fluid is forced or filtered through membranes when there is a difference in pressure on the two sides. For example, filtration occurs across the capillary walls because the hydrostatic pressure within the capillary is greater than that in the surrounding interstitial fluid area. Small molecules pass with the fluid out of the capillary lumen, but the large molecules of plasma protein remain. These pressures are diagrammed in Fig. 9-5, p. 162.

Pinocytosis. Proteins and fats sometimes enter cells by the interesting process of pinocytosis (Fig. 9-3). The word means "cell drinking." It does not mean the cell itself is engulfed; rather, as these large molecules become attached to the cell's outer surface, the cell membrane forms a pocket and encircles them. This creates an invagination, or incupping, on the cell surface, from which the engulfed material is eventually released into the cell cytoplasm. Apparently this is the mechanism by which fat, for example, is absorbed from the small intestine (Fig. 3-5, p. 36).

ELECTROLYTES

Because the electrolytes play such a prominent role in the control of water balance in the body, it will be well to discuss them in greater detail. They may be considered in four important aspects: (1) *measurement* of electrolytes in body fluids, (2) electrolyte *composition* of body fluids, (3) electrolyte *balance* within fluid compartments, (4) electrolyte *control of body hydration.*

Measurement of electrolytes

The chemical activity of a solution is determined by the concentration of electrolytes (charged solutes) in a given volume of the solution. Concentration is a function of volume, since the degree of concentration indicates the number of particles or charges in a unit volume. It is the *number* of particles in a solution, not the *weights* of the various particles, that is the important factor in determining chemical combining power. Electrolytes are dynamically active chemicals; the ions that are released when the electrolyte enters into solution carry charges of electrical energy, and each particle contributes chemical combining power to the whole according to its *valence,* not its weight. Therefore, electrolytes are measured according to the total number of particles in solution rather than total weight.

The unit of measure commonly used is an *equivalent,* with hydrogen as a reference point. One equivalent of a substance is equal to the combining power of one gram of hydrogen. Since small amounts are

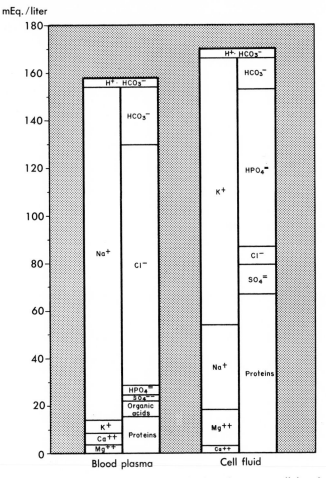

Fig. 9-4. Electrolyte distribution in extracellular fluid and in intracellular fluid. (From James L. Gamble: *Chemical anatomy, physiology and pathology of extracellular fluid,* Cambridge, Mass., 1954, Harvard University Press.)

usually in question, most physiologic measurements are expressed in terms of *milliequivalents.* One milliequivalent (mEq.) is equal to the chemical combining power of one milligram of hydrogen. The term milliequivalent refers to the *number of ions* (cations and anions) in solution, as determined by their concentration in a given volume. This measure is expressed as the number of milliequivalents per liter (mEq. /L.).

Electrolyte composition of body fluids

Electrolytes are distributed in the body water compartments in a definite pattern, which has great physiologic significance. This distribution pattern (the pattern of

relative positions and concentrations) provides the overall regulation of water shifts and balances, as well as the basis of respective tissue functions.

The comparative profiles of electrolyte distribution are shown in Fig. 9-4. Several electrolyte characteristics of each major fluid compartment are important to note and remember.

Extracellular fluid (ECF). Ionized sodium (Na^+) is the main cation in extracellular fluid. Sodium provides about 90% of the total base concentration (or about 45% of the total electrolyte concentration) in the body water outside the cells. Its concentration here is much greater than inside the cells. The sodium in the extracellular fluid provides the primary osmotic force that maintains the water volume necessary for the cell environment. The amounts of the other cations (K^+, Ca^{++}, Mg^{++}) in the extracellular fluid are relatively small.

Ionized chlorine (Cl^-) is the main anion in extracellular fluid. Chloride provides the main balancing anion in the extracellular fluid. It is present in particularly high concentration in gastric secretions as a constituent of hydrochloric acid, and in interstitial lymph.

The extracellular fluid also contains the variable anion bicarbonate (HCO_3^-), the fixed anions phosphate ($HPO_4^=$), sulfate ($SO_4^=$), and protein, together with various organic acids (such as lactic acid and pyruvic acid). A fixed anion is one that is not destroyed by the metabolic processes for example, Cl^-, $PO_4^=$, $SO_4^=$. Because they are not destroyed metabolically, the fixed anions are excreted in the urine. A variable or unfixed anion is one that is converted during metabolism to other chemical forms; for example, bicarbonate is converted to carbon dioxide and water, which are used in various metabolic processes. Organic anions are similarly converted and used. The variable ions do not have to be excreted in the urine, since they do not cause the kidney to perform work in selecting them for passage in the urine.

Protein is in the plasma portion of the extracellular fluid. If the electrolyte profiles of interstitial and plasma portions of the extracellular fluid are compared, it will be noted that they are the same, except for one important difference. The extracellular fluid protein is in the plasma portion only. These are the plasma proteins present in the blood vessels that provide the colloidal osmotic pressure necessary to maintain the integrity of blood volume.

Intracellular fluid. Ionized potassium (K^+) is the main cation in the intracellular fluid. The relative concentrations of ionized sodium and potassium in the intracellular fluid are the reverse of those in the extracellular fluid. Ionized potassium is concentrated within the cells where it provides a

major osmotic force for maintaining the necessary water volume inside the cell. Most of the cellular potassium is free. However, a significant amount—about one-third—is bound with the cell protein. Therefore, when cell protein is broken down, as in tissue oxidation or extensive tissue destruction, more potassium is freed and influences fluid shifts.

Phosphate ($HPO_4^=$) is the main anion in the intracellular fluid. Because of the significant role of phosphate in cell metabolism in the various energy-producing chains and pathways for glucose oxidation, a much greater concentration of this anion is found inside the cells than outside.

The quantity of protein in the cell fluid is three or four times greater than that in the extracellular plasma. Again, this is not surprising because of the greater protoplasmic mass in tissue cells, and the important work of protein synthesis constantly going on in each cell. Together with phosphate, then, protein constitutes a major cellular anion.

Electrolyte balance within fluid compartments

Biochemical and electrophysical laws demand that in a stable solution the number of positively charged particles must equal the number of negatively charged particles. In other words, the solution must be electrically neutral. When shifts and losses occur, compensating shifts and gains follow to maintain electroneutrality.

Such a balance does indeed exist in body fluids, as can be seen by adding up the respective concentrations of cations and anions in each fluid compartment expressed in mEq. (see Table 9-2).

Electrolyte control of body hydration

As indicated, ionized sodium is the chief cation of extracellular fluid and ionized potassium is the chief cation of intracellular fluid. These two electrolytes, with the others present in smaller amounts, exercise control over the amount of water to be retained in any given compartment. The usual bases for these shifts in water from one compartment

Table 9-2. Balance of cation and anion concentrations in extracellular fluid (ECF) and intracellular fluid (ICF), which maintains electroneutrality within each compartment

		ECF		ICF	
Cation	Anion	Cation (mEq./L.)	Anion (mEq./L.)	Cation (mEq./L.)	Anion (mEq./L.)
Na^+		142		35	
K^+		5		123	
Ca^{++}		5		15	
Mg^{++}		3		2	
	Cl^-		104		5
	$HPO_4^=$		2		80
	$SO_4^=$		1		10
	Org. acids		5		
	Protein		16		70
	HCO_3^-		27		10
Totals		155	155	175	175

to another are changes occurring in the *extracellular* concentrations of these electrolytes. The terms *hypertonic dehydration* and *hypotonic dehydration* refer to the electrolyte concentration of the water *outside* the cell, which in turn causes a shift of water into or out of the cell.

Hypertonic dehydration. In the extracellular fluid, when water loss exceeds electrolyte loss, the extracellular fluid becomes hypertonic to the intracellular fluid (the osmotic pressure of the extracellular fluid is higher than that of the intracellular fluid). The imbalance in osmotic pressures causes water to shift from the cell into the extracellular fluid spaces. This situation could occur from either excess water loss or water restriction. Clinical manifestations include severe thirst, hot, dry body (especially the tongue), vomiting, disorientation, and scanty and concentrated urine.

Hypotonic dehydration. When large amounts of water are added to the extracellular fluid without the addition of sufficient electrolytes to maintain the normal density of the solutions, the extracellular fluid becomes hypotonic to the intracellular fluid. This type of imbalance in osmotic

pressures causes a compensatory shift of water from the extracellular fluid into the cell. The result is a dangerous shrinking of the extracellular fluid, especially the blood volume. Renal blood flow is impaired, and swelling of cells (cellular edema) occurs. This serious situation could result either from over-zealous hydration of patients (giving too much plain water without accompanying electrolytes) or from losses of both water and electrolytes and replacement with water only. Clinical manifestations include progressive weakness without thirst or decreased urine output. Also, the hematocrit reading and the red blood cell count are elevated because of concentration of the blood.

Influence of protein on internal fluid shifts

Protein influences the internal shifting of body water in three areas. These are the water exchange across capillary walls, water exchange across cell walls, and lymph drainage of tissue water.

Water exchange across capillary walls. The plasma proteins exert a tremendous colloidal osmotic pressure within the capillaries which pulls fluid and solutes from the interstitial spaces into the blood. This maintains the necessary plasma volume. About 70% of this total colloidal osmotic pressure comes from the albumin, which is present in a greater quantity than any other plasma protein; the remaining 30% is from the presence of globulins and fibrinogen. Because the molecules of the plasma proteins are for the most part too large to pass through the capillary wall, they exert a constant osmotic pull on the interstitial fluid. However, this osmotic pull is balanced by an opposite outward thrust (hydrostatic pressure) of the blood within the capillary. This blood pressure tends to push fluid *out* of the capillary lumen into the interstitial fluid. Throughout the length of the capillary—from the end at which it emerges from the arteriole to the end at which it merges into the venule—these two forces play against one another in an intricate and subtle opposition that produces an exquisite balance. At the arteriole end of the capillary, the hydrostatic pressure predominates just enough to filter some water and solutes (including salts and a small amount of protein) out into the tissue fluids. By the time the blood has reached the venous end of the capillary, it has lost so much water that the relative osmotic pull of the plasma proteins within

its lumen has risen considerably. Meanwhile, the opposing hydrostatic outward thrust has diminished because the fluid is just that much farther from the heart, which sent it on its way. The balance topples to the other side; water and solutes are drawn through the wall of the capillary into its lumen.

The statement of this equilibrium of pressures was first proposed in 1895 by E. H. Starling, and is now called *Starling's law of the capillaries*, or the *capillary fluid shift mechanism*. This equilibrium is one of the body's most important homeostatic mechanisms to maintain fluid balance. The diagram illustrating this fluid shift (Fig. 9-5) should be studied carefully.

The blood enters the capillary from the arteriole under a hydrostatic pressure from the heart beat of about 45 mm. mercury, which is the intracapillary blood pressure. Working against this pressure is the colloidal osmotic pressure of the protein molecules (approximately 25 mm. of mercury) and a small amount of resisting tissue turgor of the capillary wall (approximately 5 mm. of mercury). If the total of these resistant pressures (30 mm. of mercury) is subtracted from the blood pressure of 45 mm. of mercury, a net filtration pressure at the arteriole end of the capillary is 15 mm. of mercury.

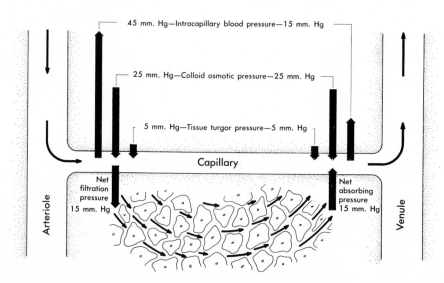

Fig. 9-5. The fluid shift mechanism. Note the balance of pressures which controls the flow of fluid.

Under this thrust, the water with its small amount of diffusible solutes (glucose, amino acids) goes out into the interstitial spaces to bathe the cells.

As the capillary flow continues to the venule end, the protein molecules that are too large to pass through the capillary wall accumulate, and maintain the colloidal osmotic pressure at about 25 mm. of mercury; but the blood pressure (from the cardiac impulse) has diminished to about 15 mm. of mercury. The balances are now reversed; the colloidal osmotic pressure exceeds the blood pressure, a net absorbing pressure of 15 mm. of mercury now prevails, and water is drawn back into the vascular compartment. The constant operation of this mechanism maintains the plasma volume and provides the transfer fluid environment to serve the cell's needs.

Water exchange across cell wall. In much the same way that the plasma proteins provide colloidal osmotic pressure which helps to maintain the integrity of the extracellular fluids, the cell protein (protoplasm) helps to provide the osmotic pressure that maintains the integrity of the intracellular fluid. Added to the osmotic pressure from the cell protein is the osmotic pressure provided by the intracellular ionized potassium. Balanced against the total intracellular pressure from these two sources is the osmotic pressure outside the cell, which is maintained by ionized sodium. As a result of the balance between the intracellular and the extracellular osmotic pressures, water and nutrients flow in and water and metabolic wastes flow out through the cell membrane.

Lymph drainage of tissue water. Protein in the lymphatic fluid provides a further means of removing excess water from the tissue spaces. During periods of relative inactivity of tissue, the capillaries are adequate to drain away the water that remains after exchanges. In an active organ, however, such as a contracting muscle, more water is produced. Here, the lymphatic vessels help to carry off the excess water, averting the accumulation of fluid (edema) in the interstitial spaces. The severe leg edema

seen in elephantiasis is a result of the cutting-off of this lymph circulation. A parasitic worm lodges in the lymph vessel and obstructs it, these fluids accumulate, and the leg swells.

ROLE OF THE GASTROINTESTINAL TRACT

In considering total fluid and electrolyte balance in the body, it is easy to lose sight of the vast importance of the gastrointestinal secretions in maintaining that balance. Water from the plasma, containing ions in patterns that vary according to numerous factors, is converted by the appropriate sections of the gastrointestinal tract into digestive secretions. These secretions, which are produced daily, function progressively throughout the alimentary system in the processes of digestion and absorption. They circulate constantly between plasma and secreting cells. Finally, in the distal portion of the intestine, most of the water and electrolytes are reabsorbed into the plasma to circulate again.

These fluids should be considered according to the sheer magnitude of the gastrointestinal secretions, and the serious results of fluid loss from the upper or the lower portion of the gastrointestinal tract.

Magnitude of the gastrointestinal secretions. Seldom realized are the enormous quantities of water and electrolytes secreted daily into the gastrointestinal tract. As indicated in Table 9-3, the total amount of fluid participating in the gastrointestinal circulation has been variously estimated from 7,500 to 10,000 ml. daily. The distribution of this total volume in the various secretions should be noted.

Because of the large quantities of fluid that are returned into the plasma, only from 100 to 150 ml. of water is left for fecal elimination.

The approximate total volume of the gastrointestinal secretions is 8,200 ml. while the total blood volume in the average sized adult is only 3,500 ml. The blood volume is less than half that of the gastrointestinal fluids. It is no wonder, then, that imbalances

Table 9-3. Approximate total volume of digestive secretions produced in twenty-four hours by adult of average size*

Saliva	1,500 ml.
Gastric	2,500
Bile	500
Pancreatic	700
Intestinal	3,000
Total	8,200 ml.

*From Gamble, J. L.: Chemical anatomy, physiology and pathology of extracellular fluid, ed. 6, Cambridge, Massachusetts, 1954, Harvard University Press.

Table 9-4. Approximate concentration of certain electrolytes in digestive fluids (mEq./L.)

	Na⁺	K⁺	Cl⁻	HCO₃⁻
Saliva	10	25	10	15
Gastric	40	10	145	0
Pancreatic	140	5	40	110
Jejunal	135	5	110	30
Bile	140	10	110	40

in gastrointestinal circulation, if allowed to go uncorrected, rapidly lead to serious consequences.

In addition, a surprisingly large amount of key cations and anions is present in the gastrointestinal tract. Table 9-4 shows the distribution of these electrolyes.

If the relative ionized potassium values of the various gastrointestinal secretions are compared, the *total* quantity of gastric ionized potassium is two to five times that of the blood serum. In the rest of the gastrointestinal tract, ionized potassium concentration is equal to that of the extracellular fluid. Also, there are large amounts of ionized sodium in the gastrointestinal fluids. These total approximately 1,000 mEq. per day, which is about one-third of the total body sodium. An adequate diet supplies sufficient amounts of these two cations—from 75 to 100 mEq. (3 to 4 gm.) of potassium and from 130 to 250 mEq. (8 to 15 gm.) of salt.

The gastrointestinal fluids are held in *isotonicity* (equality of osmotic pressure due to ion equilibrium) with the extracellular fluid compartment. When water is drunk without solutes or accompanying food, electrolytes and salts enter the intestine from the extracellular fluid. If a hypertonic solution or food is ingested, additional water is drawn into the intestine from the extracellular fluid. In each instance, water and electrolytes are shifted from compartment to compartment to maintain solutions in the alimentary tract isotonic with the extracelluar fluid. This law of isotonicity has many clinical implications. For example, what would happen if a patient on gastric suction drank water; or if a patient being maintained by tube feeding were given his formula too rapidly, at too concentrated a dilution? In the first case, the water would cause the stomach to produce more secretions containing electrolytes; the electrolytes would in turn be lost in the suctioning. The plasma, from which the electrolytes are supplied, would be gradually depleted of them and unable to supply these essential nutrients to tissue cells. In the second case, the hypertonic solution being given by tube would cause a shift of water into the intestine, which would rather rapidly shrink the vascular volume of the extracellular fluid.

Upper and lower gastrointestinal losses. It is not surprising, because of the large amounts of water and electrolytes involved, that loss of gastrointestinal secretions is the most common cause of clinical fluid and electrolyte problems. The biochemical problem differs according to whether the upper or the lower portion of the alimentary tract is involved. For example, in persistent vomiting, much fluid and hydrochloric acid is eliminated, and dehydration, a potassium deficit, and alkalosis result. In prolonged diarrhea, large amounts of water, sodium, chlorine, and bicarbonate are lost. As sodium losses continue, sodium is shifted from the plasma and interstitial fluid to replace it, and potassium then moves out of the cells to replace the extracellular sodium. The loss of potassium is compounded by the triggering of the aldosterone mechanism, a hormonal device for the conservation of sodium, and more potassium is eliminated in the process (see Fig. 9-8, p. 169).

ROLE OF THE KIDNEYS

The major responsibility for regulating the water and electrolyte balance in the body falls to the kidney. This marvelous organ is central to the successful operation of many other organs and tissues. In his delightful book, *From Fish to Philosopher*, Homer Smith places the kidney in a primary position in the body's hierarchy of parts. He states:

It is no exaggeration to say that the composition of the body fluids is determined not by what the mouth takes in but by what the kidneys keep: they are the master chemists of our internal environment. . . . Recognizing that we have the kind of internal environment we have because we have the kind of kidneys that we have, we must acknowledge that our kidneys constitute the major

foundation of our physiological freedom. Only because they work the way they do has it become possible for us to have bones, muscles, glands, and brains. Superficially, it might be said that the function of the kidneys is to make urine; but in a more considered view one can say that the kidneys make the stuff of philosophy itself.[1]

The basic anatomy and physiology of the kidney should be reviewed carefully in terms of water and electrolyte balance. The kidney's functional unit, the *nephron*, is particularly well adapted in structure for this vital regulatory role (Fig. 9-6). There are two significant aspects of this role: (1) the nephron's basic functions, for which it is uniquely structured, and (2) the hormonal homeostatic mechanisms involved in renal control of water and electrolyte conservation and excretion.

Functions of the nephron

In the cortex of each kidney there are about one million minute, finely structured, functioning units called nephrons. The tremendous capacity of these units to select, reject, conserve, and eliminate is demonstrated over and over again, as they cleanse the blood fifteen to eighteen times every day. Filtration, tubular reabsorption, and secretion are the three basic functions involved in this overall control process.

Filtration. Filtration has been defined (p. 158) as one of the ways in which water and certain solutes move across capillary walls as the result of pressure differences on either side. Because the intracapillary fluid pressure is greater than the interstitial fluid pressure, water and small freely diffusible molecules pass out of the capillary through its wall into the surrounding interstitial fluid and thence into the absorbing capsule of the renal tubule. In the nephron, several structures are especially adapted to facilitate this initial filtration process. These structures are the arterioles, and the cells in the walls of the glomerules and the capsule.

Afferent and efferent arterioles. The head of the nephron consists of a cuplike structure called Bowman's capsule, which holds the glomerulus (a tuft of branching capillaries). The afferent (entering) arteriole is relatively large. As it breaks up into its many branching capillaries it offers a narrowing stream bed, which effectively slows down the renal blood flow to promote filtration. The loops of the capillary tuft join again, to form a single vessel, the efferent (leaving) arteriole, which is of smaller diameter than the afferent arteriole. This offers resistance to flow, and produces additional backward pressure to favor filtration.

Further control is added by the ability of the uniquely muscular afferent and efferent arterioles to constrict or dilate independently of one another, according to blood pressure requirements. For example, when the blood pressure is lower, the afferent arteriole may dilate and efferent arteriole constrict to provide additional pressure favoring filtration. If the blood pressure is high, this reaction may be reversed.

Cells in walls of glomerulus and capsule. The glomerulus and the receiving tubular capsule are lined with long, thin, flat cells especially structured to provide optimum filtration and absorbing surfaces. Resistance to flow is therefore minimized and filtration occurs readily.

Tubular reabsorption. After water and

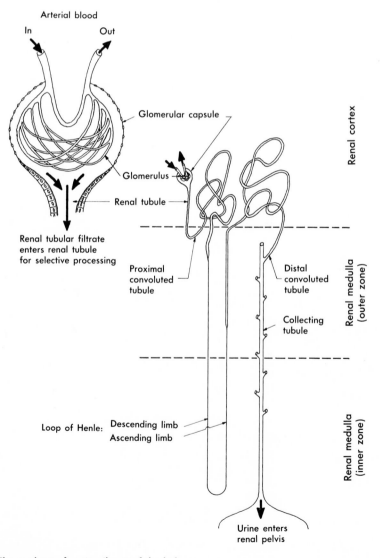

Fig. 9-6. The nephron—functional unit of the kidney.

filterable solutes are filtered from the blood via the glomerulus into the receiving capsule, they pass in turn through the three portions of the tubule in which selective reabsorption takes place. These areas are the proximal tubule, the loop of Henle, and the distal tubule. It is in these areas that the nephron carries on its highly selective process of reabsorbing needed materials and rejecting others for eventual elimination. In this process, the nephrons perform several tasks. They control the amount of water in the body and the electrolyte level, they excrete various electrolytes as waste products, and they excrete excess metabolic materials.

Amount of water in the body. By varying the amount of water retained or eliminated, the nephrons effectively control and guard the total fluid volume. This control is largely regulated in turn by certain hormones, such as the antidiuretic hormone (ADH, vaso-

pressin) from the pituitary. Indirect control is also exerted by aldosterone. These two important homeostatic mechanisms are discussed on pp. 168-170. As the result of the renal tubular control of hydration, 99% of the water filtered is recovered and returned into the bloodstream to be reused.

Levels of electrolytes in the body. The nephrons also have the task of maintaining various electrolyte blood levels within normal ranges. The integrity of the concentration of certain electrolytes, especially of sodium and potassium, is necessary for delicate fluid-electrolyte and acid-base balances throughout the body. The control of sodium concentration illustrates the adaptation of the nephron's structure and function to the maintenance of the proper supply of electrolytes. Two interesting mechanisms are involved. One is the aldosterone mechanism, which is periodically triggered by a threat-

TO PROBE FURTHER
Renal reabsorption of sodium by the countercurrent system

The reabsorption of sodium is continuously carried on in the nephron as one of its most significant tasks in reclaiming this vital electrolyte. The reabsorption of sodium occurs between the two limbs of the loop of Henle, and is believed to involve a *countercurrent system* of active transport. This countercurrent theory, advanced by Wirz* and now widely held, contributes a significant step in the knowledge of renal function and physiology. As the fluid that has passed through the distal convoluted tubule flows through the portion of the loop of Henle that descends into the inner zone of the renal medulla, much of its water passes out into the interstitial fluid, while the sodium moves on into the ascending limb of the loop of Henle. From this site, the sodium is actively transported out of the ascending limb into the interstitial fluid of the medulla, then back into the descending limb by means of a series of sodium pumps. The result is a progressive increase in sodium concentration (and therefore in the osmolarity) of the urine in all structures from the inner to outer portions of the renal medulla. The net effect is to conserve water and concentrate the urine in the distal collecting duct as it passes through this hyperosmolar section of the medulla on its way to the renal pelvis. The total system that controls levels of osmolarity has come to be known as the *countercurrent multiplier of concentration*. These relationships are shown in Fig. 9-7.

---

*Wirz, H.: Kidney, water, and electrolyte metabolism, Ann. Rev. Physiol. **23**:577, 1961.

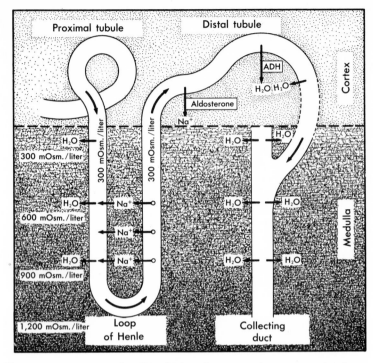

Fig. 9-7. Countercurrent system of sodium (Na) and water exchange operating between the two limbs of the loop of Henle.

ened loss of sodium. The other is a continuous, active transport process that involves a countercurrent system against the usual osmotic pressure gradient. This system makes use of the sodium pump.

Excretion of various metabolites as waste products. The waste products excreted by the nephrons include such materials as urea and excess ketones, which the nephrons selectively reject and discard, thus preventing their harmful accumulation in the blood.

Excretion of excess metabolic materials. The nephrons excrete harmful excess loads of otherwise beneficial metabolic materials. Glucose, for example, is a beneficial product of the metabolism of carbohydrates. Normally it is not excreted but is conserved for use. However, in uncontrolled diabetes, the glucose accumulates in the blood to harmful levels, and the kidney then begins to excrete these excesses.

Secretion. A third major function of the kidney involved in control of fluid and electrolytes, especially as related to acid-base balance, is secretion. Control of acidity is effected by secretion of hydrogen ions and ammonia from the blood. This function is further detailed in the general discussion of acid-base balance on p. 173.

Hormonal control of water and electrolyte balance

The two hormonal mechanisms designed to guard the body's water and electrolytes and to maintain their state of equilibrium are the antidiuretic hormone (ADH) mechanism, and the aldosterone mechanism. These mechanisms function to protect the integrity of the blood volume and to maintain adequate circulation despite real or threatened deprivation of water or sodium.

ADH mechanism. The antidiuretic hormone secreted by the posterior lobe of the pituitary gland acts mainly in the distal collecting tubule. It stimulates the reabsorption of water according to body need. Excess secretion of the hormone may be

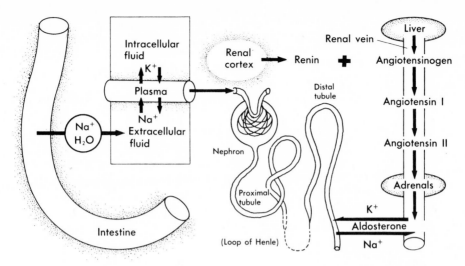

Fig. 9-8. The aldosterone mechanism which conserves sodium in exchange for potassium and causes increased reabsorption of water.

triggered by a real or apparent loss of body water. The actual loss of body water, as in hemorrhage, engages the ADH mechanism in an effort to conserve water. In certain situations, such as congestive heart failure, the body water is not actually diminished, but is shifted from the circulating plasma into the interstitial extracellular fluid spaces by the diminished action of the heart. Included in this general reduction of plasma flow to all organs is reduction of plasma flow to the kidney. The kidney interprets this diminished plasma flow to mean that the body is deprived of water, and the ADH mechanism is set in motion in an effort to conserve water for the total body.

The mechanism by which ADH is released from the pituitary is believed to be mediated by changes of the osmotic pressure in the plasma that bathes the hypothalamus. It is further believed that in the hypothalamus there are pressure-sensitive centers called *osmoreceptors* (volume receptors). Their precise location within the hypothalamus is not known. Various stress reactions inducing shock stimulate release of the hormone to guard water and electrolytes.

Aldosterone mechanism. A second important hormone that governs the renal control of water and electrolyte balance is the aldosterone mechanism. This mechanism is primarily a sodium-conserving device, but in carrying out this function it also exerts a secondary control over the diuresis of water. Therefore, it essentially restores the volume of extracellular fluid and of circulating blood in times of stress and threatened loss. The operation of the aldosterone mechanism involves a specific cycle of events (Fig. 9-8):

1. When sodium intake is decreased, or sodium is lost, or body fluid volume is contracted, the renal cortex forms the enzyme *renin* and secretes it into the blood via the renal vein. In the blood, renin acts upon its specific substrate from the liver, *angiotensinogen,* to form *angiotensin I,* which in turn is converted to *angiotensin II.* The latter is an active pressor substance that increases the force of the heartbeat, constricts the arterioles, and diminishes renal blood flow.

2. Angiotensin II stimulates secretion of aldosterone by the adrenals. Aldosterone then causes retention and reabsorption of sodium, and therefore of water; improved renal circulation follows. A secondary result of aldosterone activity is a potassium loss in the tubular ion exchange for sodium.

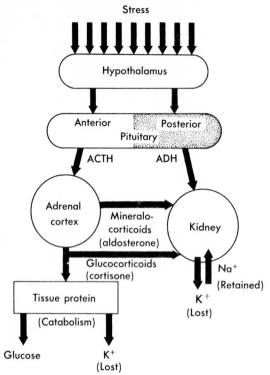

Stress

Hypothalamus

Anterior   Posterior
       Pituitary
  ACTH   ADH

Adrenal
cortex   Mineralo-
            corticoids   Kidney
            (aldosterone)

         Glucocorticoids   Na⁺
         (cortisone)   (Retained)

Tissue protein   K⁺
                                 (Lost)
(Catabolism)

Glucose   K⁺
               (Lost)

Fig. 9-9. Hormonal response to stress.

3. Aldosterone is operative chiefly in the distal renal tubule. It can increase reabsorption up to 98% as in shock, because of lowered blood volume. Shock shrinks the total fluid compartment; less fluid therefore circulates through the kidneys, and reabsorption of greater quantity is needed to supply the deficit.

Aldosterone release may also be stimulated by ACTH, a hormone secreted by the anterior pituitary in response to body stress. Both ADH and aldosterone mechanisms may be activated by stress situations such as bodily injury or surgery. The relationship of these hormones to stress is illustrated in Fig. 9-9.

Clinical applications

Many applications of these fluid and electrolyte balance principles may be discovered in daily clinical nursing practice. The following are questions concerning clinical situations which should be reviewed care-

fully to try to work out the chain of successive events that produce serious water and electrolyte imbalances. The linear diagrams of these triggering chains are given at the end of this chapter on pp. 176-178.

1. What accounts for the edema of starvation?
2. Why would cellular dehydration result from drinking sea water?
3. Why does potassium depletion occur in prolonged diarrhea?
4. Why would oliguria occur and why is there a danger of potassium depletion following surgery?
5. What is the danger of trying to hydrate a patient (one with diarrhea, for example) with plain water?
6. Why should patients on gastric suction not be allowed to have water in liquid or solid form?
7. Which is preferable for a gastric lavage—plain water or isotonic saline solution? Why?
8. Why are salt tablets supplied for men working at the open hearth in a steel mill? What is the danger of satisfying their thirst only with water?

Additional clinical applications center around postgastrectomy problems, edema in congestive heart failure, ascites in advanced liver disease, and renal disease such as the nephrotic syndrome. These specific situations are discussed in greater detail in Unit IV, Nutrition in Medical-Surgical Nursing.

ACID-BASE BUFFER SYSTEM

Water and electrolytes are involved in a second area that has broad physiologic implications—the *acid-base buffer system*. This system is essential to the maintenance of an optimal acid-base balance throughout the body. In order to understand the physiologic buffer systems, the answers to the following questions will be considered:

1. What is the difference between an acid and a base?
2. What is a buffer?
3. What ratio should exist between acids and bases if the buffer system is to successfully offset changes in the ion-

ized hydrogen concentration in the extracellular fluid?

4. What role do the kidney and lung play in maintaining the acid-base balance in the extracellular fluid?
5. What are acidosis and alkalosis?

Definitions of acid and base

A substance is *more or less* acid, according to the degree of its concentration of ionized hydrogen. Its degree of acidity is expressed in terms of pH. The symbol pH is derived from a mathematical term. It is the negative logarithm expressed as an exponential *p*ower of the *H*ydrogen ion concentration. If the pH of a solution is 5, its hydrogen ion concentration is 10^{-5}. The hydrogen ion concentration in pure water is 10^{-7}; therefore, the pH of pure water is 7. A pH of 7 is the neutral point between an acid and an alkaline (base). Substances with a pH *lower* than 7 are *acid*. (Since the pH is the *negative* logarithm, the higher the hydrogen ion concentration, the lower the pH). Substances with a pH above 7 are *alkaline*.

Acids. An acid may be defined as a compound that has enough hydrogen ions to give some away. When in aqueous solution, an acid releases hydrogen ions. The following are some examples of acids and their donation of ionized hydrogen when in aqueous solution:

$$H_2CO_3 \rightarrow H^+ + HCO_3$$
$$HCl \rightarrow H^+ + Cl$$
$$H_2SO_4 \rightarrow 2H^+ + SO_4$$
$$H_3PO_4 \rightarrow 2H^+ + HPO_4$$

Bases. A base possesses *few* hydrogen ions. It therefore takes up ionized hydrogen. The following are examples of bases:

$$OH^- + H^+ \rightarrow H_2O$$
$$HCO_3 + H^+ \rightarrow H_2CO_3$$
$$OH^- + H_2CO_3 \rightarrow H_2O + HCO_3$$

Buffers

The word *buffer* comes from a Middle English root meaning "to protect from blows." In the 17th century it referred to a coat of armor. In chemistry, a buffer is a mixture of acidic and alkaline components, which protects a solution against wide variations in its pH, even when strong bases or acids are added to it. A solution containing such a protective mixture is called a *buffered solution*. A buffer protects the acid-base balance of a solution by rapidly offsetting changes in its ionized hydrogen concentration. It works by protecting against either added acid or base.

Protection against added acid. If a strong acid is added to a buffered solution, the base partner of the acid-base buffer reacts with the added acid to form a weaker acid. The acidity of the total solution is effectively lowered toward (or to) the starting point. Formula 9-1 shows the reaction when hydrochloric acid is added to a buffered solution. The H^+ donated by the hydrochloric acid is taken up by the bicarbonate to form a weaker acid.

Protection against added base. If a strong base is added to a buffered solution, the acid partner of the buffer donates ionized hydrogen, which combines with the intruder to form a weaker base and restores the pH to the starting point. Formula 9-2 shows the reaction that occurs if sodium hydroxide is added to a buffered solution.

The human body contains many buffered solutions, including those that involve hemoglobin, oxyhemoglobin, protein, and the disodium hydrogen phosphate-sodium dihydrogen phosphate (Na_2HPO_4-NaH_2PO_4) system. Its main buffer system is the relatively weak carbonic acid-sodium bicarbonate (H_2CO_3-$NaHCO_3$) system. The

(strong acid)		(base-buffer)		(weaker acid)		(salt)	
HCl	+	$NaHCO_3$	$\rightarrow$	H_2CO_3	+	NaCl	(9-1)
hydrochloric acid		sodium bicarbonate		carbonic acid		table salt	

(strong base)		(acid-buffer)		(weaker base)		(water)	
NaOH	+	H_2CO_3	$\rightarrow$	$NaHCO_3$	+	H_2O	(9-2)
sodium hydroxide		carbonic acid		sodium bicarbonate		water	

body selects this as its principal buffer system for two reasons: (1) the raw materials for the production of carbonic acid (CO_2 + H_2O = H_2CO_3) are readily available and, (2) the lungs and kidneys can easily adjust to ratio alterations between carbonic acid and the base bicarbonate, sodium bicarbonate.

Buffer system ratio in the extracellular fluid

The normal pH of the extracellular fluid is 7.4, with a normal range from 7.35 to 7.45. Maintenance of the pH within this narrow range is necessary to sustain the life of cells. The carbonic acid-sodium bicarbonate buffer system is able to make an effective contribution to the stabilization of the extracellular fluid at this pH because the base bicarbonate partner in this buffer system is about twenty times as abundant as the carbonic acid. This 20:1 base to acid ratio is normally maintained even though the absolute amounts may fluctuate during compensation periods from the normal concentrations of 27 mEq./L. of base bicarbonate and 1.35 mEq./L. of carbonic acid. As long as the 20:1 ratio is maintained, the extracellular fluid acid-base balance is held constant (Fig. 9-10).

Roles of the lungs and kidneys

The lungs and kidneys guard the body's acid-base balance by regulating the supply of components of the carbonic acid-sodium bicarbonate buffer system. According to the body's immediate need each of these two organs conserves or releases substances that are essential to the production of either base or acid. This permits the buffer system to perpetuate the necessary 20:1 base to acid ratio.

Lungs. The lungs ultimately control the body's supply of carbonic acid. Carbonic acid is formed from carbon dioxide and water:

$$CO_2 + H_2O \rightarrow H_2CO_3$$

Changes in rate and depth of breathing alter the amounts of carbon dioxide that

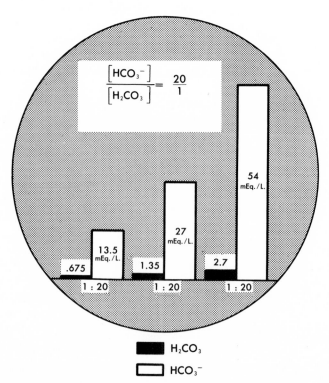

Fig. 9-10. The base to acid ratio of 20:1 maintains a constant normal blood pH of 7.4.

enter the body, which effectively control the level of carbonic acid in blood and tissues. When the blood level of sodium bicarbonate goes down, the lungs expel excess carbon dioxide; this decreases the quantity of raw material available for the production of carbonic acid, and the ratio of base to acid in the buffer system is restored to 20:1.

Kidneys. The kidneys maintain the base bicarbonate component of this buffer system. In the renal tubule, hydrogen ions are secreted; in an ion exchange with hydrogen, sodium is recaptured, and returned to the blood stream. The sodium is combined with HCO_3^- to form sodium bicarbonate (Na HCO_3).

The kidney also conserves base by eliminating extra hydrogen ions, through the production and excretion of ammonia (NH_4):

$$NH_3 + H^+ \rightarrow NH_4$$
$$\updownarrow$$

from
deamination
of
amino acids

ACIDOSIS AND ALKALOSIS

The key concept that has enabled investigators to understand the clinical states of acidosis and alkalosis is ionized hydrogen *concentration*. It was not possible to develop adequate therapy for these states as long as they were thought of merely as conditions in which the blood was "more acid" or "more alkaline." *In acidosis, the ionized hydrogen concentration is above normal. In alkalosis, ionized hydrogen concentration is below normal.* Either of these abnormal states initiates compensatory responses of the buffer system, lungs, and kidneys, which cause body fluids to accept, to release, or to excrete ionized hydrogen. Increases and decreases in ionized hydrogen concentration are therefore modified so that the pH is not significantly changed from its normal range of 7.35 to 7.45. Failure of either the lungs or the kidneys to carry out their functions results in acidosis or alkalosis. If the failure is predominantly related to the pulmonary system, the clinical result is called respira-

tory acidosis or respiratory alkalosis. If the failure is chiefly related to the renal system, the resultant clinical state is called metabolic acidosis or metabolic alkalosis.

Respiratory acidosis

Cause. Diseases that interfere with normal breathing impede the release of carbon dioxide from the lungs. The retained carbon dioxide combines with water and forms carbonic acid. The carbonic acid level may rise to twice normal. In addition, the carbon dioxide combining power in the serum is increased by the presence of the carbon dioxide which was retained by the lungs.

Pulmonary compensation. The lung attempts to increase ventilation in order to expel excess carbon dioxide. It is often prevented from doing so by the same pulmonary disease that initiated the retention of carbon dioxide.

Renal compensation. Two compensatory responses take place in the kidney. First, increased ionized hydrogen is secreted by the renal tubule and exchanged for sodium; the sodium is combined with HCO_3 to form sodium bicarbonate ($NaHCO_3$), and is returned to the bloodstream. This elevates the base bicarbonate component in this buffer system. Second, increased quantities of ammonia are formed so that more ionized hydrogen is excreted.

Clinical examples. The exchange of oxygen and carbon dioxide occurs at the alveolo-capillary membrane. A variety of diseases that affect the lung involve this membrane, and therefore contribute to the development of respiratory acidosis. These include emphysema, bronchiectasis, asthma, pulmonary edema, bronchial pneumonia, and congestive heart failure. A similar effect may follow administration of inhalation anesthesia to a patient whose pulmonary function is marginal or weak. Respiratory acidosis may also occur because of paralysis of respiratory muscles as in poliomyelitis.

Respiratory alkalosis

Cause. The primary cause of respiratory alkalosis is excess carbon dioxide output, which in turn is caused by hyperventilation. The decrease in available carbon dioxide lowers the production of carbonic acid, and the ionized hydrogen concentration, therefore, falls (pH rises). In addition, because less carbon dioxide is available, carbon dioxide combining power is diminished.

Pulmonary compensation. The lung cannot initiate efforts to compensate for respiratory alkalosis, as it is directly involved in the cause; however, the decreased carbonic acid level in the extracellular fluid tends to gradually depress respiration.

Renal compensation. The major task of compensation falls to the kidneys, where tubular ionized hydrogen formation is suppressed so that sodium bicarbonate is excreted. Ammonia formation is also diminished, so that further sodium is excreted.

Clinical examples. Common causes of respiratory alkalosis are the hyperventilation syndrome (brought about by hysteria or acute anxiety); hyperpnea (labored breathing) in response to hot weather, high altitude, or fever; or excessive breathing forced upon a patient by a poorly adjusted mechanical respirator. Respiratory alkalosis may also result from overstimulation of the respiratory center in the brain; this may be brought about by salicylate (aspirin) poisoning (a frequent occurrence in children), or by meningitis or encephalitis.

Metabolic acidosis

Cause. In certain metabolic disorders, the blood may contain an excess of specific metabloic organic acids (ketones, lactic acid). Part of the bicarbonate in the buffer system is displaced by these acids, and the ionized hydrogen concentration rises.

Pulmonary compensation. In order to reduce the carbonic acid level, the lungs attempt to expel carbon dioxide by deep, pauseless breathing (air hunger or Kussmaul breathing). Kussmaul breathing is characteristic of diabetic acidosis, for example.

Renal compensation. The renal tubule increases its secretion of hydrogen ions which are exchanged for sodium. The sodium is returned to the blood as sodium bicarbonate.

Ammonia production rises, taking up ionized hydrogen and excreting it in the urine.

Clinical examples. It is interesting to trace (as in Fig. 25-2, p. 489) the chain of events, for example, that characterizes states of fluid and electrolyte imbalance in diabetic acidosis. These potentially disastrous consequences are brought about because, in these situations, the body cannot properly metabolize blood glucose and turns for its energy to the catabolism of protein and fat.

A similar metabolic situation prevails in starvation when the body turns to its own body stores of protein and fat to supply its needs. In states of accelerated metabolism such as thyrotoxicosis, when increased metabolic demand rapidly depletes carbohydrate stores, the body burns protein and stores, producing ketosis. Gastrointestinal problems may also produce metabolic acidosis. For example, although initial vomiting may cause metabolic alkalosis due to loss of gastric hydrochloric acid, prolonged vomiting frequently causes metabolic acidosis as the inability to eat results in decreased carbohydrate intake, glycogen depletion, burning of body protein and fat, and finally ketosis. Severe diarrhea may induce acidosis because large amounts of bicarbonate (HCO_3) and sodium (Na), as intestinal contents are swept away. Chronic and acute renal diseases may contribute to metabolic acidosis as the kidney becomes unable to compensate in the face of excess ionized hydrogen concentrations.

Metabolic alkalosis

Cause. Metabolic alkalosis is characterized by a fall in ionized hydrogen concentration (rise in pH), due primarily to an increase in bicarbonate. Such an excess of bicarbonate may be caused by excretion or loss of large amounts of ionize hydrogen, by excessive intake of bicarbonate, or by decrease in potassium stores: as ionized hydrogen and sodium move into the cell to replace lost potassium, the extracellular fluid concentration of ionized hydrogen is reduced.

Pulmonary compensation. The decreased

ionized hydrogen concentration (increased pH) gradually suppresses ventilation; the lungs tend to conserve carbon dioxide which increases the production of carbonic acid.

Renal compensation. The renal tubule suppresses secretion of ionized hydrogen, which allows sodium bicarbonate to be excreted rather than reabsorbed. Ammonia production is reduced, so that more base is excreted. The excretion of various acid metabolites is also reduced.

Clinical examples. Loss of ionized hydrogen and chlorine, as in initial vomiting, induces metabolic alkalosis. The same ions are lost in excessive gastric suction, or when the proximal intestine is obstructed, as by pyloric stenosis. Conditions that involve potassium depletion also induce alkalosis, as ionized hydrogen and sodium move into the cells to replace lost potassium. This reduces the extracellular fluid hydrogen concentra-

tion. Such conditions include lack of potassium intake, gastrointestinal loss of potassium, or ACTH (adrenocorticotrophic hormone) therapy. (ACTH induces renal tubular reabsorption of sodium in an ion exchange for potassium, and, therefore, potassium is excreted.) Excess intake of alkali powders or sodium bicarbonate, as in long-term ulcer therapy, may also contribute to alkalosis.

In all states of acid-base imbalance, two basic rules of treatment apply. First, the primary cause of the acidosis or alkalosis is treated. Second, efforts are made to aid the various compensatory responses of the lungs and kidneys. Each of these therapeutic attempts calls for careful and continuous adjustment. The summary diagram (Fig. 9-11) of the acid-base buffer system involving all four clinical situations (respiratory acidosis and alkalosis, metabolic acidosis and alkalosis) should be reviewed.

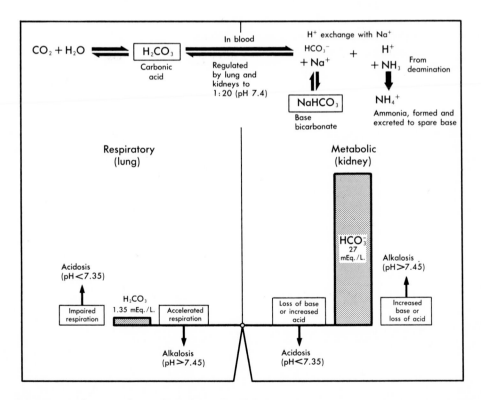

Fig. 9-11. Carbonic acid to sodium (base) bicarbonate buffer system. Note the types of clinical situations that lead to respiratory acidosis and alkalosis and to metabolic acidosis and alkalosis.

Answers to questions on p. 170

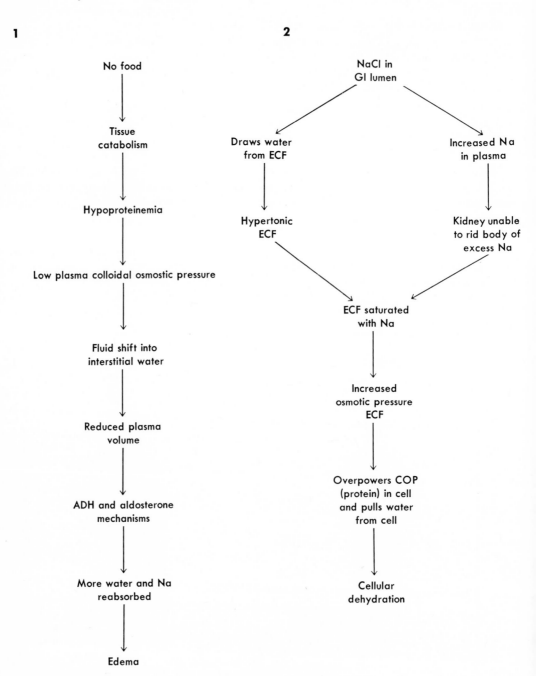

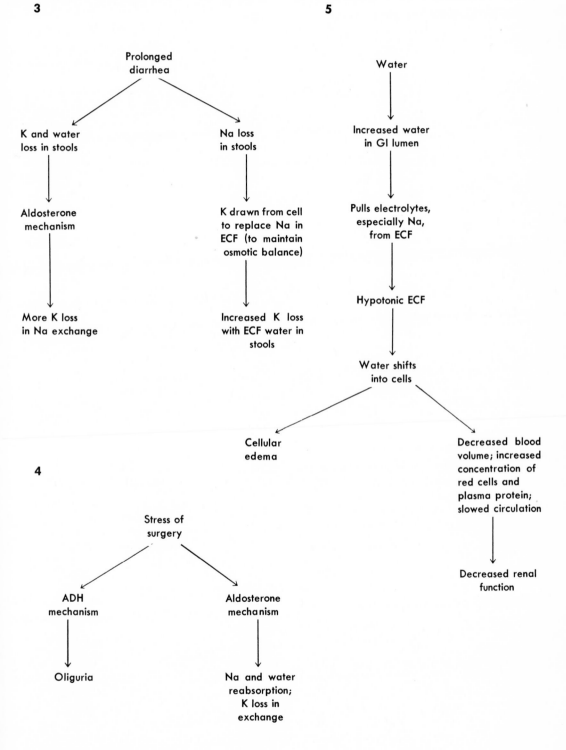

6

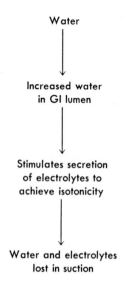

Water

↓

Increased water
in GI lumen

↓

Stimulates secretion
of electrolytes to
achieve isotonicity

↓

Water and electrolytes
lost in suction

7 Isotonic saline solution is better than plain water for gastric lavage. Same principle as in No. 6.

8

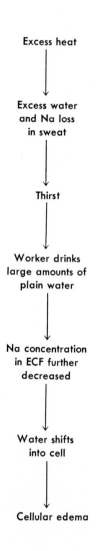

Excess heat

↓

Excess water
and Na loss
in sweat

↓

Thirst

↓

Worker drinks
large amounts of
plain water

↓

Na concentration
in ECF further
decreased

↓

Water shifts
into cell

↓

Cellular edema

GLOSSARY

acid (L. *acidus,* sour) a substance that is sour to taste and neutralizes base substances. Acids are essentially ionized hydrogen donors—in solution they provide H ions.

acidosis a disturbance in acid-base balance in which there is a reduction of the alkali reserve. Acidosis may be caused by an accumulation of acids (as in diabetic acidosis) or by an excess loss of bicarbonate (as in renal disease).

active transport the movement of solutes in solution (for example, products of digestion such as glucose) across a membrane *against* the usual pressure gradient. Movement against pressure requires energy, which is supplied by the cell. Sometimes an additional transporting substance is required such as the sodium pump for absorbing glucose, and the intrinsic factor (IF) for absorbing vitamin B_{12}.

ADH antidiuretic hormone, secreted by the anterior pituitary gland in response to body stress. It acts upon the renal tubules (chiefly the distal tubule) to cause reabsorption of water. The ADH mechanism is the body's primary water-conserving mechanism and is therefore essential to life; see also *vasopressin.*

aldosterone potent hormone of the cortex of the adrenal glands which acts upon the distal renal tubule to cause reabsorption of sodium in an ion exchange with potassium. The aldosterone mechanism is essentially a sodium-conserving mechanism, but indirectly conserves water also as water reabsorption follows the sodium reabsorption.

alkalosis a disturbance in acid-base balance in which there is a reduction of the acid partner in the buffer system, or an increase in the base. In either case, the necessary 20:1 ratio between base and acid is upset by an increase in the relative amount of base.

angiotensin (Gr. *angeion,* vessel; L. *tensio,* stretching, pressure) A pressor substance produced in the body by interaction of the enzyme renin, produced by the renal cortex, and a serum globulin fraction, angiotensinogen, produced by the liver. Successive products are formed by the interaction—angiotensin I and II. Angiotensin II is the active pressor substance which increases arterial muscle tone and triggers the production of aldosterone by the adrenal gland. Angiotensin I and II, therefore, are key products in the cycle of the aldosterone mechanism.

anion an ion that carries a negative electrical charge.

base a chemical substance which is capable of neutralizing acid by accepting hydrogen ions from the acid. A synonomous term is *alkali.*

base bicarbonate in the term "base-bicarbonate" the word "base" refers to *any* base that might be combined with bicarbonate. In the main buffer system of the human body, this base is sodium bicarbonate.

buffer a mixture of acidic and alkaline components, which, when added to a solution, is able to protect the solution against wide variations in its pH even when strong acids and bases are added to it. If an acid is added, the alkaline partner reacts with it to counteract its acidic effect. If a base is added, the acid partner reacts with it to counteract its alkalizing effect. A solution to which a buffer has been added is called a buffered solution.

capillary fluid shift mechanism the process which controls the movement of water and small molecules in solution (electrolytes, nutrients) between the blood in the capillary and the surrounding interstitial area. Filtration of water and solutes out of the capillary at the arteriole end, and reabsorption at the venule end are accomplished by shifts in balance between the intracapillary hydrostatic blood pressure and the colloidal osmotic pressure exerted by the plasma proteins.

carbonic acid (H_2CO_3) the acid partner in the carbonic acid- base bicarbonate buffer system in the body.

cation an ion that carries a positive electrical charge.

colloidal osmotic pressure (COP) pressure produced by the protein molecules in the plasma and in the cell. Because proteins are large molecules they do not pass through the separating membranes of the capillary cell walls. Thus, they remain within their respective compartments, exerting a constant osmotic pull which protects vital plasma and cell fluid volumes in these compartments.

compartment the collective quantity of material in a given type of tissue space in the body. For example, in speaking of body water, the physiologist calls all the water in the body which is outside of cells the extracellular fluid compartment (ECF). In like manner, he calls all the water in the body which is inside of cells the intracellular fluid compartment (ICF).

diffusion (L. *diffundere,* to spread or pour forth) the process by which particles in solution spread throughout the solution and across separating membranes from the place of highest solute concentration to all surrounding spaces of lesser solute concentration.

electrolyte (Gr. *electron,* amber [which emits electricity if it is rubbed] + *lytos,* soluble) a chemical compound which, in solution, dissociates by releasing ions. (An ion is an atomic particle that carries a positive or a negative electrical charge.) The process of dissociating into ions is termed ionization.

filtration (Medieval L. *filtrum,* felt used to strain liquids) passage of a fluid through a semipermeable membrane (a membrane permeable to water and small solutes, but not to large molecules) as a result of a difference in pressures on the two sides of the membrane. For example, the net filtration pressure in the capillaries is the difference between the outward-pushing hydrostatic force of the blood pressure and the opposing inward-pulling force of the colloidal osmotic pressure exerted by the plasma proteins retained in the capillary.

hydrostatic pressure the pressure exerted by a liquid upon the surfaces of the walls that contain it. Such pressure is equal in the direction of all containing walls. In body fluid balance, hydrostatic pressure usually refers to the blood pressure, which, together with the plasma proteins, maintains fluid circulation and volume in the blood vessels.

hypertonic dehydration loss of water from the cell as a result of hypertonicity (excess solutes, hence greater osmotic pressure) of the surrounding extracellular fluid.

hypotonic dehydration increase of water in the cell (cellular edema) at the expense of extracellular fluid, as a result of hypotonicity (decreased solutes, hence diminished osmotic pressure) of the extracellular fluid surrounding the cell. A dangerous shrinking of the extracellular fluid (especially blood) volume follow.

interstitial (L. *interstitium,* standing between) spaces or interstices between the essential parts of an organ that comprise its tissue. For example, interstitial fluid is the fluid that occupies the spaces between the cells of a body tissue. This interstitial fluid is freely exchanged, and in balance, with the vascular fluid (fluid in blood and lymph vessels) that services the tissue area.

ion (Gr. *iōn,* to wander) a molecular constituent of one or more atoms that is a free-wandering particle in solution. An ion carries a positive or a negative electrical charge. Ions carrying positive charges are called cations; those carrying negative charges are called anions.

isotonic (Gr. *isōs,* equal; *tonos,* tone, tension) having the same tension or pressure. Two given soltuions are isotonic if they have the same osmotic pressure and therefore balance each other. For example, the law of isotonicity operates between the gastrointestinal fluids and the surrounding extracellular fluid. Shifts of water and electrolytes in and out of the gastrointestinal lumen are controlled to maintain this state of isotonicity.

milliequivalent the unit of measure used for electrolytes in a solution. It is based on the number of ions (cations and anions) in solution, as determined by their concentration in a given volume, not the weights of the various particles. The term refers to the chemical combining power of the solution, and is expressed as the number of milliequivalents per liter (mEq./L.).

nephron (Gr. *nephros,* kidney) the structural and functional unit of the kidney. The nephron includes the renal corpuscle (glomerulus), the proximal convoluted tubule, the loop of Henle, the distal convoluted tubule, and the collecting tubule (which empties the urine into the renal medulla). The urine passes into the papilla and then to the pelvis of the kidney. Urine is formed by filtration of blood in the glomerulus and by the selective reabsorption and secretion of solutes by cells that comprise the walls of the renal tubules. There are approximately one million nephrons in each kidney.

osmosis (Gr. *ōsmos,* a thrusting) the passage of a solvent such as water through a membrane that separates solutions of different concentrations. The water passes through the membrane from the area of lower concentration of solute to that of higher concentration of solute, which tends to equalize the concentrations of the two solutions. The rate of osmosis depends upon (1) the difference in osmotic pressures of the two solutions, (2) the permeability of the membrane, and (3) the electric potential across the membrane.

pH symbol used in chemistry to express the degree of acidity or alkalinity (the concentration of H^+) of a solution. It is mathematically based upon the negative logarithm expressed as an exponential power (pH = *p*ower of *h*ydrogen ion concentration). Therefore, the acidity of a solution varies inversely with the figure expressing it—the smaller the pH number, the greater the degree of acidity. A neutral solution (pure water) has a pH of 7.0. Solutions with a lower pH are acid; those with a higher pH are alkaline. The blood buffer system maintains the blood at a pH of 7.4.

pinocytosis (Gr. *pinein,* to drink; *kytos,* cell) the absorption of large molecules (products of digestions such as fat substances by engulfing them directly into the cell cytoplasm.

renin (properly pronounced rěnin. This word is often mispronounced rěnin. It may then be confused with *rennin,* an enzyme from a calf's stomach, used to sour milk to make cheese or puddings.) A protein substance formed in the renal cortex, which, in response to blood pressure changes, is secreted to act as an enzyme on its specific substrate, angiotensinogen, to form angiotensin I and II. Angiotensin II is a powerful vasoconstrictor. Angiotensin II also stimulates the adrenal glands to produce aldosterone which causes reabsorption of sodium by the distal renal tubule, thus holding water and maintaining the plasma volume.

solute a dissolved substance; particles in solution.

valence (L. *valens,* powerful) the power of an

element or a radical to combine with (or to re-place) other elements or radicals. Atoms of various elements combine in definite proportions. The valence number of an element is the number of atoms of hydrogen with which one atom of the element can combine.

vasopressin (ADH) a hormone secreted by the anterior pituitary gland, which acts upon the distal renal tubule, causing the reabsorption of water. The result is diminished urinary output; hence the term, *antidiuretic hormone* (ADH).

References
Specific
1. Smith, Homer W.: From fish to philosopher, Garden City, N. Y., 1961, Anchor Books, Doubleday & Co., Inc.

General

Anthony, C. P.: Fluid imbalances, formidable foes to survival, Amer. J. Nurs. 63:75, 1963.

Anthony, C. P.: What makes fluids flow? Amer. J. Nurs. 56:1256, 1956.

Ashley, F. L., and Love, H. G.: Fluid and electrolyte therapy, Philadelphia, 1954, J. B. Lippincott Co.

Bard, P.: Medical physiology, ed. 11, St. Louis, 1961, The C. V. Mosby Co.

Best, C. H., and Taylor, N. B.: The physiological basis of medical practice, ed. 8, Baltimore, 1966, The Williams & Wilkins Co.

Bland, J. H.: Clinical metabolism of body water and electrolytes, Philadelphia, 1963, W. B. Saunders Company.

Brooke, C. E., and Anast, C. S.: Oral fluid and electrolytes, J.A.M.A. 179:792, 1962.

Brooks, S. M.: Basic facts of body water and ions, New York, 1960, Springer Publishing Co., Inc.

Cannon, W. B.: The wisdom of the body, New York, 1932, W. W. Norton & Company, Inc.

Davenport, H. W.: The ABC of acid-base chemistry, ed. 4, Chicago, 1958, University of Chicago Press.

Drummond, E., and Anderson, M.: Gastrointestinal suction, Amer. J. Nurs. 63:109, 1963.

Elkington, J., and Danowski, T.: The body fluids, basic physiology and practical therapeutics, Baltimore, 1955, The Williams & Wilkins Co.

Farr, H.: Fluid and electrolyte balance with special reference to the gastrointestinal tract, Amer. J. Nurs. 54:826, 1954.

Fielo, S. B.: Teaching fluid and electrolyte balance, Nurs. Outlook 13:43, 1965.

Fluid and electrolytes, Chicago, 1960, Abbott Laboratories.

Frohman, I.: The adrenocorticosteroids, Amer. J. Nurs. 64:120, 1964.

Gamble, J. L.: Chemical anatomy, physiology and pathology of extracellular fluid, ed. 6, Cambridge, 1954, Harvard University Press.

Ganong, W. F.: Review of medical physiology, Los Altos, Calif., 1963, Lange Medical Publications.

Goldberger, E.: A primer of water, electrolyte and acid-base syndromes, ed. 2, Philadelphia, 1962, Lea & Febiger.

Grollman, A.: Diuretics, Amer. J. Nurs. 65:84, 1965.

Hardy, J. D.: Fluid therapy, ed. 2, Philadelphia, 1962, Lea & Febiger.

Harper, H. A.: Review of physiological chemistry, ed. 11, Los Altos, Calif., 1967, Lange Medical Publications.

Hill, F. S.: Practical fluid therapy in pediatrics, Philadelphia, 1955, W. B. Saunders Co.

Krehl, W. A.: The potassium depletion syndrome, Nutrition Today 1:20, 1966.

Krehl, W. A.: Sodium: A most extraordinary dietary essential, Nutrition Today 1:16, 1966.

Lowe, C.: Principles of parenteral fluid therapy, Amer. J. Nurs. 53:963, 1953.

Programmed instruction: potassium imbalance, Amer. J. Nurs. 67:343, 1967.

Scholander, R. F.: The wonderful net, Sci. Amer. 196:96, 1957.

Smith, H.: From fish to philosopher, Garden City, N. Y., 1961, Doubleday & Company, Inc. (Natural History Library, Anchor Books).

Smith, H. W.: Principles of renal physiology, New York, 1956, Oxford University Press.

Snively, W. D., Jr.: Sea within—the story of our body fluids, Philadelphia, 1960, J. B. Lippincott Co.

Snively, W. D., Jr.: Toward a better understanding of body fluid disturbances, Nurs. Forum 3:1, 1964.

Statland, H.: Fluid and electrolytes in practice, ed. 3, Philadelphia, 1963, J. B. Lippincott Co.

Strauss, M. B.: Body water in man, Boston, 1957, Little, Brown and Company.

Weisberg, H. F.: Water, electrolyte and acid-base balance, ed. 2, Baltimore, 1962, The Williams & Wilkins Co.

Welt, L. G.: Clinical disorders of hydration and acid-base equilibrium, ed. 2, Boston, 1959, Little, Brown and Company.

Wolf, E.: The nurse and fluid therapy, Amer. J. Nurs. 54:831, 1954.

CHAPTER 10

Digestion, absorption, and metabolism

Thus far in this study, each of the fundamental nutritional components has been examined separately, and each has been considered with respect to its particular role in human nutrition. At the same time that the components have been separated in order to consider them in detail, the all-important concept of *the interrelatedness of the nutrients* has been emphasized. This has been largely a biochemical study, although it has certainly not been exclusively biochemical, since such matters as the clinical significance of each nutrient and its availability in foods have also been considered. In addition, other aspects have been considered that must be understood if the individual is to receive the correct balance of needed nutrients.

In this chapter the body's use of nutriment will be looked at in still another way—from the point of view of the anatomy and physiology of the organs that digest and absorb nutrients. Once the body receives nutrients, how does it go about converting them into forms it can use? The physiologic process can be separated into components, and can only be understood as one recognizes that it consists of three events: digestion, absorption, and metabolism. Again, however, because the process of analysis is a necessity for the human mind, each of these phases will be considered separately, even though analysis as such does not characterize nature. All the while that these three processes are being studied separately they are actually functioning as a digestion-absorption-metabolism continuum—*a dynamic unit*.

The question of why this intricate complex of biochemical and physiological activities is necessary may be asked at this point. Two reasons are apparent. First, food as it naturally occurs (and as man consumes it) is not a single component, but is a mixture of substances. If these substances are to be induced to release their energy for use, they must be separated into their components so that each component may be handled by the body as a separate unit. Second, because in most instances the still simpler chemical units that make up these nutrient components are still unavailable to the body, some additional means of changing their form must follow. The intermediate units must be broken down, simplified, regrouped, and rerouted. This exceedingly complex chemical work must take place because man is the most highly organized and intricately balanced of all organisms whose life is developed and sustained in an internal chemical environment. This view of the human body as an integrated physiochemical organism is basic to an understanding of human nutrition.

To achieve this picture of the digestion-absorption-metabolism process as a whole, the general principles related to each phase should be noted. The student should then be able to follow the fate of food components as they travel together through the successive parts of the gastrointestinal tract and into the body cells. For reference, these

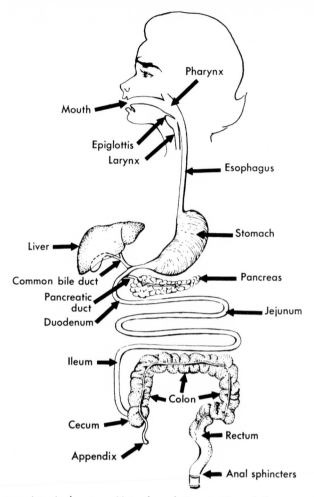

Fig. 10-1. The gastrointestinal system. Note the relative position of the successive parts. (From Stacy, R. W. and Santolucito, J. A.: Modern college physiology, St. Louis, 1966, The C. V. Mosby Co.)

respective components of the gastrointestinal tract and their relative position in the over-all system should be carefully reviewed (Fig. 10-1).

DIGESTION
Basic principles of digestion

Digestion achieves the initial preparation of food for use by the body. Two basic types of action are involved: (1) mechanical or muscular activity, which produces gastrointestinal motility, and (2) chemical or enzymatic activity, which results from gastrointestinal secretions. The cells and glands of the gastrointestinal tract also secrete mucus and water and electrolytes.

Gastrointestinal motility. Mechanical digestion takes place through a number of neuromuscular, self-regulatory processes. These actions work together to move the food components along the alimentary tract at a rate that is optimum for digestion and absorption of nutrients.

Four types of muscle in the stomach and intestine contribute to this motility: (1) a layer of circular, contractile rings that break up, mix, and churn the food particles, (2) longitudinal muscles which help to propel the food mass along, (3) sphincter muscles which act as valves (the pyloric, ileocecal, and anal valves) to control passage of material to the next segment of the intestine,

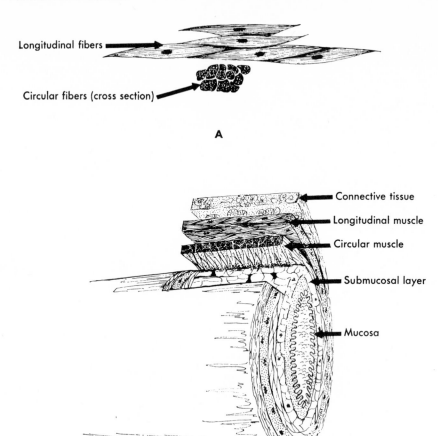

Longitudinal fibers

Circular fibers (cross section)

A

Connective tissue

Longitudinal muscle

Circular muscle

Submucosal layer

Mucosa

B

Fig. 10-2. Layers of smooth muscle in the intestinal wall. **A,** Microscopic appearance of muscle tissue. **B,** Arrangement of layers of muscle. (From Stacy, R. W. and Santolucito, J. A.: Modern college physiology, St. Louis, 1966, The C. V. Mosby Co.)

and (4) a thin, mucosal layer of smooth muscle that can raise intestinal folds to increase the absorbing surface. The interaction of these four types of muscle produce two general types of movement: (1) a general muscle tone or tonic contraction, which ensures continuous passage and valve control, and (2) periodic, rhythmic contractions which mix and propel the food mass. These alternating muscular contractions and relaxations that force the contents forward are known by the term *peristalsis.* The layers of smooth muscle making up the gastrointestinal wall are shown in Fig. 10-2.

Specific nerves regulate these muscular actions. A complex, interrelated network of nerves within the gastrointestinal wall, the *intramural nerve plexus,* extends from the esophagus to the anus. The intramural plexus controls muscle tone of the gastrointestinal wall, regulates the rate and intensity of periodic muscle contractions, and coordinates the various movements (Fig. 10-3).

Gastrointestinal secretions. Food is digested chemically by the action of a number of secretions. Generally these secretions are of four types:

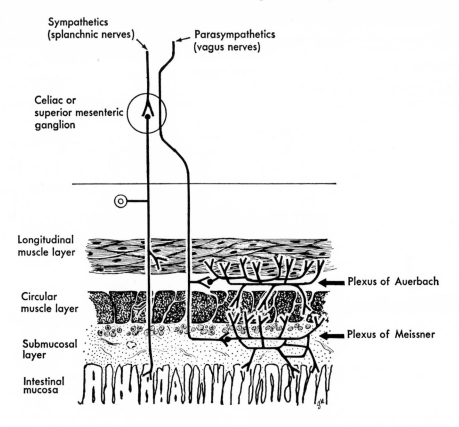

Fig. 10-3. Innervation of the intestine, showing the plexus of Auerbach and the plexus of Meissner. (From Stacy, R. W. and Santolucito, J. A.: Modern college physiology, St. Louis, 1966, The C. V. Mosby Co.)

1. Enzymes—specific in kind and quantity for the degradation of a given nutrient
2. Hydrochloric acid and buffer ions—to produce the pH necessary for the activity of given enzymes
3. Mucus—for lubrication and protection of the gastrointestinal tract
4. Water and electrolytes—in quantities sufficient to carry or circulate the organic substances

There are several kinds of cells and glands that produce these secretions. There are single mucous cells on the epithelial surface, called *goblet cells,* which act alone. In the small intestine there are *multicellular tubular glands,* such as the simple pits lined with goblet mucous cells (crypts of Lieberkühn). Enzymes and hydrochloric acid are secreted by the deeper, branched *gastric glands.* In addition, there are complicated *glands outside the gastrointestinal tract,* such as the salivary glands, the pancreas, and the liver. These secrete enzymes and bile from organized secretory cell structures called *acini,* which feed into ducts that empty into the gastrointestinal lumen. The secretory action of these various special cells or glands may be stimulated locally by the presence of food, by sensory nerve stimuli, or by hormones specific for certain foods.

Digestion in the mouth and esophagus

Mechanical digestion. Mastication (biting and chewing) begins the breaking up of food into smaller particles. The teeth and other oral structures are particularly suited for this function. The incisors cut; the molars grind. Tremendous force is supplied by the jaw muscles—55 lbs. of muscular pressure is applied through incisors, and 200 lbs. is applied through the molars. Mastication makes it possible for an enlarged surface area of food to constantly be exposed to enzyme action, and the fineness of the food particles eases the continued passage of material through the gastrointestinal tract.

Swallowing of the mixed mass of food particles and its passage down the esophagus are accomplished by peristaltic waves controlled by nerve reflexes. In the usual upright eating position, gravity aids this movement down the esophagus. However, for a bed patient in a prone position, it is more difficult. At the point of entry into the stomach, the gastroesophageal constrictor muscle relaxes to allow food to enter, then constricts again to prevent regurgitation of stomach contents up into the esophagus. (When regurgitation does occur, through failure of this mechanism, the patient feels it as "heartburn.") Clinical conditions such as cardiospasm, caused by failure of the constrictor muscle to relax properly, or hiatus hernia (protrusion of the stomach into the thorax through an ab-

normal opening in the diaphragm, which allows food to be held in the outpouched area) hinder normal food passage at this point.

Chemical or secretory digestion. Three pairs of salivary glands—parotid, submaxillary, and sublingual—secrete a serous material containing *ptyalin,* an enzyme specific for starches, and a mucous material that lubricates and binds the food particles. These salivary secretions amount to 1,000 to 1,500 ml. per day. They usually are slightly acid (pH about 6.8). However, they may range around neutrality (pH from 6.0 to 7.0). Stimuli such as sight, smell, taste, and touch—and even the thought of likes or dislikes in foods—greatly influence these secretions.

Because food remains in the mouth only a short time, starch digestion by ptyalin is relatively unimportant, as it is terminated by the acid medium of the stomach. Secretions of mucous glands that line the esophagus aid in swallowing and movement of the food mass toward the stomach.

Digestion in the stomach

Mechanical digestion. The major parts of the stomach are shown in Fig. 10-4. Muscles in the stomach wall provide three

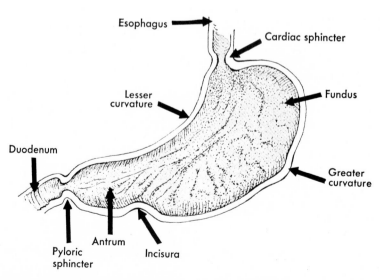

Fig. 10-4. Major parts of the stomach. (From Stacy, R. W. and Santolucito, J. A.: Modern college physiology, St. Louis, 1966, The C. V. Mosby Co.)

basic motor functions of the stomach: storage, mixing, and slow, controlled emptying. As the food mass enters the stomach it lies against the stomach walls, which can stretch outward to store as much as one liter. Gradually, local tonic muscle waves increase their kneading and mixing action as the mass of food and secretions moves on toward the region of the pyloric antrum at the distal end of the stomach. Here, waves of peristaltic contractions reduce the mass to a semifluid chyme. Finally, with each peristaltic wave, small amounts of chyme are forced through the pyloric valve. This pyloric pump controls the emptying of the stomach contents into the duodenum by constrictive action of the sphincter muscle (the pyloric valve), and by controlling the rate of propulsive peristaltic activity in the antrum. This control releases the acid chyme slowly enough so that it can be buffered by the alkaline intestinal secretions.

Chemical or secretory digestion. About 2,000 ml. of gastric secretions are produced daily. Two basic types of gland in the stomach wall—the gastric and pyloric glands—secrete materials that act on specific nutrients.

Gastric gland secretion. Gastric glands are located in the upper portion of the stomach and the wall of the body and fundus. They secrete enzymes, hydrochloric acid, and some mucus. These gastric glands are tubular and are lined with secreting cells.

The *chief cells* (also called the *adelomorphous cells*) secrete pepsinogen, which is activated by previously formed pepsin and

TO PROBE FURTHER
"Executive monkeys"

Interesting data concerning the relationship of emotional states to gastric hypersecretion and the development of peptic ulcer disease were obtained from the now classic experiments of Brady and his associates* performed on monkeys.

In the first experiment, an electrical shock was applied to the animals' feet. The animals were taught that, by pressing a lever at regular intervals, they could avoid this shock. After a long period of such testing, the animals incurred gastric hypersecretion, excessive acid rise, and resulting duodenal ulcers with perforation.

In the second experiment, two monkeys were placed together in a test situation like the first. Each was supplied with a lever to press. This time, however, the lever for Monkey A did not control the shock. The lever of Monkey B, if pressed on schedule, prevented the shock to both. Monkey A soon learned that he had no control over his situation and incurred no gastric hypersecretion. But Monkey B—the "executive" who had to make the decisions for both of them—did incur gastric hypersecretion.

Although complicating factors in the experiments make simple cause-and-effect conclusions impossible, the observations raise interesting speculation. They may suggest that the greater the controlling power one has over the lives and fortunes of others, the worse off he is physically. And perhaps, if we consider the "executive syndrome" repeatedly observed in the driving "organization man in the gray flannel suit" of our industrial age, we may conclude that not all monkeys are in cages. Or is it that we build cages for ourselves, of another sort?

*Brady, J. V.: Ulcers in "executive monkeys," Sci. Amer. **199:**95, 1958.

hydrochloric acid, to form the active enzyme pepsin. A highly acid medium (pH approximately 2.0) is required for this enzyme activation. Pepsin begins the enzymatic breakdown of proteins to smaller polypeptides. The *parietal cells* secrete the necessary hydrochloric acid. *Mucous cells* secrete mucus, which helps to protect the gastric mucosa, and to give body and cohesiveness to the food mass. Other enzyme-secreting cells produce small amounts of a specific gastric lipase, tributyrinase, which acts on the tributyrin in butterfat; this is a relatively minor activity.

The *pyloric glands* secrete additional thin mucus. Surface *goblet cells* produce a thicker, more viscous mucus, which coats and protects the stomach wall. When irritation occurs, a still greater quantity of mucus is produced.

Stimuli for all of these secretions are twofold.

1. Nerve stimulus is produced in response to sensation, to food taken in, and to emotions. For example, in response to anger and hostility, secretions increase. Fear and depression decrease secretions and inhibit blood flow and motility as well.

2. Hormonal stimulus is produced in response to the entrance of food into the stomach. Certain stimulants, especially coffee, alcohol, and meat extractives, cause the release of *gastrin* from mucosal glands in the antrum, which in turn stimulates the parietal cells to secrete more hydrochloric acid. When the pH reaches 2.0, a feedback mechanism stops secretion of the hormone to prevent excess acid formation. Another hormone, *enterogastrone*, produced by glands in the duodenal mucosa, counteracts excessive gastric activity by inhibiting acid and pepsin secretion and gastric motility.

Digestion in the small intestine

Up to this point, the digestion of food consumed has been mainly mechanical, delivering to the small intestine a semifluid chyme made up of fine food particles mixed with watery secretions. Chemical digestion has thus far been limited. Starch was slightly attacked by ptyalin in the mouth

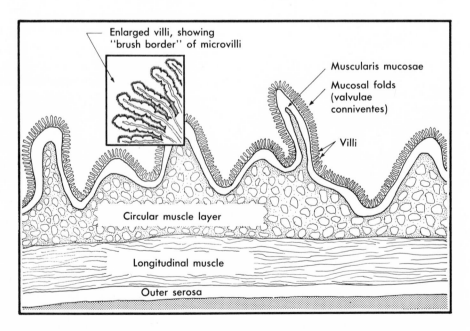

Fig. 10-5. Intestinal wall. Note the arrangement of muscle layers and the structures of the mucosa which increase the surface area for absorption—mucosal folds, villi, and microvilli.

but this action was quickly terminated by stomach acid. The breakdown of complex proteins to polypeptides has been barely begun in the stomach by the action of pepsin; but even this is not vital, since a full enzyme system for the digestion of proteins is available in the small intestine. Therefore, the major task of digestion (and of absorption which follows) occurs in the small intestine. Its structural parts, its synchronized movements, and its array of enzymes are highly developed for this all-important final task of mechanical and chemical digestion.

Mechanical digestion. The structural arrangement of the intestinal wall is shown in the diagrammatic section in Fig. 10-5.

Finely coordinated intestinal motility is

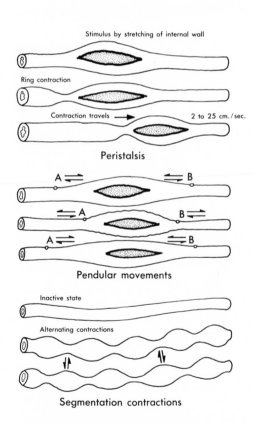

Stimulus by stretching of internal wall

Ring contraction

Contraction travels →   2 to 25 cm./sec.

Peristalsis

A   B

A   B

A   B

Pendular movements

Inactive state

Alternating contractions

Segmentation contractions

Fig. 10-6. Types of movement produced by muscles of the intestine: peristaltic waves from contraction of deep circular muscle; pendular movements from small local muscles; and segmentation rings formed by alternate contraction and relaxation of circular muscle.

achieved by the three basic layers of muscle: (1) the thin layer of smooth muscle in the mucosa (muscularis mucosa) with fibers extending up into the villi, (2) the circular muscle layer, and (3) the longitudinal muscle next to the outer serosa. Under the control of the nerve plexus, of wall stretch pressure from food present, or of hormonal stimuli, these muscles produce several types of movement that aid mechanical digestion (Fig. 10-6):

1. Segmentation rings from alternate contractions of circular muscle progressively chop the food mass into successive boluses. This action constantly mixes the food materials with secretions.

2. Longitudinal rotation by the long muscle running the length of the intestine rolls the slowly moving food mass in a spiral motion, mixing it and exposing new surfaces for absorption.

3. Pendular movements from small local muscle contractions sweep back and forth and stir chyme at the mucosal surface.

4. Peristaltic waves, produced by the contraction of deep circular muscle, propel the food mass slowly forward. The intensity of the waves may be increased by food intake or by the presence of irritants. In some cases this causes long, sweeping waves over the entire length of the intestine.

5. Motion of the villi also aids mechanical digestion. Alternating contractions and extensions of mucosal muscle fibers constantly agitate the mucosal surface. This action stirs and mixes chyme that is in contact with the intestinal wall and exposes additional nutrient material for absorption. A specific hormone, *villikinin,* is released from the upper intestinal mucosa when it is bathed by chyme entering from the proximal gastrointestinal tract. Villikinin stimulates these contractions, which in turn constantly shorten and lengthen the intestinal villi.

Chemical or secretory digestion. Since the major burden of chemical digestion falls upon the small intestine, this portion of the alimentary tract secretes a large number of enzymes, each of which is specific for one of the fundamental types of nutrient. These important specific enzymes are secreted from the intestinal glands and the pancreas.

A. Intestinal glands in the mucosa (crypts of Lieberkühn)
 1. Fat—intestinal lipase converts fat to glycerides and fatty acids
 2. Protein
    a. Enterokinase converts the inactive precursor trypsinogen to active trypsin.
    b. Amino peptidase removes from polypeptides the terminal amino acids that contain a free amino (NH_4) group, by attacking the peptide bond.
    c. Dipeptidase converts dipeptides to amino acids.
    d. Nucleosidase converts nucleosides to a purine or a pyrimidine base, and pentose sugar.
 3. Carbohydrate—disaccharidases (maltase, lactase, sucrase) convert maltose, lactose, and sucrose to their constituent monosaccharides (glucose, fructose, and galactose).

B. Pancreas
 1. Fat—pancreatic lipase converts fats to glycerides and fatty acids
 2. Protein
    a. Trypsin causes initial breakdown of proteins and polypeptides to smaller polypeptides. It also activates chymotrypsinogen to chymotrypsin.
    b. Chymotrypsin breaks down proteins and polypeptides to smaller polypeptides
    c. Carboxypeptidase removes carboxyl (COOH) terminal amino acid from polypeptidases
    d. Nucleases convert nucleic acids (RNA and DNA) to nucleotides

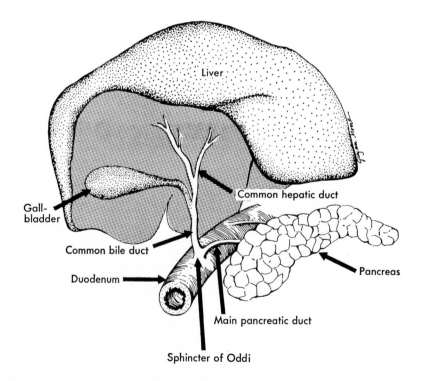

Fig. 10-7. Organs of the biliary system and the pancreatic ducts. (From Stacy, Ralph W. and Santolucito, John A.: Modern college physiology, St. Louis, 1966, The C. V. Mosby Co.)

3. Carbohydrate—pancreatic amylase converts starch to disaccharides

Mucous glands. In addition to enzymes, large quantities of mucus are secreted by intestinal glands (Brunner's glands) located immediately inside the duodenum. This secretion protects the mucosa from irritation and digestion by the highly acid gastric juices, which enter the intestine at this point. Emotions inhibit these mucous secretions and are an important factor in the production of duodenal ulcers. Additional mucous cells on the mucosal surface or in intestinal glands continue to secrete mucus as they are touched by the food mass to provide lubrication and protection of tissues. The combined secretions of the mucous glands of the intestine and pancreas

Table 10-1. Summary of digestive processes

Nutrient	Mouth	Stomach	Small Intestine
Carbo-hydrate	Starch $\xrightarrow{\text{Ptyalin}}$ Dextrins		*Pancreas* Starch $\xrightarrow{\text{Amylase}}$ (Disaccharides) Maltose and sucrose *Intestine* Lactose $\xrightarrow{\text{Lactase}}$ (Monosaccharides) Glucose and galactose Sucrose $\xrightarrow{\text{Sucrase}}$ Glucose and fructose Maltose $\xrightarrow{\text{Maltase}}$ Glucose and glucose
Protein		Protein $\xrightarrow[\text{Hydrochloric acid}]{\text{Pepsin}}$ Polypeptides	*Pancreas* Proteins, polypeptides $\xrightarrow{\text{Trypsin}}$ Dipeptides Proteins, polypeptides $\xrightarrow{\text{Chymotrypsin}}$ Dipeptides Polypeptides, dipeptides $\xrightarrow{\text{Carboxypeptidase}}$ Amino acids *Intestine* Polypeptides, dipeptides $\xrightarrow{\text{Aminopeptidase}}$ Amino acids Dipeptides $\xrightarrow{\text{Dipeptidase}}$ Amino acids
Fat		Tributyrin (butterfat) $\xrightarrow{\text{Tributyrinase}}$ Glycerol Fatty acids	*Pancreas* Fats $\xrightarrow{\text{Lipase}}$ Glycerol Glycerides (di-, mono-) Fatty acids *Intestine* Fats $\xrightarrow{\text{Lipase}}$ Glycerol Glycerides (di-, mono-) Fatty acids *Liver and gallbladder* Fats $\xrightarrow{\text{Bile}}$ Emulsified fat

total about 4,200 ml. daily (3,000 ml. from intestinal glands and 1,200 ml. from the pancreas).

Hormonal stimulus for secretions. The hormone *secretin,* produced by the mucosa of the upper part of the small intestine, stimulates the pancreatic secretions, and regulates their pH so that they are maintained at the alkalinity that is necessary to stop the acidic enzyme activity of chyme entering from the stomach. The unprotected intestinal mucosa alone could not withstand this high degree of acidity. The resultant

alkalinity of the medium also provides the pH (8.0) that is optimum for pancreatic enzyme activity.

Bile. Another important aid to digestion and absorption in the small intestine is bile, since it is an emulsifying agent for fats. Bile is produced by the liver, and is concentrated and stored by the gallbladder. When fat enters the duodenum, the hormone *cholecystokinin* is secreted by intestinal mucosa glands, and stimulates the gallbladder to contract and release bile. From 600 to 700 ml. of bile is produced

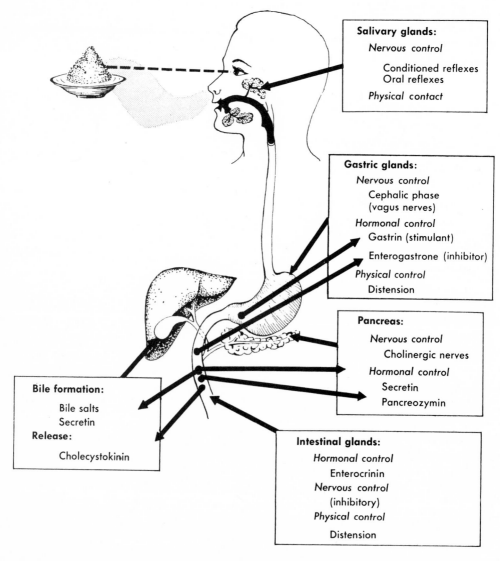

Fig. 10-8. Summary of factors influencing secretions of the gastrointestinal glands. (From Stacy, R. W. and Santolucito, J. A.: Modern college physiology, St. Louis, 1966, The C. V. Mosby Co.)

daily, and provides for the repeated circulation of bile salts in the enterohepatic circulation (see Fig. 3-4, p. 35).

The organs of the biliary system and the pancreatic ducts are illustrated in Fig. 10-7. A summary of these digestive processes is given in Table 10-1. Many factors influence the various secretions of the gastrointestinal tract. Control by hormone, by nerves, and by physical contact is summarized in Fig. 10-8.

ABSORPTION

After digestion of the food nutrients is complete, the simplified end-products are ready to be absorbed. These end-products include monosaccharides such as glucose, fructose, and galactose from carbohydrates; fatty acids and glycerides from fats, and amino acids from proteins. Also liberated are vitamins and minerals. Finally, with a water base for solution and transport, plus necessary electrolytes, the total fluid food mass forms the material that is involved in a constant, life-sustaining, gastrointestinal circulation.

The absorptive powers of the gastrointestinal circulation may be visualized in terms of the total fluid volume handled daily (Table 10-2).

Small intestine

Surface structures. Viewed from the outside, the serosa of the intestine appears smooth. But the inner mucosal surface is quite different. There are three types of convolutions and projections which are progressively smaller in size. These mucosal folds, villi, and microvilli increase the inner surface area some 600 times over that of the outer serosa! These special structures of the mucosal surface of the small intestine, plus the contracted length of the live organ (21 to 22 feet), combine to produce a tremendously large absorbing surface. The remarkable potential of the luminal surface of the small intestine is a total absorbing surface area as large as or larger than half a basketball court!

Fig. 10-5 (p. 188) should be referred to again to compare the three structures that enlarge the absorptive surface of the luminal serosa.

Mucosal folds. Easily seen by the naked eye are heaped-up folds along the mucosa surface, like so many hills and valleys in a mountain range.

Villi. Closer examination by light microscope reveals small finger-like projections, the villi, covering these convoluted folds of mucosa. These villi further increase the area of the exposed surface. To receive the absorbed nutrients, each villus has an ample vascular network that involves venous and arterial capillaries and central *lacteals*. Lacteal is the special name given to a lymphatic vessel in the small intestine. It is like any other lymphatic vessel in structure and function. It receives this special name because the chyle that fills it during digestion looks like milk.

Microvilli. An electron microscope fo-

Table 10-2. Daily absorption volume in human gastrointestinal system

	Intake (liters)	Intestinal absorption (liters)	Elimination (liters)
Food ingested	1.5		
Gastrointestinal secretions	8.5		
Total	10.0		
Fluid absorbed in small intestine		9.5	
Fluid absorbed in colon		.4	
Total		9.9	
Feces			.1

cused upon the surface of a single villus brings to view extremely numerous minute surface projections. This vast array of microvilli covering the edge of each villus is called the "brush border," because they look like bristles on a brush. At the base of the brush border is the basement membrane.

All three of these mucosal surface structures function as a unit for the absorption of nutrients. Although the small intestine is popularly thought of as the lowly "gut," it is actually one of the most highly developed, exquisitely fashioned, specialized tissues in the human body!

Mechanism of absorption. Absorption is accomplished by the small intestine by means of a number of processes, including passive diffusion, active ferrying, energy-driven transport, and penetration by engulfment.

Passive diffusion (osmosis) through epithelial membrane pores. Where no opposing pressure exists, molecules small enough to pass through the capillary membranes diffuse easily into the capillaries of the villi, in the direction of pressure flow, in quantities that represent their concentration or electrochemical gradient. For example, electrolytes diffuse in and out of the intestinal lumen as electrochemical need demands, and water molecules flow back and forth as osmotic pressures vary (p. 157).

Carrier-mediated diffusion. Ferry systems carry molecules across the epithelial cells and basement membrane of microvilli into the capillary circulation of villi. Molecules too large to traverse membrane pores must be helped through the barrier of the cell wall. If the pressure gradient is from greater to lesser, a molecule of another nutrient combines with the large molecule to provide a vehicle which carries the large molecule through the barrier.

For example, the stomach secretes the highly specialized ferry called intrinsic factor (IF), that is required to carry the very large molecule of vitamin B_{12} out of the intestinal lumen into the circulating blood. If the stomach fails to secrete IF,

the large vitamin B_{12} molecule lacks the ferrying molecule, and cannot enter the blood. Lacking vitamin B_{12}, the red blood cells cannot mature normally, and pernicious anemia results (p. 103).

Energy-dependent active transport. Even against a pressure gradient, nutrient molecules must cross the intestinal epithelial membrane to feed hungry tissue cells. Such work requires extra machinery and energy. This need is supplied by a mechanism that physiologists have come to call a pump,* which continuously picks up the waiting molecules and carries them across the membrane. Energy to operate the pump is supplied from the cell's metabolism. The sodium pump which transports glucose molecules is an example of this fascinating mechanism (Fig. 2-3, p. 18).

Engulfing (pinocytosis). Some even larger macromolecules require still another means of reaching the tissue circulation outposts in the villi. In these instances, epithelial cells of the villi act like amebae or leukocytes and ingest foreign particles. A small portion of the edge of the cell, on coming in contact with the material to be transported, dips inward (invaginates), engulfs the particle, and opens to swallow the particle into the interior of the cell. The particle is conveyed through the cytoplasm to the opposite side of the epithelial cell which borders on the capillary lumen. Here, the particle is discharged into the intracapillary blood. Occasionally whole proteins are absorbed by pinocytosis. This

---

*The use of the word *pump* for this type of mechanism may be confusing at first. It must be remembered that what makes a pump *pump* is the *threat of vacuum.* A pump pulls material from one place to another by the exercise of negative pressure. The pump is able to suck material from one place to another because the new site *cannot endure the absence of material.* It is from this characteristic that biochemists and physiologists have adopted the name *pump.* The avidity of the empty site for something to fill its space provides the power to move the molecules across membranes. A biochemical "pumping mechanism" is one that works by pulling a fresh molecule in, to fill a place that has been emptied by the removal of a molecule that was formerly present.

mechanism is probably also involved in the absorption of neutral fat droplets (chylomicrons) and their transportation into the lacteals of the villi (Fig. 9-3, p. 158).

Routes of absorption. After their absorption by any of these processes, each of the nutrient components from carbohydrates and proteins enters the portal blood system and travels to the body tissues. Only fat is unique in its route. After enzymatic processing in the cells of the intestinal lumen, the fat is largely converted into esterified lipids. These molecules are small enough to pass between the cells of the intestinal mucosa and into the lymph vessels in the center of the villi. From these, they flow into the larger lymph vessels of the mesentery and finally enter the common portal blood flow at the thoracic duct. Exceptions are the medium and short chain fatty acids, which are absorbed directly into villi blood circulation. However, most commonly consumed fats are made up of long-chain fatty acids, which travel the lacteal route.

Large intestine (colon)

The main absorption task remaining for the large intestine is that of taking up water. However, related factors are involved, such as the absorption of sodium and other minerals, absorption of some vitamins and amino acids, the action of intestinal bacteria, the collection of nondigestible residue, and the formation and elimination of feces.

Water absorption. Within a twenty-four-hour period, about 500 ml. of remaining isotonic chyme leaves the ileum (the last portion of the small intestine) and enters the cecum (the pouch at the start of the large intestine). The *ileocecal valve* exerts important control over passage of the semiliquid chyme. Normally, the valve remains closed. With each peristaltic wave, however, it relaxes briefly to allow a small amount of chyme to squirt into the cecum. This control mechanism holds the food mass in the small intestine long enough to ensure adequate digestion and absorption of vital nutrients. Such timing is necessary because

no digestive enzymes are secreted by the colon.

The chyme continues to move slowly through the large intestine, aided by mucus secretion from glands in the colon, and by muscle contractions. Segmentation contractions mix the residue mass and aid absorption by exposing more of the mass to the mucosa. Long muscles produce peristaltic waves to propel the mass forward. The major portion of the water in the chyme (from 350 to 400 ml.) is absorbed in the proximal half of the colon; only from 100 to 150 ml. remains to form and aid in elimination of the feces.

Studies with test meals[1] indicate that the food residue mass moves through the large intestine at a gradually slowing pace. Usually, the test meal, having traversed the 21 to 22 feet of small intestine, starts to enter the cecum about four hours after it is consumed. About eight hours later it reaches the sigmoid colon, having traveled through the large intestine for a distance of about 3 feet! In the sigmoid colon, the mass descends still more slowly toward the anus. Even seventy-two hours after the meal has been eaten, as much as 25% of it may still remain in the rectum!

Mineral absorption. Electrolytes, principally sodium, are transported into the blood stream from the colon. From 20 to 70% of ingested calcium is eliminated in the feces, as is from 80 to 85% of ingested iron, a considerable amount of phosphates, and some carbonate.

Bacterial action—vitamin absorption. Bacteria in the colon are closely associated with a number of vitamins. At birth, the colon is sterile, but very shortly thereafter intestinal bacterial flora is well established. The adult colon contains large numbers of bacteria, the predominant species being *Escherichia coli.* Great masses of the bacteria are passed in the stool. The colon bacteria synthesize vitamin K and some vitamins of the B complex (especially biotin and folic acid) which are absorbed from the colon in sufficient amounts to meet the daily requirement.

Although vitamin B_{12} (cyanocobalamin) is also synthesized by intestinal bacteria, it is not absorbed from the large intestine. What factor, secreted by the gastric mucosa, necessary for B_{12} absorption and present in the small intestine, is not present in the large intestine? (See p. 103.) Since the large intestine lacks this cofactor, the vitamin cannot be transported through the wall of the colon, and is eliminated in the feces.

Other bacterial action. Intestinal bacteria also affect the color and odor of the stool. The brown color represents bile pigments, which are formed by the colon bacteria from bilirubin. Thus, in conditions where bile flow is hindered, the stools may become clay-colored or white. The characteristic odor results from amines, especially indole and skatole, formed by bacterial enzymes from amino acids.

Gas, or flatus, formed in the large intestine contains hydrogen sulfide or methane produced by the bacteria. Gas formation, however, is attributable not so much to specific foods per se as to the state of the body that receives them. Many foods have been labeled gas formers, but in reality such classifications have little or no scientific basis.[2]

Residue. Since man, unlike herbivorous animals and some insects such as the termite, has no microorganisms or enzymes to break down cellulose, this plant product remains after digestion and absorption as

Table 10-3. Intestinal absorption of some major nutrients

Nutrient	Form	Means of absorption	Control agent or required cofactor	Route
Carbohydrate	Monosaccharides (glucose and galactose)	Competitive Selective Active transport via sodium pump	— — Sodium	Blood
Protein	Amino acids	Selective	—	Blood
	Some dipeptides	Carrier transport systems	Pyridoxine (pyridoxal phosphate)	Blood
	Whole protein (rare)	Pinocytosis	—	Blood
Fat	Fatty acids	Fatty acid-bile complex (micelles)	Bile	Lymph
	Glycerides (mono-, di-)		—	Lymph
	Few triglycerides (neutral fat)	Pinocytosis	—	Lymph
Vitamins	B_{12}	Carrier transport	Intrinsic factor (IF)	Blood
	A	Bile complex	Bile	Blood
	K	Bile complex	Bile	From large intestine to blood
Minerals	Sodium	Active transport via sodium pump	—	Blood
	Calcium	Active transport	Vitamin D	Blood
	Iron	Active transport	Ferritin mechanism	Blood (as transferritin)
Water	Water	Osmosis		Blood, lymph, interstitial fluid

residue. Cellulose contributes important bulk to the diet and helps form the feces. The feces contain about 75% water and 25% solids. The solids include cellulose, bacteria, inorganic matter (mostly calcium and phosphates), a small amount of fat and its derivatives, some mucus, and sloughed-off mucosal cells.

Some major features of nutrient absorption in the intestines are summarized in Table 10-3.

METABOLISM

The various absorbed nutrient components, including water and electrolytes, are carried to the cells as raw materials to produce a myriad of substances needed by the body to sustain life. Metabolism encompasses the total, continuous complex of chemical changes that determine the final use of the individual nutrients.

Purposes. Each of these chemical processes is purposeful, and all are interdependent. The processes are designed to fill two essential needs: (1) to produce energy, and (2) to maintain a dynamic equilibrium between the building-up or breaking-down of tissue. The controlling agents in the cells are the cellular enzymes, their coenzymes (many of which are B vitamins), other cofactors, and hormones.

Interrelationships. The main features of cell metabolism of the fundamental nutrients and of some vitamins and minerals are summarized in the diagram in Fig. 10-9. This summary diagram should be studied carefully. Here some of the important relationships between individual components which work together to comprise the whole can be visualized. All in all, it is an exciting biochemical system. By it, the human body works to develop, sustain, and protect its most precious possession—life itself.

GLOSSARY

absorption (L. *ab,* away + *sorbere,* to suck in) the process by which digested food materials pass through the epithelial cells of the alimentary canal (mainly of the small intestine) into the blood or lymph. A number of variables influence absorption—the chemical nature of the nutrient, the cell membrane, and electrochemical pressure differences between the solutions in the intestinal lumen and in the mucosal cells. Therefore, different absorptive mechanisms may be used—simple osmosis or passive diffusion, energy-dependent active transport, or direct ameba-like engulfing (pinocytosis).

acini (L. *acinus,* grape) groups of secretory cells

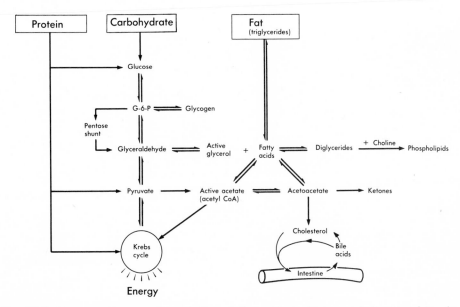

Fig. 10-9. Summary diagram of metabolism of the nutrients. Note metabolic interrelationships of carbohydrate, protein, and fat.

in glands such as the salivary glands, the pancreas, and the liver. These organized clusters of cells are called acini because their shape resembles that of a bunch of grapes. Their secretions of enzymes and bile feed into ducts that empty into the gastrointestinal lumen.

Brunner's glands mucus-secreting glands in the duodenum, which provide mucus to protect the mucosa from irritation and erosion by the strongly acid gastric juices entering from the stomach. Emotional tension and stress inhibit these mucus secretions—a large factor in duodenal ulcer formation.

chief cells special cells in the lining of the tubular gastric glands, which secrete pepsinogen. Previously formed pepsin and hydrochloric acid in the stomach convert the inactive pepsinogen to the active enzyme pepsin, which begins the breakdown of protein to polypeptides.

crypts of Leiberkühn (Gr. *kryptein,* to hide) tubular glands of the intestine which secrete intestinal juice. These special secretory organs open between the bases of the villi. Their walls are lined with special cells which secrete digestive enzymes, water, and electrolytes.

digestion (L. *dis,* apart + *genere,* to carry; *digerere,* to separate, arrange, dissolve, digest) the process by which food is broken down chemically in the gastrointestinal tract through the action of secretions containing specific enzymes. Digestion separates complex food structures into their simpler parts, which are the chemicals needed by the body to sustain life.

enterogastrone a hormone produced by glands in the duodenal mucosa, which counteracts excessive gastric activity by inhibiting acid and pepsin secretion and gastric motility.

gastrin a hormone secreted by mucosal cells in the antrum of the stomach which stimulates the parietal cells to produce hydrochloric acid. Gastrin is released in response to entry of stimulants (especially coffee, alcohol, meat extractives) into the stomach. When the gastric pH reaches 2.0 a feedback mechanism cuts off gastrin secretion, and prevents excess acid formation.

goblet cells special single secretory cells on the mucosal surface which produce mucus. Mucin droplets accumulate in the cell, causing it to swell. The free surface finally ruptures and liberates the mucus. This mucus coats and protects the mucosa.

intramural nerve plexus (L. *intra,* within; *murus,* wall; *plexus,* a braid) a network of interwoven nerve structures within a particular organ. The action of smooth muscle layers comprising the gastrointestinal wall is controlled by such a network of nerve fibers. The interlacing of short nerve fibers in the muscle layers forms the *plexus of Auerbach;* in the submucosal layer, a similar network forms the *plexus of Meissner.*

Together, these systems regulate the alternating muscular contractions and relaxations which produce the synchronized waves of motion along the gastrointestinal tract.

microvilli minute surface projections that cover the edge of each intestinal villus. They are visible only through the electron microscope. This vast array of microvilli on each villus is called the brush border. The microvilli add a tremendous surface area for absorption.

mucus a viscid fluid secreted by mucous membranes and glands, consisting mainly of mucin (a glycoprotein), inorganic salts, and water. Mucus serves to lubricate and protect the gastrointestinal mucosa, and to help move the food mass along the digestive tract.

parietal cells (L. *paries,* wall) cells of the gastric glands in the fundus of the stomach which produce hydrochloric acid.

secretin a hormone produced in the mucous membrane of the duodenum in response to the entrance of the acid contents of the stomach into the duodenum. Secretin in turn stimulates the flow of pancreatic juice, providing needed enzymes and the proper alkalinity for their action.

villikinin a hormone produced by glands in the upper intestinal mucosa in response to presence of chyme entering the intestine. Villikinin stimulates alternating contractions and extensions of the villi. This motion of the villi constantly agitates the mucosal surface, which stirs and mixes the chyme, and exposes additional nutrient material for absorption.

References
Specific
1. Menguy, R.: Motor function of the alimentary tract, Ann. Rev. Physiol. **26:**227, 1964.
2. Report, Joint Committee of the American Dietetic Association and the American Medical Association: Diet as related to gastrointestinal function, J. Amer. Diet. Ass. **38:**425, 1961.

General
Best, C. H., and Taylor, N. B.: The physiological basis of medical practice, ed. 8, Baltimore, 1966, The Williams and Wilkins Co.

Bogert, L. J., Briggs, G., and Calloway, D.: Nutrition and physical fitness, ed. 8, Philadelphia, 1966, W. B. Saunders Co.

Cantarow, A., and Trumper, M.: Clinical biochemistry, ed. 6, Philadelphia, 1962, W. B. Saunders Co.

Clifton, J. A.: Intestinal absorption and malabsorption, J. Amer. Diet. Ass. **39:**440, 1961.

Danielsson, H.: Influence of bile acids on digestion and absorption of lipids, Amer. J. Clin. Nutr. **12:**214, 1963.

Davenport, H. W.: Physiology of the digestive

tract, Chicago, 1961, Year Book Medical Publishers.

Dragstedt, L. R.: Why does not the stomach digest itself? J.A.M.A. 177:758, 1961.

Ganong, W. F.: Review of medical physiology, Los Altos, Calif., 1963, Lange Medical Publications.

Guyton, A. C.: Textbook of medical physiology, ed. 3, Philadelphia, 1966, W. B. Saunders Co.

Harper, H. A.: Review of physiological chemistry, ed. 11, Los Altos, Calif., 1967, Lange Medical Publications.

Ingelfinger, F. J.: Gastrointestinal absorption, Nutrition Today 2:2, 1967.

Kleiner, I. S., and Orten, J. M.: Biochemistry, ed. 7, St. Louis, 1966, The C. V. Mosby Co.

Miller, D., and Crane, R. K.: The digestion of carbohydrates in the small intestine, Amer. J. Clin. Nutr. 12:220, 1963.

Nasset, E. S.: Role of the digestive tract in the utilization of protein and amino acids, J.A.M.A. 164:172, 1957.

Stacy, R. W., and Santolucito, J. A.: Modern college physiology, St. Louis, 1966, The C. V. Mosby Co.

Wilson, T. H.: Intestinal absorption, Philadelphia, 1962, W. B. Saunders Co.

Wiseman, G.: Absorption from the intestine, New York, 1964, Academic Press, Inc.

APPLIED NUTRITION
IN PUBLIC HEALTH

Public health nursing presents the alert and skilled nurse with a unique opportunity —indeed, even a responsibility—to apply her knowledge of the science of human nutrition.

These scientific principles are not applied abstractly in a vacuum. They have meaning only in terms of *people*—people in families, people in communities, people in various work situations, people in financial distress, people with housing problems, people with deeply ingrained habits and customs, people with differing religious and cultural backgrounds—young people, old people, fat, thin, ill, well, discouraged, happy, clean, not so clean, educated, and illiterate people. The nurse will come to know many kinds of people in many places and with many needs. Each is a human being with unique dignity and pride and worth.

Therefore, knowledge alone is not enough. In her work with the individual, the family, and the community, the nurse will need to feel human compassion and concern and will need to employ practical guides, insights, appreciations, and skills in order to apply her knowledge in a useful and helpful manner. The chapters in this study unit will help to provide a background on which the nurse will be able to draw, as she tries to fill these human needs.

First, because some efforts to help people are hindered by their food fads or by their belief in false claims about foods, the chapter on "Food Misinformation" compares myths and magic to scientific facts.

Second, to guard against diseases that are spread by improper handling of food, the chapter on "Protecting the Food Supply," describes the problem, and suggests ways of guarding food throughout its journey from producer to consumer.

Third, because cultural forces so strongly influence the meanings of food and its use in the family, the chapter on "Cultural, Social, and Psychological Influences on Food Habits" provides a frame of reference for work with individual families.

Fourth, because knowing and doing are two different things, and because money spent for food is a large part of any family budget, the chapter on "Family Diet Counseling: Food Needs and Costs" offers tools and techniques, methods and materials for the effective delivery of sound nutrition education.

Finally, because in some pockets of extreme poverty in communities in the United States or in less developed countries the added factor of gross deficiency diseases may be encountered, the chapter on such conditions briefly pictures the classic examples of malnutrition.

CHAPTER 11

Food misinformation

Every year millions of dollars are spent by zealously health-conscious Americans as they respond to the claims of self-styled "scientists" who offer panaceas for ills. The panacea may be a pill, pellet, book, lecture, special food, or food supplement. Often the message is couched in garbled, pseudo-scientific jargon which seems to the unwary to indicate knowledge. But the pitch is usually the same—a glibly worded advertisement that appeals more to the emotion than to the intellect. The result is an immense "health food" industry. Surrounding that industry are satellite personalities who capitalize upon the insatiable anxiety of people about their health, through lectures and publications full of half-truths or outright error.

At one time or other, and with great frequency in some communities, the worker in the health professions will confront these barriers to sound health teaching. The nurse needs to know the nature and extent of food faddism, to understand why it exists, and to have a clear concept of the harm it may do. She needs to be able to identify, among the people she serves, the risk groups who may be particularly vulnerable to the bogus authority of the food fad salesman. She will want to determine effective countermeasures to his enticing misstatements.

The first step is to understand the problem of food misinformation as objectively as possible. The term "as objectively as possible" is used because if everyone is entirely honest with himself he will probably acknowledge that there is some vestige of superstition about foods lying deep within him. Perhaps, as Dr. Frederick Stare[1] of Harvard University has suggested, most people gullibly accept certain myths because they (like primitive peoples) secretly suspect there is something magical in nearly every kind of food. As the nurse scrutinizes her own beliefs and the beliefs of others, she will find it helpful to ask some fundamental questions:

1. What is a food fad or food myth?
2. What are some examples of these fallacies? How do they hold up in the light of nutritional science?
3. What harm is there in fads?
4. Why do faddists and quacks exist?
5. Who is especially vulnerable?
6. What can be done to prevent fallacies about nutrition from harming patients?

DEFINITIONS

Food fads. The word "fad" is a shortened form of an old word, *faddle* (it is retained today in the phrase "fiddle-faddle"), meaning "to play with." A fad is something one "plays with" for awhile. A fad is any popular fashion or pursuit, without substantial basis, that is followed enthusiastically. Most fads are short-lived; but some persist, and a few eventually become incorporated into a society's customs or mores.

Food fads are scientifically unsubstantiated beliefs about certain foods, which may persist for a time in a given community or society. Some may be perfectly harmless.

Others have more serious implications concerning the health and welfare of their followers.

Food faddist. A food faddist is one who follows such food customs for a time. Usually, he does so with exaggerated fervor, as do some enthusiasts for molasses, wheat germ, yogurt, and so on. He may be an individual faddist, whose practice may have its basis in an acute or chronic psychological problem. Or the faddist may be a member of a group which has accepted some rigid, stereotyped dietary practice in the belief that it will improve health or cure disease.

Food myths. The word *myth* comes from the Greek word *mythos* meaning "story" or "fable." The Greeks applied it to the vast array of stories that accumulated through the centuries about their gods and goddesses—their mythology. A myth is a traditional legend without a determinable basis of fact; it is an invented story, idea, or concept. Food myths are unproved stories or beliefs about food which are accepted uncritically, or are used to justify one's own desires, interests, or practices.

Over the years, many myths have developed around foods. Current myths that have been identified by the U. S. Food and Drug Administration center upon food and disease. To a large extent, they represent a reactionary response to advances in scientific agriculture and food technology (see p. 205).

Quack. The word *quack,* as used in this sense, has an interesting history. It is a shortened form of "quacksalver," a term invented centuries ago by the Dutch, to describe the pseudo doctor or professor who sold worthless salves, "magic" elixirs, and cure-all tonics. He proclaimed his wares, like a barker, in a patter that skeptical people compared to the quacking of a duck. The quacksalver made much loud noise but had no real medical ability or knowledge.

In medicine, nutrition, and allied fields, a quack is a fraudulent pretender who claims to have skill, knowledge, or qualifications which he does not possess. His motive is usually money. By a cruel hoax, he feeds upon the physical and emotional needs of people. The food quack exists because food faddists exist.

The food quack can usually be recognized by four aspects basic to his method of operation:

1. He uses the direct sales approach to promote the sale of his special food products. Although he may start by appealing to the gullible in a comparatively mild way, eventually his lectures, writings, and special products are foisted on the unwary at extravagant prices. The buyer of such products becomes persuaded that he should ignore the advice of the reputable physician and nutritionist, in favor of self-diagnosis and treatment.

2. The quack makes exaggerated claims. He promises that his treatment will cure or prevent all diseases.

3. The quack warns his customers against American agriculture and established food distributors; he creates distrust in all scientific technology.

4. He uses emotionally convincing double-talk which is full of half-truths and misinterpretations. Often he quotes out of context leading medical and nutritional authorities, to support his claims. He is usually a charming person, with a flair for words and a clever wit.

Food misinformation. To misinform is to give false or misleading information. Food misinformation is a statement about food, which is not based upon, or is not in agreement with scientific evidence. False information may have arisen out of a traditional fallacy, or it may represent a belief in magic or folklore. It may be built upon outright lies, more subtle half-truths, innuendos, and inferences that are the stock-in-trade of the ingenious quack.

Scientific nutritional concepts. Opposed to food misinformation is the body of nutritional concepts that have been built on scientific evidence. Scientifically sound concepts are the result of persistent research and testing over many decades. They represent organized, tested knowledge. The scientific, or problem-solving method, here as in all other branches of modern learning, involves four steps:

1. Recognizing that a problem exists, identifying the problem, and determining some desirable goals in relation to it
2. Gathering all possible pertinent data, background knowledge, and principles; and on the basis of this information forming a hypothesis (an educated guess) about the solution to the problem
3. Testing this hypothesis under controlled conditions, which entails isolating the pertinent variables and studying one variable at a time; usually a large number of cases must be observed in detail before valid results accrue
4. Evaluating these test results; and, if the hypothesis seems to be borne out, applying the results to a much larger population, while continuing to observe critically for errors that may become apparent only with time and broad application over a wide range of circumstances

Whenever one is confronted with questionable food information from a quack or a faddist, it is highly legitimate to ask, "What is your evidence?"

MYTHS AND FADS VS. SCIENTIFIC FACT
Basic food myths

It is an intriguing test of one's own beliefs to notice how some sample myths appear in the light of facts that have been amassed by scientific observers. Four basic food myths, which occur in many different disguises, have been identified by the American Medical Association and the Federal Food and Drug Administration. Each one is compared with scientifically tested facts.

Myth: all disease is due to faulty diet. The proponents of this myth contend that certain chemical imbalances in the body are the cause of disease, and that these imbalances are directly due to improper or inadequate diet. Since it is impossible for the average person to eat an adequate diet, according to the myth, he must supplement it with whatever product is being sold at the time. The product in question usually contains a long list of ingredients, including those labaled as "mysterious substances as yet unknown to nutritional scientists."

Here, for example, is the colorful "line" of one such food supplement salesman, as tape recorded by an investigator employed by the Food and Drug Administration: "You eat food to make blood. You send down junk, your body will be junk. Your body will wind up in the junk pile. You send down vital elements that are needed, you're okay. Whenever you get your body normalized, you won't have no condition. You can't even take a cold. I don't care how you're exposed to freezing temperature, wet feet and cold feet, you'll never take it if you get your blood stream up to par."[2] And, of course, according to the salesman, the only way to "get your blood stream up to par" was to take large numbers of the special pills he was selling.

FACT. Disease, by and large, is caused by many sorts of variation from normal states, such as inherited defects; and by any of a host of agents such as microorganisms and parasites. A large number of these causes of disease have no specific etiologic relationship to nutrients.

The few classic nutritional deficiency diseases such as scurvy, rickets, pellagra, kwashiorkor, and a small number of others, have been well studied by medical science. Although they are still a major health problem in some impoverished parts of the world, they are seen less often in the United States because of increased nutritional knowledge and abundant food supply. Officials of the Food and Drug Administration, and of the American Medical Association have stated that the American food supply is "unsurpassed in volume, variety, and nutritional value,"[3] making it actually difficult not to obtain a nourishing diet. Only in the extreme instances of poverty pockets in the United States population do these deficiency diseases exist. Even in such areas, the problem is usually one of economics, social alienation, education, or rejection of middle class health values—not of food availability per se.

Myth: soil depletion causes malnutrition. People who believe this myth argue that the soil has lost its vitality from long overuse, and that crops grown on it are deficient in nutrients. Moreover, the chemical fertilizers used in agriculture only "poison" the land and its crops. The only salvation is so-called organic farming, and eating the "natural" foods thus produced.

FACT. Both scientists and farmers have repeatedly observed that if a soil lacks minerals and other materials necessary for plant growth, the plant simply will not grow. Poor soil affects only the *quantity* of food grown on it, not the *quality*. Extensive, controlled tests indicate these two facts:

1. Fertilizing the soil significantly increases the yield, not the nutritive content, of the food grown on it.[4]
2. The kind of fertilizer used—commercial chemical mix or organic manure—makes no difference in the food's nutritional composition.[5]

It is a magnificient achievement of American agriculture to have met as well as it has two advancing pressures: (1) a rapidly growing population—demographers predict there will be approximately 400 million people by the year 2000—and (2) an even more rapidly shrinking amount of farmland as cities and suburbs spread over soil once used to grow food. The purpose that dominates agrarian research and the development of chemical fertilizers is to increase the yield of available land.

Myth: food processing destroys the nutritive value of food. This myth is extensively promoted by food supplement exponents. They insist that such products as white bread and flour, refined cereals, canned foods, and even pasteurized milk are worthless or inferior because processing has removed their natural vitamins and minerals. They even lament that cooking causes further nutritive loss and advocate the use of raw foods, often liquefied in a blender. Some promote the sale of special cookware (at inflated prices) because they claim that certain utensils, especially aluminum, slowly poison the body.

FACT. Three false premises in this myth are refuted by scientific observations:

First, modern food processing methods are scientifically developed and highly controlled to preserve or restore nutritional values in foods. Processing times, temperatures, and quality are rigidly controlled in the canning and freezing of vegetables and fruits in order to preserve the nutrients that are present. Enrichment of grain products restores, and in some instances even increases, their natural vitamin and mineral content. United States food enrichment laws in general have been a primary factor in almost eliminating from the American population deficiency diseases that were once prevalent. A clinical case of ordinary vitamin D-deficiency rickets, for example, is now hard to find, largely because milk has been fortified for some years with 400 I.U. of vitamin D per quart. These food enrichment regulations are under constant study so that correlate current practice can be coordinated with developing scientific knowledge. One result of such continuing study is the new body of F.D.A. regulations concerning vitamin and mineral additions to foods (see p. 238).

Second, the nutritive qualities of vitamins and minerals as they occur naturally in foods do not differ from those that are synthetically produced in a laboratory and added to food. Categorically and unequivocally, *a vitamin is a vitamin.*

Third, aluminum is a trace element in the human body and widespread in nature. There is no evidence to indicate that these trace amounts are harmful, or that the amounts that may be ingested in food that has been cooked in an aluminum utensil significantly increases the total amount in the body. Extensive use of aluminum cookware, even in quantity cookery in governmental and industrial food service installations, has produced none of the harmful effects claimed by promoters of this myth. Statements by the American Cancer Society, the U. S. Public Health Service, and the American Medical Association's Council on Foods and Nutrition declare that there is absolutely no scientific basis for such a claim.

Myth: the United States population suffers from widespread subclinical deficiencies requiring supplements of vitamins and minerals. Many times in advertisements one hears or reads about "that tired feeling" or "tired blood" or vague aches and pains, for which the advertiser has blamed dietary deficiencies. The very vagueness of this myth makes it difficult to refute. It is particularly appealing to the anxious person who constantly worries about his health, and who fears that there must be something wrong with him which the doctors simply haven't been able to detect. Such a person accepts the claims of the vitamin or tonic salesman and purchases his product, perhaps because it provides the emotional support he needs. The vitamin is his placebo.

FACT. The word *subclinical* is a general, nonspecific term given to conditions for which there are no observable symptoms. It can be used in almost any context, depending upon the purposes of the user. It is therefore rather meaningless in itself, and if used by an irresponsible person it may be misleading. Moreover, every normal person occasionally experiences such vague feelings of fatigue of being worn-out or achy. There is no more reason for attributing temporary tiredness to a dietary deficiency, than for ascribing it to any of a variety of life situations. Should such feelings persist, the patient should consult a qualified physician for competent examination and individually indicated treatment. He will prescribe supplementary vitamins and minerals only if he finds that they are needed by the patient. If the physician does not write such a prescription, a sound, normal diet including a variety of foods will supply ample amounts of the essential nutrients.

Fallacious claims by food faddists

Types of claims. Food faddists make exaggerated claims for certain types of food. These claims fall into four basic classifications:

1. Certain foods will cure specific conditions.
2. Certain foods are harmful and should be omitted from the diet.
3. Special food combinations are very effective as reducing diets and have special therapeutic effects.
4. Only "natural foods" can meet body needs and prevent disease.

Basic error. If these claims are examined carefully, the reader will notice that each one focuses upon foods per se, not upon the chemical components in them—the nutrients—which are the actual physiological agents of life and health. *It is the nutrients, not specific foods as such, that have specific functions in the body.* Each of these nutrients may be found in a number of different foods. *People require specific nutrients, never specific foods.*

Examples of food fads. A number of food fads have flourished from time to time. The following are a few examples and the fallacies they represent.

1. Milk and fish form a harmful combination and should never be eaten together.

FACT. Both milk and fish are excellent foods, alone or together. Only if either milk or fish is contaminated or spoiled by improper handling or lack of refrigeration, may difficulty be encountered.

2. Pasteurized milk is a "dead milk" and should be replaced by raw milk.

FACT. The process of pasteurization may destroy a small amount of vitamin C. But the quantity of vitamin C in cow's milk is so small that it makes no significant contribution to the human diet, and its destruction by pasteurization is therefore not important. Control of microorganisms by pasteurization, and the prevention of the spread of disease by this means far outweigh any imagined dietary loss.

3. Citrus fruits such as oranges and

lemons make the body acid, or produce "acid stomach."

FACT. Hydrochloric acid, secreted by the parietal cells in gastric mucosal glands, forms the normally acid medium of the stomach. Citrus fruits have no influence on this secretion. As they undergo metabolism by the body, almost all fruits form an alkaline, not an acid, residue.

4. Onion and garlic will cure a cold; or will purify the blood.

FACT. No such powers are inherent in either food—unless, of course, copious use of such pungent partners so isolate one socially as to free him from viral contagion! Extension of the superstition that garlic has an effect on the blood is the basis on which the quack is able to sell "garlic pills" to cure high blood pressure.

5. Yogurt, blackstrap molasses, honey and other such "wonder foods" assure good health.

FACT. Yogurt is merely a fermented, cultured form of milk; it has no mysterious additional properties. It costs more than plain milk. Blackstrap molasses is a syrup formed in the process of refining sugar. It contains vitamins and minerals; but so do many, many other foods in more common use. Honey is simply a form of sugar (fructose). Some have claimed any number of unfounded curative properties for honey combined with vinegar.

6. Oysters, olives, lean meat, and raw eggs enhance sexual potency and fertility.

FACT. Perhaps the notion that there is a connection between lean meat and potency had its origin in the primitive belief that eating certain foods gave the consumer the characteristics of the thing eaten. Hence, lean meat (animal flesh) was supposed to arouse animal passions. Such folklore has no basis in fact. There is no food that has any effect on sexual potency.

7. Grape juice, tomato juice, beets are strong blood builders.

FACT. The nutrients necessary to the production of red blood cells are protein and iron, neither of which these foods supply. Presumably, this superstition arises from the color of these foods: they, like blood, are red.

8. Fish, celery, and nutmeg are good brain foods; raw beef juice is good nerve food.

FACT. No food as such builds any specific tissue. Again, it is the specific nutrients in foods that are required for the building of specific tissue. Nervous tissue, including brain tissue, is built and repaired from amino acids contained in protein, and protein is, of course, found in many foods.

9. Gelatin in large amounts builds strong fingernails.

FACT. Gelatin is an incomplete protein, which alone builds nothing. Nail formation is influenced by many other factors such as general body nutrition, disease, environment, and local nail care.

10. Seaweed or kelp products are important dietary supplements that prevent serious iodine deficiency.

FACT. The small amount of iodine needed by the body is supplied in iodized table salt, which is commonly used in the American diet, and in seafood. To spend money on seaweed because it provides additional iodine is sheer waste.

11. Special food combinations are highly effective as reducing diets. Examples of such odd combinations are bananas and skimmed milk, lamb chops and pineapple, steak and spinach, or just eggs and more eggs.

FACT. A weight reduction program is successful only when calorie intake is smaller than caloric output (energy expenditure). For optimum nutrition during such a program, the diet must contain a wisely balanced group of nutrients. These faddish reducing combinations do not.

12. Special foods influence pregnancy and lactation by marking the child, by tainting breast milk, or by increasing milk production. Examples of such taboos and unfounded notions about the need for special foods are:

  a. Strawberry birth marks on infants are caused by strawberries eaten by the mother during her pregnancy.

b. Cravings for specific foods or for clay or cornstarch, indicate physical needs of the gestating woman.
c. Beer increases lactation.
d. Foods such as cabbage, chocolate, and onions taint breast milk and produce gastrointestinal upsets in the nursing infant.

FACT. It is not specific foods that are needed for optimum maternal nutrition, although increased amounts of specific nutrients may be required. No food can mark the developing fetus. No food taints breast milk. The lactating mother does not need beer, although she may well need to increase her total daily fluid intake. Each of the beliefs listed here is unfounded.

DANGERS OF FOOD FADS

Why should the nurse be concerned about food faddism and food quackery? What harm may they do? Essentially, food fads involve four basic dangers, which concern all members of the health professions.

Dangers to health. Self-diagnosis and self-treatment are always dangerous. When they are based on questionable sources, the dangers are multiplied. By following such a course, a person with a real illness may fail to secure proper medical care. Many anxious patients who have cancer, diabetes, or arthritis have been misled by quacks who fraudulently claimed that they had a cure for these diseases, and have postponed effective therapy until the chance of cure was gone.

Money spent needlessly. Some of the foods and supplements used by faddists are harmless; but many are expensive. All money spent for useless food is wasted. When dollars are scarce, the family may neglect to buy foods that will fill its basic needs, in order to purchase a "guaranteed cure."

Lack of knowledge of scientific progress. Misinformation spread by charlatans hinders the development of our society along lines that have been opened by scientific progress. The superstitions that are perpetuated by quacks counteract sound health teaching in the minds of many persons.

Distrust of food market. Erroneous teaching concerning food and health breeds public suspicion and distrust of the common food market and of food technology and agriculture in general. The many new food products make possible the multitude and variety of standard quality food items in out grocery stores. They provide an abundant choice of interesting, palatable, and attractive sources of nutrients. Yet, food faddists and food quacks would have people rely upon health food merchants to fill their nutritional needs. Those who do so may also be robbed of the esthetic values inherent in foods that have positive worth.

REASONS FOR EXISTENCE OF FOOD FADDISM

In the face of unprecedented advances in the knowledge available to scientists, why should some lay persons be addicted to such unsound and wasteful practices? Perhaps several reasons may be considered. They relate to both group culture pressures and individual human needs. These reasons include the rapid scientific and technological advances, the population increase, the growth of the American economy, the communications media, individual emotional needs, and lack of general health education.

Scientific advances. The very rapidity of technical advance in itself has contributed to the problem. As medical knowledge has increased, most acute diseases have come under control.

Everyone is familiar with the statement: *During the first half of this century there was a dramatic increase in human longevity.* This has been stated many, many times. Do people feel its impact? Do people who live in the second half of the twentieth century sense the profound change that the promise of longevity has made in the human psyche?

The statement has more meaning when it is realized that the change was not so much a lengthening of the lifespan of those individuals who survived the acute diseases of childhood and the dangers of childbirth, as it was a remarkable rise in the *total number of persons who lived to reach old age.* Today, most people take it for granted that the average man and woman can reasonably expect to live to the age of seventy. Yet this is the most exciting news that has ever come out of man's endeavors. This one fact created in the peoples of developed countries, within a single generation, a new attitude toward life: people *expect* to live.

A woman, if she plans to marry, does not carry in the back of her mind a haunting dread of the possibility that she may die if she has a child. If a woman is pregnant, she does not have to grope about for ways of facing a haunting terror that her baby will quite probably die before his or her fifth birthday. With the exception of persons with specific genetically transmitted diseases, such fears as these hardly enter the consciousness of healthy-minded young people today. Yet, a single example of what life was like in all former centuries, even for rather well-off professional people, shows how different their expectations were. It gives a gauge by which the change in human attitudes can be measured that has resulted from the conquering of acute disease and of the high rate of deaths in childbirth. The composer Johann Sebastian Bach, who even in his own day was famous and successful, and who came from vigorous stock, had twenty children from his two wives. His first wife died young, after bearing the first seven children. Of those twenty children, only 10 survived their infancy, and this infant death rate was not unusual. The effect that the nearness of death had upon people's thoughts and feelings will become clear after considering how often and how deeply this man, who was the respected friend of princes, knew grief.

The mastery, in the Twentieth Century, of most of the diseases that killed mothers and young children pushed the thought of death far into the background of the average person's consciousness. Taking its place has been an eager determination to live. Most Americans today are looking for ways to ensure that each will get his full share of happiness while he is alive and that he will live out his full measure of years.

Americans are fully aware through their popular press that this change had come about through the application of scientific principles to biologic problems. They therefore look to science to give them still more of this good thing, life. Unfortunately the alteration has been so swift that public education has not had time to catch up. Even young persons whose total education has been within the scientific era do not always apply scientific principles to all phases of their lives. Persons educated before World War II, or those who attend schools where teaching is less than optimal, are sometimes unable to perceive the relationship between the glittering achievements of science and the sober step-by-step work of physiology, pathology, and calculus. Without having gone through those painstaking steps, thousands have felt themselves to be emotionally converted to science as they might be converted to a belief in magic if they saw proof that it worked. Such enthusiasts are easily duped by any hoax that masquerades in pseudoscientific jargon, and that offers glib explanations which sound as though they were scientific. Thus, faith in the results of science is distorted into gullibility toward pseudoscience.

Such converts turn toward pseudomedicine for quack cures. And they turn toward the propaganda of the food faddist for the same reason—there is a real basis for believing that nutrition is related to health. New knowledge of nutrition has yielded undeniable evidence of the role of proper diet in disease prevention and in the maintenance of sound health. What the food quack does *not* mention is that nutrition is a relatively infant science. More reliable information about food and its production, composition, and functions in maintaining health has been discovered within the past four decades than was established in all man's previous history. But the true scientist is far from ready to make the glib assertions and the broad promises of the quack.

Food technology advances. Together with the increased knowledge of nutritional science has come a revolution in food technology. The American food supply 'has become almost transformed by new methods of food preservation, processing, distribution, packaging, and transportation. The food quack points to these new processes with suspicion. He knows and uses the psychologic basis for building a wall of distrust in that which is new and unfamiliar.

The human mind maintains its stability by means of an equilibrium between eagerness for the new and distrust of the unfamiliar. Professional workers respect this equilibrium. The same sort of balancing activity goes on in the mind of the doctor as he assesses the value of a new drug. His interest is aroused by the claims of the manufacturer, by the reasonable way in which the pharmacological chemist has worked out a respectable hypothesis, by the convenience of a new form of administration, by attractive packaging, which tends to help his patients accept the treatment. But his trained skepticism is also aroused. He asks whether the new agent is effective. The doctor has been taught the tests to apply in making an informed judgment. He knows when to take advantage of the new, and when to rely upon the old.

Less well trained persons often do not know. Many intelligent people are unfavorably impressed or are calmly unimpressed by gaudy packaging and extravagant claims. The trouble starts when this healthy conservatism is outbalanced by superstitious clinging to the old, for one reason only—simply because it is familiar.

The notion that people in those mythical "good old days" enjoyed better food, and better nutritional health, than people do today is nonsense. Rates of death and disease were far higher then and the average chance of living out the full human life span was much less. The present food supply exceeds that of any past time in terms of nutritive value, safety, stability, variety, convenience, attractiveness, and availability. Basic research in food technology has enabled the prudent shopper in the community food market to procure good food of high quality for family health and enjoyment.

Population increases. Population explosions the world over have focused attention on the amounts of food that will be needed to sustain the increasing numbers of people. The pressure to develop more and better means of food production distribution has led to revolutionary changes in agriculture. It has been necessary to increase the efficiency of agricultural workers through new techniques, and to increase the yield of farmland by the intelligent and economical use of chemicals. These developments are an example of the application of technological advance to the fulfillment of pressing human need. Yet the food quack seizes the opportunity created by tensions that mount as people are forced to change old habits to accommodate the population rise. He plays on the food neurotic's anxiety, and makes his profit.

American economic growth. Oddly enough, America's great economic growth has also contributed to food faddism. By and large, food faddism with its many special foods and gadgets is a costly practice, one that only a relatively affluent society can maintain. Today's worker has more money than any worker in history. Automation has given him more leisure time in which to seek new interests; those who are so inclined will spend much of this time in seeking for foods that will fill some imagined need. And there are some persons who feel that to require a special food is to prove that one has a higher status than ordinary people. Appeals to each of these peculiarities have been used by clever promotors to enhance their products.

Mass communication media. Through television, radio, and public press, a health-conscious culture has been developed in America. Public awareness of medical advances, of nutrition's role in health, and of food technology has created a general desire for more information. This very desire for information provides a fertile soil for the growth of faddism. Some of the statements of faddists are honest errors of misguided zeal. Some statements made by quacks are deliberately deceptive.

Emotional needs. Very real contribution to food faddism arises from the emotional needs of people. Food has emotional value for the average person. Everyone knows this from personal experience. People today live in a world of many pressures. This era has been called the age of anxiety. Sometimes these anxieties are converted into an exaggerated concern for health, and attachment to certain food practices may result.

In human societies, especially where scarcity of food is not a problem, food assumes significance far beyond fulfillment of hunger as a basic drive. Eating together symbolizes social acceptance, friendliness, cultural identification, prestige, and position. Eating with one's peers, and the exclusion of those who do not rank with the peer group, may even be a form of weapon. Foods are used as bribes or rewards. From infancy, foods mean love, comfort, pleasure, and protection. In the anxious adult, these associations may form the basis of compulsive drives to overeat. Faddism appeals to such human emotional values and drives. Quackery makes direct capital of them.

Lack of general health education. In many instances, faddism has grown because nurses, nutritionists, and physicians have failed to communicate sound information about relationships between food and health. Sometimes health workers have not been sufficiently person-centered to appreciate the emotional value of foods. Sometimes, by being rigidly fact-centered, they have repelled rather than appealed to those persons who are vulnerable to fads. Although the information given must be scientifically grounded, the importance of a balance between intellect and emotion must not be ignored. The professional medical person is often depicted as a sterile, cold personality, perhaps more concerned with maintaining his own professional status than with meeting the needs of people. If this image is contrasted with the warmly sympathetic, soothing tones of the pseudo-professional food quack, it is no wonder that many frightened or anxious persons reject the first, and accept the latter.

Groups vulnerable to food faddism

Food fads appeal especially to certain groups of people with particular needs and concerns. Among these are the middle-aged, the elderly, the adolescent, the obese, and people whose living depends on their physical appearance.

Fear of the changes that come about as youth and potency wane leads many middle-aged persons to grasp at exaggerated claims that some purchasable product will restore their vigor.

When in pain and discomfort, perhaps facing chronic illness, the elderly patient may respond to the hope that the food quack holds out for a sure cure. Desperately ill and lonely people are an easy prey for a cruel hoax.

Figure-conscious girls and muscle-minded boys frequently respond to advertisements that glowingly depict a crash program for attaining the perfect body. Young people, particularly those who are lonely, but also many who have exaggerated ideas of glamor, hope to achieve peer group acceptance by these means.

One of the most disturbing health problems in America today is obesity. It is often most frustrating to treat. Obese persons, faced with a bewildering barrage of propaganda advocating diets, pills, candies, wafers, and devices, are likely to succumb to fads.

People in the public eye—entertainers and athletes—are often prey to those who make false claims that certain foods, drugs, or dietary combinations will enable them to retain the physical appearance and strength on which their careers depend.

These groups are vulnerable for obvious reasons. There seems to be no segment of the population, however, that is completely free from food faddism's appeal. Particularly in metropolitan areas, large groups of faddists present a constant array of misinformation that hinders the efforts of the members of the legitimate health professions to raise the community standards in nutrition.

ANSWERS TO THE PROBLEM

What is the answer to the problems associated with food faddism, misinformation, and outright quackery? What can workers in the health professions do? What *should* they do? At least six courses of action merit consideration:

1. Members of the health professions must assess their own attitudes and habits. No one can teach another until he has first examined his own position. Instruction based on personal conviction, practice, and enthusiasm will achieve far more than teaching that says, in effect, "Do as I say, not as I do."

2. Sound facts must be obtained from reliable sources. Two types of background knowledge are vital. (1) The health worker must have facts that will accurately controvert specific items of misinformation, and that will clearly explain why a certain product is worthless, harmful, inflated in price, or cannot have the effects claimed for it. One must have facts about people involved in a given instance of fraud, or in a specific kind of fraud. One must avoid making broad generalizations or vague charges; effective counteraction is necessarily based on knowledge of the adversary. (2) The worker must also have facts concerning human nutritional physiology, and about the scientific approach to the solution of health problems. The health worker must have facts about food technology, agricultural methods, and other related data, since these facts are tools. To have them at her command, the worker must keep up with relevant research, be alert to scientific discoveries, and to the constant developments in the practices of applied science.

3. The health worker must recognize the basic human needs involved in nutrition. The nurse must observe in herself and others how psychological and cultural factors affect food habits. She cannot effectively combat false information unless she considers the emotional needs that are symbolically fulfilled by foods, by the eating of food, and by the rituals with which everyone surrounds the eating of food. As she plans a program of nutritional education for a group or for a single patient, these emotional needs must be respected. Everyone has them. They are part of life. The power that foods and eating rituals possess for filling those needs should be welcomed. That power should be used intelligently and worked into the health worker's program. Foods should not be disparaged as a mere "crutch." Even when the nurse has reason to believe that her patient is using food as a crutch for an ailing emotional adjustment, she should consider its value. A wise teacher has put it well. "We must avoid 'breaking crutches' without offering alternative support." This should be remembered particularly when a patient falls within one of the categories that is especially vulnerable to food faddism.

4. The health worker must be alert to community opportunities and resources. Any opportunity that arises within a community should be taken to present sound health information to groups or individuals, formally and informally. The worker should know what community resources are available, such as a local or state university agricultural extension service, volunteer health agencies, clinic and hospital facilities, federal, state, county, and city public health departments, professional health organizations. Workshops, conferences, meetings, classes, clinics, demonstration projects, displays, exhibits, bulletins, newsletters, and many other channels are excellent devices for promoting sound nutritional concepts. Skill in communication is essential to success in using these devices. Clarity in speech and writing is all-important. Monotony should be avoided and the worker should possess a well disciplined imagina-

tion. Without this, the message will not convince.

5. Young people should be taught to think scientifically. While very young, children may be introduced to the problem-solving approach to everyday situations. Children are naturally curious. A child often seeks evidence to support statements with which he is confronted. Far too often the system of education fails to develop this spirit of inquiry. Children can learn early that it is valuable to ask legitimate questions such as, what do you mean, how do you know, and what is your evidence.

6. The health worker should know the work of responsible legal authorities and support them in their direct dealing with quacks. The Federal Food and Drug Administration is charged with the legal responsibility for controlling the quality and safety of all food and drug products marketed in this country. Every worker in the health professions should know of this organization and its work, and should relay to it information about illegal food handling, or food quackery.

James L. Goddard, M.D., who was commissioner of the Food and Drug Administration from 1966 to 1968, used science and law enforcement in a sensible and tough team approach to protect the consumer. K. L. Milstead who was the former commissioner's special assistant made the following encouraging statement: "Through scientific research, improved regulations, vigorous enforcement, and expanding educational programs, we expect to eliminate nutritional quackery as a major health and economic problem within the next five years. And this includes the false and misleading promotion of products for weight control which has become the most serious type of nutritional quackery today."[3]

Other governmental, professional, and private organizations provide additional resources for consumer education. The Federal Trade Commission exerts control of consumer products. The U. S. Department of Agriculture maintains a broad program of research, regulation, and education. The Agricultural Extension Services extend this department's work into communities. A group of scientists form the Food and Nutrition Board of the National Research Council, which studies human nutrient requirements and recommends standards and guidelines.

On a world-wide basis, the Food and Agriculture Organization and the World Health Organization, divisions of the United Nations, help to raise living standards, attack the problem of insufficient food for the world's increasing population, and contribute to general nutritional health. Two other United Nations agencies, UNESCO and UNICEF, also work in the area of world nutrition.

Professional organizations, such as American Nursing Association, National League of Nursing, the Food and Nutrition Council of the American Medical Association, and the American Dietetic Association, provide additional educational resources through their printed materials and local group activities.

An important private foundation, The Nutrition Foundation, Inc., of which Dr. Charles G. King is executive director, provides an important service through research, publication, and education.

References
Specific
1. Stare, F. J.: Sense and nonsense about nutrition, Harper's Magazine **229**:66, 1964.
2. Bell, Joseph N.: Let 'em eat hay, Today's Health, Sept., 1958.
3. Milstead, K. L.: Science works through law to protect consumer, J. Amer. Diet. Ass. **48**:187-191, 1966.
4. Maynard, L. A.: Effect of fertilizers on the nutritional value of foods, J.A.M.A. **161**:1478, 1956.
5. Beeson, K. C.: Effects of fertilizers on nutrition quality of crops and health of animals and man, Plant Food Journal **5**:7, 1951.

General
Beeuwkes, A. M.: Characteristics of the self-styled scientist, J. Amer. Diet. Ass. **32**:627, 1956.
Beeuwkes, A. M.: Food faddism and the consumer, Fed. Proc. **13**:785, 1954.
Conference on Quackery, Science **134**:1057, 1961.

Deutsch, R. M.: The nuts among the berries, New York, 1961, Ballantine Books, Inc.

Editorial: Facts about drugs and devices for weight reducing, J.A.M.A. 171:1731, 1959.

Editorial: Quackery in the field of nutrition, Amer. J. Public Health 42:997, 1952.

Editorial: Vitamins—good or bad? J.A.M.A. 173: 1831, 1960.

Engel, R. W.: Food faddism, Nutr. Rev. 17:353, 1959.

Food facts talk back: food information—fallacies and facts, Chicago, 1957, The American Dietetic Association.

Huenemann, R. L.: Combating food misinformation and quackery, J. Amer. Diet. Ass. 32:623, 1956.

Jalso, S. B., and others: Nutritional beliefs and practices, J. Amer. Diet. Ass. 47:263, 1965.

King, C. G., and Sipple, H. L.: Educational and economic hazards imposed by faddists, Fed. Proc. 13:794, 1954.

Krehl, W. A.: Nutritional advice—a problem and a challenge, Amer. J. Clin. Nutr. 10:365, 1962.

Larrick, G. P.: The nutritive adequacy of our food supply, J. Amer. Diet. Ass. 39:117, 1961.

Millman, M.: Can drugs reduce weight? Amer. J. Nurs. 55:308, 1955.

Mitchell, H. S.: Don't be fooled by fads, In: Food: the yearbook of agriculture, Washington, D. C., 1959, U. S. Dept. of Agriculture.

Mitchell, H. S.: Nutrition books for lay readers: a guide to the reliable and unreliable, Library J. 85:710, 1960.

Mott, M. A.: Better business bureaus fight food faddism, J. Amer. Diet. Ass. 39:122, 1961.

Nelson, E. M.: Control of nutrition claims under the Food, Drug, and Cosmetic Act, Fed. Proc. 13:790, 1954.

New, P. K., and Priest, R. P.: Food and thought: a sociologic study of food cultists, J. Amer. Diet. Ass. 51:13, 1967.

Olson, R. E.: Food faddism—why? Nutr. Rev. 16: 97, 1958.

Queries and minor notes: nutritive value of black-strap molasses, J.A.M.A. 146:1088, 1951; Yogurt, J.A.M.A. 146:221, 1951.

The role of nutrition education in combatting food fads, New York, 1959, The Nutrition Foundation, Inc.

Rosenberg, R. S.: Nutritional claims in food advertising, J. Amer. Diet. Ass. 32:631, 1956.

Sebrell, W. H.: Food faddism and public health, Fed. Proc. 13:780, 1954.

White, P. L.: Book review: Taller, H.: Calories don't count, New York, 1961, Simon & Schuster, J.A.M.A. 179:828, 1962.

White, P. L.: A close look at nutri-bio, Today's Health 40:16, 1962.

White, P. L.: How good are the 900-calorie formula diets? Today's Health 39:5, 1961.

White, P. L.: Who treats arthritis? J.A.M.A. 163: 942, 1957.

CHAPTER 12

Protecting the food supply

America's present food supply is one of the best in the history of man. The abundance is the result of an increasing application of scientific knowledge to a vast heritage of fertile acres.

However, the rapid growth of the population is increasing the demand for food at the same time that it is reducing the available farming land. Every year, hundreds of thousands of acres of rich farm soil are sacrificed to the spread of cities and suburbs. The agricultural sections are pushed farther and farther away from the consumers who are crowded into the cities, where virtually no food can be grown. This means that foods must be hauled greater distances than ever before. It is one more factor that poses a problem of food preservation. But there are many additional reasons why there is never freedom from the threat of food spoilage and waste, or from disease carried by food either by microorganisms and parasites, or by the poisons used to combat them. Therefore, to maintain this abundant harvest and ensure its safety and high quality, safeguards within the agricultural, chemical, and food industries are imperative.

In considering ways of protecting the food supply, knowledge of four factors is important: (1) food-borne disease agents, (2) protection of food during handling from farm to table, (3) means of food preservation, and (4) control agencies to ensure food safety and quality. This study should be focused upon the following questions:

1. What agents of disease may be spread by food?

2. How is food guarded during production from spoilage and harmful agents?
3. How is food preserved for continuing use?
4. What agencies control food safety and quality?

Human ecology and nutrition. Many advances have been made in hygiene, sanitation, and preventive medicine, in man's struggle to protect himself from the pathogenic organisms that are constantly present in his environment, and are transmitted by contaminated food and water. Epidemiologic studies of the classic triad of host, agent, and environment, and the interactions between them have led to valuable knowledge of how to control the environment and make it more healthful. All of these problems are by no means solved. Even scientific advances sometimes create new difficulties. Everyone is cognizant of air pollution and radioactivity which are by-products of superb technical achievements. The study of man's relation to his environment—human ecology—has arisen out of his awareness of pressing needs. Constant vigilance is necessary to control the diseases that result when that relationship is disturbed.

FOOD- AND WATER-BORNE DISEASE AGENTS

The agents of disease carried by food or water may be classified in three main categories: (1) pathogenic organisms, which carry disease to man, usually by the fecal-oral route through contaminated food and water, or through unsanitary food handling,

(2) natural poisons in certain plants and animals, and (3) man-made chemical contaminants.

Pathogenic organisms

The organisms pathogenic to man that are transmitted through his food or water are parasites, bacteria, and viruses.

Parasites

A number of protozoa and helminths inhabit man's intestinal tract. The term *helminth* means "worm," but medical workers usually use it to indicate pathogenic worms. Two types of worm are of serious concern in conjunction with food: (1) *nematodes,* or roundworms, of which the trichina worm found in pork is an example, and (2) *cestodes,* or flatworms, such as the common tapeworms of beef and pork.

Trichina worm (Trichinella spiralis). The trichina worm is transmitted through unsanitary garbage eaten by hogs. The larvae become embedded in the pork muscle. If man eats such infested meat, the organism grows and multiples in his intestinal tract, then moves into muscle tissue, and causes fever and intense pain. In some fatal cases of trichinosis, millions of encysted larvae have been found in the muscle tissue at the time of autopsy. Two measures are imperative to prevent trichinosis: (1) Underdone pork should never be eaten. It should be cooked thoroughly until the meat is all white, and no pink color remains. (2) Hog food sources must be controlled. Garbage must be cooked before it is fed to hogs. Laws in all states now ban the feeding of uncooked garbage to swine.

Tapeworms. The beef tapeworm, *Taenia saginata,* and the pork tapeworm, *Taenia solium,* are transmitted by the fecal-oral route, usually in the form of mature eggs in segments of the worm. These cysts are eaten by cattle in sewage-polluted pastures or by hogs in polluted garbage. The larvae develop in the animal's intestine, then encyst in the muscle. If man eats the infected meat raw or rare, the adult tapeworm matures in his intestine and continues its re-productive cycle. Important controls are prevention of sewage pollution of pastures, sanitary hog-raising operations, and to avoid eating rare beef and underdone pork.

Amebae. Although numerous harmless amebae normally inhabit man's intestinal tract, some are highly pathogenic. The most widely known pathogenic species is that which causes amebic dysentery—*Entamoeba histolytica* (Gr. *ent,* inside; *histo,* tissue; *lytic,* dissolving). The name indicates its mode of attack. The organisms are ingested as cysts in contaminated food or water. In the intestine, the cysts grow into adult forms which produce tissue-destroying enzymes that enable the organism to burrow into the intestinal lining and cause ulcers. Occasionally such embedding may be deep enough to produce intestinal rupture, and the patient may die of resulting peritonitis. The amebae may also enter the intestinal lymph vessels and blood vessels, and travel to liver, lungs, brain, and other organs, where they may localize and form large, destructive abscesses.

Transmission is entirely by the human fecal-oral route. Man is the reservoir, the carrier, and the passer. Fecal contamination of food and water is caused by soiled, unwashed hands, and by flies. Carriers who are food handlers contaminate food and utensils. Leaking sewers may pollute water supplies. Control obviously centers upon strict sanitation measures and personal hygiene.

Bacteria

Two terms that relate to bacterial sources of food-borne disease need to be distinguished. These terms are food infection and food poisoning.

Food infections (bacterial). Food infections result from the ingestion in food of large amounts of viable bacteria, which multiply inside the host (man) and cause infectious disease. Each specific disease is caused by a specific organism. Because incubation and multiplication of the bacteria take time, symptoms of food infection develop relatively slowly, usually twelve to twenty-four hours or more after the infected food has been eaten.

Salmonellosis. The typhoid and paratyphoid bacilli, which infect man, belong collectively to the genus *Salmonella.* They produce various infections (salmonellosis) of the intestinal tract. Some, such as the typhoid bacillus, also invade the blood and cause general infection. The genus is named for the American bacteriologist and veterinarian, Daniel E. Salmon, who in 1885 first isolated from a pig a species of the organisms that infects animals. Man is sometimes involved indirectly in the animal infection chain by eating infected meat or meat products (pork and poultry). However, the types of salmonella that are chiefly responsible for human disease are *S. typhi* and *S. paratyphi.* They are largely restricted to man, and they spread either directly or indirectly from person to person.

Salmonellae are rod-shaped bacteria that resist cold and survive for long periods in soil, ice, water, milk, and foods. Since they do not form spores, they are easily killed by being boiled for five minutes or by pasteurization. Drying and direct sunlight also kill them. The organisms grow easily in simple, common foods such as milk, custards, egg dishes, salad dressings, and sandwich fillings. Seafoods from polluted waters may also be a source of infection.

Immunization practices and regulations controlling the sanitation of community water and food supplies have reduced the incidence of typhoid fever to rare outbreaks. However, paratyphoid organisms continue to frequently infect food. As is true of most species that cause enteric infections, transmission of the several Salmonella species that cause paratyphoid fever (enteric fever) is by the oral-fecal route, through careless, unsanitary handling of foods and utensils. One carrier may infect a large number of persons at one meal, by preparing a dish ahead of time and leaving it in a warm room for several hours, which would incubate the bacilli. The resultant cases of gastroenteritis may vary in intensity from mild diarrhea to severe attacks.

Shigellosis. Bacillary dysentery (shigellosis) is caused by rod-shaped bacteria of the genus *Shigella.* The organism is named for the Japanese physician, Kiyoshi Shiga, who was the first to discover a species of the organism during an epidemic in Japan in 1898. Shigellosis is usually confined to the large intestine and may vary from mild transient intestinal disturbance (as is most common in adults) to fatal dysentery (as occurs more often in young children).

The Shigella organisms grow easily in foods, especially in milk, which is a common vehicle of transmission to infants and children. The boiling of food and water or the pasteurization of milk kills the organisms; but the food or milk may easily be reinfected subsequently through unsanitary handling by a carrier. The several species that may cause shigellosis are spread in much the same way as are those that produce salmonellosis—by feces, fingers, flies, milk, and food and by articles handled by unsanitary carriers.

Cholera. Chiefly an Asiatic disease, cholera is caused by *Vibrio comma* (also called *Vibrio cholerae*), an organism that resembles *Salmonella* in many respects. It also is a nonspored bacillus which may be easily killed by boiling, pasteurization, and disinfectants. Transmission is from person to person in the same manner as that of Salmonellae. Attacks of cholera are usually more severe than attacks of salmonellosis; diarrhea, prostration, and emaciation often proceed rapidly to death unless treatment is given in time.

Food- and water-borne epidemics are common in Asiatic countries. In the Nineteenth Century, five such epidemics originating in Asia swept through western countries and killed millions of persons. Some of these epidemics even reached the United States. It is only because of the alertness of public health agencies and continuous environmental sanitation that most countries of Europe and America are free of cholera today.

Brucellosis. Milk from infected cows or goats may transmit the coccobacilli that cause brucellosis (undulant fever). The genus *Brucella* was named for Sir David Bruce, a British-Australian physician who, working in Malta in 1887, discovered the organisms in goats and in British soldiers who had drunk the goats' milk. The disease in man is characterized by intermittent fever that recurs daily over a period that may vary from days to years, with general malaise, aching and stiffness of the back and joints. In mild forms it may be regarded as "intestinal flu."

Brucella organisms may be transmitted in the milk of goats or cows or through cuts or scratches on the skin of persons who work with infected animals. Thus, butchers, slaughterhouse workers, stock raisers, and veterinarians are particularly exposed. The disease is prevented by using only pasteurized milk and other dairy products, and by avoiding contact with infected animals.

Leptospirosis. (Gr. *leptos*, thin [literally, stripped]; L. *spira*, coil.) The genus *Leptospira* is so named because it is the smallest and most delicately formed of the spirochetes (spiral-shaped bacteria). The organisms are transmitted to man mainly in polluted water—by drinking it, or by swimming or wading in it and acquiring the organisms through cuts or scratches on the skin. Infected animals that may pollute streams include dogs, cattle, swine, mules, rats, and many wild animals. The disease in man, characterized by high fever and intense, hemorrhagic jaundice and hepatitis, was originally called Weil's disease, after Adolf Weil, a German physician. It is common among persons who work in foul, watery places such as trenches in wartime, poorly built mines, sewers, rice fields, and the like, where urine-polluted water and rats abound. It may also occur, however, in persons who do not enter such situations, but who ingest food or water which has been polluted, usually by rats.

Careful storage of foods in the home, general cleanliness in housekeeping, and constant control of rats are obvious measures for the prevention of leptospirosis.

Tularemia. The bacterial genus *Pasteurella*, named for Pasteur, includes one species that occasionally causes food-borne disease in man. The organism is *P. tularensis,* named for Tulare county in California where it was first observed. The disease is commonly called tularemia. It is popularly known as rabbit fever, because it is frequently transmitted to rabbit hunters, trappers, and handlers (market men and housewives) from wild rabbits that have been infected by ticks, fleas, lice, or other insects that carry the microorganism. Such an infectious disease of animals, usually transmitted by arthropods, is called a *zoonosis.* Man may accidentally enter the animal-insect-animal transmission cycle. Tularemia resembles plague, although it is much milder. It is characterized by focal ulcers at the site of infection, recurrent fever, prostration, myalgia, and headache.

Restrictions against the sale of wild rabbits has sharply reduced the incidence of tularemia. Caution should be exercised in eating rabbits of wild or unknown origin.

Escherichia coli infections. Several *Escherichia coli* species normally inhabit the human gastrointestinal tract in enormous numbers. The bacterial genus *Escherichia* was named for a German physician, T. Escherichia, who first studied them. *Escherichia* are widely distributed in nature. The species that normally inhabits the human colon receives the name *E. coli* from its location in man. Ordinarily, *E. coli* cause their host no difficulty; but certain strains produce enteritis, especially in infants. Babies' formulas prepared under unsanitary conditions are the usual route of infection.

Clostridium perfringens food infection. *Clostridium perfringens,* the bacterium that causes gas gangrene when it infects deep wounds, is also capable in certain circumstances of inducing gastrointestinal illness. Rarely is the illness fatal, and then only in elderly, debilitated patients. Its symptoms are usually mild—diarrhea, acute abdominal cramping, nausea, and headache. Most patients recover in twenty-four hours, or at most within a few days.

The *C. perfringens* spores are in soil, water, dust, refuse—everywhere. They are resistant to drying, heat, cold, chlorination, and irradiation. Some heat-resistant strains can survive in boiling water for more than six hours. In cold storage tests, some spores survived at least six months in frozen raw beef.

The organism multiplies in cooked meat and meat dishes held for extended periods at warming temperatures or at room temperature. A number of outbreaks of clostridia infection from food eaten in restaurants, college dining rooms, and school cafeterias have been reported. In each case, cooked meat was improperly handled in preparation and refrigeration. Control rests principally upon careful preparation and adequate cooking of meats, prompt service, and immediate refrigeration at sufficiently low temperatures.

Food poisonings (bacterial toxins). Food poisoning is caused by the ingestion of bacterial toxins that have been produced in the food by the growth of specific kinds of bacteria before the food is eaten. The powerful toxin is ingested directly, and symptoms of food poisoning therefore develop rapidly, usually within one to six hours after the food is eaten.

Staphylococcal food poisoning. Of the bacterial food poisonings observed in the United States, staphylococcal food poisoning is by far the most common. Powerful preformed toxins in the contaminated food produce illness within one to six hours after ingestion. The manifestations appear suddenly. There is severe, cramping, abdominal pain, with nausea, vomiting, and diarrhea, usually accompanied by sweating, headache, and fever. There may be prostration and shock. Recovery is fairly rapid, however, and the symptoms subside within twenty-four hours. The amount of toxin ingested and the susceptibility of the individual eating it determine the degree of severity.

The source of contamination is usually a locus of staphylococcal infection on the hand of a worker preparing the food. Often it is only a minor infection, considered harmless or even unnoticed by the food handler. Custard or cream-filled bakery goods are particularly effective culture beds for staphylococci and are common carriers of the toxins formed during their growth. Other foods that often support the development of staphylococci are processed meats, ham, tongue, cheese, ice cream, potato salad, sauces, chicken and ham salads, and combination dishes such as spaghetti and casseroles. The toxin causes no change from the normal appearance, odor, or taste of the food, so the victim is not warned.

A careful food history is necessary to determine the source of the poisoning. If possible, portions of the food are obtained for bacterial examination. Few bacteria may be found, for heating kills these organisms but does not destroy the toxin they produce.

Prevention of staphylococcal food poisoning rests upon enforcement of three practices:

1. Strict observance by food handlers of the rules of hygiene
2. Careful and immediate refrigeration of all perishable foods
3. Reheating foods only immediately before serving; not allowing them to stand long periods at room temperature

Education of food handlers, an on-going activity of many public health departments, is vital to the prevention of food poisoning incidents in the community (Fig. 12-1).

Botulism. Serious, often fatal food poisoning results from ingestion in food of the toxin produced by the bacteria *Clostridium botulinum*. Depending upon the dose of toxin taken and individual response, the illness may vary from mild discomfort to death within twenty-four hours. Mortality rates are high. Nausea, vomiting, weakness, and dizziness are initial complaints. Progressively, the toxin irritates motor nerve cells and blocks transmission of neural impulses at the nerve terminals (myoneural junction); gradual paralysis follows. Sudden respiratory paralysis with airway obstruction is the major cause of death.

C. botulinum spores are widespread in soil throughout the world. These spores may be carried on harvested food to the

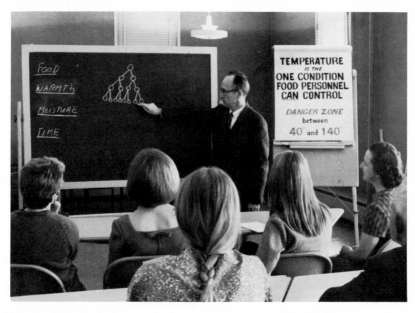

Fig. 12-1. Food handler's class taught by sanitarian in a city health department. Instruction is provided for personnel involved in preparing and serving food for public use, as a means of maintaining a safe food supply.

TO PROBE FURTHER
"Ptomaine poisoning"—a misnomer

A misnomer is a misapplied name or designation. It is an error in naming a person or thing. Such an error has crept into common usage, as a term used by laymen for food poisoning—the use of the word *ptomaine.* There is no such thing as "ptomaine poisoning" in man.

The word ptomaine comes from the Greek word *ptoma,* meaning "dead body." Ptomaines are members of a large class of basic nitrogenous substances, some of them highly poisonous, which are produced during putrefaction of animal or plant protein. They are easily detectable by the deteriorated appearance of the material almost to a liquid state and by the powerful, obnoxious odor they produce. Food in such a condition is hardly human fare!

The word ptomaine is therefore erroneously used when it is applied to other common food infections or poisonings, such as salmonellosis or staphylococcal intoxication.

canning process. Like all Clostridia, this species is anaerobic (develops in the absence of air), or nearly so. The relatively anaerobic environment in the can, and canning temperatures (above 80° F.) provide good conditions for toxin production. The development of high standards in the commercial canning industry has eliminated this source of botulism, but a few cases still result each year from the eating of carelessly home-canned foods. Since boiling for ten minutes destroys the toxin (not the spore), all home canned food, no matter how well preserved it is considered to be, should be boiled *at least* ten minutes before eating.

Viruses

Illnesses produced by viral contamination of food are few in comparison with those produced by bacterial contamination of food. These include upper respiratory infections and viral infectious hepatitis.

Common upper respiratory infections. Persons infected with viruses that produce diseases of the upper respiratory tract such as colds and influenza often transmit these illnesses through foods. They may, with soiled hands, handle unwrapped foods in stores or cafeterias; or they may sneeze or cough over them.

Viral infectious hepatitis (virus A). Acute viral hepatitis, an inflammatory disease of the liver, is caused by either of two strains of virus: Virus A causes infectious hepatitis (IH); Virus B causes serum hepatitis (SH). Virus B has been found only in blood, and is transmitted only by parenteral inoculation (intravenous transfusion of infected blood; or injection with a contaminated needle). Virus A is usually transmitted by the fecal-oral route common to food- and water-borne diseases. Explosive epidemics have occurred in towns, schools, and other communities after fecal contamination of water, milk, or food. Shellfish contaminated by living in polluted water have been a source of several outbreaks. Continuous vigilance in maintaining community controls of water, milk, and food supplies, and stringent personal hygiene and sanitary practices by food handlers are essential to the prevention of infectious hepatitis.

Fungus toxins (mycotoxins)

Crop damage by molds has long been an economic problem. Only recently, however, has it been demonstrated that foods may be contaminated by toxins that are produced by molds (fungi). Such toxins are called mycotoxins (Gr. *myco*, fungus; L. *toxicum*, poison). Several toxins formed by fungi have been studied.

Aflatoxins. First found in peanut meal fed to poultry, aflatoxins were extracted and found to be produced by strains of *Aspergillus flavus*, a common storage mold. The name *aflatoxins* comes from the abbreviation *A. flavus*. Isolation and identification of four aflatoxins was accomplished in 1963.

TO PROBE FURTHER
Alimentary toxic aleukia (ATA)

An extreme example of food poisoning caused by mycotoxins occurred in grain-producing areas of the Soviet Union during World War II.* Because of the wartime shortage of farm workers, large crops of grain had to remain in the fields during the winter snows. Alternate freezing and thawing in the early spring produced excellent conditions for growth of soil fungi on the grain. As a result, the grain became highly toxic to animals and human beings, and produced a syndrome of profound bone marrow suppression and decrease in white blood cells (aleukia). Large numbers of persons became ill and many death resulted. Incidents such as this have stimulated new research concerning mold toxins in foods.† Undoubtedly others will be discovered.

---

*Jaffe, A. Z.: Toxin production in cereal fungi causing toxic alimentary aleukia in man. In Wogan, G. N., ed.: Mycotoxins in foodstuffs, Cambridge, 1965, Massachusetts Institute of Technology Press, p. 77.
†Wogan, G. N.: Current research on toxic food contaminants, J. Amer. Diet. Ass. 49:95, 1966.

Apparently the toxins are produced immediately after harvesting and early in the storage period. Rapid drying, improved storage conditions, and possible use of fungicides would be important control measures.

Natural food poisons

Certain plants and animals contain poisonous substances that occasionally cause human illness or death. Most of these toxic substances are poisonous alkaloids, such as strychnine, atropine, scopolamine, and solanine. Some organisms, for unknown reasons, are toxic at one season of the year and not at others; some plants produce toxic substances at one point in their growth cycle and not at others. Man has been cognizant for centuries of some of these toxic plants and animals; others have been recognized, and their toxins isolated, only recently. A few examples of these organisms which are poisonous as food are listed in the following sections.

Poisonous plants

Cottonseed. A toxic pigment, *gossypol,* contained in cottonseed, has created problems in preparing protein-rich food supplements for use in combating protein malnutrition throughout the world. Procedures for removing the toxin from cottonseed meal during processing have been devised, and efforts are being made to develop strains of the plant that do not contain gossypol.

Soybeans. A trypsin inhibitor in *raw* soybeans is responsible for a toxic substance contained in them. Fortunately, this substance is destroyed by heat and is therefore easily inactivated by cooking.

Cycad nuts. Plants of the genus *Cycas,* common in tropical and subtropical areas, are intermediate in appearance between ferns and palms. Many species have a thick, unbranched, columnar trunk bearing a crown of large, leathery, pinnate leaves. The nuts are sometimes eaten in times of extreme need, as during famine; they were investigated in Guam as a possible cause of a disease of the nervous system, *amyotrophic lateral sclerosis* (ALS), observed in persons who had eaten them. In 1960, they were found to contain the active toxin, *cycasin,* which was isolated and chemically identified. The toxin is now removed from the nuts by a washing process before they are eaten.

Potatoes. The green part of sprouting white potatoes contains sufficient amount of the toxic substance solanine to cause gastroenteritis, jaundice, and prostration. Solanine is a poisonous, narcotic alkaloid. Usually it is removed with the peel before the potato is cooked.

Mushrooms. Certain species of mushroom belong to the poisonous genus *Amanita.* Wild mushrooms should be strictly avoided as food. A number of edible species of mushrooms are grown commercially.

Rhubarb leaves. The large amount of oxalic acid contained in rhubarb leaves causes illness. These leaves should not be used as leafy greens for cooking and eating. Edible leafy greens are spinach, chard, mustard, turnip, and a few others.

Fava bean. Favism is the name given to a severe form of hemolytic anemia produced by the ingestion (or by the inhalation of pollen) of fava beans *(Vicia faba)* in persons sensitive to them. This sensitivity is caused by a genetically controlled deficiency of the enzyme glucose-6-phosphate dehydrogenase in the shunt pathway (see Hexose Monophosphate Shunt, p. 24) for glucose oxidation normally found in the red blood cell. This genetic trait was first observed in certain members of the Mediterranean (Sicilian and Sardinian) and African populations, and has more recently been noted in about 10% of Negroes in the United States. The same genetic trait provides some protection against falciparum malaria. It is a good example of an evolutionary genetic adaptation of a population group to a disease process. Susceptible individuals also react to antimalaria drugs such as primaquine, and to the analgesic, phenacetin, in the same way that they react to fava beans.

Wild plants. Hemlock, wild parsnip,

monkshood, foxglove, and deadly night-shade are a few of the many wild plants known to be poisonous. Occasionally they are mistaken for harmless plants they resemble and are inadvertently eaten.

Poisonous animals

Puffer fish. The puffer fish (family *Tetra-odontidae*) is so named because it is capable of inflating its body with water or air until it forms a globe. It has a gland containing a powerful neurotoxin, *tetraodon-toxin,* which causes death soon after ingestion. Nonetheless, the puffer fish is considered a delicacy in the Orient, and chefs take pride in their ability to remove the gland with great care before cooking the fish. This game of chance brings death from *tetrao-dontoxin* poisoning to a number of persons each year whose chefs' knives slipped!

Clams and mussels. During the summer months, certain species of clam and mussel in waters along the Pacific Coast from Alaska to California feed on marine organisms, plankton, which infect the fish and produce a toxic alkaloid similar to strychnine. At this season, the eating of these fish can be fatal.

Herring. At different seasons in various locations, herring apparently become poisonous as human food. Poisonings have been observed from herring caught in the waters around Cuba and Tahiti from May to October, and in waters around the New Hebrides Islands in the South Pacific, from April to July. Just what accounts for these seasonal changes is not known.

Barracuda. Observations have been made of seasonal poisoning from barracuda. In Florida, in the spring and summer of 1954, four outbreaks of poisoning were traced to the eating of barracuda.

Food spoilage

Food-borne disease and economic waste may also be caused by general food spoilage. Food may deteriorate or become contaminated by chemical or physical changes, by microbial growth, or by contact with insects or rodents.

1. Chemical spoilage may be due to oxidation. Fats may become rancid and fruits may be discolored. Hydrogen gas formation in canned foods may cause cans to swell. Enzymatic activity causes color changes and a haylike flavor in old frozen vegetables.

2. Physical spoilage may be manifested as granulation, as in honey or ice cream. (While granulation does not spoil honey in the sense that it becomes harmful as food, this change in its appearance and texture makes it unacceptable to many consumers.) Sunlight destroys the riboflavin content of milk.

3. Microbial spoilage may be caused by bacteria, yeasts, or molds. Souring of milk, contamination of cooked food that has been held too long before eating, mold growth on bread, and rotting of fruits and vegetables may present problems of disease control and economic loss.

4. Animal and insect spoilage. Food storage problems are constantly presented by insects and rodents (Fig. 12-2). Hairs, droppings, fragments of insects, and disease organisms may be deposited. Rigorous vector control programs are carried on by public health officials.

Radioactivity in foods

Many communities are concerned with the extent of food contamination by radioactive fallout from nuclear weapons testing. Even if testing of weapons is halted, peacetime uses of atomic energy will release small amounts of radioactive materials into the environment. The benefits that are to be gained by the use of atomic energy, in contrast to its biological cost, demand scientific and philosophical study.

Vegetation may be contaminated directly or through the soil, and animals, especially cattle, can become contaminated both directly and through their forage and water. Man, in turn, ingests radioactivity in milk (strontium^{90}) and meat, and their products.

Monitoring systems reveal that present radiation levels are far below those permissible in the human life span. Radioactivity

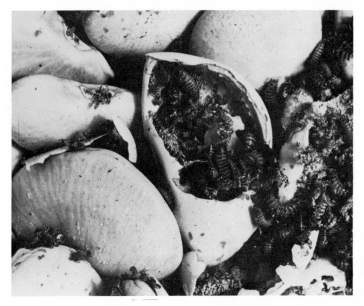

Fig. 12-2. Food spoilage in lima beans by insects. Protecting stored food against insects, molds, and rodents is a constant activity of agricultural experts. (USDA photograph.)

in foods is checked extensively and continuously by the FDA, the Public Health Service, and the Atomic Energy Commission. Their current findings do not warrant government action, or changes in habits of buying or preparing foods.

FOOD ADDITIVES
Man-made chemicals

A number of chemicals have been developed by the agricultural and food processing industries to protect and preserve food. They have contributed in large measure to the unprecedented quantity and quality of America's present food supply. These man-made chemicals, which are used in scientifically controlled amounts, may be intentional or incidental (adventitious) additives.

Intentional food additives

In the past two decades, chemicals intentionally added to foods have to an increasing degree become vital components of the food supply. The great variety and quality of marketed items would be impossible without them.

The use of additives has been a major factor in the rapid evolution of the corner grocery store into the supermarket. The change that has swept the food marketing system during the last twenty-five years is rooted in a deeper social revolution and in scientific advance. Among the reasons for development and use of food additives are the following:

1. Because of the unprecedented population growth, more food must be produced. However, this greater quantity must be produced on less land, and it is more important than ever before that food be preserved and protected from waste and spoilage.

2. New and widely publicized discoveries have increased the food purchaser's awareness of nutritional needs, and have impressed her with the importance to health of a well-balanced diet. Specific foods are enriched or fortified to help supply these needs.

3. There is an increased desire for variety in foods, and creativity in cooking. Foods from local and distant places provide great variety in choice. New types of foods, and a range of uniformly high quality in-

gredients, make cooking in the average American kitchen the creative art enjoyed by most housewives.

4. The increasing complexity of family life, and the number of working wives and mothers have created a need for convenience foods that are nutritious, appealing, and require little time for preparation.

5. People want to be assured of safe, high quality food. Wholesome food for her family is the concern of every normal mother. Most Americans are aware that their health depends upon an adequate supply of fresh, or properly preserved foods. Efforts of the food industry to protect the American food supply are backed by laws governing food production, processing (including the use of intentional additives), and sale.

Purposes served by food additives. Intentional additives may be grouped according to the purpose they serve in a particular food.

Addition of specific nutrients. Certain foods have proved to be good carriers for factors essential to sound nutrition. To other foods, nutrients have been added to replace those removed in processing. Examples include the addition of iodine to salt, of ascorbic acid to many fruit juices, of vitamin D to milk, vitamin A to margarine, and B vitamins (thiamine, niacin, riboflavin) and iron to cereal products. As a result of enrichment, controlled in many instances by enrichment laws, deficiency diseases such as goiter and pellagra have largely been eliminated from the American population. The enrichment of bread and corn meal has been an important factor in the almost total disappearance of pellagra in the southern United States. The addition of vitamin D to milk has made rickets rare in this country.

Production of uniform sensory properties. The esthetic value of food is enhanced by such sensory properties as color, flavor, aroma, texture, and general appearance. No matter how nutritious a food may be, if it is unappealing in appearance, taste, aroma, or texture, it often goes uneaten. In their natural state, samples of a given food may vary widely in color and flavor, according to the season or locality in which they are harvested, or to the species. Natural and synthetic flavoring agents, colorings, preservatives, and texturing materials add appeal and characteristic uniformity to common food products.

An interesting example of color control is the addition of bleaching agents to processed flour. Small quantities of natural pigments in freshly-milled wheat flour give it a yellowish color which many persons find less attractive than pure white. Such flour also lacks the qualities necessary to make the elastic stable dough necessary for making bread of the texture that is preferred by the majority of Americans. Natural aging and ripening permit the development of these desirable characteristics, and for years long aging was the only way millers and bakers could make desired products. Natural aging, however, was time-consuming, costly, and wasteful. Deterioration and infestation from insects and rodents took a great toll. About 1915, a process for bleaching flours was discovered, and a little later a method for accelerating its maturation was found. Today, bleaching and maturing agents produce consistently high quality products for immediate use. Without these agents, quality cakes, breads, and cake mixes as they are known today could not exist.

Standardization of functional properties. A number of additives enhance and standardize the functional properties of given goods. In this class are emulsifiers, stabilizers, moisture retainers, thickeners, binders, dough conditioners, anticaking agents, jelling agents, and others. Many of the common foods would be impossible or far more difficult to prepare without such additives.

Preservation of food. Many agents are added to food to help maintain it at its best, long past the peak of harvest time or the time of processing. Salt and certain curing agents preserve meat and make possible a variety of meat products. Antioxidants prevent discoloration of fruits and rancidity of fats. Antimycotic agents, such as mold in-hibitors, and bacterial control agents, such as "rope" inhibitors, preserve bread and other baked products. Sequestrants (L. *sequester,* a depositary) set apart, in an inactive form, trace substances in foods which would otherwise interfere with its processing. For example, in fats, sequestrants combine with trace minerals such as iron and copper and prevent their catalytic action, which would hasten oxidation—the cause of rancidity in fats. Sequestrants also inactivate certain minerals in the water that is used in making soft drinks. This prevents turbity caused by the minerals settling out during processing.

Control of acidity or alkalinity. The acidity or alkalinity of foods often affects their flavor, texture, and the cooked product. Various acids, alkalis, buffers, and neutralizing agents are used to achieve the desired balance or flavor. For example, acids contribute flavor to candy and help prevent a grainy texture. The flavor of many soft drinks is modified by the addition of acid. Acids and alkalis constitute leavening agents such as baking powder. In making butter, alkali is added to sour cream so that it will churn properly, and yield a satisfactory flavor.

Some common examples of intentional food additives are listed in Table 12-1. All of these chemicals are carefully tested, and their use is controlled, under strict laws which are administered by the Food and Drug Administration (p. 229).

Incidental (adventitious) food additives

The chemicals used in American agriculture have made possible the tremendous advances in food production that are required to meet the demands of a growing population. Today's farmer uses chemicals to control a wide variety of destructive insects (Fig. 12-3), to kill weeds, to control plant diseases, to stop fruit from dropping prematurely, to make leaves drop so that harvesting will be easier, to make seeds sprout, to keep seeds from rotting before they sprout, and many other purposes related to increased yield and improved marketing qualities.

Pesticide residues in food. The use of agricultural chemicals brings hazard as well as gain. Recognition of the necessity for control led to the initial Federal Food, Drug, and Cosmetic Act of 1938, which established procedures for setting safe limits (tolerances) on the amount of pesticide residues permitted on crops. More workable

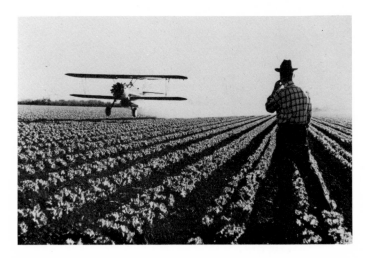

Fig. 12-3. Spraying lettuce fields by plane. The use of insecticides in modern agriculture has enabled farmers to produce increasing crop yields to supply population needs. (Shell photograph, U. S. Dept. of Agriculture.)

Table 12-1. Some examples of intentional food additives

Function	Chemical compound	Common food uses
Acids, alkalis, buffers	Sodium bicarbonate	Baking powder
	Tartaric acid	Fruit sherbets
		Cheese spreads
Antibiotics	Chlortetracycline	Dip for dressed poultry
Anticaking agents	Aluminum calcium silicate	Table salt
Antimycotics	Calcium propionate	Bread
	Sodium propionate	Bread
	Sorbic acid	Cheese
Antioxidants	Butylated hydroxyanisole (BHA)	Fats
	Butylated hydroxytoluene (BHT)	Fats
Bleaching agents	Benzoyl peroxide	Wheat flour
	Chlorine dioxide	
	Oxides of nitrogen	
Color preservative	Sodium benzoate	Green peas
		Maraschino cherries
Coloring agents	Annatto	Butter, margarine
	Carotene	
Emulsifiers	Lecithin	Bakery goods
	Mono- and diglycerides	Dairy products
	Propylene glycol alginate	Confections
Flavoring agents	Amyl acetate	Soft drinks
	Benzaldehyde	Bakery goods
	Methyl salicylate	Candy; ice cream
	Essential oils; natural extractives	
	Monosodium glutamate	Canned meats
Non-nutritive sweeteners	Saccharin, calcium and sodium cyclomates	Diet packed canned fruit
		Low calorie soft drinks
Nutrient supplements	Potassium iodide	Iodized salt
	Vitamin C	Fruit juices
	Vitamin D	Milk
	Vitamin A	Margarine
	B vitamins, iron	Bread and cereals
Sequestrants	Sodium citrate	Dairy products
	Calcium pyrophosphoric acid	
Stabilizers and thickeners	Pectin	Jellies
	Vegetable gums (carob bean, carrageenin, guar)	Dairy desserts and chocolate milk
	Gelatin	Confections
	Agar-agar	"Low calorie" salad dressings
Yeast foods and dough conditioners	Ammonium chloride	Bread, rolls
	Calcium sulfate	
	Calcium phosphate	

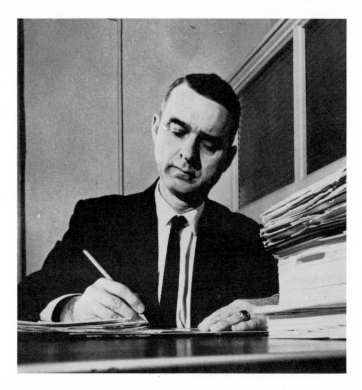

Fig. 12-4. A USDA chemist carefully reviews a manufacturer's application for a pesticide approval and registration. Every page of the stack of supporting data submitted will be studied in determining whether the product meets rigid registration requirements. (USDA photograph.)

and realistic controls were established by a 1954 amendment, which gave the FDA greater responsibility and authority for controlling chemical residues in food. Today, the FDA directs a far-reaching pesticide control program in two phases: (1) requirement for initial approval, and (2) continued surveillance.

Initial approval of a chemical for use. Any chemical for which an agricultural use is planned is subjected by the manufacturer to several years of development and controlled testing before it is submitted to the FDA to be approved for use (Fig. 12-4). The FDA, if it grants its approval, also sets the tolerances under which the chemical must be used. A tolerance is granted only on definite proof, by pharmacological tests, that the residues are safe at levels greatly exceeding those remaining on the food. The tolerance amount is always set at the lowest level that will accomplish the agricultural

purpose, even if larger amounts would still be safe.

Enforcement through continued surveillance. The FDA enforces the laws governing use of pesticides in three ways—through public education, sampling of field produce and market basket studies.

PUBLIC EDUCATION. FDA inspectors and laboratory scientists keep in constant touch with producers, growers, county agents, insect control specialists, pesticide dealers, and agriculture stations. They learn the nature of pest problems in all localities throughout the United States. They observe which pesticides are being recommended and used in different localities, and what violations may be most likely. All known violations are acted upon immediately.

OBJECTIVE SAMPLING OF FIELD PRODUCE. In all states crops are periodically sampled at random, and inspected at producing, shipping, and destination points. A large number of samples are taken to ensure reliable results. Tests are sometimes conducted on the spot, in mobile trailer laboratories. If excessive residues of harmful chemicals are found, the goods are seized and, if necessary, destroyed. As a result of this sampling program, most growers are careful to comply with directions and laws governing the use of pesticides.

MARKET BASKET STUDIES. In 1961, annual surveys of pesticide residues in the total diet of persons living in the United States were begun, as an additional check on the chemical safety of food consumed. Since he eats more than almost any other American, the 19-year-old boy was selected as the reference person. Each year, in five regions and thirty cities of the United States, a list of the food that would be eaten by a 19-year-old boy over a two-week period is made out by nutritionists. All food on the list is purchased in local markets and prepared for the table. After the prepared food has been grouped into 12 classes to facilitate analysis, the foods of each group are homogenized, and a composite sample is examined by highly sensitive laboratory tests for a number of pesticide residues. The test results are compared with the daily intake levels jointly set as acceptable by the United Nations Food and Agriculture Organization and the World Health Organization Expert Committee. These studies have indicated that the amounts of pesticide residues in foods as consumed are far below the currently acceptable levels. This reassuring information supplements the data from field sampling.

FOOD PROTECTION FROM FARM TO TABLE

From producer to consumer, modern devices and practices protect food and ensure its quality and safety. Little does the average consumer realize how much is involved in providing him with the variety of appealing foods that are available today.

Crop control and protection. Before a specific crop is sown, the seed is selected from the improved strains that are con-

stantly being developed and tested in agricultural research units. While the crop is growing, it is protected from damage by numerous insect, plant disease, and weed control measures. The U. S. Department of Agriculture operates an alert plant disease forecasting program, similar to the weather forecasts supplied by the Weather Bureau, so that farmers can plan for crop protection.

Harvesting. The eating quality of many foods depends upon their being harvested rapidly at the right moment in their development. Quality also depends upon getting them immediately from the field to the processor. Mechanization has speeded most harvesting processes (Fig. 12-5). For example, large machines move through lettuce fields and, in one complex operation, harvest the lettuce, wrap each head individually in film, and box it. It is then ready to be picked up by a side truck and transported to the wholesale market under refrigeration.

Transportation. Modern refrigeration design and equipment in trucks, trailers, and railroad cars have reduced losses of fresh produce. For overseas shipment, refrigerated trailer vans ("fishybacks") are driven to dockside and the entire trailer van container is lifted aboard ship and carried to its destination as a unit. Opening of the van and handling of its contents during transfers en route are eliminated. For example, Florida grapefruit arrives at Swiss markets intact and in excellent condition. Better loading patterns and newer fiberboard boxes have also prevented much bruising and damaging during transportation.

Milk and meat protection. Because milk and meat are particularly susceptible to contamination by harmful microorganisms, special laws govern their production and marketing.

Milk production. The modern dairy industry is founded upon many years of experience and research, which have built dependable safeguards into milk processing to ensure high quality. Rigidly enforced government ordinances regulate the handling of milk from farm to consumer.

Disease in milk-producing cows is eradi-

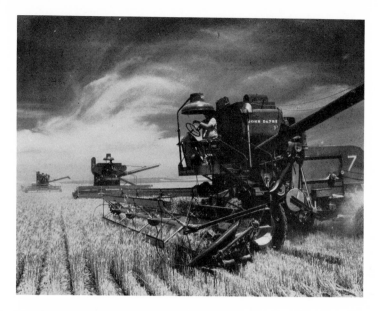

Fig. 12-5. Grain harvest on large midwestern farm, using modern mechanized equipment. (USDA photograph.)

cated by veterinary programs under government control. For example, bovine tuberculosis, brucellosis, and mastitis are quickly eliminated by constant, sensitive testing and vaccination, and by the isolation and treatment of affected cows. Personnel and equipment involved in care and milking of the animals and in the handling of the milk are required to pass rigid health and sanitation inspections.

Cows are usually milked by machines, which pipe the milk to storage tanks without exposure to contaminating dust and insects. In these refrigerated tanks, the milk is cooled quickly to about 38° F. and held at that temperature throughout a brief storage period and while it is being transported in refrigerated tank trucks to the dairy.

At the processing plant, the milk is first subjected to a vacuum treatment which removes objectionable flavors that may have resulted from certain grasses, or from wild onions, for example, that have been eaten by the cow. Next it is pasteurized, by any of several legal heat treatments. For example, the milk can be held at 145° F. for thirty minutes, or at 161° F. for fifteen

seconds. Pasteurization destroys disease-producing organisms that might be present in the milk, and also kills bacteria that could grow during storage under refrigeration. It renders milk and milk products not only safe for consumption, but also less likely to spoil during storage and marketing.

Homogenization is usually associated with pasteurization. By this treatment, the fat globules are reduced in size and evenly dispersed, so that the cream does not separate from the milk. Vitamin D is added, to compensate for the lack of this vitamin in milk. The standard supplement is 400 I.U. per quart. Finally, the milk is packaged and is kept refrigerated until it is delivered to the consumer. At each step, the production, processing, marketing, and delivery of milk is constantly regulated and supervised by law enforcement agencies. These include at the Federal level, the U. S. Public Health Service, the U. S. Department of Agriculture, and the Food and Drug Administration; at the state level, the state departments of health and agriculture; and at the local level, city and county governments.

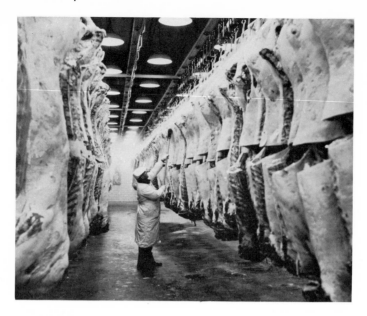

Fig. 12-6. Meat inspection and grading. A U. S. Department of Agriculture meat grader marks the quality grade on beef carcasses at an Omaha, Nebraska packing plant. (USDA photograph.)

Meat production. The circular, purple stamp-mark placed on meat and poultry that has passed government inspection are the consumer's guarantee of a safe, wholesome product. Under the Meat Inspection Act of 1906 and the Poultry Products Inspection Act of 1957, the Consumer and Marketing Service of the U. S. Department of Agriculture closely controls the commercial marketing of meat and poultry. Highly qualified inspectors scrutinize meat production and marketing in every detail. They are concerned with sanitation of the processing plant, inspection of animals at the stockyard before slaughter, immediate examination of the carcass and internal organs, and inspection during meat processing, curing, canning, and smoking. They also regulate disposal of condemned material, the marking and labeling of products, and inspection of imported meat (Fig. 12-6).

Meat is a large item in American diets, and the meat and poultry industries of the United States the world's largest. It is a credit to the high standards and vigilant efforts of producers and government alike that the American family is assured of safe, high quality meat products.

Storage. Tremendous amounts of food are stored each year for consumption by market animals, by the population of our country, and for shipping overseas. Well-built storage facilities are constantly checked for temperature and humidity. The stored food is protected from harm by insects, fungi, mold, bacteria, and rodents through the rigid application of control measures.

Marketing. Safeguards applied in the supermarket continue to protect food for the consumer. Temperature and humidity controls keep the food in optimum condition until it is purchased. Inspection of perishables maintains high standards. Specific codes regulate the handling and temperatures of frozen foods. Rotation of shelf goods maintains the freshness of canned and packaged stocks. Sanitary handling and facilities ensure the cleanliness of food.

Home care. The final steps in the protection of food for the family are the responsibility of the homemaker. Unless she handles the products intelligently, the industry's efforts to supply her with safe, high quality food is wasted as far as her family is concerned. She should first select foods of the best quality she can afford, either from the market or from the farm. The alert homemaker will purchase sound, fresh produce and will look for reliable grades in processed food, reading labels carefully. At home, she will store foods promptly under proper conditions of space, ventilation and refrigeration. She will use each within the recommended storage periods. Finally, she will prepare and serve the food, and will care for leftovers, by methods that protect their natural goodness and food value, and that avert spoilage.

FOOD PRESERVATION

To keep seasonal excess quantities for later use, to enable foods to withstand transportation to distant places, and to protect them from spoilage and contamination, various methods of food preservation have been developed.

Drying. Perhaps the oldest known method of preserving food is drying. Removing most of the moisture from highly perishable fruits and vegetables, for example, halts the growth of bacteria contained in them, and extends the period in which they are edible. Drying is a *bacteriostatic* method of preservation. Fresh grapes rot quickly. But for many centuries, grapes have been preserved by making them into raisins, by a method that is essentially unchanged even today. The fruit is laid out on open racks and dried in the sun. Since primitive times, men have preserved meat and fish by drying, and have added smoking, salting, and curing to the process.

Newer forms of dried foods include such items as skimmed milk and eggs. Impetus was given to the exploration of drying processes by the successful development of field rations used by soldiers in World War II, and by the obvious convenience of such products both to the consumer and to the marketer. Properly dried foods lose none of their nutrients, are light to handle, occupy far less storage space than fresh, and are exceedingly simple to prepare. In this busy era, and in homes with limited storage space, these are important advantages. An entire new branch of the food industry has been developed to prepare and market an array of instant foods—potatoes, tea, coffee, fruit juice, sauces, soups, and substitutes for coffee cream. The list of such items grows daily.

Canning. Canning is a *bactericidal* method of food preservation. It destroys bacteria with heat. The history of the canning process is a story of man's response to the pressure of crisis and of his persistent ingenuity in finding a solution. The story begins in France.

In the late 1700's, France was burdened by wars with England, Prussia, Austria, and Spain and with revolution at home. By 1795, more French soldiers were dying from malnutrition and scurvy than from bullets. In desperation, the five man French Directory offered a prize of 12,000 francs to the patriot who could find a way to preserve food long enough so that it could be transported to the front. An obscure French citizen, Nicolas Appert, took the offer seriously. Until then, he had drifted in and out of a number of jobs involving food and drink. He had been chef, pickler, preserver, candy maker, wine maker, brewer, and distiller. In response to this challenge, he began to work in earnest. For fourteen years he experimented with methods and materials. In 1810, he succeeded in preventing food from spoiling by packing it in an airtight container. He was awarded the prize by the French Minister of the Interior. In 1811, Appert published an account of his method, *L'art de conserver, pendant plusieurs années, toutes les substances animales et végétales* (The Art of Preserving for Several Years All Animal and Vegetable Substances). Appert knew, from long trial and error, that heat applied to food sealed in an airtight container prevented spoilage. But he did not know why. It was not until 1857 that another Frenchman, Louis Pasteur, demonstrated chemically that spoilage was caused by microorganisms, which Appert's canning method destroyed. Although Appert did not know that microorganisms existed, he stated the two essentials that have long been proved valid, and are still followed: (1) complete cleanliness in the process, and (2) a permanent seal on the container to exclude air.

From France, Appert's method immediately spread to England, where in 1810, Peter Durand developed and patented a container made of iron and tin. The word canister, from the Greek word *kanastron,* meaning "basket of reeds," was then used in England for the reed baskets that held tea, coffee, spices, or fruit. Durand called his crude container a metal canister.

In 1819, canning reached America. William Underwood, in Boston, began using cumbersome glass jars with sealed cork stoppers; in 1839 he substituted the metal canisters. His workmen shortened the word to "can," and the slang term shortly became accepted as the official name. It has remained to label a giant modern food industry.

Modern "tin" cans are not actually made of tin. They are thin sheets of specially prepared steel, coated with tin by dipping or electroplating. Today's canning plant, with its sanitary, automated production line and sophisticated quality controls, is a far cry from Appert's crude beginnings. But the hermetically sealed container, filled under sanitary conditions and sterilized by heat, still preserves food by destroying microorganisms.

Freezing. Although ancient tribes living in cold climates no doubt learned that meat and fish could be held in frozen form for long periods, quick freezing came into being only in the 1920's when Clarence Birdseye first applied rapid freezing methods to fish for commercial purposes. In 1927, the process was extended to vegetables, and the frozen food industry began to grow. Frozen precooked food was first offered for sale in the late 1940's. Today, more than 700 frozen items are found in supermarkets and more are yet to come.

Freezing destroys many microorganisms and inhibits the growth of others. Because frozen foods are not sterile, they must be handled as perishables from the time they are processed until they are eaten. The mo-

ment they are thawed, bacteria begin to multiply. This is no problem with such frozen foods as vegetables and meats, which are cooked in the same way as fresh foods. However, precooked frozen foods are exposed to greater hazards of contamination during processing so that it is necessary to take extra precautions at all stages of preparation. Competition in the food industry, however, and vigorously enforced codes based on bacteriologic standards have resulted in the availability of safe, nutritious, and flavorful frozen prepared foods. The two factors that have proved important in the control of microorganisms and in the maintenance of high quality in the frozen product are time and temperature. Rapid, sanitary food preparation, followed immediately by quick freezing, controls bacterial growth and prevents damage to the cell walls, which would break down the texture. Quick freezing is made possible by the use of liquid nitrogen ($-320°$ F.) or fluidized-bed freezers. After the initial quick freezing, it is imperative that the food be stored at a low temperature, and used before expiration of the recommended storage time. Most frozen food should be held a $0°$ F. or lower; $-10°$ F. is better.

New methods of food preservation. Two new methods that represent attempts to combine the best features of freezing and drying, and one method that is based on the pharmacological destruction of microorganisms are already in commercial use; a fourth is in an advanced phase of practical application, but is still being extensively tested.

Freeze-drying. Piece-form foods such as fruits and seafoods are kept frozen while they dry in a vacuum. This retains the original size and shape of the food but greatly reduces its weight. A freeze-dried strawberry is the same size as the fresh strawberry, but weighs only one-sixteenth as much. This lightness is an advantage in handling and transportation. Because vacuum drying by piece is a costly method of water removal, it is usually restricted to high-cost foods such as meats and seafoods, or to special military situations. At the present stage, foods processed by this technique are less excellent in taste, and meet with less acceptance than do quick-frozen or canned foods.

Dehydrofreezing. Fruits and vegetables are first dehydrated to about 50% of their original weight and volume, but not until their quality is impaired, then frozen. The quality of dehydrofrozen foods is usually equal to that processed by the standard quick-freezing methods. They have the advantages of lighter weight and less bulk and, therefore, they cost less to package, freeze, store, and ship. Foods that have been satisfactorily dehydrofrozen include potatoes, carrots, peas, apples, apricots, berries, and cherries. They are used chiefly in commercially prepared combinations, as vegetables in soup or fruits in pies.

Use of antibiotics. In 1955 and 1956, the U. S. Food and Drug Administration approved the use of chlortetracycline and oxytetracycline for the preservation of raw poultry. Tolerance levels were established in 1959 for chlortetracycline in preserving certain kinds of raw fish and shellfish. Since about 10% of the population of the United States are sensitive to various drugs, the addition of antibiotics to foods must be carefully controlled. Only small amounts of the antibiotic may be employed. Residues in tissues are destroyed in cooking. Used under specified conditions, these antibiotics significantly increase retention of quality in fresh poultry and fish during storage.

A food-grade antibiotic (from 10 to 20 ppm) is added to the ice-slush that chills cleaned and dressed poultry carcasses (Fig. 12-7). Usually the poultry remains in this solution from one to two hours, and then is drained and packaged for shipment to retailers. Antibiotics are a constituent of preservative dips for fresh fish fillets, of refrigerated brines in which dressed whole fish are held in fishing vessels, and in ice used to refrigerate fish during transport, processing, and marketing. The feed of agricultural animals is supplemented with antibiotics, to stimulate growth and to treat disease. Many crop sprays contain antibiotics. When properly used in any of these ways, antibiotics have not been shown to constitute a hazard to human health.

Irradiation. Ionizing radiation offers a method of food preservation that has been

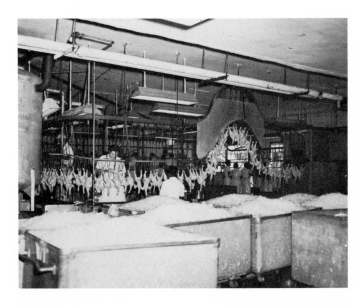

Fig. 12-7. Poultry processing. Interior view of the production line showing preserving ice-slush in foreground. (USDA photograph.)

developed only in the past two decades. It was first approved by FDA in 1963 for use on canned bacon and bulk wheat, largely on the basis of extensive test data submitted by the U. S. Army Quartermaster Research Organization and others. Gamma radiation was used to kill insect life in bulk wheat; the electron beam was used to sterilize bacon. Irradiation under approved processes does *not* cause the food to become radioactive, or to retain radioactivity that may have lingered in it from previous exposure.

Radiation, in its simplest terms, means the sending of energy from a source to an absorbing substance. Heat and sunlight are forms of radiation. In relation to radiation of food, however, the term is most often used to refer to the sending of electromagnetic x-rays or gamma rays, both of which have a shorter wave-length than heat or light rays. These rays are used together with electrons, given off by a radioactive isotope or other radioactive substance. The use of x-rays, gamma rays, or electrons on food kills bacteria, inactivates some enzymes, and destroys insects. Cobalt[60] has been used as a source of gamma radiation. When used in food processing, the radioactive isotope is sealed in a container that allows only the gamma rays to penetrate and radiate. Electron beams are best secured from man-made generators which accelerate electrons by high voltage electrical fields.

Aside from high costs, there are two problems in developing a practical food irradiation process. First, the radiation changes the characteristics of the food. Radiation high enough to completely sterilize food sometimes causes undesirable changes in flavor, appearance, and texture. Cooked meats, normally brown or gray, turn pink, lettuce wilts, egg whites thin, and baked products are reduced in volume. Second, there is the problem of safety. Thorough study, however, has now resulted in techniques that render safe levels and kinds of irradiation. Controlled gamma rays, such as from cobalt[60], do not produce radioactive elements in foods.

Although not yet applied on a commercial scale, irradiation will no doubt be used extensively for food preservation in the near future. It may be employed not only to sterilize certain foods (4,500,000 rads destroys *Clostridium botulinum,* the most resistant spoilage bacterium), to give them an indefinite shelf life, but also in smaller quantities (100,000 to 500,000 rads) to control other forms of spoilage, such as the sprouting of potatoes and onions, and to kill insect eggs that have been deposited on fruit, vegetables, and grain. Such smaller doses of irradiation, combined with refrigeration, may greatly increase the preservation and storage life of perishables.

CONTROL AGENCIES TO PROTECT FOOD SAFETY AND QUALITY

A number of government and private agencies and professional organizations are constantly at work to ensure the safety and high quality of food. Among them are the organizations introduced in the previous chapter (p. 214) in relation to their work concerning food misinformation.

Foremost among concerned groups in the U. S. Department of Health, Education and Welfare are the Food and Drug Administration and the Public Health Service; in the U. S. Department of Agriculture, there are the Agricultural Research Service and the Consumer and Marketing Service. Also acting to protect the consumer are the Federal Trade Commission and the National Bureau of Standards.

Food and Drug Administration

The broad and vital work of the Food and Drug Administration serves as an example of the protection of the food supply by government control. In essence, the FDA is a law enforcement agency, charged by Congress to ensure, among other things, that the food supply is safe, pure, and wholesome. It seeks to carry out its responsibility through scientific research and public education as well as by surveillance and enforcement.

Food standards. Section 401 of the Federal Food, Drug, and Cosmetic Act is designed "to promote honesty and fair dealing in the interest of Consumers." It directs the Secretary of Health, Education, and Welfare to establish, for any food he deems necessary, regulations governing definition and standard of identity, reasonable standard of quality, and standards of fill of container. The food label must indicate these standards, and must tell what is in the package. It must not be false or *misleading* in any particular.

Standards of identity. Reference standards have been established for a number of common foods such as jams, jellies, macaroni, noodles, mayonnaise, salad dressing, catsup, and cheese. A ratio of ingredients (or percentage of constituents) is established as specifically identifying that food item, and any food bearing that name on the label and sold as such must have been prepared exactly by that standard. On such identified foods, there is no requirement to list the ingredients, as they are named in the standard. For many less common foods, no standards of identity have been established, and the label must list all of the ingredients *in the order of their predominance* in the food.

Single copies of the complete text of these standards may be obtained without charge from the FDA.

Standards of quality. For a number of canned fruits and vegetables, minimum standards have been set concerning such properties as tenderness, color, and freedom from defects. If such a fruit or vegetable is safe for human consumption but does not meet these standards, its label must carry a specific statement of the characteristic in which it is defective; for example, "broken parts," "excessive peel," or other indication.

Standards of fill of container. For many foods, standards of fill have been established to protect the consumer against slack fillings. These are especially necessary for products that settle after filling such as cereals, or for products that consist of a number of pieces packed in a liquid such as fruit cocktail. The legal standards ensure that no air, water, or space is sold as food, and that the container fits the food.

Standards for enriched products. Standards are set for enrichment of flour, cereals, margarine, and other foods with specific quantities of vitamins and minerals. Any such product labeled "enriched" or "fortified" must contain precisely the specified amount of added nutrients.

Safe use of food additives. The many intentional food additives that make possible our wide variety of food products must first be approved for use by the FDA. The bureau frequently checks currently sold products to make certain that processors are following the rules that ensure the safety of the product.

Safe limits for pesticide residues in food. The amount of chemical residue from sprays and dusts applied to crops, that may safely remain on food, is carefully set as a tolerance limit by FDA scientists. FDA field inspectors check food shipments to see that these limits are observed. Market basket tests assure that food as consumed by the day-to-day buyer does not contain pesticide residues in excess of tolerance.

Nutritional misinformation. The FDA wages a continual campaign against food quackery and misinformation. Thousands of persons spend millions of dollars yearly on food supplements they do not need, some of which may be harmful. In the previous chapter on Food Misinformation this problem is discussed in detail.

Interstate food shipments and food imports. FDA officials constantly inspect food establishments and processing plants to see that standards of sanitation, food safety, and quality are maintained. Samples of foods shipped from one state to another are examined for purity and quality. Food imported from other countries is checked to see that it complies with United States law.

Check on food contamination in disasters. In cooperation with local and state officials, the FDA inspects food that has been damaged by flood, hurricane, fire, or

TO PROBE FURTHER
New FDA regulations: "truth in packaging" laws

The Fair Packaging and Labeling Act. A law enacted in 1966, which took effect in July, 1967, initiated the procedures for bringing into being new regulations requiring fuller and more prominent information in the labels of packaged foods. After initial publication of these proposed regulations, and consideration of written comments and objections that were subsequently filed, the new provisions were adopted in September, 1967.

Five basic regulations concerning label information have been specified:[*]
1. A statement of the food's identity must appear on the principal display panel in bold type.
2. The name and address of the manufacturer, packer, and distributor must be conspicuously stated.
3. A statement of the net contents must appear in concise standard measure. No qualifying terms, such as "giant quart," or "jumbo pound," may appear.
4. A statement listing ingredients, when required, must appear in type of legible size, on a single panel of the label. The common names of the ingredients must appear in decreasing order of predominance.

Dietary foods regulations. The new regulations also involve proposals for special diet foods, with particular reference to vitamin and mineral supplementation and low calorie foods.[†] At the time this textbook goes to press, it is anticipated that these proposals may become effective upon completion of hearings and amendments, probably in early 1969.

1. Vitamins and minerals:
    a. The following statement is proposed for use on all vitamin and mineral supplements: "Vitamins and minerals are supplied in abundant amounts by the foods we eat. The Food and Nutrition Board of the National Research Council recommends that dietary needs be satisfied by foods. Except for persons with special medical needs, there is no scientific basis for recommending routine use of dietary supplements."
    b. It is proposed that the National Research Council's recommended dietary allowances for seventeen vitamins and minerals replace the outmoded, misleading, and frequently abused concept of "minimum daily requirement."
    c. It is proposed that eight classes of food which may be fortified with vitamins and minerals be stated, and that the specific elements and amounts that may be used in these foods be clearly stipulated. These food groups are (1) pastes (macaroni products), (2) whole milk (fluid and powdered) for drinking, (3) fluid skimmed milk and fluid low fat milk for drinking, (4) fruit juices and drinks, (5) fruit products for infants, (6) processed cereals, (7) salt, and (8) formulas for infant feeding.

---

[*]Friedelson, I.: Fair packaging: synopsis of food packaging and labeling regulations, F.D.A. Papers 1:21, 1967.

[†]FDA proposes major overhaul of dietary food regulations, FDA report on enforcement and compliance, Food and Drug Administration, U. S. Department of Health, Education, and Welfare, Washington, D.C., July, 1966, p. 3.

d. It is proposed that extravagant, deceptive promotion of "shotgun" multivitamin and mineral supplements that serve no dietary need be prohibited. It is also proposed that specific required and optional elements and their amounts be indicated. In multivitamin products, six ingredients are to be required (vitamin A, vitamin D, ascorbic acid, thiamine, riboflavin, niacin or niacinamide), and five others are to be optional (vitamin E, vitamin B_6, folic acid, panthothenic acid, vitamin B_{12}). In mineral supplements, calcium and iron are to be required; phosphorus, magnesium, copper, and iodine are to be optional.

2. Low calorie foods:
   a. It is proposed that use of the term "low calorie" on labels be restricted to those foods that contain fifteen or fewer calories per serving.
   b. It is proposed that use of the term "lower in calories" be limited to those foods that contain at least 50% fewer calories than their ordinary food counterpart. Such comparison of calories in equivalent servings is to be clearly stated on the label. Any non-nutritive ingredients, such as artificial sweeteners or added bulk, are to be declared.

other disaster, and assists in the removal of contaminated items from the market.

Education of consumers. The Division of Consumer Education of the FDA carries on an active program of consumer protection through education and public information. Many excellent materials are prepared and distributed to individuals and student and community groups. Consumer specialists work through all FDA district offices.

Scientific research. As a basis for all its activities, in a world of burgeoning technology, the FDA scientists constantly seek to provide a background of evaluation through their own research (Fig. 12-8). That they discharge this responsibility in a notable manner was formally recognized in 1956, by the presentation to them of the Lasker Award, with the statement that the FDA is "both a scientific institution and a federal law enforcement agency."

The extent of the task discharged by the FDA was indicated by John W. Gardner, Secretary of Health, Education, and Welfare, at the dedication of the new FDA building in Washington, D.C., on November 23, 1965: "The FDA serves as the public's protector against contamination, fraud,

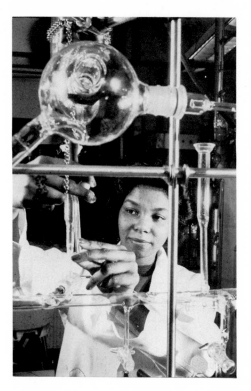

Fig. 12-8. Research in food chemistry. A chemist in the U. S. Department of Agriculture's Agricultural Research Service makes an adjustment on a molecular still used in a project to aid in the manufacture of dry milk. (USDA photograph.)

impurity, and hazards in the products on which our lives depend. . . . The products regulated under FDA laws account for about a fourth of what American families spend each year. They account for over $100 billion worth of the annual commerce of the United States. Nearly 70% of FDA's total commitment is to protect the food supply of this nation."

References
General

Agar, E. A., and Dolman, C. E.: Type E botulism, J.A.M.A. **187**:538, 1964.

Beacham, L. M.: Food standards, F.D.A. Papers **1**(6):4, 1967.

Bird, K.: Freeze-dried foods, Marketing Research Report No. 617, Washington, D. C., 1963, U. S. Department of Agriculture.

Brooke, M. M.: Epidemiology of amebiasis in the United States, J.A.M.A. **188**:519, 1964.

Burr, H. K., and Elliott, R. P.: Quality and safety in frozen foods, J.A.M.A. **174**:1178, 1960.

Cannon, P. R.: Why we have a safe and wholesome food supply, Amer. J. Public Health **53**:626, 1963.

Coerver, R. M.: One man's meat, Amer. J. Nurs. **58**:690, 1958.

Comar, C. L.: Radioactivity in foods, J.A.M.A. **171**:119, 1959.

Dack, G. M.: Food poisoning, Chicago, 1956, University of Chicago Press.

Despaul, J. E.: Food poisoning microorganisms—a study of characteristics and methods of detection with particular emphasis on *Clostridium perfringens*, Washington, D. C., 1964, Government Printing Office.

Despaul, J. E:. The gangrene organism: a food-poisoning agent, J. Amer. Diet. Ass. **49**:185, 1966.

Dolman, C. E.: Botulism, Amer. J. Nurs. **64**:119, 1964.

Duggan, R. E., and Dawson, K.: Pesticides: a report on residues in food, F.D.A. Papers **1**(5):4, 1967.

Dunning, G. M.: Radioactivity in the diet, J. Amer. Diet. Ass. **42**:17, 1963.

Eadie, G. A., and others: Type E botulism, J.A.M.A. **187**:496, 1964.

Ebbs, J. C.: New horizons for food, J. Amer. Diet. Ass. **39**:101, 1961.

Fine, S.: F.D.A.'s Dallas district: an incident in Laredo, F.D.A. Papers **1**(5):9, 1967.

Food additives: what they are, how they are used, Washington, D. C., 1961, Manufacturing Chemists Association, Inc.

Food and Drug Administration: Facts for consumers: food additives, F.D.A. Pub. No. 10, Washington, D. C., 1964.

Food and Drug Administration: Facts for consumers: food standards, F.D.A. Pub. No. 8, Washington, D. C., 1964.

Food and Drug Administration: Facts for consumers: pesticide residues, F.D.A. Pub. No. 18, Washington, D. C., 1963.

Food and Drug Administration: Read the label, F.D.A. Pub. No. 3, Washington, D. C., 1963.

Food Protection Committee, Food and Nutrition Board, National Research Council, Washington, D. C., Selected Publications. Chemicals used in food processing, Pub. 1274, 1965; An evaluation of public health hazards from the microbiological contamination of foods, Pub. 1195, 1964; Food packaging materials—their composition and uses, Pub. 645, 1958; Radionuclides in foods, Pub. 988, 1962.

Friedelson, I.: Fair packaging: synopsis of food packaging and labeling regulations, F.D.A. Papers **1**(8):21, 1967.

Frobisher, M., and others: Microbiology for nurses, Philadelphia, 1964, W. B. Saunders Co.

Halstead, B. W.: Poisonous fishes, Public Health Reports **73**:302, 1958.

Hodges, R. E.: The toxicity of pesticides and their residues in food, Nutr. Rev. **23**:225, 1965.

Kemp, G. E., and others: Foodborne disease in California with special reference to *Clostridium perfringens (welchii)*, Public Health Reports **77**:910, 1962.

Kingma, F. J.: Establishing and monitoring drug residue levels, F.D.A. Papers **1**(6):8, 1967.

Larrick, G. P.. The role of the Food and Drug Administration in nutrition, Amer. J. Clin. Nutr. **8**:377, 1960.

Lovell, R. T., and Flick, G. T.: Irradiation of Gulf Coast area strawberries, Food Technology **20**:99, 1966.

Milk Borne Diseases, Nurs. Times **62**:1676, 1966.

Milstead, K. L.: Science works through law to protect consumers, J. Amer. Diet. Ass. **48**:187, 1966.

Most, H.: Trichinellosis in the United States, J.A.M.A. **193**:871, 1965.

Nelson, E. M.: The philosophy of food fortification, J. Amer. Diet. Ass. **30**:984, 1954.

Patterson, M. I., and Marble, B.: Dietetic foods, Amer. J. Clin. Nutr. **16**:440, 1965.

Polk, L. D.: Nursing responsibilities in a Salmonella outbreak, Nurs. Outlook **13**:56, 1965.

Protecting our food: yearbook of agriculture, 1966, Washington, D. C., 1966, U. S. Government Printing Office.

Report: Analysis of pesticide residues, F.D.A. Papers **1**(5):17, 1967.

Robinson, H. E., and Urbain, W. M.: Radiation preservation of foods, J.A.M.A. **174**:1310, 1960.

Roe, R. S.: F.D.A. and the food industry. III. Regulations, tolerances, and technology, Food Technology 16:66, 1962.

Roe, R. S.: Pesticide regulatory activities of the Food and Drug Administration, Amer. J. Public Health **55** (Part II):36, 1965.

Setter, L. R.: Radioactive contamination of foods, J. Amer. Diet. Ass. **39**:561, 1961.

Shelton, R. L.: The changing concept of food sanitation, F.D.A. Papers **1**(8):12, 1967.

Smillie, W. G., and Kilbourne, E. D.: Preventive medicine and public health, ed. 3, New York, 1963, The Macmillan Co.

Strong, D. H., and others: Survival of *Clostridium perfringens* in starch pastes, J. Amer. Diet. Ass. **49**:191, 1966.

Tarr, H. L. A.: Control of bacterial spoilage of fish with antibiotics, First International Conference on Antibiotics in Agriculture, National Academy of Sciences, National Research Council, Pub. No. 397, 1956.

Thatcher, F. S.: Food-borne bacterial toxins, Canad. Med. Ass. J. **94**:582, 1966.

Thomas, M. H., and Calloway, D. H.: Nutritional value of dehydrated foods, J. Amer. Diet. Ass. **39**:105, 1961.

Vaughn, R. H., and Stewart, G. F.: Antibiotics as food preservatives, J.A.M.A. **174**:1308, 1960.

Ward, G. M., Johnson, J. E., and Wilson, D. W.: Deposition of fallout cesium-137 on forage and transfer to milk, Public Health Reports **81**:639, 1966.

Ward, J. C.: The functions of the Federal Insecticide, Fungicide, and Rodenticide Act in the United States, Amer. J. Public Health **55** (Suppl.):27, 1965.

Welch, H.: Problem of antibiotics in foods, J.A.M.A. **170**:2093, 1959.

Werrin, M., and Kronich, D.: Salmonella control in hospitals, Amer. J. Nurs. **66**:528, 1966.

Wogan, G. N.: Current research on toxic food contaminants, J. Amer. Diet. Ass. **49**:95, 1966.

Wogan, G. N., editor: Mycotoxins in foodstuffs, Cambridge, 1965, Massachusetts Institute of Technology Press.

CHAPTER 13

Cultural, social, and psychological influences on food habits

In public health work, as in other aspects of their professional activities, nurses and nutritionists are confronted constantly with the fundamental question of why people eat what they eat. The health professions are concerned with the nutritional needs of persons and families in communities. They know that food is necessary to sustain life and health. But they also recognize that man eats for many reasons other than physical sustenance, and that he seldom eats in order to supply his body with the good nutrition that they may propose. Food has many meanings, and a person's food habits are intimately tied up with his whole way of life.

Important as a sound knowledge of the science of human nutrition is, it is not enough to provide the nurse with the means of carrying out her function in relation to persons. It is only the beginning. Unless this knowledge is applied realistically to persons in their unique life situations with their particular cultural conditioning, the nurse does not help them. Indeed, she may even create barriers and problems rather than help find solutions.

Consider the example of the public health nurse working with a family whose income is relatively limited, and which is faced with several health problems involving inadequate nutrition. The nurse knows the necessity of an adequate and safe food supply. She knows food values, the nutrients, and their functions in the body. She can outline a well-balanced family meal pattern that will assure all these nutritional essentials. She proceeds with great enthusiasm to accomplish this for the mother, telling her and her family to eat three good, square meals a day, which *everyone* should have for health.

But must everyone have three meals a day? Why not two meals a day, or five, or six? Why orange juice and egg only for breakfast? Why meat only for dinner? Why dinner only in the evening? Perhaps this particular family has different eating habits. Failing to recognize or explore this family's cultural variation, in spite of her good intentions the nurse may have unconsciously confused *biological necessity* (which her plan surely does not represent) with *cultural patterning*, which her plan does represent—the pattern of *her own* cultural background. Perhaps the nurse persists in her plan against the family's resistance. She remains unperceptive of this family's uniqueness, and continues to project her own cultural values. When *her* plan for the family fails, she is likely to label them "unco-operative," and so describe them in her report, still unaware that the problem is her own, not the family's.

Perhaps this is an extreme and unlikely example. But it is just such failures to find the means of helping that have made it necessary for there to be greater awareness on the part of the health care professions of the human factors which operate in a human being's response to health and illness.

Traditionally, medical care has been

based upon the physical and biological sciences. A knowledge of these is essential, of course, if one is to understand disease and care for persons who are ill. However, complexity is increasing from two points of view. Throughout the world, societies are becoming more complex with the intermingling of cultures and exchange of health workers across cultural boundaries. The study of disease processes, and the growing concept of preventive medicine prove increasingly the need to understand the social and cultural aspects of human behavior, and especially to analyze human responses to health care.

This need is strikingly evident in the area of nutrition, and is of increasing interest and concern to the nurse. If she is thoughtful, if she knows her patients' basic nutritional needs or deficiencies, yet observes differences in their ways of eating and their strong emotional responses to proposed changes in habits, she asks herself questions. Why do people eat what they eat? Why do they choose one food and reject another? What accounts for the total complex of behaviors that constitute food habits?

Food habits, like other forms of human behavior, are the result of many personal, cultural, social, and psychological influences. Studies in the behavioral sciences—anthropology, sociology, and psychology—have contributed much insight concerning the bases of these habits. Perhaps everyone tends to be somewhat ethnocentric—centered in his own culture—so that he views his own way as the best or right way. The habits of another who differs from him are looked on as foreign or wrong or superstitious or stupid. If people are honest enough to recognize their own biases, many of the misconceptions that prevent understanding other people can be cleared away. Such misconceptions hinder the nurse's ability to give her patients sensitive, constructive care.

In the last analysis, it is the cultural and sociopsychologic factors in the individual patient that will prove most influential in his nutritional behavior. In each patient, these factors are interwoven into a behavioral complex. In order to study them, each will be looked at separately.

CULTURAL INFLUENCES
The concept of culture

A century-old definition by E. B. Taylor describes culture as "that complex whole which includes knowledge, belief, art, law, morals, custom, and any other capabilities and habits acquired by man as a member of society." Modern anthropologists have enlarged the definition of culture to include the entire way of life of a people. Margaret Mead states that culture involves not only the more obvious and historical aspects of man's communal life (his language, religion, politics, technology, and so on), but also all the little habits of everyday living such as preparing and serving food, caring for children, feeding them and lulling them to sleep. Often the most significant thing that can be known about a culture is what it takes for granted in daily life.

These many facets of a man's culture are *learned*. Gradually, as the child grows up within a given society, the slow process of conscious and unconscious learning of values, attitudes, habits, and practices takes place through the conscious and unconscious influence of parents, teachers, and other enculturating agents of his society. Whatever is invented, transmitted, and perpetuated—his socially acquired knowledge and habits—man learns as part of his culture. These become internalized and entrenched.

Function of culture

The culture of a people develops over a long period. It is partly the result of this people's *adaptation to its environment*. The environment may be harsh and hostile, and the way of life developed by this people is what has enabled them to survive. Sometimes the changing of these habits by an outsider who does not understand these adaptations may upset this balance with nature. It will then do more harm than good. This has been the case when some health workers have tried to impose Western culture and habits upon people in other parts of the world, without prior study and appreciation of established customs. Such programs have failed for this reason.

The culture of a people also develops as a means of *interpreting common (and sometimes terrifying) life experiences,* such as birth, death, illness, disease, sex, and phenomena of nature. Rituals, taboos, totems, habits, and practices develop to explain, placate, or protect, and to establish human and environmental relationships. A certain poisonous plant, for example, may have become taboo as a food because the tribal ancestors observed that it caused death.

Food in a culture

Food habits are among the oldest and most entrenched aspects of many cultures. They exert deep influence on the behavior of the people. The cultural background determines what shall be eaten, as well as when and how it shall be eaten. There is, of course, considerable variation; and both rational and irrational, beneficial and injurious customs are found in every part of the world. Nevertheless, by and large, food habits are based upon food availability, economics, or symbolism. Included among these influential factors are the geography of the land, the agriculture practiced by the people, their economy and market practices, and their history and traditions.

Cultural determination of what is food. Items considered to be food in one culture may be regarded with disgust, or may actually cause illness in the persons of another culture. In America, milk is valued as a basic food; in many other cultures it is rejected with revulsion as an animal mucous discharge. In the Philippines, the Ifugao tribesmen of northern Luzon are famous for adapting their steep mountain terrain to the production of rice by forming multiple, narrow, terraced, dry rice fields (Figs. 13-1 and 13-2) in which they grow a major portion of this staple food (an example of overcoming geographic barriers to food pro-

duction). They are also known for their enjoyment of other dietary items which they prize, such as dragon flies and locusts— which they boil, dry, and grind into a powder. Crickets, flying and red ants, beetles, and water bugs are fried in lard.

The use of the staple item, bread, is another example. Many a diet-obsessed American rejects bread. In a Greek home, bread is the main food. It is *the* meal. All other foods are considered accompaniments to bread, and are eaten between bites of bread. So strong is the place of bread in the diet throughout much of the Middle East, that in Egypt wives have been divorced because they seldom provided fresh bread for their husbands.

Religious aspects of culture also control food rejection and use. Pork is unacceptable as food for a Moslem or an orthodox Jew; any meat is unacceptable for the Seventh Day Adventist; the strict Hindu or Buddhist eats no meat, and even the liberal Hindu may not eat beef. In his youth, Ghandi is said to have intellectually agreed that beef was a good food for human use and he therefore ate some. But his Hindu culture and rejection of beef was so deeply ingrained and internalized that the food made him violently ill.

Appetite for specific food. Foods acceptable for one meal may be rejected for another meal. For example, the main breakfast food in a Greek home may be bread and cheese; in Europe, a sweet roll; in America, ham and eggs. Inhabitants of different regions within a country also vary in their choices. In America, the Westerner would probably have fried potatoes at breakfast with his ham and eggs; the Southerner would consider potatoes a dinner food and have grits (a porridge made with coarsely ground white corn) for breakfast instead; the New Englander is fond of pie for breakfast.

How and where food is eaten. In a highly urban, industrialized society such as America, in which value is placed on action, speed, and productivity, lunch for the businessman may be a quick snack which he

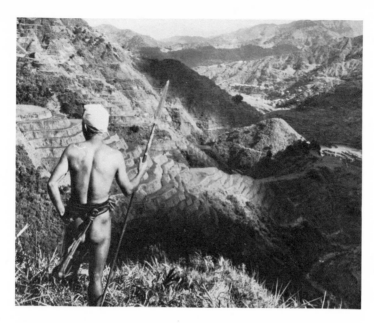

Fig. 13-1. An Ifugao tribesman of Banawe, in the Philippines, looks out across the terraces of his people. The rice terraces of the Ifugao mountain tribe have existed for 3,000 years and are carefully tended by each succeeding generation. (FAO photograph.)

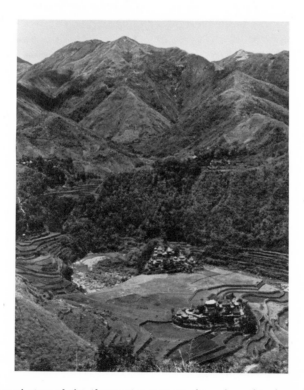

Fig. 13-2. A general view of the Ifugao rice terraces shows how they have been shaped out of the mountain face. The villages of the tribespeople in the valley are made up of stilt houses.

eats while standing at a lunch counter. Even the form of food is geared for quick eating—fruit in juice form, and meat in a sandwich. To the Spanish or Latin American merchant, such a lunch is unthinkable. His less tensely paced culture allows him to close his shop for two hours in the middle of the day while he enjoys a leisurely meal and siesta at home with his family.

Appropriate occasion for specific foods. The force of dietary patterning is seen in the Thanksgiving turkey, the Easter ham, and until recently (and still for strict observers) the Friday fish. Times of religious observance, such as Lent, call for specific food patterns. Food becomes an integral part of transmitting and teaching many aspects of one's particular culture.

Symbolism of food in a culture

Within every culture, there are certain foods that are deeply imbued with symbolic meaning. These symbols are related to major life experiences from birth through death, to religion, to politics, and to general social organization. (In the following examples, many foreign food names are mentioned. These terms are explained in the section of this chapter on Cultural Food Patterns, p. 257).

Major life experiences. The birth of a child is observed in many cultures by a meal that symbolizes a general celebration of the beginning of life. It is an occasion for feasting; or, in some cultures, for offering special foods to one or more deities. Soon after birth, a baptism or dedication ceremony may be followed by a special family meal. Birthdays are celebrated with special foods—in modern America, with a cake decorated with candles. Stages of the young person's development are often observed by special food uses. At a coming-of-age ceremony such as the Bar Mitzvah for Jewish boys at the age of thirteen, honey cake and wine, canapes, strudel, knishes, and piroggen are generally served. Puberty rites in other cultures often involve the eating of special foods. Graduation ceremonies marking levels of attainment in educational,

occupational, religious, or social life may require special feasting, or, in some cultures or instances, fasting.

Weddings are especially surrounded with symbolic foods. The bride's cake and the wedding reception are common in Western culture. Family feasting often lasts for several days in other cultures, where it is the eating of special foods together that seals the marriage pact.

Pregnancy is attended by many food symbols, taboos, and practices. Certain foods may be avoided in the belief that they will mark the infant. Certain foods may be denied the pregnant woman in the belief that she will contaminate the food supply. For example, in the Zulu tribe of South Africa the pregnant woman may not go near the cattle enclosure or drink any milk from the cows, because of the belief that she will exert an evil influence on the prized herd. In rural Southern United States and some other areas, pica (the eating of clay or of starch) is sometimes practiced by pregnant women, who profess strong cravings for it.

In many cultures the death of a member of the group involves food use symbolizing the general fact that each individual life has its end. In one group, food may be buried with the body to sustain the departed on his journey to the hereafter. In another group, food may be the main expression of sympathy, sorrow, or support for the bereaved, and many offerings of food are brought to the home by neighbors. A special funeral supper may be a part of the mourning prescribed in still another group.

Religion. Food symbolism plays a large role in most religions of the world. From early times ceremonies and religious rites surrounded acts pertaining to fertility and the harvest seasons. Food gathering, preparing, and serving followed specific customs, and commemorated special events of religious significance. Many of these customs remain.

Among the Jewish people, a number of special feast or fast days commemorate sig-

Table 13-1. Jewish holidays and associated foods

Holiday	Month	Event	Traditional foods
Rosh Hashanah (New Year)	September or October	Beginning of Jewish New Year (Tishri 1)	Honey, honey cake, carrot tzimmes
Yom Kippur	September or October	Day of Atonement	Fast day (total)
Sukkoth	October	Feast of Booths, Harvest festival; symbolizes booths in which Israelites lived on flight from Egypt and wilderness wanderings	Kreplach or holishkes (chopped meat wrapped in cabbage leaves) Strudel
Chanukah	December	Feast of Lights; celebrates heroic battle of the Maccabees for Jewish independence (165 B.C.) Home festival with candles	Grated potato latkes, potato kugel
Chamise Oser b'Sh'vat	January	Festival of the Trees (Arbor Day); blossoming time of trees in Palestine	Bokser (St. John's Bread) fruits, nuts, raisins, cakes
Purim	March	Feast of Esther; celebrates downfall of Haman and deliverance of Hebrews by influence of Queen Esther to King Xerxes of Persia	Hamantashen (three cornered pastry), apples, nuts, raisins
Passover (Pesach)	April	Festival of Freedom; celebrates escape of Israelites from Egyptian slavery	Seder meal; matzoth and matzoth dishes, wine, nuts
Shevuoth	May	Feast of Weeks (Pentecost); celebrates the day Moses received Ten Commandments on Mt. Sinai	Cheese blintzes, cheese kreplach, dairy foods

nificant events in their history (Table 13-1) and are a means of teaching cherished beliefs and traditions to the children. The Jewish New Year, Rosh Hashanah occurs in September or October and begins the Hebrew calendar of holidays. At this time it is customary to serve apple slices dipped in honey, signifying the yearning for a sweet and happy year. Carrots in some form are served to signify the wish for prosperity in the coming year. A carrot tzimmes is usually served. Perhaps the two most significant holidays that follow in the Jewish calendar are Yom Kippur (Day of Atonement), the high holy day of fast, which comes in September or October; and Pesach (Passover), which occurs in April. On the evening before the fast day, Yom Kippur,

no highly spiced or seasoned foods are served. At the end of the fast, the *Kiddush* (the blessing over wine) is observed, followed by a special meal of Sabbath dishes such as stuffed herring (gefüllte fish), noodle soup, poultry, vegetables, salad, fruit, and strudel. Observance of Passover, usually celebrated for eight days in April, commemorates the liberation of the Israelites from Egyptian bondage. This feast has come to play an important role in the democratic struggle for human dignity for many peoples of the world, to strengthen conviction that justice and freedom for all men may yet prevail on the earth. The holiday begins with a highly symbolic family meal on the evening before the Passover—the Seder, at which each food eaten signifies a

TO PROBE FURTHER
The Seder, beginning of the Jewish Passover

On the eve of Passover Week, perhaps the most beloved of all the Jewish festivals, a special ceremonial meal is held in Jewish homes to commemorate the deliverance of the Israelites from Egyptian bondage. This symbolic meal is called the Seder, which means "order"; the word refers to the prescribed order of the Passover service. Each item of the table setting and each food used has special significance.

Candles—ancient symbol for enlightment, or human consciousness growing out of prehuman darkness

Ke'arah—the seder plate, containing the symbolic objects used for the ceremony

Betzah—roasted egg, symbol of an offering; the shape, without beginning or end, signifies eternal redemption and liberation of all mankind

Zeroa—roasted lamb or chicken bone, symbol of the paschal lamb, sacrificed the night of Passover in the Temple

Morar—bitter herb (grated horseradish) symbol of the bitter life of the Hebrews in bondage

Karpas—green vegetable (parsley, lettuce, or watercress) dipped in a dish of salt water and eaten as a relish; symbolizes the manner of leisurely eating enjoyed by free men in olden times

Kharoses—mixture of chopped nuts, apples, cinnamon, and wine; symbol of the mortar and clay used by the ancient Israelites in making bricks when they toiled under Pharaoh

Three matzoth—(1) bread of poverty eaten by the afflicted Israelites; (2) symbol of haste in which Israelites fled from Egypt—the dough had not leavened because they could not tarry, (3) symbol of ancient ceremonial custom, The Feast of Unleavened Bread

Arba Kosos—wine goblet for each person, from which four cups of wine are drunk, symbolizing the four expressions in the Bible relating to redemption

Cup of Elijah—extra goblet left for Elijah, the herald of the messianic era

Hard-cooked eggs and salt water are passed to each person at the feast, as an entrée to the main meal, symbolic of mourning for the destruction of the Temple. The eggs also symbolizes Life, the perpetuation of existence.

specific aspect of the historical deliverance.

Among the Moslem people, a month of fasting during Ramadan (the ninth month of the Islamic lunar calendar, thus rotating through all seasons) has replaced the Jewish fast day, Yom Kippur. The fourth pillar of Islam is fasting. "O ye who believe! Fasting is prescribed to you as it was prescribed to those before you, that ye may ward off evil," commands the Koran. Ramadan was chosen for the sacred fast because it is the month in which Mohammed received the first of the revelations that were subsequently compiled to form the Koran, and also the month in which his followers first drove their enemies from Mecca in A.D. 624.

During the month of Ramadan, Mohammedans all over the world observe rigid daily fasting, taking no food or drink from dawn to sunset. Nights, however, are often spent in gay feasting. First, an appetizer is

TO PROBE FURTHER
Id al-Fitr, the post-Ramadan festival

Traditionally, in Moslem countries, at the conclusion of Ramadan, Islam's holy month of prayer and fasting, wealthy merchants and princes hold public feasts for the needy. This is the festival of Id al-Fitr.

Over the years, many delicacies have been served to symbolize the joy of return from fasting, and the heightened sense of unity, brotherhood, and charity which the fasting experience has brought to the people. Among the foods served are chicken or veal, sautéed with eggplant and onions, then simmered slowly in pomegranate juice and spiced with turmeric and cardamom seeds. The highlight of the meal usually is kharuf mahshi, a whole lamb (symbol of sacrifice) stuffed with a rich dressing made of dried fruits, cracked wheat, pine nuts, almonds, onions, and seasoned with ginger and coriander. The stuffed lamb is baked in hot ashes for many hours, so that it is tender enough to be pulled apart and eaten with the fingers.

At the conclusion of the meal, rich pastries and candies are served. These may be flavored with spices or flower petals. Some of the sweets are taken home and savored as long as possible as a reminder of the festival.

taken, such as dates or a refreshing drink. A popular modern beverage is a sherbetlike liquid made from dried apricots, called qamar-al-deen ("moon of religion"). After this appetizer, the family enjoys an "evening breakfast"—the iftar. At the end of Ramadan, a feast lasting up to three days climaxes the observance. Special dishes mark this joyous occasion. There are delicacies such as thin pancakes dipped in powdered sugar, savory buns, and dried fruits.

Among the Christian people of the world, there is prescribed the six-week fast period of Lent that precedes Easter. There is a special light-meal pattern and abstinence from meat, in symbolic preparation of the spirit to observe the holy season of Easter, which commemorates the death and resurrection of Christ. Throughout the year, the Communion meal (the Lord's Supper, the sacrament of the Mass) involves symbolic use of foods. Bread is taken as the body of Christ, broken and offered for men, and wine is taken as the blood of Christ, shed in sacrificial redemption for men. For the Christian, the simple line of the Lord's

Prayer, "Give us this day our daily bread," the saying of grace at mealtimes, and the offering of thanks at harvest time all relate food to faith.

Many of the religous rituals associated over the years with the preparation and use of food result not only from symbolic meaning but also from wisdom regarding possible contamination and spread of disease. For example, the Jains, members of an ascetic religious sect founded in India in the sixth century by a Hindu reformer as a revolt against the caste system, eat their meals before sunset to avoid the possibility of insect pollution in their food. They avoid root vegetables because such foods carry on their skins organisms that proliferate in the earth.

Politics. Food use has had political significance in man's history, as well as religious significance. In India, the fasts of Ghandi wielded tremendous political power, which contributed enormously to that country's achieving independence from Great Britain. The Boston Tea Party was concerned with important interrelationships between food, economics, and a budding nation's political views. Tea was considered to be an almost essential commodity by the American colonists, and English taxes on tea stimulated the politics of American independence.

SOCIAL INFLUENCES
The concept of social organization

Sociology may be defined in simplest terms as the study of group life. It is concerned with man's group behavior, the numerous activities, processes, and structures by which his social life goes on. Through the discipline and methods of sociology human behavior is understood in terms of social phenomena. Such fields and problems as social change, urbanism, rural life, the family, the community, race relations, crime, and delinquency are studied.

This broad behavioral science has many implications for nursing and nutrition. Two aspects of social organization that particularly concern a nurse are class structure and value systems.

Class structure. The structure of a society is largely formed by groupings according to such factors as economic status, education, residence, occupation, or family. Within a given society, many of these groups exist, whose values and habits vary. These subgroups within a larger culture are called subcultures. They may be established on the basis of region, religion, age, sex, social class, occupational group, or political party. Within these subgroups there may be still smaller groupings with distinguishing attitudes, values, and habits—the community juvenile gang, the college fraternity, the industrial executives, the Army officers, the families in a given neighborhood, or the nurses in a hospital hierarchy. A person may be a member of several subcultural groups, each of which influences his values, attitudes, and habits.

Social class, especially, influences value systems, responses, and behavior patterns. Social classes may be considered as comprising those persons having similar community status, responsibilities, and privileges. In America, social classes are less distinct and rigid than in some countries. For example, class barriers clearly separate the aristocrat from the commoner in Great Britain, and a severe caste system characterizes the Hindu population of India. Nonetheless, social classes are present in America and do influence behavior. One study of an American urban community reported the presence of six social layers.[1] Perhaps this is a fair sample and may roughly serve as a model, although current social change is effecting some lessening of these distinctions:

1) Upper-upper class—old-line community aristocrats
2) Lower-upper class—the newly rich of the community
3) Upper-middle class—professional persons, business owners, executives
4) Lower-middle class—tradesmen, white collar workers, some highly skilled workers
5) Upper-lower class—skilled and semiskilled workers
6) Lower-lower class—laborers, some unassimilated foreign groups

These class lines are often blurred, and movement from class to class occurs. Essentially, the distinctions are based on the related factors of income, occupation, education, and residence.

A later study, at Yale University[2] in 1950, identified five classes in the community of New Haven, Connecticut. This stratification may have been typical of similar United States cities of 250,000 population at that time. Using an Index of Social Position based on area of residence, occupation, and education (including a sampling of income and behavior patterns regarding books and periodicals read, radio and television programs heard and viewed, organization and club memberships), the researchers found the comparative results shown in Table 13-2.

The democratic and equalitarian philosophy of American society, and the humanitarian ideals on which members of the health professions have been nurtured, combine to make the reality of class differences

Table 13-2. American urban social class structure (New Haven study, 1950)*

Class	Occupation	Residence	Education	Social life	Popula-tion (percent)
1	Inherited wealth; business and professional leaders	"The best"	College graduation; famous private schools	Private clubs; family cliques; exclusive organizations	3
2	High managerial positions; professions; live well but no great wealth	"Better" residence areas	College graduation; graduate professional study	Family; church; clubs; community and professional organizations	9
3	Small businessmen; office and sales workers; skilled workers	"Good" residential areas	High school graduation; business school; 1 to 2 yrs. college	Family; low prestige churches; lodges	20
4	Semi-skilled factory industrial workers	Scattered	Older members: elementary school Young adults: high school	Family; neighborhood; labor unions; public places	50
5	Semi-skilled factory hands and unskilled laborers	Tenements, cold-water flats	Lower grades of elementary school	Family; flat; street; neighborhood; social agencies	18

*Hollingshead, A. B., and Redlich, F. C.: Social class and mental illness, New York, 1958, John Wiley and Son.

difficult to accept. Yet the differences do exist, and they probably influence the approach to patients, relationships with them, and the outcome of those relationships more than the nurse may be aware or care to admit.

Value systems. Another important aspect of a society's social organization is its value system, which develops as a result of its history and heritage. Values held in America, for example, stem largely from its relatively recent pioneer history. The majority of American settlers were from rigidly Puritan backgrounds. Their highest values were placed upon industry, self-denial and self-control, work, will-power, cleanliness, honesty, responsibility, and initiative. These values became intensified because the survival of the settlers often depended upon the exercise of these characteristics. Pleasure and entertainment were considered to have secondary value at best, and in most instances were held by the settlers who

lived through the most difficult pioneer periods to be unworthy or even evil.

Jurgen Reusch[3] has identified four basic premises on which the present American value system is based: *equality, sociality, success,* and *change.* All of these values influence attitudes toward health care and food habits. The placement of a high value on equality leads health workers to establish standards of quality health care for all people. The high respect accorded to sociality builds peer group pressures and status-seeking within social groups. Foods may be accepted because they are high-status foods, or rejected because they are low-prestige foods. The esteem in which success is held often leads persons to measure life in terms of competitive superlatives. They want to set the best table, to provide the most abundant supply of food for the family, and to have the biggest eater, and therefore the fattest, of any baby in the neighborhood. The value that is placed upon change leads families or individuals to seek constant variety in their diets, to be geared for action, and to seek quick-cooking, conveniently prepared foods. In response to such market demands, food technologists are producing an increasing array of food products each year.

Food and social factors

The food habits of people in any setting are highly socialized. These habits perform significant social functions, some of which may not always be evident to the persons who have such habits.

Social relationships. Food is a symbol of sociability, warmth, friendliness, and social acceptance. The breaking of bread together binds a group. From the earliest Christian era, such custom enriched fellowship and became the symbol of the Communion meal. "And they, continuing daily with one accord, breaking bread from house to house, did eat their meat with gladness and singleness of heart" (Acts 2:46).

Similar use of food for binding fellowship is seen in the honor reception, the wedding breakfast, the political party banquet, and the serving of food to visitors. Very early socialization was observed once in a young child who offered his little friend his "sucking thumb" for awhile! From the first hours of life, eating is not a solitary experience. It is a matter of two people—a feeding adult and an eating newborn.

An extreme example of the social function of food is seen in the practice of the mountain Arapesh, a Papuan people of New Guinea. With great effort, sometimes in groups of six families, they clear small plots for gardens, often at long distances from their homes. They raise animals for food and they hunt game. But none of this is ever for themselves! Each person gives the product of his labors to other members of the group, frequently traveling great distances over mountain trails to do so. The worst thing an Arapesh man can do is keep some of his produce for himself. The entire process of food production, gathering, and consumption is a means of social

warmth and intercourse. By American standards, this practice might be called highly inefficient and even irrational, for about one-third of the tribe's time is spent in traveling the difficult terrain for the purpose of feeding others. But for these warm, happy people it is a source of group fellowship and strength. And which of these basic values is more important?

Persons involved in social relationships. People tend to accept food more readily from those persons viewed as friends or allies. People most enjoy eating with those persons to whom they feel close. New foods from persons who seem congenial are acceptable. Advice about food is accepted from persons who are considered to be authorities, and with whom is felt a warm relationship. For example, people are more willing to take such counsel from the family doctor than from the more remote nutritionist. People tend to distrust food given them by strangers and outsiders. Emotional feelings about people are transferred to their food. The more alien the authority figure, the more he is considered to be unconcerned, and it is more likely that his food suggestions will be considered as outlandish, or perhaps even harmful.

Maternal role. Food is symbolic of motherliness. In the family, the early feeding process is the vehicle of much conscious and unconscious learning between mother and child. The mother teaches what is acceptable as food, when to eat, how much to eat, and why it is eaten. Many mothers are unaware that they impart their own likes and dislikes to their children. Yet how often statements about food are prefaced with the words, "My mother always . . ."!

A mother's self-esteem is deeply involved in feeding her family. She feels it necessary to be confident that she has done the right thing for them as a mother. Depending on her education, she decides who is an authority to advise her about child feeding. If she is relatively unsophisticated and has little education, she is likely to view her own mother and her neighbors as her best guides. If she has somewhat more education she perhaps accepts more readily the advertising of business concerns as the greatest authority. Mothers with middle-class or better education place most faith in a professional medical authority. Under the stress of emergency, however, most mothers of all educational levels are likely to turn to the recognized health worker for advice about food for a sick infant.

Status foods. Status is often sought in terms of food. A person may build a reputation as a gourmet. In order to accomplish this, he may eat, and become expert with respect to exotic foods (which he secretly may not enjoy), simply as a means of gaining prestige among his peers. (Compare the enthusiast for opera, who attends every first-night performance, and knows who designed every high fashion gown worn by the women in the audience, but is ignorant of what opera is being performed or what artists are singing lead roles.) High prestige foods such as roasts or steaks are usually served for dinner when guests are invited, and lower prestige foods such as hamburger or liver are rarely served. For some social groups, forms of bread vary in status. White bread is preferred to dark bread. In some social groups, purchased bread has higher status that homemade biscuits; in others, the reverse is true.

Food in family relationships. Eating together as a family group builds closeness and family solidarity. Food habits that are most closely associated with family sentiments are the most tenacious throughout life. The role of each family member is most clearly illustrated to the child as the family eats together. Long into adulthood, certain foods trigger a flood of childhood memories, and these foods are valued for reasons totally apart from any nutritional value.

Certain meals have more family significance than others. In America, breakfast and lunch may be rather impersonally served, and eaten by various family members at individual times. Dinner is more family-centered and its pattern is more complex. Its foods are often more symbolic. Changes in one's food habits or the introduction of new foods may tend to be more acceptable at breakfast or lunch than at dinner. Strong religious factors associated with food also tend to have their origin and reinforcement within the family meal circle.

Economic factors. People tend to eat foods that are readily available to them, and that they can afford. Family income, community sources of food, and market conditions influence food habits and ultimate food choices.

Social problems and food habits

Among the many effects of rapid social change, with the uprooting and displacing of persons and families, are changes in the food habits of millions of persons.

Poverty. In large urban centers, growing numbers of persons who are members of minority groups live in slums, where they are unassimilated and often disregarded by the mainstream of a sophisticated, affluent society. They are unprepared for earning a living in industry's automated age, and are often frightened, insecure, and lonely. Many persons from such nearby places as Puerto Rico, Cuba, and Mexico, or from some areas of the United States such as the rural South, have made their way to the cities, where they hoped to find a new life. Instead, they sometimes find obstacles that they cannot surmount, and live a marginal existence at best. Inadequate housing is attended by problems related to cooking, refrigeration, storage, and sanitation. Malnutrition, broken spirits, and hostility often result.

Family disintegration. Abject poverty for some workers and increased affluence for others, has resulted from industrialization and changing urban-suburban living patterns. These newly emerging patterns appear to have contributed to changes in family patterns and values. An increasing number of families seldom gather for meals; in such families, the reinforcement of group unity and stability that was formerly felt from eating together is lost. Children who are left to shift for themselves incur erratic eating habits, and tend to fill their stomachs with a diet that is nutritionally inadequate. The increased number of teen-age marriages, often between young people with limited means of support and little knowledge of food preparation or of child feeding, may lead to poor food choices and poor eating habits.

Alcoholism. Alcoholism is frequently associated with poor nutrition. Both the addict and his family may be adversely affected. If the wage-earner is addicted, he or she may spend a great portion of the family's small income for alcohol; inadequate funds remain for feeding the family. The alcoholic who does not deprive others of food frequently damages his own health by obtaining in alcohol the mere calories requisite for direct energy expenditure. He neglects to eat a proper diet that would supply the many other nutrients his body needs and malnutrition results.

PSYCHOLOGIC INFLUENCES
Social psychology—understanding dietary patterns

Social psychology is the most recent o the behavioral sciences. It began in the last part of the Nineteenth Century and combines concepts from psychology and sociology. This discipline is concerned with social interaction in terms of its effect upon individual behavior, and with the social influences and determining factors of individual perception, motivation, and action. How does a particular individual perceive a given situation? What basic needs motivate his action and response? What social factors surround his particular action? Social psychologists are particularly interested in the effect of culture on personality, the socialization of the child, differences in individuals and groups, group dynamics, group attitudes and opinions, and leadership. The detailed individual case study is much used as a research method.

The science and methods of social psychology have made important contributions to medical, nursing, and allied health care, especially to problems of human behavior under stress. Intensive study has been made of the psychosocial aspects of physical disability, aging, obesity, problems attending surgical procedures such as mastectomy, gastrectomy, and colostomy; and those related to chronic diseases such as peptic ulcer.

It must be borne in mind by the nurse that deep psychological connotations lead to exceedingly sensitive areas in the individual's total structure as a person capable of meeting life and carrying out his responsibilities. While the nurse should know that such connections exist, she will need to use her knowledge to avoid mistakes and to better understand the depth of the roots of the problems she will encounter. However, she will recognize the limits beyond which she would be unwise to dig. Foods-as-symbols may lead the psychiatrist to discoveries of which the nurse should be aware in general; but she would be no better equipped to treat those psychologic aspects by *direct* attack than to operate on a perforated ulcer.

Food and psychologic factors

Individual behavior patterns including those related to eating are the result of many interrelated psychosocial influences and factors. Factors that are particularly pertinent to the shaping of food habits are motivation and perception.

Motivation. People are not the same the world over. People of differing cultures are not motivated by the same needs and goals. Even primary biological drives, such as hunger and sex, are modified in their interpretation, expression, and fulfillment by many cultural, social, and personal influences. The kinds of food sought, prized, or accepted by one individual at one time and place may be violently rejected by another individual living in different circumstances. In the person existing in a state of basic hunger or semistarvation, the whole perception and motivation is concerned with food. Such a person thinks, talks, and dreams about food. Under less severe circumstances, however, the concern for food may be on a relatively abstract level, and may involve symbolism that is associated with other levels of need.

Maslow[4] has developed a useful concept of a hierarchy of human needs, wants, and strivings. He indicates that only as each level of need is met is the individual able to progress to the next level of experiences and awareness. He describes five levels that operate in turn, each building upon the prior ones:

1. Basic physiologic needs—hunger, thirst
2. Safety needs—physical comfort, security, protection
3. Love, affection, "belongingness" needs —giving and receiving affection
4. Self-esteem, status, recognition needs —sense of self-worth, strength, self-confidence, capability, adequacy
5. Self-actualization—self-fulfillment, creative growth

Although these levels overlap and vary with time and circumstance, Maslow's concept of such hierarchy can help the nurse to understand patient needs and to plan health care accordingly.

Perception. Perception is the process of adding meaning to what is taken in through the senses. It is perception that enables people to create a relatively stable environment out of an otherwise chaotic assortment of sensory impressions. Perception also limits understanding. Each phenomenon that the outer world offers is perceived through social and personal lenses. In every experience of a person's life, what he perceives is a blend of three factors: (1) the external reality, (2) the message of the stimulus that is conveyed by his nervous system to the integrative centers where thinking and evaluation go on, and (3) the interpretation that each person puts upon each datum of experience. A host of subjective elements such as hunger, thirst, hate, fear, self-interest, values, and temperament influence response to the phenomena that are presented by the outer world. Those responses are called behavior.

The philosopher Justus Buchler[5] has suggested the term *proception* as being more accurate. By proception, Buchler means all one's past relations to one's world, one's accumulated experience, and the future toward which his past and present propel him. The individual acquires this direction from his native temperament, his culture, his cumulative habit, his situation, and his emotional character. In short, proception is the total process of relevant behavior, from input to act. The procept opens and closes the gate to the percept.

This concept relates significantly to health education. Allport[6] states that health workers are highly selected, well-educated, specialized persons who tend to be intellectualizers, abstract thinkers, and less emotionally dependent than uneducated persons are upon the surrounding environment. But the people for whose health they assume certain responsibilities usually do not think abstractly, particularly under the stress of illness, anxiety, and pain. The responses of such persons to attempts at health education may vary from over-reaction to repression. The patient who is repressing his response to the health worker's efforts may seem to us to be turning a deaf ear to the message. However, if the nurse concludes that the patient is deliberately excluding her message, *her* perception is at fault. The patient wants to know and understand. Deep within all men is a basic desire for meaning. Every person searches for meaning in all his life experiences including illness, suffering, and death. It is an important part of the nurse's task to shape her instructions to the patient's proception. It is she who must be sensitive to the individual patient at his particular stage of development. She must respect him as a unique being if she is to help him to find the answers in his search for meaning.

It is this dimension that makes a nurse's work profound. She cannot impose on her patients mechanical routines of sanitation, hygiene, and nutrition born of her own antiseptic cultural values. Patients will not carry them out if they are presented in this way. The nurse must look *at* her own spectacles, and not just *through* them. At the same time she must also look *at* and *through* the spectacles of her patients. This takes skill and a nurse must care enough to work at it. Only as she attains a higher level of perception will she realize that glib answers fail. In the last analysis, persons learn because they sense an urgent need to know. They learn because their curiosity is aroused. They learn by exploring, making mistakes and correcting them, testing, verifying. *All of these things the individual must do for himself.* This is true of our own learning. It is true of the learning we desire for our patients. We cannot change or shorten or avoid the process.

Diet and behavior—psychodietetics

Emotional responses to food stem from many sources. The practices and relationships that surrounded one's early infant feeding experiences build lasting emotional responses. Cultural and family conditioning, religious, and economic factors all mold the adult's behavior with respect to food.

Food feeds the psyche as well as the body. Several areas of psychological significance give symbolic meaning to foods:

Milk. Of all commonly used foods, milk is perhaps imbued with more psychological meaning than any other. To many persons milk symbolizes security and comfort. This is especially likely to be true if the individual's early relationships with the mother figure were satisfactory. At the same time, milk may mean dependence and helplessness, particularly in periods of stress. For example, ulcer patients on prolonged treatment of milk every few hours may find in such routine a socially accepted form of symbolic regression. In fact, the ulcer itself may in part stem from an inner dependent-independent conflict and a fear of success.

Sex-related attitudes. Certain foods, such as meat and bread, carry masculine meanings. They connote the paternal role of hunter, provider, and acceptor. These notions about meat have been traced by anthropologists to the beliefs of primitive tribes. Meat was (and still is in many cultures) considered the only food that would make a warrior strong and courageous. A plethora of traditions about the magic power of meat and blood is known to anthropologists. Warriors are forbidden to eat any food but meat. In certain cultures a youth to be initiated into the warrior group may have to drink tiger's blood, or eat bear's meat, or eat the flesh of a sacred animal. Some of this ancient tradition has been handed down to modern times in every culture. In some cultures it has been modified by the wish of the group to eradicate ferocity; therefore, eating meat is forbidden. In America, the tradition that strong men eat meat has been fostered until modern times by frontier history. The survival of the pioneers depended on their physical energy, strength, activity, and aggression. Meat has been the center of the meal, both in terms of menu planning and money expended. In modern industrial America, it remains the main concern of the wife that she have a strong husband and active children. Though she may know that eggs are nutritionally equal to meat (actually better in ideal amino acid combination), eggs never quite make the grade as a meat substitute. They are offered only as a last resort. The housewife's attitude toward a given food market may be based upon the quality of meat it sells.

Vegetables and fruits carry feminine meanings. They connote the maternal role of the one who feeds and gives. This symbolic concept also has a fascinating anthropologic history. When early human beings first settled down after a purely nomadic and hunting existence to an agricultural life, it was women who tilled the fields, while men continued to hunt and fight. The supremacy of the male is bound up with his belief in the "feminine weakness" represented by "mere" fruits and vegetables. The less educated (and the less psychologically developed) a man is, the more likely he is to scorn fruits and vegetables on emotional grounds—though he usually is totally unaware of the reason for his preference, and attributes it simply to the taste of the food itself.

Fruits are most feminine in meaning. The apple for the teacher, the gift basket, grapes, and peaches and cream symbolize love, beauty, sexuality, esteem, and luxury. The reproductive notion is basic in the word fruition, the bearing of fruit. Vegetables carry ideas related to even more primitive and earthy aspects of femininity—vegetate, vegetation. Fruits and vegetables are seasonal, ripe, bright-colored, and pleasantly shaped.

Age. Milk and strained foods, sometimes necessary components of a therapeutic diet for the adult, are considered infant foods and may be rejected, particularly by the person who is uncertain that he has genuinely attained adult status. Such a person may be of any chronological age.

In the latency period, the child's food horizon widens. As he leaves home for school, he encounters new foods and is given greater freedom of choice. He also compares his family's food to that of his peers and begins to learn the social status of foods. Certain foods, such as peanut butter, becomes labeled as child food and are promoted as such by advertisers.

During adolescence, the tenacious struggle for selfhood ensues. Not only clothes, late hours, driving, and dating, but also foods become battlegrounds between the generations. The teenager periodically adopts food fads, exhibits intense likes and dislikes, and displays enormous appetite. His obsession with his body image is basically a sexual problem. It may take the form of muscle-building foods for boys or figure-control diets for girls.

Adulthood brings certain ideas of food privileges. Foods such as olives, shrimp, and gourmet dishes may be considered adult. Drinks such as coffee, tea, or alcohol are reserved in most groups for adults.

Reward foods. Sweets are often used to bribe children; they are given as rewards for good behavior, and are withheld for bad behavior. This pattern may carry over into adulthood. In a moment of self-pity a person may think, "Life has deprived me of my fair reward; therefore, I shall eat chocolate cream pie." Sometimes unusual foods, special ways of preparation, or rare delicacies become symbolic rewards or punishment.

Illness. Illness is a period of psychologic repercussion. During illness, some degree of regression usually manifests itself. The patient may become picky and finical about his food and make frequent special demands. Poor appetite may compound the feeding problem. The patient, more than the well person, needs to be involved in the selection of his food. The same person who, while well, cares little about the style of food service, may as a patient find that his appetite is surprisingly dependent on esthetic appeal in preparation and service.

CULTURAL FOOD PATTERNS

A number of different cultural food patterns are represented in American community life. Many have contributed characteristic dishes or modes of cooking to American eating habits, and in turn many of the food habits of these subcultures have been Americanized. Traditional foods tends to be used more consistently by the older members of the families, while the members of younger generations may use such foods only on special occasions or holidays. Nonetheless, these traditional food patterns have strong meanings and serve to bind families and cultural communities in close fellowship. A few representative cultural food patterns are given here. The unique characteristics of each should be noted. It should be remembered that among persons of all cultures, individual tastes vary, geographic patterns within a country vary, and economic factors make for wide differences, as does the educational level.

Jewish food pattern

Adherence to Jewish dietary food laws varies among the three basic groups within Judaism: Orthodox—strict observance; Conservative—nominal observance; Reform—less ceremonial emphasis and minimal observance of the general dietary laws. This body of laws is called the rules of kashruth, and food selected and prepared accordingly is called kosher food. Both words come from the Hebrew word *kāsher,* meaning "right" or "fit." The basis of these laws is primarily self-purification and a means of service to God, although they probably also had some hygienic or ethical foundation in their inception. Most of these rules relate to ordinances given to the ancient Hebrews as recorded in the Old Testament books of the law (Leviticus and Deuteronomy) and to the Jewish traditions accumulated through the ensuing centuries. These were collected and interpreted in the Talmud, a body of laws set down in the Fourth to Sixth Centuries B. C.

Since the original Hebrew religion was centered in practices of animal sacrifice, and the blood had special ritual significance, the present day dietary laws apply specifically to the selection, slaughter, preparation, and service of meat, to the combining of meat and milk, to fish, and to egg.

Food restrictions

1. The only meat allowed is the meat of cloven hoofed quadrupeds that chew a cud (cattle, sheep, goat, deer), and only the forequarters may be used. The hind quarter may be eaten only if the Sinew of Jacob (hip sinew of the thigh) is removed (Leviticus 11:1-8, Deuteronomy 14:3-8, Genesis 32:33).

2. Chicken, turkey, goose, pheasant, and duck may be eaten (Leviticus 11:13-19).

3. Ritual slaughter follows rigid rules based upon minimal pain to the animal and maximal blood drainage. This process of preparing kosher meat involves several steps. The meat is soaked in water in a special vessel. It is then rinsed and thoroughly salted with coarse salt. It is placed on a perforated board tilted to permit blood to flow off, and the meat is left to stand for an hour. After it has drained thoroughly it is washed three times before being used in cooking.

4. No blood may be eaten as food in any form, as blood is considered synonymous with life (Genesis 9:4, Leviticus 3:17 and 17:10-14, Deuteronomy 12:23-27).

5. No combining of meat and milk is allowed. This prohibition is based upon the oft-repeated Old Testament command, "Thou shalt not seethe a kid in its mother's milk." (Exodus 23:19, 34:26; Deuteronomy 14:21). Milk or milk food (cheese, ice cream) may be eaten just before a meal, but not for six hours after eating a meal that contains meat. In the Orthodox Jewish home it is customary to maintain two sets of dishes, one for serving meat meals and the other for serving dairy meals.

6. Only those fish with fins and scales are allowed; no shellfish or eels may be eaten (Leviticus 11:9-12; Deuteronomy 14:9-10). Fish of the type permitted may be eaten with either dairy or meat meals.

7. No egg that contains a blood spot may be eaten. Eggs may be taken with either dairy or meat meals.

8. There are no special restrictions on fruits, vegetables, or cereals.

Foods for special occasions

Many of the traditional Jewish foods are related to the different festivals of the Jewish calendar. These holidays and associated foods are summarized in Table 13-1.

Special Sabbath dishes. In Orthodox Jewish homes, no food is prepared on the Sabbath, which begins at sundown on Friday and ends when the first star becomes visible Saturday evening. Foods are prepared on Friday and held for use on the Sabbath. A long-honored custom is that of inviting a guest (an orach) to share the Sabbath meals, as a remembrance of the Biblical injunction, "For you were once strangers in the land of Egypt." (Exodus 22:20). A few of the special Sabbath dishes follow:

1. Challah—a special loaf of white bread shaped as a twist or a beehive coil; used at the beginning of the meal after the Kiddush (the blessing over wine)

2. Gefüllte (gefilte) fish (Ger. "stuffed fish")—first course of the Sabbath eve meal; fish fillet, chopped, seasoned,

and stuffed back into the skin or minced and rolled into balls

3. Cholent (chulent, or shalet)—a one-dish meal of meat and vegetables, usually beef, potatoes, dried beans, onion, and chicken fat
4. Kugel—a sweet pudding seasoned with spices, raisins, and almonds
5. Tzimmes—carrot pudding made as a main dish with white and sweet potatoes, beef, and onion; may also be a sweet carrot pudding made with honey and spices; prunes may be used instead of carrots.

Other representative foods

1. Bagel—doughnut-shaped hard yeast roll
2. Blintzes—thin filled and rolled pancakes
3. Borscht (borsch)—soup of meat stock, beaten egg or sour cream with beets, cabbage or spinach; served hot or cold
4. Bubke—coffee cake
5. Farfel—grated noodle dough or crumbled matzoth, used in soup
6. Kasha—buckwheat groats (hulled kernels), used as a cooked cereal or as a potato substitute with gravy
7. Knaidlach or kloese—dumplings, served with chicken soup
8. Knishes—pastry filled with ground meat
9. Latkes—pancakes (potato *latkes* especially popular)
10. Lox—smoked, salted salmon
11. Lukshen—noodles
12. Matzo—flat, unleavened bread
13. Strudel—thin pastry filled with fruit and nuts and rolled, then baked

Greek food pattern

In the close-knit, traditionally organized life of the Greek family, food and the ceremonial aspects of meals constitutes a primary value. In many Greek homes, the meal is a family ritual. A blessing is said or sung, and hospitality is extended to guests. Everyday meals are simple, but holiday meals are the occasion for serving a great variety of delicacies. Bread is always the center of every meal, indeed it is *the* meal, with other foods considered accompaniments to it. Bread is eaten between bites of other food. During religious holidays such as Lent there are fast days of meat free meals with large use of vegetables.

Food groups

Milk. A relatively small amount of milk is used as a beverage by adults, who usually take this food in the form of yogurt. Children drink hot boiled milk sweetened with sugar. Cheese is a favorite food; varieties include feta, a special white cheese made from sheep's milk and preserved in brine; and two hard, salty cheeses, caceri and cephalotyri.

Meat. Lamb is the favored meat. Little beef, but some pork and chicken, are taken. Frequent use is made of organ meats, and of fresh fish. Eggs are sometimes taken as a main dish, but not at breakfast. Some characteristic meat dishes include:

1. Kreas souvlas, barbecued lamb; brizoles, broiled lamb or pork chops; yiouvarlakia—meat balls and rice with egg-lemon sauce or tomato sauce
2. Mousaka—alternate layers of fried potato, eggplant or squash, cheese, cooked ground meat in spiced tomato sauce, covered with thin pastry and baked
3. Ketta vrasti—boiled chicken, eaten hot or cold
4. Psari scharas—broiled fish with olive oil and lemon sauce seasoned with chopped parsley and mustard
5. Psari plake—baked fish with tomatoes, onions, parsley, and olive oil.

Vegetables. Vegetables are usually cooked until very soft, and are seasoned with meat broth or tomato with onions, olive oil, and parsley. Vegetables are often the main dish. Large amounts of many varieties are eaten. Fresh vegetables are preferred. Combination salad of thinly cut raw vegetables with a simple dressing of olive oil and vinegar or lemon juice is used often. Many legumes (beans, peas, lentils, and chick peas) are eaten; often a meal is made of cooked dried beans served with olives and pickles. Characteristic vegetable dishes include:

1. Yiachni—chopped onion browned in olive oil, vegetable added with tomato and seasonings, simmered until soft
2. Dolmathes—meat and rice mixture rolled in cabbage or vine leaves, steamed, served with egg sauce
3. Paragemista—stuffed vegetables such as eggplant, zucchini, green peppers, tomatoes
4. Tiganita—fried vegetables served with garlic or tomato sauce
5. Fasolia yiachni—dried beans cooked with tomatoes and onions

Fruits. Large amounts of fruit are eaten. Peeled raw fruit is an everyday dessert.

Bread and cereals. Bread made of plain wheat flour, water, salt, and yeast is an indispensable part of every meal. It is preferred plain without a spread of butter, jam, or jelly. Dark breads are used by some families. Wheat products such as noodles, macaroni, and spaghetti may be used plain or with meat and tomato sauce. Rice is commonly used. The following are some characteristic cereal dishes:

1. Pilafi—rice to which, after it has been browned in butter, broth or water is added, and simmered until the liquid is absorbed
2. Tyropetta and spanacopetta—cheese pie and spinach pie; thin layers of pastry brushed with olive oil alternating with layers of cheese and egg mixture or cheese and spinach
3. Pastitsio—alternating layers of noodles, macaroni, or spaghetti with tomato sauce containing meat and spices, and cheese, covered with thick white sauce, bread crumbs, more cheese and baked
4. Macaronia me kima—macaroni with meat-tomato sauce
5. Kritharaki—cooked cereal made of flour and water; formed into grains shaped like rice added to cooked meat

Desserts. Desserts other than raw fruit are usually served on special occasions such as holiday meals. Some of these characteristic dishes include:

1. Tsoureki—an Easter holiday bread similar to coffee cake, shaped in a braid and glazed with fruit and nuts
2. Baklavas—many layers of very thin pastry brushed with butter and sprinkled with nuts, sugar, and spices, cut in diamond shapes and baked, served with syrup
3. Loukoumathes—batter of plain flour, yeast, water, dropped in deep fat and fried, served with honey and cinnamon
4. Melomacarona—short dough (flour, oil, orange juice, soda, sugar) filled with mixture of nuts, sugar, and spices, sealed and baked, dipped in syrup and sprinkled with nuts
5. Risogalo—rice custard sprinkled with cinnamon

Italian food pattern

The sharing of food and companionship is an important part of the Italian pattern of life. Meals are associated with much warmth and fellowship, and special occasions are marked by the sharing of food with families and friends. Leisurely meals are customary, with a light breakfast, the large main meal in the middle of the day, and a small evening meal. Bread and pasta are the basic Italian foods. On religious fast days, such as Fridays, Lent, and the period of Advent before Christmas, pasta is prepared with meatless sauces or with fish.

Food groups

Milk. Milk is seldom used alone as a beverage. Frequently it is consumed with coffee in a mixture of about half coffee and half milk. Cheese, however, is a favorite food. Parmesan and romano are hard grating cheeses used in cooking; ricotta and mozzarella are two soft Italian cheeses used in cooking or with bread.

Meat. Chicken baked with oil or in tomato sauce, is used often. Beef and veal are used as meat balls, meat loaf, cutlets, stews, roasts, and chops. Roasted or fried Italian pork sausage is common. A number of Italian cold cuts are famous—salami, mortadella (bologna-type sausage), coppa (peppered sausage), and prosciutto (Italian cured ham). Many kinds of fish are used. Fresh fish are preferred, but some canned fish such as tuna, sardines, anchovies, and special salted codfish are used also. Some characteristic meat dishes are pollo alla cacciatora (chicken browned in olive oil, then simmered in wine and tomato sauce), scaloppina di vitello (thin, floured strips of veal browned in olive oil and simmered in sauce flavored with wine and herbs), Italian meat balls with spaghetti, and baccalà (dried salted codfish, soaked several days, browned in olive oil and simmered with tomato sauce and herbs).

Vegetables and fruit. Favorite vegetables include zucchini and other squash, broccoli, spinach, eggplant, escarole and other salad greens, green beans, peppers, and tomatoes. Tomatoes are used in sauces either whole or as paste, or they are puréed. Vegetables are usually cooked in water, drained, and seasoned with olive oil, or with oil and vinegar. A combination salad of greens such as escarole, chicory, lettuce, endive, and romaine, seasoned with a simple dressing of olive oil, vinegar, garlic, salt, and pepper is called insalata.

Fruit. Fresh fruit in season is taken as dessert.

Bread and cereals. Bread is present at every Italian meal as a highly regarded principal food. It is made in loaves of many shapes. Each shape is characteristic of a different Italian province. All Italian breads are made of wheat flour, and are white, crusty, and substantial. Some rice and corn meal are used in special dishes. For example, risotto alla Milanese is a dish made of rice cooked in broth with saffron, parmesan cheese, onion, and mushrooms. Polenta is a thick, yellow cornmeal mush sometimes made into a casserole with sausage, tomato sauce, and cheese.

A basic item in the Italian food pattern is pasta. This term is used for all of the wheat products made into various shapes and forms such as spaghetti, macaroni, and egg noodles. Pasta is served in many ways. Spaghetti is commonly used with a characteristic tomato sauce and cheese, or with added meat balls or fish. Special dishes of pasta of various kinds filled with meat mixtures are served on holidays—ravioli, lasagna, manicotti, tortellini, and cannelloni. A dry red or white wine is usually served also.

Soups. Thick soups often serve as the main food for lighter meals. Minestrone is made with vegetables, ceci (chick peas), and pasta. Pasta e fagioli is a substantial bean soup.

Seasonings and basic cooking method. Herbs and spices characteristically used in Italian dishes include oregano, rosemary, basil, saffron, parsley, and nutmeg. Garlic is used often, as are wine, olive oil, tomato purée, salt pork, and cheese. The basic processes of Italian cooking of main dishes are the initial browning of the seasonings in olive oil, adding meat or fish for browning also, then covering with liquid such as wine, tomato sauce, or broth and simmering slowly on low heat for several hours.

Puerto Rican food patterns

Indigenous tropical vegetables and fruits form the base of the Puerto Rican food pattern. Almost everyone eats the main food, viandas (compare the English word "viands"), which are starchy vegetables and fruits such as plantain and green banana. The two other staples of the diet are rice and beans. Milk, meat, yellow and green vegetables, and other fruits are used in limited quantities.

Food groups

Viandas. The many kinds of vianda eaten every day include piche verde (green banana), platano verde (green plantain), platano maduro (ripe plantain), batata blanca (white sweet potato), batata amarilla (yellow sweet potato), ñame blanco (white yam), panapen (breadfruit), yautia (tanier), and yuca (cassava). Viandas are cooked in many ways. Usually codfish and onion are added, and, if income permits, some avocado and hard-boiled eggs are also added. This dish is called serenata. A soup containing vianda and meat is called sancocho.

Rice. A large proportion of the daily calories is obtained from rice. Most Puerto Ricans eat about seven ounces daily. The rice is usually cooked in salted water and seasoned with lard (arroz blanco—white rice). Other dishes prepared with rice include arroz con habichuelas, rice stewed with beans and sofrito (a sauce of tomatoes, green pepper, onion, garlic, salt pork, lard, herbs); arroz con pollo, rice with chicken, seasoned with olives, red peppers, and sofrito; arroz con dulce, a dessert made with rice, sugar, and spices; and asopao, a thick soup of chicken and rice.

Other cereal grains. Some wheat is used in the form of bread, noodles, and spaghetti. Oatmeal and cornmeal mush may be added if income permits.

Beans. Legumes used include chick peas, navy beans, red kidney beans (preferred), and dried peas. Usually they are boiled until tender and cooked with sofrito.

Meat. Most Puerto Rican families cannot afford meat, although pork and chicken are used when income allows. The only animal protein that the majority can buy is dried codfish.

Milk. Low-income groups can afford little milk. Most of that which is taken is boiled and used with coffee (cafe con leche). Some cocoa and chocolate are used in the same way.

Vegetables and fruits. Small amounts of other vegetables are used by the Puerto Rican people. Many tropical fruits are available. Puerto Rico is the home of the acerola, the tiny, sour West Indian cherry, which looks like a miniature apple and has the highest quantity of ascorbic acid known to be contained in any food (about 1,000 mg. per 100 gm.). Other fruits include oranges, pineapples, grapefruits, papayas, and mangos.

Meal pattern. In most homes a typical day's food would include coffee with milk for breakfast, a large plate of viandas with codfish for lunch, and rice, beans, and viandas for dinner. If income permits, egg or oatmeal may be added to the breakfast, some meat to dinner, and some fruit may be taken between meals. This simple daily diet is in contrast with a holiday meal such as that enjoyed at Christmas time—whole pig roasted on a spit (lechon asado), blood sausage, green bananas or plantains cooked in the ashes, rice, pasteles (plantain dough filled with chopped pork, sofrito, olives, raisins, and boiled peas), rice pudding, and wine, beer, or brandy.

An effort is being made by the government to improve the diet of the Puerto Rican people, by listing the basic foods everyone eats (rice, beans, viandas, codfish, lard, sugar, coffee) and suggesting things that need to be added, such as milk in the form of goat's milk or dry milk, meat and egg, yellow and green vegetables, and fresh native fruit.

Mexican food pattern

A blending of the food habits of the Spanish settlers and native Indian tribes formed the basis for the present food patterns of the people of Mexican heritage who now live in the United States (chiefly in the Southwest). Three foods are fundamental to this pattern—dried beans, chili peppers, and corn. Variations and additions may be found in different localities or among those of different income levels.

Food groups

Milk. Very little milk is used. A small amount of evaporated milk may be purchased for babies.

Meat. Because of its cost, little meat is taken. Beef or chicken may be eaten two or three times a week. Eggs also are used only occasionally, and fish rarely.

Vegetables. Corn (fresh or canned) and chili peppers are the main vegetables. Chicos is steamed green corn dried on the cob. Pasole is similar to whole grain hominy (lime-treated, hulled whole kernels). Chili peppers provide a good source of vitamin

C. They are usually dried and ground into a powder. Pinto beans or calice beans are used daily. They may be reheated by frying (refried beans), or they may be cooked with beef, garlic, and chili peppers (chili con carne).

Fruits. Depending upon availability and cost, oranges, apples, bananas, and canned peaches are used.

Bread and cereals. For centuries corn has been the basic grain used as bread and cereal by the Mexican people. Masa, (dough) is made from dried corn, which has been heated, soaked in lime-water, washed, and ground wet, to form a mass of the consistency of putty. This dough is formed into thin, unleavened cakes and baked on a hot griddle to make the typical tortilla. Wheat is now replacing corn for making tortillas. Unless the wheat flour is enriched, the calcium which is a dietetically important constituent of the lime-treated corn is lost to the Mexican diet. Cornmeal gruel, or atole, is served with hot milk. Rice cooked in milk may be used as a dessert. Oatmeal, a popular breakfast cereal, is eaten by those who can afford it.

Beverage. Large amounts of coffee are used. In many families coffee is given to young children.

Seasonings. Chili pepper, onion, and garlic are used most frequently. Occasionally other herbs may be added. Lard is the basic fat.

Chinese food pattern

Traditional Chinese cooking is based on three principles: (1) the natural flavors must be enhanced, (2) the texture and color must be maintained, and (3) undesired qualities of foods must be masked or modified. Like the French, Chinese cooks feel that refrigeration lessens natural flavors. They select the freshest possible foods, hold them the shortest possible time, then cook them quickly at a high temperature in small amounts of liquid or fat. By these means natural flavor, color, and texture are preserved. Vegetables are cooked just before serving, so that they are still crisp and flavorful when eaten. The only sauce that

may be served with them is a thin, translucent one, perhaps made with cornstarch. A thick gravy is never used. To mask some flavors or textures or to enhance others, foods that have been dried, salted, pickled, spiced, candied, or canned may be added as garnishes or relishes.

Food groups

Milk. Very little milk, and limited amounts of cheese, are used.

Meat. Pork, lamb, chicken, duck, fish, and shellfish are used in many ways. Eggs and soybeans (soybean curd and milk) add to the protein content of the Chinese diet. Some characteristic dishes include egg roll, a thin dough spread with meat and vegetable filling, rolled and fried in deep fat; egg foo yung, an omelet of egg, chopped chicken, mushrooms, scallions, celery, and bean sprouts; and sweet and sour pork, pork cubes fried, then simmered in a sweet-sour sauce of brown sugar, vinegar and other seasonings. Chow mein is an American invention. It is a mixture of meat, celery, and bean sprouts served over rice or noodles and seasoned with soy sauce.

Vegetables. Cooked by the characteristic method described, vegetables such as cabbage, cucumbers, snow peas, melons, squashes, greens, mushrooms, bean sprouts, and sweet potatoes are made into many fine dishes.

Fruit. Usually fruits are eaten fresh, without addition; but pineapple and a few others are sometimes used in combination dishes.

Bread and cereals. Rice is the staple grain used at most meals.

Seasonings. Soy sauce is a basic seasoning. Almonds, ginger, and sesame seeds are also used. The most frequently used cooking fats are lard and peanut oil.

Beverage. The traditional beverage is unsweetened green tea.

Japanese food pattern

Japanese food patterns are in some ways similar to Chinese. Rice is a basic constituent of the diet, soy sauce is used for seasoning, and tea is the main beverage.

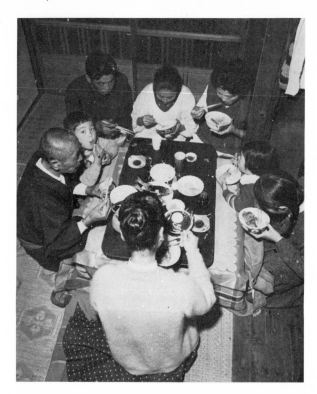

Fig. 13-3. Japanese family at dinner. The evening meal consists of rice, vegetables, pickles, and seafood. Sometimes chicken is prepared. The favorite dish is sashimi, pieces of raw fish dipped in soy sauce. (WHO photograph by T. Takahara.)

However, there are some characteristic differences. The Japanese diet contains more seafood, especially raw fish. A number of taboos prohibit certain food combinations, or the use of certain foods in specific localities or a specific times. Some of these taboos are associated with religious practices such as ancestor veneration.

Food groups

Milk. Little milk or cheese is used. Some evaporated or dried milk may be added in cooking or given to babies.

Meat. On these islands, where no city is far from the ocean, the main animal protein source is seafood. Many varieties of fish and shellfish are served such as raw squid or octopus. Other unusual saltwater fare are eels, abalone, globefish (puffer fish); more familiar to the Westerner are crab, shrimp, mackerel, carp, and salmon.

Families living inland, especially, may also eat rabbit, chicken, and occasionally beef or lamb. Eggs are a source of additional protein.

Vegetables. Japanese menus include many vegetables, usually steamed and served with soy sauce. Pickled vegetables are also well liked.

Fruit. Fresh fruit is eaten in season. A tray of fruit is a regular course of the main meal.

Bread and cereals. While rice is the staple grain, some corn, barley, and oats are served, and white wheat bread is coming into increasing use in Japanese cities.

Meal sequence

A specific sequence of courses is followed at most meals. A dinner is served in this order: green tea, unsweetened; some appetizer such as soy or red bean cake, a raw fish (sashimi) or radish relish (komono); broiled fish or omelet; vegetables with soy sauce; plain steamed rice; herb relish; fruits in season; a broth base soup (shirumise), and perhaps more unsweetened green tea. Typical dishes include tempura (batter fried shrimp) and aborakge (fried soybean curd). Sukiyaki is as American as chow mein. It is a mixture of sautéed beef and vegetables served with soy sauce. Soybean oil is the main cooking fat.

References
Specific

1. Warner, W. L., and Lunt, P. S.: The social life of a modern community, New Haven, Conn., 1941, Yale University Press.
2. Hollingshead, A. B., and Redlich, F. C.: Social class and mental illness, New York, 1958, John Wiley and Son.
3. Ruesch, J. and Batesen, G.: Communication, New York, 1951, W. W. Norton & Company, Inc. pp. 94-134.
4. Maslow, A. H.: Motivation and personality, New York, 1954, Harper & Bros. (See also Maslow's Toward a psychology of being, Princeton, 1962, D. Van Nostrand Co.
5. Buchler, J.: Nature and judgment, New York, 1955, Columbia University Press.
6. Allport, G. W.: Perception and public health. In Katz, A. H., and Felton, J. S., editors: Health and the community, New York, 1965, The Free Press.

General

Adams, R. N.: Nutrition, anthropology, and the study of man, Nutr. Rev. 17:97, 1959.
Adolph, W. H.: Nutrition in the Near East, J. Amer. Diet. Ass. 30:753, 1954.
Babcock, C. G.: Food and its emotional significance, J. Amer. Diet. Ass. 24:390, 1948.
Bennet, J. W., Smith, H. L., and Passin, H.: Food and cultures in Southern Illinois—a preliminary report, Amer. Soc. Rev. 7:645, 1942.
Boni, A.: The talisman Italian cook book (translated and augmented by Matilde Pei), New York, 1955, Crown Publishers.
Brözek, J.: Nutrition and psyche, with special reference to experimental psychodietetics, Amer. J. Clin. Nutr. 3:101, 1955.
Burgess, A.: Nutrition and food habits, Int. J. of Health Education 4:55, 1961.
Cantoni, M.: Adapting therapeutic diets to the eating patterns of Italian-Americans, Amer. J. Clin. Nutr. 6:548, 1958.
Cussler, M., and de Give, M. L.: 'Twixt the cup & lip, New York, 1952, Twayne Publishers.

Fathauer, G. H.: Food habits—an anthropologist's view, J. Amer. Diet. Ass. 37:335, 1960.
Favorite recipes from the United Nations, U. S. Committee for U.N., Washington, D.C., 1960.
Goldston, I.: Nutrition from the psychiatric viewpoint, J. Amer. Diet. Ass. 28:405, 1952.
Hacker, D. B., and Miller, E. D.: Food patterns of the Southwest, Amer. J. Clin. Nutr. 7:224, 1959.
Hee, M. W.: Ways of using milk in the Chinese Dietary, J. Amer. Diet. Ass. 30:788, 1954.
Heller, C. A.: The Diet of some Alaskan Eskimos and Indians, J. Amer. Diet. Ass. 45:425, 1964.
Hughes, H. H.: No eggs for breakfast, Amer. J. Nurs. 57:470, 1957.
Jourard, S. M.: How well do you know your patients?, Amer. J. Nurs. 59:1568, 1959.
Judd, J. E.: Century-old dietary taboos in the 20th century Japan, J. Amer. Diet. Ass. 33:489, 1957.
Kaufman, M.: Adapting therapeutic diets to Jewish food customs, Amer. J. Clin. Nutr. 5:676, 1957.
Knutson, A.: Human behavior factors in program planning, Pub. Health Reports 70:1129, 1955.
Korff, S. I.: The Jewish dietary code, Food Technology 20:76, 1966.
Lee, D.: Cultural factors in dietary choice, Amer. J. Clin. Nutr. 5:166, 1957.
Loeb, M. B.: Aboriginal influences in Southern diet, Pub.. Health Reports 70:920, 1955.
Loeb, M. B.: The social functions of food habits, J. Amer. Acad. Appl. Nutr. 4:1, 1951.
Longman, D. P.: Working with Pueblo Indians in New Mexico, J. Amer. Diet. Ass. 47:470, 1965.
Macgregor, F. C.: Uncooperative patients, some cultural interpretations, Amer. J. Nurs. 67:88, 1967.
Manning, Mary Louise, The psychodynamics of dietetics, Nursing Outlook 13:57, 1965.
Mayer, J.: The nutritional status of American Negroes, Nutr. Rev. 23:161, 1965.
McCabe, G. S.: Cultural Influences on Patient Behavior, Amer. J. Nurs. 60:1101, 1960.
Mead, M. and Wolfenstein, M., editors: Childhood in contemporary cultures, ed. 1, Chicago, 1955, University of Chicago Press.
Mead, M.: Cultural patterning of nutritionally relevant behavior, J. Amer. Diet. Ass. 25:677, 1949.
Mead, M.: Dietary patterns and food habits, J. Am. Diet. Ass. 19:1, 1943.
Mead, M.: Understanding cultural patterns, Nurs-Outlook 4:260, 1956.
Mitchell, H. S., and Jaffe, N. F.: Food patterns of some European countries: background for study programs and guidance of relief workers, J. Amer. Diet. Ass. 20:676, 1944.
Montagu, M. F. A.: Nature, nurture, and nutrition, Amer. J. Clin. Nutr. 5:237, 1957.
Murdock, G. P.: Anthropology and its contributions to public health, Amer. J. Public Health 42:7, 1952.
Phillips, M. G., and Dunn, M. M.: Toward better

understanding of other lands and other people: their folkways and foods, Nurs. Outlook 9:498, 1961.

Pumpian-Mindlin, E.: The meanings of food, J. Amer. Diet. Ass. 30:576, 1954.

Queen, G. S.: Culture, economics, and food habits, J. Amer. Diet. Ass. 33:1044, 1957.

Roberts, L. J.: A basic food pattern for Puerto Rico, J. Amer. Diet. Ass. 30:1097, 1954.

Saunders, L.: Cultural differences and medical care: the case of the Spanish-speaking people of the Southwest, New York, 1954, Russell Sage Foundation.

Simoans, F. J.: The geographic approach to food prejudices, Food Tech. 20:42, 1966.

Torres, R. M.: Dietary patterns of Puerto Rican people, Amer. J. Clin. Nutr. 7:349, 1959.

Valassi, K. V.: Food habits of Greek Americans, Amer. J. Clin. Nutr. 11:240, 1962.

Wellin, E.: Cultural factors in nutrition, Nutr. Rev. 13:129, 1955.

CHAPTER 14

Nutritional education

In the previous chapter the question of why people eat what they eat was explored. This question is fundamental to understanding people's food habits. Cultural, social, and psychological factors shape the patterns of attitudes, beliefs, and values that govern food habits of groups and individuals.

The second question fundamental to success as effective health professionals is, *how can insights contributed by the behavioral sciences be used to improve family and community nutrition?* What principles must guide health education work with individuals, families, and communities? How can these principles be applied in practical ways, so that people can be reached and helped to meet their health needs through improved food habits? What methods, approaches, and materials may be most effective?

In the search for answers, there are four aspects of nutrition education and applied community nutrition that should be considered: (1) the relationship of cultural forces to changes in food habits, (2) the teaching-learning process, (3) health teaching in nursing, and (4) community nutrition education. Throughout all of these ramifications of the problem, one underlying concept is essential. The health workers themselves must become imbued with a concept of *change* if their efforts are to succeed. Life—always a dynamic process—and learning—which is manifested in terms of changed behavior—are in essence based upon the principle of change. Biologically and educationally, to be static is to be dead. To be alive is to be willing to change. The

more eager people are to change in ways that lead to improvement for themselves and others, the more they are alive.

CULTURAL FORCES AND FOOD HABIT CHANGE

Many examples could be cited to demonstrate the power of social and cultural forces in determining food behavior. Three studies clearly illustrate the far-reaching implications of these forces in efforts to reach people needing health care. Two of these studies were in other cultures; one was made in an American community. Experiences of workers in a health center serving a Zulu community in the Union of South Africa, and those of workers in a child welfare clinic in West Bengal, India, reveal the strong and intimate relationships that exist between cultural forces and health practices; hence the necessity for health personnel to know and understand those forces. Kurt Lewin's classic wartime study of food habits in a midwestern U. S. community defined the social and economic forces that channel food from source to consumer, and identified the various "gatekeepers" who control those channels.

A health program among South African Zulus

Dr. John Cassel's[1] study of health habits in a community of Zulu tribesmen in southwestern Natal, South Africa, underscored two principles important to health education. (1) The more central and strongly integrated segments of a culture, especially those closely related to moral codes governing interpersonal conduct, resist change. Other segments, made up of persons who are less deeply concerned with such codes, are more open to change. (2) The health team that works *in*—not apart from—the community, and that integrates health education and disease prevention activities with curative aspects of health practice can produce desirable changes in the beliefs of persons, and can alter their habits in ways that will improve health and general living standards.

In 1940, when the Polela Health Centre organized its first multidiscipline teams, each consisting of a family physician, a family nurse, and a health educator, health conditions in the African community described in this report were extremely poor. Infant and crude mortality rates were high. Eighty percent of the people bore marks of malnutrition, and epidemics were common. After only ten years of operation, the health program's results were evident. The infant mortality rate had been greatly reduced by the improved nutritional state of the babies, the incidence of such malnutrition diseases as pellagra and kwashiorkor had fallen from twelve or more cases a week to fewer than twelve a year, and epidemics of infectious diseases were better controlled.

Re-education for better nutrition. Since severe malnutrition was the major health problem, the Health Centre based its program on re-education for better nutrition. The first step was a detailed survey of existing dietary habits, an analysis of factors behind these habits, and a study of current attitudes and beliefs about food. The team learned that the tribe subsisted on a monotonous diet which was composed principally of maize (corn), with some dried beans, little or no milk, occasional potatoes or pumpkins in season, and large quantities of beer brewed from millet (sorghum). Factors that contributed to malnutrition were eroded soil, extreme poverty (money was earned by migrant labor in distant cities), traditional ideas about foods, ignorance of food values and of the body's needs for food, inefficient use of available

resources, and cooking methods that destroyed much of the nutritional value of the product.

After analysis had led the team to a clear understanding of the community's needs, the workers approached the problem of changing the ingrained food habits of the people. They began with activities aimed at creating awareness of needs and increasing interest in possible dietary changes. Informal group discussions in the Zulu language were held in key homes. Other homes throughout the community were visited periodically. Subjects discussed were food values, ideas about digestion, fetal nutrition, how the body is nourished, comparison of the people's poor diet with the better diet of their ancestors, and available but unused food resources. The members of the community agreed upon three changes: (1) the addition of vegetables, to be grown in home gardens, (2) the addition of eggs, by overcoming negative but not strongly entrenched economic and cultural notions concerning the bad effects of this food, and (3) the addition of milk from the tribe's prized herds of cattle.

General results of the program. Under the impetus of continued group discussions, demonstrations, and instructions, the first two of these aims were accomplished with little difficulty. To induce these people to take milk in any form, including curd or cheese, proved to be a far more complex problem. According to their ancient and deep-seated religious belief, the link between a man and his ancestors was his cattle. The members of the tribe strove to maintain their cattle at all costs, even though the size of the herd exceeded food and pasture resuorces. Only by doing so could a man retain the good will of his ancestors; and only his ancestors' beneficence could ward off misfortune, ill health, and harm. Cattle were also prized as an index of wealth and as payment of the bride price necessary to obtain a wife and to seal the marriage contract. Only the kin group of the male head of a household could use milk from his cattle. Since a menstruating or pregnant woman had power to bewitch the cattle, milk was excluded from the diet of all girls past puberty. A double prohibition fell upon a married woman. She was a woman, and she lived in her husband's family as a "foreigner" to his kin group, to his ancestors, and hence to his cattle and their milk. This was, of course, particularly unfortunate for the married woman during her childbearing years, when nutritional demands are especially pronounced.

It was soon evident that factual knowledge about the nutritional value of milk, especially for pregnant and lactating mothers who were a major health concern, could not change so deep a system of cultural and religious beliefs. Another way had to be found. The need was met, ingeniously, by the introduction of powdered milk! This, the people readily accepted, calling it "meal" or "powder," and consuming it in large quantities.

Numerous social and economic problems remained to be solved at longer range. Methods of agriculture and stock-raising needed to be improved, and there were other difficulties beyond the scope of the health program. But the inclusion in the diet of more vegetables, eggs, and milk was a beginning, and its value was reflected in improved maternal and child health.

This experience serves to emphasize that health conditions in a community do not exist in isolation. They are bound up in a network of economic, political, ecologic, and cultural factors and must be approached in such a context.

A health program among West Bengal Indians

In 1947, the province of Bengal, which had been developed in northeast India while that country was under British rule, was divided between India and East Pakistan. West Bengal, whose population was largely Hindu, became a part of India; East Bengal, largely Moslem, was absorbed into the newly-created, divided country of Pakistan. The personal experience of Dr.

D. B. Jelliffe,[2] in a rural welfare clinic in West Bengal, reinforces the need to know the cultural pattern of a community in relation to foods and illness, and to work within this cultural pattern to find effective ways of meeting health needs. In describing his experience, Dr. Jelliffe emphasized three important principles of health education. (1) People will accept new knowledge about health and nutrition only to the extent that the new information can be amalgamated into existing patterns of custom and belief. (2) Cross-cultural exchanges are mutually beneficial. People of less highly industrialized cultures can learn from health workers, but the workers also can learn much from other cultures that will enrich their own. (3) Interest in individuals of other cultures and appreciation of the personal and social functions they perform build rapport between health workers and the families they seek to serve. Unless rapport exists between these two groups of persons, all efforts to educate are wasted.

Cultural influences. Most of the women who brought their children to the West Bengal clinic were illiterate villagers of a low socioeconomic class. They practiced the Hindu religion. The Hindu is taught that foods are to be classified in two ways. First, there is the all-important distinction between *amish* (vegetarian) and *niramish* (nonvegetarian) nutrients. Second, these mothers followed closely the ancient Indian classification of foods as *garam* (hot) and *thanda* (cold). The classification into garam and thanda is based upon properties, believed to be inherent in certain foods, which enable them to exert specific influences upon the body. Combinations of garam and thanda foods are believed to be especially harmful. Traditional Hindu medicine classifies illnesses also into those that are garam and thanda, and restricts the patient's diet accordingly. During a garam illness, one may not eat garam food, because to do so would intensify the disease; during a thanda sickness, the patient must eat no thanda food. Eggs, meat, milk, honey, and sugar are garam foods; lemon, orange, rice, water, acid buttermilk, and curd (yogurt) are thanda foods.

The health workers of Dr. Jelliffe's group had to use ingenuity in order to integrate their treatment into this system of beliefs. In treating an upper respiratory infection, the physician might want the child to increase his fluid intake and to receive ascorbic acid in the form of water and orange juice, and he might want to prescribe rice as an easily digested source of energy. But that diet would be unacceptable to the mother, because both this illness and these foods are regarded as thanda. Knowing this, the physician advised that she put a little honey in the water and juice, and that she cook the rice in milk. Since honey and milk are garam, they will neutralize the thanda of the other foods. This, the mother readily accepted, and so the health needs of the child were met.

A similar difficulty arose in prescribing for children recovering from diarrhea. Even when the child could tolerate milk, the mother did not want to give it, because both milk and diarrhea are classified as garam. Some of the Hindus avoided milk so persistently that they incurred kwashiorkor or another protein deficiency disease. Aware of these traditions, the physician would prescribe a low-residue rice gruel, and a pectin-containing apple sherbet—both thanda foods. Dilute acid buttermilk, a thanda food, was also a good choice, on two accounts. Medically, it was well tolerated and contained needed protein, and culturally, it was acceptable.

Principles of approach. Throughout this effort, the health workers in the West Bengal clinic made use of a threefold approach. (1) They made an intensive study of the cultural practices related to health. (2) They carried out an *unprejudiced* analysis of these practices, in the light of the scientific principles upon which modern western medical care is based, and in consideration of local conditions. (3) They encouraged those traditional practices that were beneficial, did not interfere with those that were harmless, and sought to overcome the harmful practices by means of persuasion and demonstration. Where it was medically important to introduce a treatment that was unacceptable on cultural grounds, they devised ways of neutralizing it, or of presenting the essential aspect of the treatment in a culturally acceptable form.

Food behavior among Midwestern United States housewives

A widely known study of food habits in America was conducted by a field staff at the Child Welfare Research Station of the State University of Iowa in 1942 under the direction of Dr. Kurt Lewin.[3] This study has given important insights into the forces that influence food habits in America and has provided a basis for the development of more effective methods of changing those habits. Combining the approaches of cultural anthropology and the quantitative methods of psychology, Dr. Lewin studied five population groups: Caucasian Americans of three income levels and two subcultural groups, Czech and Negro. He interviewed housewives to determine factors behind family food behavior. To evaluate the efficacy of methods that might be used in attempts to change food habits, he compared the responses to lectures and to group discussions.

His results led him to two conclusions. (1) Food reaches the family table from its point of origin through a series of channels. These channels are controlled at various points by "gatekeepers." The flow of food through these channels depends upon the ideas about food and the values of these "gatekeepers." (2) Changes in food habits come about more readily as a result of group discussion and decision than in response to lecture and request. It will be worthwhile to look more closely into Dr. Lewin's findings.

Channel theory

Food channels. From production point to consumer, food moves through a series of channels. A channel is a single step in the complex process of food delivery. It may refer to as simple a step as delivery of a head of lettuce from the kitchen garden to the family table. It may refer to home canning or home cooking. The channel may also be one of the many routes through which a food may be bought—a market, a wayside stand, a home delivery service. Again, a channel may be the preparation of food for sale by baking, by freezing, or by cooking and serving in a restaurant. It may be the holding of quantities of food at storage points (refrigeration plants, freezers, warehouses).

Gatekeepers. Each of these channels is governed by a "gatekeeper," who, in turn, is controlled both by psychological and cultural forces and nonpsychological forces.

Psychologic and cultural forces. Each gatekeeper—farmer, wholesale food dealer, storekeeper, housewife, or other person who controls one of the channels through which food is delivered from field to table—is more or less consciously influenced by tradition, childhood memories related to specific foods, taste preference, religious or other taboos, and beliefs or knowledge about the value or danger of specific items. Some of these psychological forces operate through the culture as a whole (such as having turkey at Thanksgiving). Others are individual matters (Mrs. Black does not like olives). Important among psychological forces are resistance (Mr. Blue refuses to eat sweets because his physician has warned him against them) and conflict. (Miss Green wonders whether to serve filet mignon when her boss comes to dinner—will he think she should show her appreciation by this special treat; or will he decide that, if she can afford this, she does not need another raise?)

Nonpsychologic forces. The gatekeepers of the food channels are also responsive to such objective pressures as the ability to raise certain foods in certain soils or under certain weather conditions, available means of transportation, the chance to buy a certain food (as a restaurant features fruits in season, a baker runs a "special" of fresh blueberry pie, or a butcher advertises a bargain in spring lamb), and available money (Miss Green counts her dimes, and decides to do miracles with beef à la stroganof; a year later, married to the chief junior executive, she serves the filet with truffles).

The main gatekeeper. Ultimately, the most significant gatekeeper in the food channel system is the individual housewife—the mother in the home. It is she who determines what food is served and in what condition it is delivered to the plate. It is she who selects, from among the many reasons that are presented to her for choosing this or that item, the set of reasons that, for her, are decisive. *The personal values of the main gatekeeper* are, in the last analysis, the key to the food habits of a family (Fig. 14-1).

The wife and mother determines *what is food.* She decides what is food for her particular family. Within this category, she decides what is food for her husband, and what is food for her children. She determines what is food for breakfast, food for lunch at home, food for lunch at school, food for family dinner on week nights, food for Sunday dinner, and food for guests, for summer, for winter, for the sick child, and for the growing boy and girl. Within her food system, a specific item (meat, milk, potato, salad, bread, egg, pie) plays various roles in relation to various family members, and in accordance with the meal pattern. If a conflict arises between the amount of money at her disposal and the meanings that foods have for her, the housewife's decisions may vary according to her response to the pressure that she considers most important.

Methods of changing food habits. Many methods have been used, and are being used, to bring about desired changes in the food habits of the American people. The approaches range from individual depth therapy, as with a disturbed child, to propaganda campaigns carried on through the mass media—radio, television, newspapers, magazines, billboards, and other advertising devices. Dr. Lewin was interested in de-

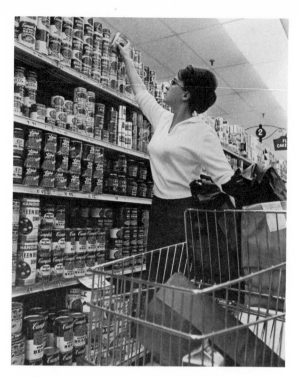

Fig. 14-1. The main gatekeeper of the family's food—the mother in the home. Her values govern her selections, and her choices determine what items come to the family table and influence the building of food habits.

tecting the most effective means by which health workers could reach and persuade people to improve their nutritional patterns. He therefore focused on the approaches that would retain the impact of personal, face-to-face meeting, while conserving the time of the health worker. These techniques were midway between individual instruction and mass methods and involved two types of group meeting—lecture-request and discussion-decision.

To test the relative effectiveness of these two group methods in bringing about a change in food habit, it was decided to attempt the introduction of a rather widely rejected type of food: organ meats, such as kidneys, heart, brains. A pair of groups were selected as the target from each of the three broad socioeconomic classes, low, middle, high. One group of each pair was approached by the lecture-request method; the other group was approached by the discussion-decision method.

Lecture-request groups. In attempting to induce the desired food habit change in the lecture-request groups, the nutritionist sought to establish motive by pointing out the relationships between nutrition and general health, and by emphasizing high food values and economic advantages in these particular meats. By detailed explanations, using charts and other devices, she told of various ways of cooking the organ meats in order to overcome aversions to odor, texture, appearance, and flavor. She concluded by handing out recipes, and requesting the group members to try them during the week.

Discussion-decision groups. In trying to persuade the members of the discussion-decision groups from each socioeconomic level, the group leader opened each meeting with a brief introductory statement. She acknowledged the difficulties involved in changing food habits, and frankly said that she hoped to gain the group's cooperation.

Table 14-1. Change of food habits in members of groups according to method used and economic level of participants*

Socioeconomic level	Group decision				Lecture			
	Low	Middle	High	Total	Low	Middle	High	Total
Number of participants	17	16	13	44	13	15	13	41
Percent of persons serving one or more of the three meats	35	69	54	52	15	13	0	10
Percent of persons serving a meat they had *hardly* ever served before	20	53	54	44	0	8	0	3
Percent of persons serving a meat they had *never* served before	13	36	50	32	0	8	0	3
Total percent of persons serving one or more of the new meats who had never used any of the three meats prior to the experiment				29†				0‡

*Lewin, K.: Forces behind food habits and methods of change. In National Academy of Sciences, National Research Council: The problem of changing food habits, Washington, D. C., 1943.
†Out of a total number of 14 participants who had never before used any of the meats.
‡Out of a total number of 11 participants who had never before used any of the meats.

The nutritionist then withdrew from the discussion, and the members of the group took it up. Step by step, they identified the problem more completely until they as a group acknowledged that it was necessary to do something about it. This led to exploration of the reasons for rejection of these particular foods. The question was then stated by the members of the group: "How can we overcome these objections?"

At this point, the group turned to the nutritionist and asked for her expert help. She now gave the same information that she had given to the lecture-request groups, but in a different manner and in a much more condensed form, and she distributed recipes. The group decided by vote to try the meats during the following week.

Results. A comparison of the results shown in Table 14-1 clearly indicates the greater effectiveness of the discussion-decision method. Perhaps the most telling contrast is that between the responses of those group members who had never before tried any of these foods. Twenty-nine percent of such participants in the discus-

sion groups used one or more of the meats in family meals for the first time after the experience described; *not one member of the lecture audience tried the meats for the first time.*

Principles for successful nutritional education

Such studies and field work, both in other cultures and in America, teach important principles with which health workers can improve their work in nutrition and in health education in general.

Knowledge of people. Health workers need to have an intimate knowledge of the people's beliefs, attitudes, values, behavior, and extent of knowledge before they attempt to introduce changes or new practices. Habits are never developed in a vacuum. All people, in every culture, have *some* knowledge of nutrition. If the health worker assumes that they know nothing, simply because their concepts differ from his, he shall only arouse their resistance to the information that he has to convey.

Understanding reasons for habits. All beliefs and practices, no matter how strange they may appear, serve psychological and social functions. If health workers hope to communicate effectively with others, they will find their path remarkably smoothed, and their results strikingly better, if they analyze the habits that people have. The habits should be evaluated objectively, and the overall pattern or system into which the customs and beliefs fit should be determined.

Identification of any customs that need to be changed. Many practices, even though they may differ from the health worker's, are beneficial and should be encouraged. Some may be harmless and need not be disturbed. Others are harmful. To overcome the harmful ones successfully, a sympathetic approach is necessary. Techniques of persuasion will have to be developed, and points must be proved by demonstration. It is useful to integrate good nutritional practices with existing habits, wherever ways can be found to do it.

Meeting individual needs. A flexible attitude that is sensitive to the needs of individuals in specific situations at specific times allows health workers to be effective. They cannot be effective if they are bound by rigid ideas. Changes cannot be brought about in others, if the health workers cling blindly to a few methods and materials that were learned at a specific time, in a specific set of circumstances, as though they were universal laws. Health workers can most successfully free others if they themselves are free to adjust, adapt, and tailor. There is always more than one way to do something; health workers should work with open systems.

Self knowledge. It is an exciting adventure for a person to study the degree to which he is culture-bound. Each person has, perhaps without realizing it, a culturally determined system of values. Success is unlikely for the person who unconsciously attempts to impose his system on the behavior of others. It's quite possible that genuine introspection on the part of health workers may lead to some major reorientation in certain areas of their own philosophy.

Involvement of key people. The leadership patterns in the community should be studied. Ways to enlist the cooperation and guidance of key individuals and families should be sought.

Main gatekeeper of the food channels. The wife and mother in the home is the main gatekeeper who ultimately determines the food habits of her family. Wives and mothers, by virtue of their feeling of responsibility for the health of the family, are probably the most open and educable members of population groups. It is also most important from the health worker's point of view that these women be reached, since they are the persons who are mainly responsible for the nutrition of children, and for the development of the food habits of persons as they grow from infancy to adulthood.

Involvement of people. Group discussions, by creating awareness of needs, help to motivate persons to action. Group decisions, because they reflect the finding of solutions by the persons themselves, usually represent a sense of identification with that solution. This sense of identification is most helpful in producing long-term results.

Communication skills. Too often people are unaware that they are speaking in a way that their hearers either misunderstand or fail to understand. Those trying to teach are then puzzled at their listeners' lack of response or at their misinterpretation. Health workers are almost sure to make this kind of error if they are not sensitive to the hearer's frame of reference and to the associated ideas that arise out of his background. The health worker needs to seek a common meeting ground, to perceive the situation as his hearer sees it, to think in the hearer's idioms, and to understand the meanings that words and actions have for the hearers. Sometimes health workers have had little or no training in educational principles or techniques. Lacking the awareness that is developed by such training, they are prone to suppose that the methods by which they were taught—lectures and demonstrations—will suffice for others. Perhaps they need to forget the textbook practices in order to look honestly and sympathetically at the situation before them.

Evaluation of results. At the end of an episode in which the health worker has tried to effect a change in the behavior of others, it is often useful simply to ask, what happened, was the teaching realistic, was it necessary, did it work and did it meet the need. Questions such as these help the health worker to appraise immediate results and to anticipate long-range effects. They may well be necessary to maintain perspective and direction.

THE TEACHING-LEARNING PROCESS

Definition of learning. Learning means *change.* There is a vast difference between a person who has *learned,* and a person who has only *been informed.* Learning must ultimately be measured in terms of changed behavior. To be valid, education must focus not on the teacher, or on the content, but on the *learner.* The teacher's primary responsibility is not to teach facts, but to educate persons. His major task is to create situations in which the person can learn, can succeed, and can develop self-direction and self-motivation.

Aspects of human personality involved in learning

The teaching-learning process involves three fundamental aspects of human personality—cognition, emotion, and will.

Cognition. Cognition is the thought process itself, by which information is grasped. Cognitions shape, and are shaped by, the terms in which the mind thinks about a given body of facts. The thought process usually starts with a diffuse sensation. This is followed by a more focused perception that leads to the construction of a concept, and to identification of specific principles involved. The total process of cognition provides the background knowledge that is the basis for reasoning and analysis. The learner senses the contribution of cognition to the learning process as, "I know how to do it".

Emotion. In each individual, specific feelings and responses are associated with given items of knowledge and with given situations. These emotions reflect the desires raised and the needs aroused. Emotions provide impetus. They create the tensions that spur a person to act. When he feels unfulfillment, lack, or need, he wants to do something about it. If the teacher understands the learner's emotions, he can direct this impetus in ways that will forward the learning process. The learner senses the contribution of emotion to the learning process as, "I want to do it."

Will. The will to act arises from the conviction that the knowledge discovered can fill the felt need and relieve the sense of tension. The will focuses our determination to act upon the knowledge received, to change an attitude, a value, a thought, a pattern of behavior. The learner senses the contribution of the will to the learning process as, "I will do it."

Principles of learning

Basic principles of learning, focused upon the learner, are individuality, contact, listening, participation, need fulfillment, and appraisal.

Individuality. Learning can only be individual. Each person, in the final analysis, must learn for himself, according to his need, in his way, in his time, and for his purpose. In order to teach, the teacher must discover who the learner is. To do this the teacher must ask questions that make clear the relationship of the learner to the problem under consideration.

Contact. Learning starts from a point of contact between prior experience and knowledge, an overlap of the new with the familiar. In order to teach a person, the teacher must know what the individual already knows, and to what past experience the present situation can be related. The process of learning must start at that point. It is the teacher, not the learner, who must find and identify this point of contact. A teacher is very likely to fail to reach and teach the individual if it is merely *assumed* that the learner is at a given point of experience and knowledge. The teacher must search for the areas of association that are present in the individual, until he is sure that he knows them. He must then relate his teaching to that point of contact.

Listening. Because learning is individual, and because it is a process which must move from a point of contact which reflects the learner's present knowledge to a desired outcome, it must involve listening—the *teacher's* listening! (Certainly, the learner must listen also; but teaching him to listen is part of the teacher's task.) The most mature teacher is the most expert listener. The listening of a fine teacher is the kind of client-centered activity that Carl Rogers[5] has called creative listening. Listening should be a skilled effort to understand a person and his situation from *his* perspective. Such listening is by no means passive. It is active concentration, an alert attempt to view the situation as the patient is experiencing it. The active listener is sensitive not merely to the words that the learner is speaking but also to the *meaning* that the learner is consciously and unconsciously communicating. There is much subsurface significance to communication. It is conveyed in tone, gesture, posture of the whole body and each of its parts, the context in which words are used, and even silences. Indeed, these aspects of the communication are often the most significant.

Participation. Since learning is an active process through which behavior changes, the learner must become involved. He must participate actively. One means of securing participation is through *planned feedback.* Feedback may take several forms. One method is to ask questions that require more than a yes or no answer. The question should elicit statements that will reveal the learner's degree of understanding and motivation. Another feedback method is to use return demonstrations by the learner under the guidance of the teacher. These usually take the form of brief periods in which procedures are practiced or skills discussed. Such guided practice develops ability, self-confidence, and security, and enables the learner to clarify his grasp of the principles involved. The third feedback method is for the learner to try the new learning outside the teacher-directed situation in the circumstances of his own life. Such trials are alternated with return visits in which the learner reviews his experiences with the teacher; the teacher answers, or helps him to answer, the questions raised and provides continued support and reinforcement.

Need fulfillment. People learn only that which they feel will be useful to them. They retain only that which they believe they need or shall need. The more immediately a person can put it to use, the more readily he grasps it. The more it satisfies his immediate goals, the more effective the learning will be. Only the intelligent and the mature put forth the effort to learn for long-term goals.

Appraisal. If the teacher accepts the premise that learning means changed behavior, he must appraise the learner's progress toward the determined goal. He must at appropriate intervals, take stock of the changes that the learner has made in outlook, attitude, and action toward the specific goal in health education. What is the learner *doing?* Careful, sympathetic questioning may reveal his blocks to learning. These may be cognitive (misunderstandings that are hindering his progress), or they may be emotional (points of negative feelings). They may also be volitional. The learner may understand (more or less) what is to be done, and emotionally he may think that it would be a fine idea to do it; but he may lack the firm will to achieve.

In addition to speeding the learning process, such person-centered concern will reveal to the health worker his own degree of progress as a teacher. It will show him whether he is communicating successfully, making contact, and making the best choices of method. It will recall to him principles that he may have glossed over. It may reveal to him significant clues to the learner's behavior, which he may have missed entirely. In the final analysis, the measure of success in teaching lies not in the number of facts transferred, but in the *change for the better that has been initiated in persons.*

HEALTH TEACHING IN NURSING

From the preceding consideration of how learning takes place, it is abundantly clear that if health teaching is to be valid, it must be patient-centered. Health teachers must focus upon the *learner*. To translate this principle into action, the role of the nurse in teaching patients about nutrition should be considered.

Definitions

First, what does not constitute nutrition teaching—or, indeed, any health teaching—should be considered. The term "health teaching" is often misused grammatically and mechanically: "Go down to Mrs. Smith's room before she leaves and health teach her about her diet." Or, "Has anyone given Mr. Jones some health teaching for his ulcer?" This attitude toward health teaching is analogous to applying a dressing with no knowledge of what might be festering beneath the surface, or administering a drug with no knowledge of what reaction might occur.

Learning is the *continuing* process of interaction between a person and his environment which leads him to *changed behavior*. Along the way, at certain points of individual and group need, this interaction is aided by helping vehicles—persons equipped by knowledge, skill, and personality to provide tools and direction according to need. These persons are called *teachers*. It is the function and the responsibility of the teacher to challenge and help motivate, to provide an atmosphere conducive to learning, to create specific learning situations, and to help provide resources as indicated. All this is done with one objective—that the learner may learn *for himself*. In the health field, the nurse is such a helping vehicle.

To help keep this larger view in mind perhaps the broader term *health education* is better than the term health teaching. Health education implies the over-all teaching-learning concept of the educative process.

Health education may be defined as the involvement of persons in their own health care and the creation of a general climate and specific situations in which persons may participate in decisions and activities concerning their health. Valid health education is based on the accurate statement of related facts which have been demonstrated scientifically, and upon the application of these facts to the protection, maintenance, and improvement of health by the patient himself, or by those responsible for his well-being.

The nurse-teacher

Health education cannot be separated from the total nursing function. It is caring and sharing. The key word that characterizes an alert and sensitive nurse-teacher is *awareness*.

1. The nurse is aware of the patient's uniqueness. She is sensitive to his culture, his social, personal needs, and physical needs.
2. She is aware of the dynamic nature of knowledge. She has a sound basis of scientific background principles, but is always flexible and open to current concepts.
3. The nurse has self-awareness. She understands that her feelings influence her ability to perceive the needs of others. She also knows the healing value of genuine care and concern for other persons.
4. She is aware of the specific skills necessary for communication and relating to others. She has identified and learned these skills, and she continues to improve them throughout her professional life. These skills include listening, perceiving, verbalizing, clarifying, analyzing, encouraging, enlarging, supporting, and sharing information.

Each of these characteristics of the sensitive nurse-teacher stems from an underlying awareness that every human being needs recognition, a sense of self-worth, and a feeling that he belongs. He needs assurance that he is making progress, and confidence that he can succeed. She tries to foster and nurture the fulfillment of these needs.

The content of health teaching

Because the nurse-teacher is not merely purveying information, but is educating persons, she derives the content of health teaching from the two sources of the specific need of persons and scientific knowledge. The specific needs of persons may arise from illness (care of a patient with a particular disease), preventing illness (positive health care), or daily living problems (concerns about physical needs and human relationships). She also needs an organized body of scientific knowledge relative to these needs of persons. These scientific principles are learned from the biological sciences, the social sciences, and the hu-

manities. They are the tools of the educated, caring nurse or nutritionist.

Basic nutrition concepts. An example of a simple statement of basic concepts for use in health education is the outline of Basic Nutrition Concepts developed by the Interagency Committee on Nutrition Education (ICNE), first published in 1964 by the Agricultural Research Service, U. S. Department of Agriculture (see below). Since this statement's appearance, various nutrition agencies have used it as a basis for in-service training of public health nurses and for teaching elementary school teachers to integrate nutrition activities into social studies and health programs. It has been used in workshops with physical education and home economics teachers, health educators, and agricultural extension work-

---

TO PROBE FURTHER
Basic concepts of nutrition*

1. Nutrition is the food you eat and how the body uses it. We eat food to live, to grow, to keep healthy and well, and to get energy for work and play.
2. Food is made up of different nutrients needed for growth and health.
   a. All nutrients needed by the body are available through food.
   b. Many kinds and combinations of food can lead to a well-balanced diet.
   c. No food, by itself, has all the nutrients needed for full growth and health.
   d. Each nutrient has specific uses in the body.
   e. Most nutrients do their best work in the body when teamed with other nutrients.
3. All persons, throughout life, have need for the same nutrients, but in varying amounts.
   a. The amounts of nutrients needed are influenced by age, sex, size, activity, and the state of health.
   b. Suggestions for the kinds and amounts of food needed are made by trained scientists.
4. The way food is handled influences the amount of nutrients in food, its safety, appearance, and taste.
   a. Handling means everything that happens to food while it is being grown, processed, stored, and prepared for eating.

---

*Interagency Committee on Nutrition Education (ICNE), Agricultural Research Service, U. S. Department of Agriculture, Nutrition Program News, September-October, 1964.

ers, in conuseling individuals who require dietary modification for the control of disease, and for countless other purposes.

Mutual activity in health teaching

In dynamic, purposive health teaching, the nurse-teacher and the patient-learner share responsibility for the outcome. Each has something to give to the teaching-learning process. The nurse gives her special knowledge and skills. The patient gives his unique personal experience with the particular problem at hand. Together, nurse and patient explore the problem and consider alternative plans for solution. Ultimately, the patient must choose a plan, and must carry out the plan of his choice by appropriately modifying his health behavior.

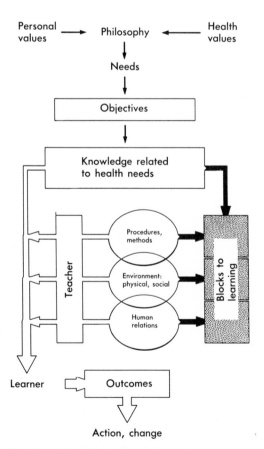

Fig. 14-2. The role of the nurse-teacher as a helping vehicle or channel in the teaching-learning process of health education.

Role of the nurse. Throughout the interview, the nurse is attempting to see the patient's world as he sees it, and to help him achieve increased insight and ability to cope with his individual situation more adequately and comfortably. The nurse acts as a helper to bridge the distance between the *health objective* (based upon the patient's needs and philosophy) and the *outcome* (the desired change in health behavior). To do this, the nurse helps the patient to understand the facts he needs to know. In so doing, she will often have to work through blocks that exist because of a variety of factors. These factors include the patient's environment (his educational level, economic resources, social conditioning, cultural habituation) and methods used by the persons around him. His wife's cooking methods, the necessity of eating lunch in a company cafeteria or bringing a lunch from home may be factors. Patients who regularly eat in a boarding school, campus dining room, boarding house, or restaurant need special consideration. There are many other human relations involved. This vital nursing function in the teaching-learning process may be visualized in Fig. 14-2.

COMMUNITY NUTRITIONAL EDUCATION
Changing concepts in community health care

The rapid changes that are occurring in population and family patterns, and in medical and allied scientific knowledge, bring with them inevitable changes in society which directly involve the teaching of nutrition to patients. These changes are reflected in shifting emphases in medical care itself. Until very recent years, stress was almost exclusively placed upon the cure or amelioration of disease by surgery and drugs. While advances in these areas continue to be made with great rapidity, there is also an increasing tendency to blend curative practices with disease-preventive, health-oriented care. Generally, a more sophisticated, affluent society knows more, has more, and asks more than a simple culture. People seek more involvement in their

own health care. As the population increases, the greater numbers of people
also demand more efficient approaches. Attempts to meet these demands have taken
many forms, including group medical practice by specialists, clustering of medical
facilities, and health insurance plans. There
has been pronounced change in the role of
the community hospital. It is rapidly emerging as the community health center of the
future. Within its environs, nutrition education is becoming recognized by professional workers and the community at large,
as an essential aspect of education for total
health.

The concept of the community health center

*The curative and preventive health sys-
tems.* Although the concept of the community health center as a focus for the coordination of curative and preventive health
care is not fully formed, it is developing as
a result of social pressures and correlated
trends in American medicine. Increasingly,
leaders in medicine and hospital administration voice these changes in direction.[4]
Project studies and pilot programs are in-

dicating the needs, and as a result the gap
between the curative and preventive health
systems is closing. These reports indicate
that the curative system (largely the professional practitioners and the hospitals) is
doing more work in home care programs,
in coordinated activities with chronic disease hospitals and nursing homes, in health
care financing, and in area-wide hospital
planning. The preventive system (largely
public health departments and other government agencies and programs) is organiz-
ing its services for the delivery of general
health care, care of the chronically ill, rehabilitation work and overall community
health planning (especially centered in
families of high-risk, low-income population groups), and in broad community
health screening programs.

Coordination of the two health systems.
The great need felt by leaders in the health
care field is for increased functional coordination between these two systems. In
some situations, this coordination may be
a blending of the community hospital and
the local health department, and it may
include parts of the local welfare agency.
In other situations, services of the two sys-

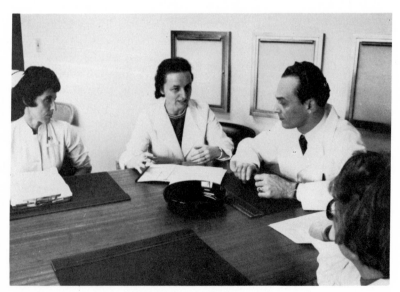

Fig. 14-3. The health team conference. The physician, nurse, nutritionist, and social worker
explore patient needs and coordinate plans for family-centered health care and education.

tems could be coordinated in activities such as home care programs, outpatient clinic services, and broad public community education programs. Such coordination would prevent much costly and inefficient overlapping and fragmentation, such as now exist in many communities. Fresh vision in planning and in program development would give needed vitality and human dignity to pressing community health needs.

Community health education center

Among the new community health centers being developed in this country is the health education center, now in the pilot phase, formed by a group of physicians in Oakland, California, the Permanente Medical Group, in conjunction with their affiliated community health facilities, the Kaiser Foundation Health Plan and Hospitals. A directing staff that serves as a model health team (physician, nurse, nutritionist and health educator) coordinates and administers a long-range program of health education. Expanded facilities, centrally located, provide space for individual staff offices and counseling rooms, small conference rooms for discussion groups, and a larger auditorium for meetings, conferences, workshops, and lectures. A library, an exhibit theater, and individual teaching machine booths are available. A long-standing activity of the medical group, its comprehensive multiphasic health screening program, has been expanded and now involves extensive data processing equipment. These data provide a broad basis for continuing research in limitless numbers of health problems. The multiphasic health screening program is a fundamental part of the expanded health education program.

Methods and approaches in the community health center

The community health center provides varied opportunities for health education and care through its facilities and personnel.

The health team. The coordinated team approach underlies the basic program of a community health center (Fig. 14-3). Under the guidance of the physician, specialists in various areas of health care work together with the patients to explore needs and provide services for family-centered health care.

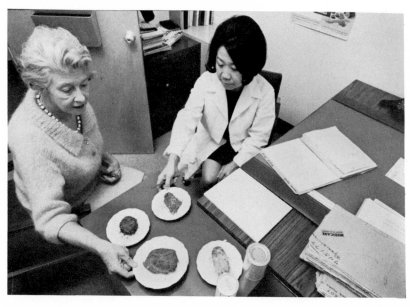

Fig. 14-4. The clinic dietitian reviews nutritional needs with a patient. She discusses dietary modifications based on a sound food plan adapted to individual requirements and desires.

Methods. The methods used include individual counseling, small discussion groups, classes, use of libraries and exhibits, and self-teaching devices.

INDIVIDUAL COUNSELING. Either by appointment or in the open clinic, according to need, individuals may have personal conferences with members of the health team, such as physician, psychologist, nutritionist (Fig. 14-4), nurse, or social worker. Instruction may be given concerning some aspect of health care as the need for such instructions becomes apparent. Dietary modification is high on the list of probabilities for such instruction. Team conferences, under the direction of the family internist and pediatrician are held in which workers in relevant disciplines explore and coordinate plans for family health care.

SMALL DISCUSSION OR DEMONSTRATION GROUPS. Studies such as those of Dr. Kurt Lewin (p. 270) demonstrate that persons are more likely to carry out a decision if they have participated in the forming of it, than if the decision has been made for them by others. Small discussion-decision groups provide opportunity for persons to explore needs, to obtain information about health care, learn whether alternatives are open to them, and gain motivation and support for action. Such discussion-decision groups are proving effective instruments for the education of persons with common health problems. Patients with diabetes, obesity, heart disease, or peptic ulcer, have found positive direction and emotional reinforcement through discussion-decision sessions. Well persons with common health interests, such as parents of young children, expectant parents (Fig. 14-5), teenagers, or older persons have taken a lively interest in learning and sharing in these ways.

CLASSES. More structured classes in subjects related to various health needs also provide needed information in such areas as prenatal care, natural child-birth, infant and child care, and family planning. Other classes may be provided for persons with heart disease, diabetes, peptic ulcer, renal disease, genetic disease, and other chronic or long-term problems. Classes in broad areas of health interest may be planned as needed. These may be in areas such as family meal planning and marketing, pre-

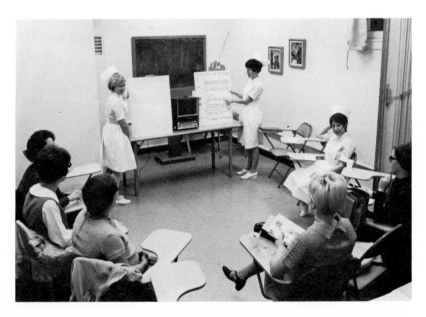

Fig. 14-5. A weekly discussion group for prenatal patients conducted by obstetrics instructors and student nurses in a community medical center. Many opportunities for health education exist in the field of maternal-child health.

ventive family health care through wise use of available comprehensive health plans and group medical practice, human relations, or current medical research in a wide variety of areas. The possibilities are as broad as the need in the individual community.

For effective teaching in such classes, the health worker will need to plan carefully. The teaching plan will include sound re-

---

TO PROBE FURTHER
Teaching plan for group instruction

I. Preparation
   A. Research the subject and make a careful study. Prepare an outline and finally reduce the kernel of the material to one sentence.
   B. Make out a teaching plan.
      1. *Aim.* Define the patient-learning goals. Make sure that this goal: (a) relates to this patient's needs, so that he can identify with it; (b) suggests teaching procedure; and (c) is a realistic one that you can attain within the class period.
      2. *Approach.* Create a learning situation that will: (a) secure attention and interest; (b) stimulate learning readiness; (c) be relevant and lead into the class topic; and (d) raise pertinent questions.
      3. *Answers.* Guide learning experiences and activities so that they: (a) secure group involvement; (b) lead to the organization of concepts; (c) provide an opportunity to explore background and alternative answers; (d) provide resurce material for analysis and discussion; and (e) allow for continuous feedback by a variety of methods.
      4. *Application.* To help each patient to apply the proffered material to his own needs: (a) summarize key points; (b) bring the group to a decision concerning a plan of action, if indicated; and (c) enable each patient to ask, specifically, "What does this mean to me?"—and to perceive the answer with clarity.
      5. *Assignment.* To secure carry-over into life situations: (a) obtain any further needed information from sources in the community; and (b) if the program involves a series of classes, propose possible feedback for next class.
   C. Prepare and check out all aids and equipment ahead of time.
II. Presentation
   A. Arrange in advance for the room, chairs, speaker's desk, displays, materials, and equipment necessary.
   B. Carry out the teaching plan
      1. *Timing.* Begin and end on time, and pace the material for balance and interest.
      2. *Group involvement.* Maintain a relaxed and permissive atmosphere. Be flexible and allow for an adjustment of the original plan as the situation warrants. Use resource people as needed.
III. Purpose fulfilled?
   A. Evaluate class results in light of its objective.
   B. Plan follow-up activity.

search and other preparation, plans for the creation of a learning situation, for the guidance of learning activities, and for helping each person who attends to apply the material to his individual situation so that he may translate what he learns into action. Various teaching aids may be planned, prepared, secured, and arranged. Equipment and classroom facilities will need to be checked. During the class the pace at which material is presented, flexibility, and group involvement will be significant factors. After the completion of each class, and of the series, a follow-up evaluation in the light of the stated objectives will be essential as the basis for planning future classes or series of classes.

LIBRARY AND EXHIBITS. Health education materials, books, pamphlets, leaflets, models, pictures, and charts in an organized health library under the care of a qualified librarian provide rich learning resources as a part of a community health center. An exhibit area, where displays of visual and graphic materials related to various aspects of health care may be presented, is another highly effective means of health education.

SELF-TEACHING DEVICES. Booths may be provided with individually operated devices such as teaching machines and recorded audio-visual materials. Persons may use these as desired to obtain new information or to review certain health care principles and practices.

Community health resources

In various forms in many types of communities, other health agencies and organizations provide opportunities and resources for community health education.

Government agencies. Public health departments conduct many service and educational activities on the local, state, and national levels. Public health nutritionists help survey community nutrition needs, plan nutrition components of community health programs (Fig. 14-6), and provide training (Fig. 14-7), consultation, and teaching materials for public health workers in other specialities such as nursing and sanitation. Public health nurses work with families through various health services, help organize and conduct clinics, and teach community health classes. Other government

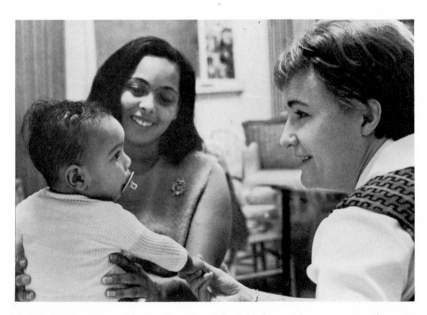

Fig. 14-6. Public health nutritionist discussing infant feeding with a young mother at a community child health conference.

health agencies working in specific community projects include those formed in response to the Economic Opportunity Act, such as VISTA (Volunteers in Service to America) and other groups operating in poverty areas, the Indian Health Program, and School Lunch Program.

Volunteer agencies. A host of volunteer health agencies, such as the American Heart Association, American Diabetes Association, and the American Cancer Society, provide educational opportunities and materials through their local chapters. In some larger urban areas, nutrition committees have classes taught by local nutritionists, nurses, and physicians. These are sometimes arranged through cooperation with the local adult evening school. There are nutrition consultation and diet counseling services provided by a staff nutritionist with educational materials developed and printed by community physicians and health workers. There are also professional workshops on specific health problems. Volunteer nutritionists and nurses also work with local chapters of the American Diabetes Association in their annual diabetes detection drives, and teach classes in the local high schools.

Specific health-interest clubs. Local chapters of organizations formed for the study and dissemination of information related to specific health problems offer support and a sharing of information to persons having such needs. These groups include the Ileostomy and Colostomy Club, TOPS (Take Off Pounds Sensibly), and Weight Watchers. Community health workers are often invited to speak at meetings of the members.

Schools, churches, civic, and fraternal groups. A number of lay organizations conduct health-related activities for groups of persons having special needs. An example is the excellent "Meals-on-Wheels" program conducted in some cities by volunteers who prepare and deliver hot meals to persons in need of such service. These are usually patients referred by the physicians of the community. They are for the most part persons who are chronically ill or who are undergoing rehabilitation, and are often elderly and alone. In rooming houses and apartment districts food is delivered by

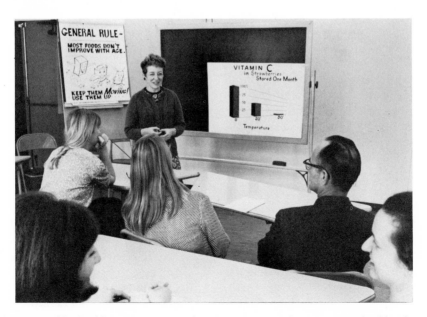

Fig. 14-7. A public health nutritionist provides many resources for community health education. Here she is helping to provide training for community health workers.

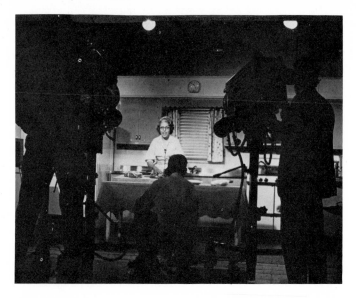

Fig. 14-8. Television provides a mass communication medium for health education. Here a nutritionist gives a demonstration on food selection and preparation. (USDA photograph.)

couriers on a regular schedule for a nominal fee. Often this courier is the only person who visits the patient for days at a time; she is awaited eagerly each day and brings more than food into the patient's life.

Professional groups. Local professional organizations—medical, nursing, dietetics—provide health education in a number of ways. They sponsor workshops, participate in mass communication through such media as radio and television (Fig. 14-8), and issue staff-written articles for publication in newspapers and magazines. A unique activity of the American Dietetics Association, for example, is the "Dial-a-Dietition" program that has been established in many urban areas. Through a telephone-answering service, persons may make inquiries about food and nutrition; dietitians return the calls and give information or clarify a confused point.

Food industry groups. A number of food industries sponsor research, provide nutrition education materials, and underwrite community nutrition projects. Among these organizations are the National Dairy Council and its affiliated state groups, and the National Livestock and Meat Board.

County interagency nutrition councils. In many counties, a nutrition council, whose members represent the various nutrition agencies in the community, coordinates the work of all of the represented groups. These nutrition councils plan and sponsor community health activities such as projects and workshops that may be carried out through the local high schools ("Food For Teen Fitness" is an example). They also develop adult conferences on nutrition, and issue teaching materials.

Information concerning nutrition education work in a community may be obtained by writing or telephoning one of the following sources:

1. Agricultural Extension Service, usually located in the state university
2. Home advisors, home economists, in district agricultural extension offices
3. Dietitians in local hospitals
4. Nutrition instructors in high schools, colleges, and nursing schools
5. Nutritionists in local health departments or clinics
6. Volunteer health agency office, the local chapter of the American Heart Association, or of the American Diabetes Association

Tests of the success of teaching about nutrition

Because health teaching involves dynamic interaction between teacher and learner, the nurse who would educate patients about nutrition and health will, at frequent intervals, reassess her own developing comprehension of the dynamics of human behavior, of growth and development, and of learning. She will evaluate, from time to time, her own growth in recognizing the needs and perceptions of persons, and her increased sensitiveness to others. Such appraisals will help to equip her with realistic self-understanding. (How does she see herself—as "the authority figure who knows best," or as the "helping vehicle of learning" who is present when needed, to guide a person's own learning?) In testing her own success as an educator in the special field of nutrition, the health professional will use the techniques of self-appraisal that have become her standbys in other aspects of nursing. These are the methods developed by such students of human interactions as Carl Rogers,[5] Jurgen Reusch,[6] and Frances Macgregor.[7] She will want to reread the findings and recommendations of these and other authorities, and consider them afresh in their application to the complex field of nutrition and the teaching of nutrition to patients and to community groups.

Key questions. To further this self-analysis, ask yourself the following key questions:

1. *Do I listen when the patient talks?* Do I listen to the patient's words? Have I become alert to the difference between "Certainly!" and "Yes, I think so . . ."? Am I sure *this* patient knows the difference between whole milk, low-fat milk, and fat-free milk? Does he know the difference between "a little sugar" and a heaping teaspoonful of sugar to a half-cup of coffee? If the patient does not speak English fluently, am I sure, from his own words, that he is certain of the information I have given him? Do I listen to the patient's inflections? Do I notice the fall of the voice that conveys reluctance, doubt, lack of faith in the therapy recommended, indifference, discouragement, revulsion, or hostility? These emotions, if not offset by stronger and more valid considerations, will negate all carefully constructed reasoning, once the patient has left the environment of the health center.

2. *Does the patient understand what I am saying?* Are the words and phrases that I use related to his experience so that he may identify with them and build upon them?

3. *Do I respect the necessity for cultural harmony?* Does my teaching conflict in any way with the patient's cultural values and conditioning? Since I know that such conflict will result in lack of confidence, and probably in rejection or confusion, do I have the imagination to find ways to integrate my knowledge with this patient's conditioning?

4. *Am I comfortable with silences that allow the patient to think through a thought raised?* Do I allow the patient to translate our conversation into his own thinking, at his own pace? Do I respect the slow thinker? Am I patient with the person who has a mind of his own, and will not change it until he sees convincing cause? Am I easily fooled by the fast thinker, who seems to agree so readily with my suggestions (but who will ignore them)? Do I recognize the various qualities of silence of each of these types of person? Do I have the poise that allows the person to go through the behind-scenes events which take place in that silence? Do I *value* the silence, because of those events—knowing that until he has gone through that inner process he cannot reach a meaningful decision?

5. *Do I accept, without approval or disapproval, what the patient says?* Have I set aside my judgmental tendencies, left behind my infantile wish to praise or blame? Do I see evidence for the maturity and freedom of my own approach, in the frankness with which patients are able to discuss with me their cravings, their aversions, or their boredom?

6. *Do I keep the conversation patient-*

centered? Do I allow him to set the direction of discussion about himself? Do I conserve the patient's energy and time (and my own time, too, for which I am responsible to others), by concentrating on the business at hand—the health of this patient?

7. *Do I reflect, without interpretation, key words and phrases expressed by the patient?* This technique, which is highly developed by the psychological counselor, is useful to the health educator insofar as it helps her to understand *precisely* what the patient is telling her. The patient who says, "I eat two eggs a day," may be relating a simple fact; or he may be telling the

health educator that he has no intention of eating eggs, and that he wants her to stop discussing that subject once for all. The obese woman who declares, "I *never* eat sweets," will make this assertion with increasing passion if she feels that she is being probed for a confession of dietary sin. The health educator who calmly restates, without interpretation, those statements which she suspects of masking an emotion-loaded situation is sometimes able to help the patient face the truth by dispelling fear or anger.

8. *Am I genuinely interested?* Do I show my interest? Do I indicate my concern by

---

TO PROBE FURTHER
The problem-solving method in nutrition education

Increasingly, efforts of leaders in nursing to develop a unique body of nursing theory have been based upon the method of problem-solving. The problem-solving method is a stepwise organization of concepts and activities directed toward the solution of specific problems. One of its essentials is the requirement for clear definitions at each step, before attempting the next phase of solution. To apply the problem-solving method to nutrition education by the nurse, the function of nursing itself will have to be defined.

The function of nursing* is to provide for a person undergoing illness, medical treatment, or the formulation of a plan for medical care, such help as he may require for the fulfillment of his needs, while encouraging him to optimum self-care. *Nursing practice* based upon this premise (clearly distinguished from medical care) must revolve around three further factors:

1. Identified patient needs—*the nursing diagnosis*
2. The plan of action, derived through consideration of needs, goals, and possible actions by patient and nurse together—*the nursing care plan*
3. Mutual exploration of results—*nursing evaluation*

Within this framework, a useful outline for a problem-solving approach for the nurse to the education of patients about nutrition, may be as follows:

Identified need	What is the specific nutrition problem in this patient?
Goal	What is the specific nutrition goal for this patient?
Background knowledge	What scientific principles are applicable to this need and goal?
Plan	What plan of nutrition improvement is organized (with the patient's participation) to meet this need and to reach this goal?
Results	What happened? Did the plan enable the patient to reach his goal? Was the goal reached completely, partially, or not at all? (If work remains to be done, the problem-solving activity is begun again, with new definitions of the need and goal.)

---

*Orlando, I. J.: The dynamic nurse-patient relationship, New York, 1961, G. P. Putnam's Sons.

looking directly at him, by my facial expression, nod of head, and tone of voice?

9. *Has my teaching been practical?* Will my suggestions prove workable for this patient in his special life-situation? Does he have the resources to carry out such a plan?

10. *Has my teaching been important?* Does this teaching really matter to the patient's health? If he makes the changes agreed upon, will they really make a difference in the outcome?

11. *If other persons are present, and I must discuss the patient with them, do I keep all communication directed to and through him?*

12. *At the end of the interview, do I leave the door open to further reflection and exploration as needed?*

Evaluate your nutrition teaching by applying these twelve tests to each program that you plan; and, in retrospect, to your daily work with individuals and groups. If you are dissatisfied with your rating, reevaluate your approach. The therapy for failure on any point can be summarized in a simple formula: *Explore more closely, with the patient, the patient's real needs.*

References
Specific

1. Cassel, J.: A comprehensive health program among South African Zulus. In Paul, B. D., editor: Health, culture and community, New York, 1955, Russell Sage Foundation, pp. 15-41.
2. Jelliffe, D. B.: Cultural variation and the practical pediatrician, J. Pediat. 49:661, 1956.
3. Lewin, K.: Forces behind food habits and methods of change. In The problem of changing food habits, Washington, D. C., 1943, National Academy of Sciences, National Research Council, pp. 35-65.
4. Clark, H. T., Jr.: Shaping the hospital for its future role, Hospitals 40:50, 1966.
5. Rogers, C.: Client centered therapy, Boston, 1957, Houghton Mifflin Company.
6. Ruesch, J., and Bateson, G.: Communication, the social matrix of psychiatry, New York, 1951, W. W. Norton and Company, Inc.
7. Macgregor, F. C.: Social science in nursing, New York, 1960, Russell Sage Foundation.

General

Babcock, C.: Attitudes and the use of food, J. Amer. Diet. Ass. 38:546, 1961.

Beeuwkes, A. M.: Educational television—nutrition's new opportunity, J. Amer. Diet. Ass. 33:477, 1957.
Burke, R. L.: Approaches to understanding leadership, J. Amer. Diet. Ass. 45:327, 1964.
Butterworth, T. H.: Learning-principles, practices, and peanuts, J. Amer. Diet. Ass. 49:15, 1966.
Cassel, J.: Social and cultural implications of food and food habits, Am. J. Public Health 47:732, 1957.
Chidester, F. H.: Programmed instruction: past, present, and future, J. Amer. Diet. Ass., 51:413, 1967.
Davis, A. J.: The skills of communication, Amer. J. Nurs. 63:66, 1963.
de la Vega, M.: New focus on the hospital as a health education center, Hospitals 40:78, 1966.
Fabun, D., editor: Communication, Kaiser Aluminum News 23, (3), 1965.
Forest, R. P.: What everyone should know about semantics, a scriptographic booklet, Greenfield, Mass., 1967, Channing L. Bete Co.
Hayakawa, S. I.: The self-concept—why we reject some ideas and accept others, J. Dent. Med. 15:3, 1960.
Heidgerken, L. E.: Teaching and learning in schools of nursing, ed. 3, Philadelphia, 1965, J. B. Lippincott Co.
Hill, M. M.: A conceptual approach to nutrition education, J. Amer. Diet. Ass. 49:20, 1966.
James, G., and Christakis, G.: New York City's Bureau of Nutrition, J. Amer. Diet. Ass. 48:301, 1966.
Jelliffe, D. B.: Cultural variation and the practical pediatrician, J. Pediat. 49:661, 1956.
Katz, A. H., and Felton, J. S., editors: Health and the community, New York, 1965, The Free Press.
Keller, M. D., and Smith C. E.: Meals on wheels: 1960, Geriatrics 16:237, 1961.
Kintzer, F. C.: Approaches to teaching adults, J. Amer. Diet. Ass. 50:475, 1967.
Mead, M.: The dietitians as a member of the therapeutic team, J. Amer. Diet. Ass. 21:424, 1945.
Mead, M.: Food habits research: problems of the 1960's, Washington, D. C., 1964, National Academy of Sciences, National Research Council, Pub. No. 1225.
McCune, H. L., and Meyer, R. T.: The bulletin board—an effective teaching aid, Nurs. Outlook 7:532, 1959.
Monteiro, L. A.: Notes on patient teaching—a neglected area, Nurs. Forum 3 (1), 1964.
Moore, A. N., and Klachko, H. W.: Problems in producing programs for auto-instruction, J. Amer. Diet. Ass. 51:420, 1967.
Moore, M. L.: When families must eat more for less, Nurs. Outlook 14:66, 1966.
New York Academy of Medicine, 1964 Health Conference Proceedings: The expanding role of ambulatory services in hospitals and health de-

partments, Bulletin of the N. Y. Acad. of Med. **41**(1), 1965.

New York Academy of Medicine, 1965 Health Conference Proceedings, Closing the gaps in the availability and accessibility of health services, Bulletin of the N. Y. Acad. of Med. **41**, (12), 1965.

New York Academy of Medicine, 1966 Health Conference Proceedings, New directions in public policy for health care, Bulletin of the N. Y. Acad. of Med. **42**, (12), 1966.

Nyhus, D.: How Medicare is affecting a public health nutrition program, J. Amer. Diet. Ass. **51**:143, 1967.

Orlando, I. J.: The dynamic nurse-patient relationship, New York, 1961, G. P. Putnam's Sons.

Pattison, M., Barbour, H., and Eppright, E., Teaching nutrition, Ames, Iowa, 1963, The Iowa State College Press.

Paul B. D., editor: Health, culture and community, New York, 1955, Russell Sage Foundation.

Pearson, J. S., and Skalitsky, M. J.: Psychodrama as a teaching aid, J. Amer. Diet. Ass. **30**:876, 1954.

Roberts, M. B.: Communicating with people. J. Amer. Diet. Ass. **30**:698, 1954.

Ruesch, J., and Bateson, G.: Communication, New York, 1951, W. W. Norton and Company, Inc., pp. 94-134.

Shapiro, I. S.: Learning more about communication, New York, 1961, National Public Relations Council.

Shapiro, L. R., Huenemann, R. L., and Hampton, M. C.: Dietary survey for planning a local nutrition program, Public Health Reports **77**:257, 1962.

Stare, F. J.: Nutrition Education via the Public Press, J. Amer. Diet. Ass. **39**:124, 1961.

Stefferud, A., editor: Food, the yearbook of agriculture, 1959, Washington, D. C., 1959, U. S. Dept. of Agriculture.

Vaughn, M. E.: An agency nutritionist looks at home health care under Medicare, J. Amer. Diet. Ass. **51**:146, 1967.

Wagner, M. G., and others: Evaluation of the Dial-a-Dietitian Program: I. Program organization, II. Impact on the community, J. Amer. Diet. Ass., **47**:381, 1965.

Walsh, E.: Nutritionists and social workers cooperate on mutual problems, J. Amer. Diet. Ass. **25**:681, 1949.

CHAPTER 15

Family diet counseling— food needs and costs

The public health nurse frequently needs to apply the basic principles of health teaching in family diet counseling. The term "counseling" is appropriate here, for if the nurse works with the family in the light of counseling principles, she will lead its various members to explore their own situation, to determine their own needs, and to find methods of meeting those needs that are best suited to their life situation and tastes.

TYPES OF FAMILIES REQUIRING COUNSELING

The families that the nurse will counsel fall into two large categories, the well family and the family that requires therapeutic modifications.

The well family. The well family is one in which no member is acutely or chronically ill from any disease that specifically requires modification of the diet as therapy. Obviously, there may be problems of overt or inapparent malnutrition such as poor dental health from lack of calcium or poor skin and flabby muscles from lack of vitamins or other essential nutrients. However, these deficits would be supplied if the diet were normal. In helping this family to understand its nutritional needs, the nurse will be most likely to encounter such problems as unawareness, lack of education, discouragement, lack of zest in life, bewilderment (particularly in the foreign-born), poverty, or food prejudices so deep-seated that they have not been dispelled by the education offered through public schools and the mass media.

The family requiring therapeutic dietary modification. This is the family in which one or more members require modification of the diet. As part of the treatment for disease, the nurse will also need to counsel the mother concerning the principles of the therapeutic diet prescribed, and the meaning of these principles in terms of food to be served. She will discuss, in terms of the total family situation, ways of fitting the patient's requirements into the family meals. As an example, the husband may have chronic heart disease and the doctor has prescribed restriction of sodium intake. The nurse may suggest that as the wife prepares the food for her family she remove the portion to be served to the husband before she adds salt to the remainder which is to be served to the family. The nurse together with the wife may also discuss ways of seasoning the husband's food with herbs, spices, or condiments that do not contain sodium. Another example is a child with diabetes. The nurse who is called upon to counsel the mother of such a child may need to take into consideration the family budget, the tastes and emotional needs of the patient's siblings, and perhaps a complex of additional factors in order to help the mother find a way to shift the diabetic child from a breakfast of pancakes and syrup to one based on egg, bacon, and orange juice or other foods

291

supplying the nutrients prescribed by the physician.

PROCEDURE FOR FAMILY DIET COUNSELING

In family diet counseling, the nurse should start by applying the initial principle of all counseling—Begin where persons are. The first step is to learn the family's situation and values, and to identify the nutritional needs. This can be accomplished by an interview in which a family nutrition history is taken. A standard form (printed or mimeographed) may be used for this purpose. Many forms have been used in such interviewing, of which the following are examples:

Twenty-four hour recall. Each member

NUTRITION HISTORY

Activity associated general day's food pattern

Name _____ Date _____

Ht. _____ Wt. Lbs. _____ Kilos _____ Age _____

Ideal Wt. _____

Referral
Diagnosis
Diet order

Members of household

Occupation

Recreation, physical activity

Present food intake

Breakfast	Place	Hour	Milk
			Cheese
			Meat
			Fish
Noon meal			Poultry
			Eggs
			Cream
			Butter,
Evening meals			margarine
			Other fats
			Vegetables,
			green
Extra meals			Vegetables,
			other
			Fruits (citrus)
			Legumes
Summary			Potato
			Bread—kind
			Sugar
			Desserts
			Beverages
			Alcohol
			Vitamins
			Candy

of the family is asked to recall every item of nutrient taken during the preceding twenty-four hours.

Food records. A record is kept for 24 hours or longer of all items eaten and drunk.

Structured schedule for meal patterns. An interview schedule is used which lists each common meal item in the cultural pattern. For example, dinner would include the entree, a starch accompaniment, a green or yellow vegetable, salad, bread, dessert, and beverage.

Activity associated general day's food pattern. Perhaps one of the simplest and most helpful methods for both the nurse and the family respondent (usually the mother) is the activity-associated general day's food pattern. Since for most people eating is related to activity or work throughout the day, making use of the association between the two gives the nurse and the mother a structure—a beginning, a middle, and an ending—and provides a series of mnemonics on which to flesh out the greater detail that will permit constructive counseling. A general form on which such an interview might be based is given on p. 292.

Diet history and analysis. Using such an interviewing schedule as the *activity-associated general day's food pattern* three basic steps may be followed in performing a family nutrition analysis.

1. A general pattern of the day's activity and food intake should be obtained. The interview may begin with questions such as, "About what time do you usually get up in the morning? After you get up do you usually have something to eat? Can you give me examples of what you might have?" When this phase has been fully explored, the mother is led slowly through the family's routine for the day. Sometimes labels for informal meals are omitted so that the informant will remember to mention food that was eaten, but not considered a meal. ("In the middle of the day do you usually have something to eat? Can you give me some examples?") Since family dinner is usually a more structured meal,

it is reviewed carefully an item at a time, from the first dish served through the main dish, the dessert, and each of the various accompaniments. With respect to each item, the questions are asked in terms of general habit—food item, form, frequency, preparation, portion, seasoning—not in terms of a specific day's food intake. Sometimes pictures, or models of portion sizes may be helpful in arriving at a clear picture of the family's general habits of food use.

2. The day's pattern should be checked by nutrient groups. A cross-check by nutrient groups helps to tally the day's use of given types of food. By referring to a cross-list of food items that have been categorized according to nutrient groups, the general use of the basic nutrients is tallied.

   a. *Protein foods*—milk, meat, fish, poultry, egg, cheese
   b. *Fruits and vegetables*—vitamin C and A sources, citrus and substitutes, deep green and yellow vegetables, raw and cooked fruits and vegetables, how cooked
   c. *Cereal grains and bread*—whole grain or enriched, forms used, frequency
   d. *Desserts and beverages*—coffee, tea, soft drinks, alcohol
   e. *Miscellaneous snack items*—candy, chips, nuts, cookies
   f. *Nutrient supplements*—vitamins and minerals

As this cross-check is made, the questions asked will reflect back to the mother her original responses concerning the frequency of use of an item by different family members and the form in which it is consumed. ("Let's see now, tell me if this is about right. You mentioned drinking milk at dinner, but not at any other time. Would you say, then, that you usually drink one glass of milk a day?") Weighted phrases such as "only one" or "plenty of," approving or disapproving tones or facial expressions, and the like should be avoided, as they tend to imply judgments, and prevent straightforward responses.

Throughout such an interview, important clues to food attitudes and values are being

NUTRITIONAL ANALYSIS SHEET

Food intake (Family member, clinic patient)	Dietary guide (Basic four food groups and main nutrient contributions of each)	Analysis of food intake
Milk group		
Meat group		
Vegetable-fruit group		
Bread-cereal group		
Miscellaneous additions		

communicated. The nurse should carefully note these, and store them in her memory for later thought and possible exploration. If the nurse's manner throughout has been interested and accepting, the information she receives should be valid and straightforward. If the nurse is judgmental and authoritarian, the mother will probably only tell her what she thinks the nurse wants to hear, not what the true situation may be.

3. The family food pattern should be analyzed by a dietary guide. Various dietary guides may be used as a measure of general nutritional adequacy. Perhaps the most familiar guide is the list known as the basic four food groups (Table 15-1). This guide groups food according to major nutrient components contributed to the daily diet, and gives the general quantity needed for nutritional adequacy in terms of numbers of servings for different ages or circumstances, such as pregnancy and lactation.

Exploration of specific modifications. By recasting the family's general food pattern into categories, the nurse may easily place the family's food intake and the basic four food groups guide side by side, so that she and the mother can analyze them together (see above). Together they may explore the possible additions or modifications needed, and discuss a plan by which these nutrients

Table 15-1. Daily food guide—the basic four food groups

Food group	Main nutrients	Daily amounts*
Milk		
Milk, cheese, ice cream, or other products made with whole or skimmed milk	Calcium Protein Riboflavin	Children under 9: 2 to 3 cups Children 9 to 12: 3 or more cups Teenagers: 4 or more cups Adults: 2 or more cups Pregnant women: 3 or more cups Nursing mothers: 4 or more cups (1 cup = 8 oz. fluid milk or designated milk equivalent†)
Meats		
Beef, veal, lamb, pork, poultry, fish, eggs	Protein Iron Thiamine	2 or more servings Count as one serving: 2 to 3 oz. of lean, boneless, cooked meat, poultry, or fish
Alternates: dry beans, dry peas, nuts, peanut butter	Niacin Riboflavin	2 eggs 1 cup cooked dry beans or peas 4 tablespoons peanut butter
Vegetables and fruits		4 or more servings Count as 1 serving: ½ cup of vegetable or fruit, or a portion such as 1 medium apple, banana, orange, potato, or ½ a medium grapefruit, melon
	Vitamin A	Include: A dark-green or deep-yellow vegetable or fruit rich in vitamin A, at least every other day
	Vitamin C (ascorbic acid)	A citrus fruit or other fruit or vegetable rich in vitamin C daily
	Smaller amounts of other vitamins and minerals	Other vegetables and fruits including potatoes
Breads and cereals		4 or more servings of whole grain, enriched or restored Count as 1 serving:
	Thiamine Niacin Riboflavin Iron Protein	1 slice of bread 1 ounce (1 cup) ready to eat cereal, flake or puff varieties ½ to ¾ cup cooked cereal ½ to ¾ cup cooked pastes (macaroni, spaghetti, noodles) Crackers: 5 saltines, 2 squares graham crackers, etc.

*Use additional amounts of these foods or added butter, margarine, oils, sugars, etc., as desired or needed.
†Milk equivalents: 1 ounce cheddar cheese, 3 servings cottage cheese, 1 cup fluid skimmed milk, 1 cup buttermilk, ¼ cup dry skimmed milk powder, 1 cup ice milk, 1⅔ cups ice cream, ½ cup evaporated milk.

may best be obtained. (See food plans at different cost levels, p. 307-315).

Inculcation of basic nutritional concepts. Using the family's general nutritional analysis as a base, the nurse may clarify or reinforce the mother's understanding of basic nutritional concepts (p. 278). A number of helpful tools, resource materials, and visual aids have been developed for use in teaching these concepts. The nurse may

Table 15–2. Examples of resource agencies for nutrition education materials

Resource agency	Location
Government agencies	
Government Printing Office	Washington, D. C.
U. S. Department of Agriculture	
Research Service	Federal Center Building
	Hyattsville, Maryland
Agricultural Extension Services	State universities
U. S. Department of Health, Education, and Welfare	
Children's Bureau	Washington, D. C.; regional offices
Federal Food and Drug Administration	Washington, D. C.; regional offices
State and local public health departments	State capitals; county seats
Professional organizations	
American Dietetic Association	620 N. Michigan Avenue
	Chicago, Illinois
American Medical Association	535 N. Dearborn Street
Council on Foods and Nutrition	Chicago, Illinois
American Home Economics	1600 20th Street, N.W.
Association	Washington, D. C.
American Dental Association	222 E. Superior Street
	Chicago, Illinois
Volunteer health organizations	
American Heart Association	44 E. 23rd Street
	New York City, New York
American Diabetes Association	18 E. 48th Street
	New York, New York
Industry-associated boards and councils	
National Dairy Council	111 North Canal Street
	Chicago, Illinois
National Livestock and Meat Board	37 South Wabash Avenue
	Chicago, Illinois
American Institute of Baking	400 East Ontario
	Chicago, Illinois
Commercial agencies (health education services)	
Food Industries	
H. J. Heinz Company	Pittsburgh, Pennsylvania
Insurance Companies	
John Hancock	Boston, Massachusetts
Metropolitan	New York City
Pharmaceutical companies	
Mead-Johnson	Evansville, Indiana
Parke-Davis	Detroit, Michigan
Ross Laboratories	Columbus, Ohio
Abbott Laboratories	North Chicago, Illinois
Science foundations	
National Academy of Sciences	2101 Constitution Avenue
National Research Council	Washington, D. C.
Nutrition Foundation	99 Park Avenue
	New York City, New York

select from materials provided by the sources listed in Table 15-2; or she may develop her own teaching materials on the basis of such guides, adapting them to this particular family's needs, abilities, and desires. Many helpful tools, such as the leaflets pictured in Fig. 15-1 and 15-2, are available from community health resources.

Follow-through plans. After the nurse and the mother have arrived at a definite plan for initial action that is expected to alter the family food pattern, the nurse will arrange with the mother for specific follow-up. This may take the form of return visits to the home, visits by the mother to the clinic or community health center, or con-

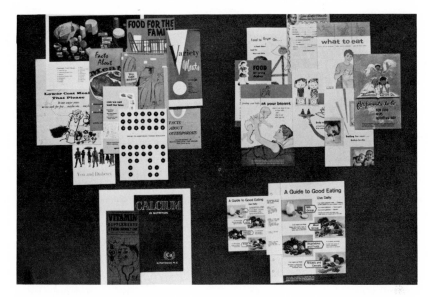

Fig. 15-1. Resources for family food guides.

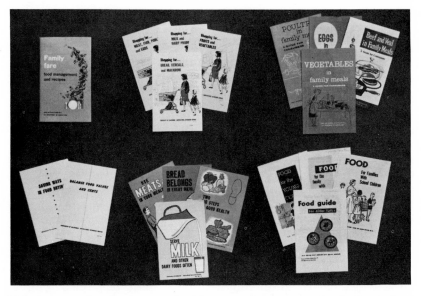

Fig. 15-2. Resources for planning wise food buying and preparation for family meals.

TO PROBE FURTHER
Further study of nutritional needs

For a more detailed study of the family's nutrition at a later time, the nurse may want to use the listings of the Recommended Daily Allowances of the Major Nutrients, published by the Food and Nutrition Board of the National Research Council.* This dietary guide gives the recommended daily allowance of the major nutrients according to age and sex, and according to special need such as pregnancy. Two additional resources the nurse may require for more detailed study are tables of food values in terms of nutrient composition and calories. Two such basic references are *Composition of Foods*,† compiled by B. K. Watt and A. L. Merrill, and *Food Values of Portions Commonly Used*,‡ by A. Bowes and C. Church.

*Food and Nutrition Board, National Research Council, Recommended dietary allowances, ed. 7, Pub. 1694, National Academy of Sciences, Washington, D. C., 1968.
†Watt, B. K., and Merrill, A. L.: Composition of foods, Agricultural Handbook No. 8, Agricultural Research Service, Washington, D. C., 1963.
‡Bowes, A. deP., and Church, C. F.: Food values of portions commonly used, ed. 10, rev. by Church, C., and Church, H., Philadelphia, 1966, J. B. Lippincott Co.

sultation as needed with other members of the health team (physician, nutritionist, social worker, or other). The nurse may continue to help the mother with meal plans, marketing, economical buying, and suggestions for preparation of specific foods. Follow-up work requires patience, persistence, and a steady recollection of the goal. Imagination and good humor are invaluable. One step must be taken at a time. Throughout the whole process of educating the family in applied nutrition, the nurse will give support, help with adjustments of the plan, provide reinforcement of prior learning, and continue to add new learning opportunities as the family's needs develop.

FAMILY FOOD ECONOMICS— NEEDS AND COSTS
Family food needs and general economy

The basic responsibility for providing nourishing meals for the family usually rests with the mother or wife. To a great extent her self-esteem is bound up in her image of herself in the role of food provider, and she spends a large proportion of her time in activities related to this function. Often she is under the pressure of con-

flict between her desire to keep her family healthy by serving an adequate and balanced supply of foods, and limitation of her financial resources for buying food.

The American housewife faces a vast array of tempting and colorful items in the supermarket, and food costs that can be bewildering. If the young wife has had little preparation for homemaking, she has even more difficulty managing to make ends meet. The average family in the U. S. spends about 20% of its income on food, or about $35 a week for a family of four (parents and two children younger than 12 years). About one-third to one-half of this money is spent for such luxury items as expensive cuts of meat, out-of-season fresh fruits and vegetables, and other special foods. Nutritious, attractive meals can be had for less. It is the need to achieve this that faces the low-income family. Often the public health nurse or the nutritionist is asked to counsel with such a family about ways to get the most nutrition from their limited food dollars. Sometimes the financial need is even more pronounced and the nurse must help plan with a family in circumstances of extreme poverty.

Table 15-3. Average quantities of food used at home per person in a week, in Washington, D. C., 1963, food consumption survey of city families at three income levels

Food items	Amount per person per week
Milk, cream, ice cream, cheese	3.1 qts. equivalent
Meat, poultry, fish	4.8 lbs.
Eggs	.5 doz.
Vegetables	5.0 lbs.
Fruits	4.3 lbs.
Grain products	2.1 lbs. flour equivalent
Fats, oils	.7 lbs.
Sugar, sweets	1.5 lbs. sugar equivalent

Baker, D., and Beloian, A.: Diets of households in Washington, D. C., Family Economics Review, June, 1967, pp. 8-11.

Table 15-4. Average money value of food used in a week, according to income after taxes, by households surveyed in Washington, D. C., 1963*

Income	Number of house- holds	Average household size† (persons)	Total value of food	Purchased food			Food received without direct expense‡
				Home use	Eaten away	Total	
Under $3,000	34	3.19	$21.23	$18.37	$0.96	$19.33	$1.90
$3,000 to $5,999	46	3.35	29.65	23.87	5.17	29.04	.61
$6,000 or more	45	3.35	37.78	30.57	6.77	37.34	.44
Not classified	26	2.22	35.94	29.63	5.72	35.35	.60
Total (averages)	151	3.29	$31.26	$25.62	$4.79	$30.41	$ .85

*Baker, D., and Beloian, A.: Diets of households in Washington, D. C., Family Economics Review, June, 1967, pp. 8-11.
†21 meals at home = 1 person.
‡Federally donated, home-produced, or received as gift or pay.

Table 15-5. Food purchases for one week for an average family of four on a moderate-cost diet*

Types of food	Cost per week
Meat, poultry, fish	$10.74
Eggs	1.23
Dairy products	4.77
Fruits and vegetables	6.50
Cereals and bakery products	4.14
Miscellaneous (fats, oils, sugars, sweets, beverages)	5.12
Total cost home food	$32.50
10 lunches away from home (children's school lunches)	3.50
Total week's food costs	$36.00
Comparative week's food costs (same family)	
Low-cost diet	$26.50
Liberal diet	41.00

*Cook, F., and Groppe, C.: Saving ways in food buying, Berkeley, California, 1967, University of California Agricultural Extension Service (adapted).

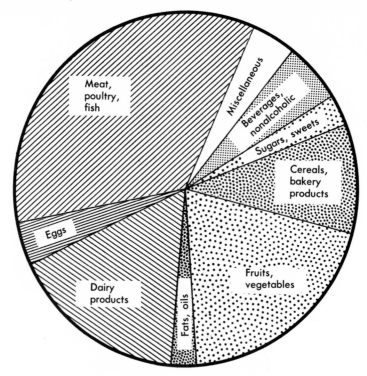

Fig. 15-3. The family food dollar, showing the relative amount of money spent on common food items. (Data from Nationwide USDA Survey, 1963-1966.)

U. S. family food use and costs

More specifically, just how much food does the average American family use and what money value does this amount of food represent? A pilot study in the Washington, D. C. area in the summer of 1963 surveyed 151 city families on three income levels.[1] During the survey week, food brought into the kitchen of these Washington households provided the amounts per person shown in Table 15-3. The money value of the food used during the survey week is indicated in Table 15-4.

The money value of food used in a week averaged about $21 in the low-income households, $30 in the middle-income group, and $38 in the high-income families.

The follow-up U. S. Department of Agriculture nationwide survey indicated that the average family divides its food dollar as indicated in Fig. 15-3.

With this division of the food dollar as a basis for reference, a survey of food prices

made in the Oakland-Berkeley, California, area in April, 1966,[2] indicated that an average Western U. S. family of four (parents under 35 years of age and 2 children under 12 years) would spend weekly on a moderate-cost diet approximately the amounts indicated in Table 15-5.

"Basic four" food bargains

The objective in wise food buying for the family is to obtain optimum nutritional value for money spent on food. The basic four food groups may serve as a guide for examples of ways in which food bargains, nutritionally speaking, may be obtained with careful planning. In Table 15-6 the food choices in the less expensive column are compared with those in the more expensive column.

Food buying guides

Today's American housewife spends more time shopping for food than she does in

Table 15-6. Bargains in the basic four food groups*

Food group	Usually less expensive, more food value for the money	Usually more expensive, less food value for the money
Milk products	Concentrated, fluid and dry nonfat milk, buttermilk, evaporated	Fluid whole milk, chocolate drink, condensed milk, sweet or sour cream
	Mild cheddar, Swiss, cottage cheese	Sharp cheddar, Roquefort or blue, grated or sliced cheese, cream cheese, yogurt
	Ice milk, imitation ice milk, imitation ice cream	Ice cream, sherbet
Meats		
Meat	Good and standard grades	Prime and choice grades
	Less tender cuts	Tender cuts
	Home-cooked meats	Canned meats, sliced luncheon meats
	Pork or beef liver, heart, kidney, tongue	Calf liver
Poultry	Stewing chickens, whole broiler-fryers, large turkeys	Poultry parts, specialty products, canned poultry, small turkeys
Fish	Rock cod, butterfish, other fresh fish in season, frozen fillets, steaks, and sticks	Salmon, crab, lobster, prawns, shrimp, oysters
Eggs	Grade A	Grade AA
Beans, peas, and lentils	Dried beans, peas, lentils	Canned baked beans, soups
Nuts	Peanut butter, walnuts, other nuts in shell	Pecans, cashews, shelled nuts, prepared nuts
Vegetables, fruits	Local vegetables and fruits season	Out-of-season vegetables and fruits, unusual vegetables and fruits, those in short supply
Vitamin A rich	Carrots, collards, sweet potatoes, green leafy vegetables, spinach, pumpkin, winter squash, broccoli, and in season canteloup, apricots, persimmons	Tomatoes, Brussels sprouts, asparagus, peaches, watermelon, papaya, banana, tangerine
Vitamin C rich	Oranges, grapefruit and their juice, cabbage, greens, green pepper, canteloup, strawberries, tomatoes, broccoli in season	Tangerines, apples, bananas, peaches, pears
Others	Medium-sized potatoes, nonbaking types	Baking potatoes, new potatoes, canned or frozen potatoes, potato chips
	Romaine, leaf lettuce	Iceberg lettuce, frozen specialty packs of vegetables
Breads, cereals	Whole wheat and enriched flour	Stone-ground, unenriched, and cake flour
	Whole grain and enriched breads	French, Vienna, other specialty breads, hard rolls
	Homemade rolls and coffee cake	Ready-made rolls and coffee cakes, frozen or partially baked products
	Whole grain or restored uncooked cereals	Ready-to-eat cereals, puffed, sugar-coated
	Graham crackers, whole grain wafers	Zwiebach, specialty crackers and wafers
	Enriched uncooked macaroni, spaghetti, noodles	Unenriched, canned, or frozen macaroni, spaghetti, noodles
	Brown rice, converted rice	Quick-cooking, seasoned, or canned rice

*Cook, F., and Groppe, C.: Balance food values and cents, Berkeley, California, 1967, University of California Agricultural Extension Service, Pub. HXT-42, pp. 6-7.

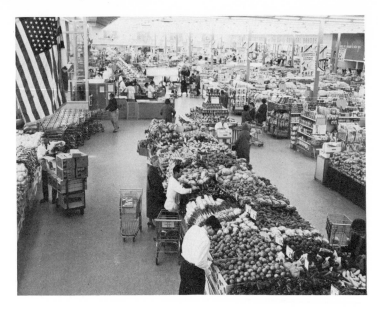

Fig. 15-4. American supermarkets such as this one in Maryland carry as many as 20,000 food and other items and do an annual volume of business ranging from $375,000 to $10,000,000. (USDA photograph.)

cooking it. Food marketing is big business, and buying food for her family may seem to the housewife to be a more intricate affair than the preparation of it at home. A large American supermarket may stock 8,000 or more different food items and more are being added daily. A single food item may be marketed in a dozen different ways at as many different prices. Frequently, in family diet counseling and in talking with patients about special, modified diets, the nurse will observe that the wife and mother places greatest stress on her need for help in food buying.

Factors affecting family food costs. A number of factors influence the way in which a family divides its food dollar. The nurse will explore these factors with the mother in helping her outline her family food plan:

1. Family income
2. The number, sex, ages, and general activities of the family members
3. Whether any part of the family food is produced or preserved at home (gardening, canning, freezing)
4. The likes, dislikes of family members; special family dishes
5. Special dietary needs of any family member
6. The time, transportation, and energy available to the mother for shopping and food preparation
7. The skill and experience the mother has in family food management (planning, shopping, storing, preparing)
8. The storage and cooking facilities in the home
9. The amount and kind of entertaining, if any, the family does
10. The number of meals eaten away from home
11. The value the family places upon food and eating

Economy buying suggestions. In each basic food group, suggestions for wise, economical buying may be explored with the mother.

Meats, fish, poultry, eggs. Since meat is commonly one of the more costly food items, considerable study should be given to how it is graded, cut, processed, and marketed. Excellent learning material is available through the local county home advisor, U. S. Department of Agriculture Extension Service.

1. The homemaker should buy cuts of meat that give the most lean meat for the money, and should avoid paying for large amounts of gristle, bone, and fat.

2. The meat grade should be checked. The lower grades provide good quality, less fat, and cost less. Meat on the U. S. market is usually graded according to quality and ratio of fat to lean. U. S. *Prime* is of excellent quality and flavor. It is tender and moist and the fat well marbelized (distributed, striated) through the lean meat. It is not often seen in markets serving the general public, since it goes mostly to the hotel and restaurant trade. U. S. *Choice* is of very good quality. It is popular because of the moderate amount of fat that is distributed through the lean portion. This is the grade usually found in most retail markets. U. S. *Good* is of good quality and is relatively tender. It is preferred by consumers who desire a lower ratio of fat to lean. U. S. *Standard* is of acceptable quality. It comes from animals under 48 months of age, and has a very thin covering of fat and high proportion of lean. It is a good buy. U. S. *Commercial* is less tender but is of acceptable quality. It comes from older animals and has less fat than the higher grades. It is often a very good buy, but is seldom seen in retail markets. It goes mostly to meat products processing plants. *USDA Utility, Cutter, and Canner* are the three lowest grades and they are used only in processed meat products.

3. The less costly meats have just as much food value as the higher cost cuts, and although they are less tender and juicy than the costlier cuts, they can be made equally tender and flavorful by cooking them slowly using methods that involve water or steam, as pot-roasting or braising.

4. Grades of ground meat that sell at lower cost should be used but the amount of fat should not be excessive. Some states (for example, California) have laws providing that all ground fresh beef may contain no more than 30% fat, and that all meat used must be skeletal meat (edible meat of striated muscle originally attached to bones). In these states no organ meats, coloring, cereal, or preservatives may be added. Specific label names indicate the following:

    a. Ground beef or hamburger—only fresh beef containing no more than 30% fat may be sold under this label

    b. Ground chuck or round—must be only chuck roast or round, with no more than 30% fat; usually contains less

    c. Pork sausage—ground pork with no more than 50% fat

5. Organ meats (liver, kidney, heart) are nutritious *bargains*. They should be used often. A good cookbook will have correct and appetizing ways of preparing them for family acceptance (for example, liver loaf [part liver, part ground beef] with Spanish sauce, stuffed and baked heart, beef and kidney pie). Other variety meats include brains, tongue, sweetbreads (thymus gland from veal or very young beef; this gland disappears with maturity), and tripe (the plain or smooth lining, especially the pocket-shaped part from the end, of the cow's second stomach).

6. Poultry should be bought as the whole bird. Usually the larger, more mature birds cost less than young broilers and fryers, and can be made equally tender by longer, moist cooking methods (braising, stewing, fricaseeing) or by pressure cooking.

7. Fish is usually a good buy as it is sold in cuts that contain little or no waste. Shellfish is more costly; fresh fish in season is less expensive.

8. Less expensive packed styles of canned fish should be used. For example, salmon species are usually priced according to color. Chinook, King, and Sockeye (Red) are deepest in color and cost more; Coho (Silver), Pink, and Chum (or Keta) are lighter colored, have less oil, and usually cost less. Tuna is packed according to the size of pieces. Fancy or solid pack (large pieces) is most expensive; chunk style is

made up of moderate-sized pieces and is moderate in price; flake or grated style consists of smaller pieces and is cheapest in price.

9. Eggs are sold according to grade and size, neither of which are related to food value. It is therefore advantageous to buy the least expensive. Egg grades are AA, A, B, and C. Differentiation into these grades is based on such qualities as firmness of the egg white, appearance, and delicacy of flavor. The AA and A grades are better for poaching, frying, and cooking in the shell; lower grades are equally good for general cooking, scrambling, and omelets. The size classifications are based on weight per dozen: Jumbo (30 oz. per doz.), Extra Large (27 oz. per doz.), Large (24 oz. per doz.), Medium (21 oz. per doz.), Small (18 oz. per doz.), Peewee (pullet eggs, 15 oz. per doz.). This classification has no relation to food value or quality. Shell color (white, brown, or speckled) varies with species and breeds of poultry and has no effect upon egg quality.

Milk, cheese. Milk and milk products are bargains in nutrition. It is hard to get enough calcium and riboflavin without including dairy products in the diet.

1. Fluid skimmed milk, buttermilk, and canned evaporated milk cost less than fresh, whole, fluid milk. So-called low-fat milks are 2% butterfat (whole milk is 4% butterfat). To make them, part of the butterfat is removed from whole milk and dry milk solids are added. Low-fat milk contains 135 calories per 8 oz. cup; whole milk contains 170 calories per cup; skim milk contains 80 calories per cup.

2. Nonfat dry milk is the best bargain of all forms. Reconstituted with water, it gives a fluid skimmed milk at less than half the cost of fresh fluid skimmed milk. Dry skimmed milk can be used in innumerable ways in cooking to add valuable nutrition.

3. Milk should be bought at the store. In most cities a family pays from 1 to 3 cents more per quart for delivery. However, some milk-delivery firms charge less than this per quart for large numbers of quarts delivered regularly.

4. Milk should be bought in large containers. Fluid milk sometimes costs less in the half-gallon or large bulk containers than in the quart container.

5. If cheese is used often it should be bought in bulk. It costs less and keeps better. Cheese standards set by the Food and Drug Administration are based upon percentage of fat and moisture. The most commonly used, cheddar cheese (American, Daisy, Longhorn), is 50% fat and 30% moisture. The spread cheeses and imported cheeses are more expensive.

6. Cottage cheese is an unripened, soft-curd cheese (80% moisture), and hence is rather rapidly perishable. It should be bought only as used to avoid waste resulting from spoilage. The buyer should not be misled by the statement on the label that a cottage cheese is low in calories. Regular recreamed cottage cheese contains not more than 4% milk fat; "low calorie" contains about 2% milk fat. The difference in calories is slight. One-half cup of regular recreamed cottage cheese provides 120 calories; the same amount of "low calorie" (partially recreamed) cottage cheese provides 100 calories.

Vegetables and fruits. Vegetables and fruits are the main sources of vitamins A and C, two nutrients found in community surveys to be most often lacking in the average American diet.

1. Fresh vegetables and fruits should be bought in season. Except for unpredictable crop shortages or surpluses, prices go through seasonal cycles according to supply. For example, citrus fruit usually costs less during the winter; fresh garden vegetables cost less during the summer, except for winter garden vegetables such as cabbage, winter squash, and sweet potatoes.

2. In buying fresh produce, pieces that are firm, crisp, and heavy for their size should be selected. Fresh vegetables and fruits that are of medium size are usually better buys than large, of which more may need to be discarded.

3. The buyer should distinguish between types of defect. Small surface defects do not affect the eating quality or food value of fruits and vegetables, and pieces so blemished may cost less. Many or deep defects cause more waste, as does decay which is even slightly evident.

4. If an item of fresh produce is sold by either weight or count, the resulting price per item should be computed by each method to find the one that costs less.

5. Fancy grades in canned vegetables and fruits should be avoided. Grading is based on shape, size, and perfection of pieces. Lower grades contain small, broken, or imperfect pieces, but are equal to higher grades in food value and are therefore good buys.

6. If family size warrants, fruits and vegetables should be bought in large cans. For example, the No. 3 cylinder can (46 fluid ounces; or 3 pounds, 3 ounces; 5¾ cups) is the "economy family size" in fruit and vegetable juices, pork and beans, and so on. It yields from 10 to 12 servings. The size of can for fruits and vegetables that is stocked in largest quantities on market shelves is No. 303 which contains 2 cups, or 4 servings. Labels should be carefully checked for servings per unit. The largest (institutional) size can, No. 10, contains from 12 to 13 cups, or 25 servings.

7. Dehydrated foods vary in price. Dried beans, peas, and lentils are excellent food buys. Specialty dried foods, such as potatoes, are usually more expensive than the fresh product.

8. Frozen vegetables and fruits are usually more expensive than fresh or canned; however, specials and large family size packages should be compared weight for weight with canned or fresh produce in season.

9. Vegetables should be cooked with care. Excess cooking water and time destroy or eliminate vitamins and minerals, and rob the vegetable of color and texture. Such unappetizing food often goes uneaten by the family, hence causes costly waste.

10. If the homemaker knows the produce man at the market, she can sometimes get good, usable produce which he has discarded on certain days as his fresh supply comes in. It will need careful checking and much cutting away of defective parts, but often it costs nothing except the time and effort in handling the crates and culling the material.

Bread, cereals. Cereals in general are bargains in nutrition. Milled cereals are now commonly enriched. Grains have earned the title "staff of life," and people in many parts of the world today subsist almost entirely on them. They are found in America markets in many forms, and are usually an economy food.

1. Grains should be bought in bulk for cheaper cost. However, adequate storage should be planned (room temperature or cool place, in tight container) to avoid waste resulting from spoilage by dust, moisture, or insects.

2. Whole grain or enriched cereal products should be purchased to ensure the content of B complex vitamins and calcium and iron.

3. Unusual forms of grain should be tried. For example, bulgur is cooked and dried wheat, with the outer bran removed and the remaining kernels cooked to the desired size. Dry, cracked bulgur keeps well in a porous container in a cool place. It has a toast-like color, is rich in wheat flavor, equal in food value to whole wheat, and makes an economical addition to family menus for variety.

4. Regular, enriched white rice should be bought. Any processing or specialty preparation increases the cost.

5. To avoid costly waste of breads and cereals resulting from careless handling, dry cereals should be stored in a cool, dry place. The package should be closed tightly after each use. For long storage of bread, it should be frozen or placed in the refrigerator.

Menu planning to save money. As an example of the economy that can be effected by food choices for family meals, two menus are compared in Table 15-7.

Table 15-7. One menu at two cost levels for family of four (father and mother 33 years of age, girl 8, boy 11)*

Meal	Menu 1 (more costly)	Menu 2 (less costly)
Breakfast	Grapefruit juice (frozen)	Grapefruit juice (canned)
	Ready-to-eat cereal (oat)	Oatmeal
	Poached eggs (large)	Poached eggs (medium size)
	Enriched English muffins	Whole wheat toast
	Butter	Margarine
	Coffee (name brand)	Coffee (store brand)
	Milk for all (fluid, nonfat)	Milk for all (concentrated)
Lunch	Onion soup (canned)	Onion soup (dehydrated)
	Tuna salad sandwiches (chunk style tuna)	Tuna salad sandwiches (grated style tuna)
	Cabbage slaw (ready-made†)	Cabbage slaw (homemade)
	Peaches (heavy syrup)	Peaches (light syrup)
	Milk for all (fluid whole for father and fluid nonfat for others)	Milk for all (concentrated)
Dinner	Cubed steaks	Individual meat loaves with potatoes and carrots
	Baked potatoes	
	Frozen carrots	
	Tossed green salad with French dressing (commercial)	Romaine salad with vinegar and oil dressing (homemade)
	Whole wheat brown-and-serve rolls	Hot whole wheat bread slices
	Butter	Margarine
	Frozen apple pie (commercial)	Baked apples
	Milk for all (whole, fluid)	Milk for all (concentrated)
	Coffee for adults (name brand)	Coffee for adults (store brand)
Total cost*	**$6.31**	**$ 4.24**
Savings:		
One day		$ 2.07
One week		14.49
One month		62.79
One year		755.55

*Cook, F., and Groppe, C.: Balance food values and cents, Berkeley, California, 1967, University of California Agricultural Extension Service, Pub. HXT-42, pp. 8-9.
†Prices based on foods purchased in a supermarket chain in the Oakland-Berkeley area on March 1, 1967.

Both menus use essentially the same foods, but the cost difference resulted from selecting the best buys in each case.

Summary of good marketing and food handling practices

Planning ahead. The homemaker should use market guides, plan general menus, keep a kitchen supply check list, and make out a market list ahead according to location of items in her regular market. Such plan-

ning helps to avert "impulse buying" and extra trips. Completely unplanned purchases account for over half of the items bought in supermarkets!

Buying wisely. The homemaker should know the market, market items, packaging, grades, brands, portion yields, measures, and food value in a market unit. She should watch for sales, and buy in quantity if it effects a saving, and if she can store and use the food. She should be cautious in selecting "convenience" foods. The added time saving may not be worth the added cost.

Storing food safely. The kitchen waste that results from food spoilage and misuse should be controlled. Food should be conserved by storing items according to their nature and utilization. Dry storage, covered containers, and refrigeration should be used as needed. After a food package has been opened and part of its contents has been consumed, the opened package with the remaining food should be kept on the front of a shelf for early use. To avoid plate waste only the amount needed by the family should be cooked, and left-overs should be used intelligently.

Cooking food well. Maximum food value should be retained, but food should also be prepared with imagination and good sense. Zest and appeal can be given to dishes by using a variety of seasonings and combinations. However much the housewife may have learned about nutrition, the members of her family usually eat because they are hungry or because the food looks and tastes good—not because it is nutritious.

FOOD PLANS ACCORDING TO FAMILY INCOME

Except perhaps for the small group of the very wealthy, most American families live under socioeconomic pressures. The problems of middle-income and low-income families differ only relatively. Health workers, if they are to provide realistic and useful assistance in health care to the individual family in these categories, will need to understand its background of economic pressures, and the types of problems that result.

Middle-income groups

General socioeconomic pressures. A number of socioeconomic pressures create problems for middle class families. Early marriage and young parenthood, incomplete education, continuing education (especially graduate and professional education), low job status, and low beginning salaries all exert financial pressures on young couples

beginning to establish their homes. In their attempts to meet these pressures, most middle-income families assume increasing debt. A study conducted in 1962-1963 by the U. S. Federal Reserve Board [3] revealed that 8 out of 10 American households in which the head was under 35 years of age owed personal debt averaging $1,000, of which $700 was installment debt; meeting payments was a problem for some. Nine of every 10 homes owned by American families in this young age group were mortgaged. This wide pattern of incurring and paying off debt is a normal part of the financial activities of the young; it becomes less important as they grow older.

Lack of preparation for family adjustments or unrealistic attitudes may also create problems for young couples. For example, the wife and mother may be a teenager, accustomed to the standard of living that characterized her parents' home, which her young husband cannot, of course, maintain. In the past, she may have had little motive or opportunity to learn skills in home and food management which would have enabled her to make optimum use of the money available. As a result the couple's small income is misused, whereas intelligently planned spending would provide better food at less cost. In the course of her professional work, particularly in the prenatal clinic, the nurse frequently encounters a bewildered and anxious young wife who welcomes sympathetic understanding and counsel in these practical areas.

As family size increases and children grow older, the food bills increase as do the other financial commitments of the family. Job insecurity and lessened income may be problems as age advances. Forced early retirement, limited pension funds, and cost of chronic illness may add to the financial problems of older families.

Family food plans. To aid the health worker in counseling with families, or in working with community groups, several *Family Food Plans* have been prepared by

Table 15-8. Moderate-cost family food plan—revised 1964

Sex-age group*	Milk, cheese, ice cream‡	Meat, poultry, fish§		Eggs	Dry beans, peas, nuts		Flour, cereals, baked goods||		Citrus fruit, tomatoes		Darkgreen and deep-yellow vegetables		Potatoes		Other vegetables and fruits		Fats, oils		Sugars, sweets	
	Qt.	Lb.	Oz.	No.	Lb.	Oz.	Lb.	Oz.	Lb.	Oz.	Lb.	Oz.	Lb.	Oz.	Lb.	Oz.	Lb.	Oz.	Lb.	Oz.
Children																				
7 months to 1 year	5	1	8	6	0	0	0	14	1	8	0	4	0	8	1	8	0	1	0	2
1 to 3 years	5	2	4	6	0	1	1	4	1	8	0	4	0	12	2	12	0	4	0	4
3 to 6 years	5	2	12	6	0	1	1	12	2	0	0	4	1	0	4	0	0	6	0	8
6 to 9 years	5	3	4	7	0	2	2	8	2	4	0	8	1	12	4	12	0	10	0	14
Girls																				
9 to 12 years	5½	4	4	7	0	4	2	8	2	8	0	12	2	0	5	8	0	8	0	12
12 to 15 years	7	4	8	7	0	4	2	8	2	8	1	0	2	4	5	12	0	12	0	14
15 to 20 years	7	4	8	7	0	4	2	4	2	8	1	4	2	0	5	8	0	8	0	12
Boys																				
9 to 12 years	5½	4	4	7	0	4	2	12	2	4	0	12	2	4	5	8	0	10	0	14
12 to 15 years	7	4	12	7	0	4	4	0	2	4	0	12	3	0	6	0	0	14	1	0
15 to 20 years	7	5	4	7	0	6	4	8	2	8	0	12	4	0	6	8	1	2	1	2
Women																				
20 to 25 years	3½	4	12	8	0	4	2	4	2	4	1	8	1	8	5	12	0	8	0	14
35 to 55 years	3½	4	12	8	0	4	2	4	2	4	1	8	1	4	5	0	0	6	0	8
55 to 75 years	3½	4	4	6	0	2	1	8	2	4	0	12	1	4	4	4	0	6	0	8
75 years and over	3½	3	8	6	0	2	1	2	2	4	0	12	1	0	3	12	0	4	0	8
Pregnant¶	5½	5	8	8	0	4	2	12	3	4	2	0	1	8	5	12	0	6	0	8
Lactating¶	8	5	8	8	0	4	3	12	3	8	1	8	2	12	6	4	0	12	0	12
Men																				
20 to 35 years	3½	5	0	7	0	4	4	0	2	4	0	12	3	0	6	8	1	0	1	4
35 to 55 years	3½	4	12	7	0	4	3	8	2	4	0	12	2	8	5	12	0	14	1	0
55 to 75 years	3½	4	8	7	0	2	2	8	2	4	0	12	2	4	5	8	0	12	0	14
75 years and over	3½	4	8	7	0	2	2	4	2	4	0	12	2	0	5	4	0	8	0	12

*Age groups include the persons of the first age listed up to but not including those of the second age listed.

†Food as purchased or brought into the kitchen from garden or farm.

‡Fluid whole milk, or its calcium equivalent in cheese, evaporated milk, dry milk, or ice cream.

§Bacon and salt pork should not exceed ⅔ pound for each 5 pounds of meat group.

||Weight in terms of flour and cereal. Count 1½ pounds bread as 1 pound flour.

¶Three additional quarts of milk are suggested for pregnant and lactating teenagers.

Table 15-9. Low-cost family food plan—revised 1964

Weekly quantities of food† for each member of family

Sex–age group*	Milk, cheese, ice cream‡ (Qt.)	Meat, poultry, fish‡ (Lb.)	(Oz.)	Eggs (No.)	Dry beans, peas, nuts (Lb.)	(Oz.)	Flour, cereals, baked goods‖ (Lb.)	(Oz.)	Citrus fruit, tomatoes (Lb.)	(Oz.)	Darkgreen and deep-yellow vegetables (Lb.)	(Oz.)	Potatoes (Lb.)	(Oz.)	Other vegetables and fruits (Lb.)	(Oz.)	Fats, oils (Lb.)	(Oz.)	Sugars, sweets (Lb.)	(Oz.)
Children																				
7 months to 1 year	4	1	4	5	0	0	1	0	1	8	0	4	0	8	1	0	0	1	0	2
1 to 3 years	4	1	12	5	0	1	1	8	1	8	0	4	0	12	2	4	0	4	0	4
3 to 6 years	4	2	0	5	0	2	2	0	1	12	0	4	1	4	3	4	0	6	0	6
6 to 9 years	4	2	4	6	0	4	2	12	2	0	0	8	2	4	4	4	0	8	0	10
Girls																				
9 to 12 years	5½	2	8	7	0	6	2	8	2	4	0	12	2	4	5	0	0	8	0	10
12 to 15 years	7	2	8	7	0	6	2	12	2	4	1	0	2	8	5	0	0	8	0	12
15 to 20 years	7	2	12	7	0	6	2	8	2	4	1	4	2	4	4	12	0	6	0	10
Boys																				
9 to 12 years	5½	2	8	6	0	6	3	0	2	0	0	12	2	8	5	0	0	8	0	12
12 to 15 years	7	2	8	6	0	6	4	4	2	0	0	12	3	4	5	4	0	12	0	12
15 to 20 years	7	3	8	6	0	6	4	12	2	0	0	12	4	4	5	8	0	14	0	14
Women																				
20 to 35 years	3½	3	4	7	0	6	2	8	1	12	1	8	2	0	5	0	0	6	0	10
35 to 55 years	3½	3	4	7	0	6	2	4	1	12	1	8	1	8	4	8	0	4	0	10
55 to 75 years	3½	2	8	5	0	4	2	0	2	0	1	0	1	4	3	12	0	4	0	6
75 years and over	3½	2	4	5	0	4	1	8	2	0	1	0	1	4	3	0	0	4	0	4
Pregnant¶	5½	3	12	7	0	6	2	12	3	4	2	0	1	8	5	8	0	6	0	6
Lactating¶	8	3	12	7	0	6	3	12	3	4	1	8	3	4	5	8	0	10	0	10
Men																				
20 to 35 years	3½	3	8	6	0	6	4	4	1	12	0	12	3	4	5	8	0	12	1	0
35 to 55 years	3½	3	4	6	0	6	3	12	1	12	0	12	3	0	5	0	0	10	0	12
55 to 75 years	3½	3	0	6	0	4	2	12	1	12	0	12	2	4	4	8	0	8	0	10
75 years and over	3½	2	12	6	0	4	2	8	1	8	0	12	2	0	4	4	0	8	0	8

*Age groups include the persons of the first age listed up to but not including those of the second age listed.
†Food as purchased or brought into the kitchen from garden or farm.
‡Fluid whole milk, or its calcium equivalent in cheese, evaporated milk, dry milk, or ice cream.
§Bacon and salt pork should not exceed ⅓ pound for each 5 pounds of meat group.
‖Weight in terms of flour and cereal. Count 1½ pounds bread as 1 pound flour.
¶Three additional quarts of milk are suggested for pregnant and lactating teenagers.

the U. S. Department of Agriculture, Consumer and Food Economics Research Division.[4] Five basic plans on different cost levels, with additional variations, are available: (1) Liberal Plan, (2) Moderate Plan, (3) Low Cost Plan, (4) Special Low Cost Plan for use in the Southeastern States, (5) Economy Plan. The Moderate and Low Cost Plans, often used to guide families of moderate income, are shown in Table 15-8 and Table 15-9.

Low-income groups— the problem of poverty

Tremendous problems exist among the poor. At times they seem almost insurmountable. It is small wonder that a "culture of poverty" develops among the poor, which too often walls them off from the rest of society more completely than would physical barriers. These families are poor not only in income, but also in other aspects of their lives. They live in dilapidated, overcrowded buildings. Their education is usually inadequate in quality and quantity, and they have little or no access to educational opportunities. As a result, they are poorly prepared for jobs and often must make a day-to-day living at unskilled labor. They are poor in opportunity for contact with middle-class and upper-class groups. Often there is little beauty in their barren lives and even less hope.

Characteristics of the poor. As a result of the extreme pressures arising from their living conditions, poverty-stricken persons and families develop attitudes and characteristics which influence their use of community health services. The health worker must understand and appreciate these characteristics if he is to work *with* these families, and if he is to avoid imposing directives *upon* them. Since imposing directives reinforces the character problems that obstruct health development, it is to be avoided as far as possible.

The traits that characterize the discouraged poor manifest themselves in many ways and in many individual forms; but experienced, sensitive workers identify them

essentially as feelings of *isolation, powerlessness,* and *insecurity.*[5]

Isolation. Strong feelings of alienation are common among the poor. In many communities, few, if any, channels of communication are open between the lowest income groups and the rest of society. Almost no opportunity exists for participation in community activities and organizations, or for any meaningful dialogue and achievement of bridges of understanding. Many poor persons respond to such alienation by further withdrawal. Feeling isolated and alone, he concludes that no one is really concerned about his situation. The hazards to his health that are inherent in poor housing and poor nutrition are compounded by alienation from the sources of help that would be available to him in his community if he were to attempt to make use of them.

Powerlessness. It is ironic that often those persons most exposed to risks and emergencies have the least resources and power for coping with them. Extreme frustration is inevitable. Many a poor person becomes overwhelmed with a sense of helplessness. Why try, he concludes, if he has no control over the situation? Why plan if he has no future different from today? In such a day-to-day struggle to exist, the dispirited poor often see little value in long-range preventive health measures.

Insecurity. Subjected to forces outside his control, the poor man has no security. A large proportion of the lowest economic class work by the day, if at all; and their unskilled labor is highly expendable. If such a person is sick and cannot work, he usually faces loss of employment rather than sick leave. In his effort to supply his family's needs, he is vulnerable to spurious schemes and enticing webs that can lead him into legal and still deeper financial problems. The impact of these pressures of insecurity and anxiety may incapacitate him. The appearance of detachment and lethargy that the health worker sees may only be a defense mechanism by which some poor persons attempt to cope with intolerable personal situations. Such an individual is so frozen with concern that he may appear to care about nothing. The coping mechanism of another poor person in the same situation may be totally different. He may respond with hostility. The openly hostile poor strike out at the helping source because they see it as part of the power structure they have come to view as towering and formidable. As part of this power structure, the source of help appears to them to be an enemy to be distrusted, rather than a friend to whom to look for help.

In such a setting, where hunger may be a constant companion, food—which has for the poor person the same deep psychological and emotional connotations that it has for all—assumes even greater meaning than it has for persons who rarely know hunger. For people in a chronic state of insecurity, food can be a very serious matter involving the total person.

Role of the health worker. How may the nurse or nutritionist work with individuals and families conditioned by years or generations of a culture of poverty? In the face of such overpowering feelings of isolation, helplessness, and insecurity, what attitudes must the health worker have if she is to help them? What methods and approaches are most likely to reach them and supply their needs?

The basic principles of learning and health teaching discussed in the previous chapter can be helpful. Several seem particularly pertinent.

Self-awareness. The nurse who has not explored her own feelings about these people, and who has not come to a realistic awareness of her own class values and attitudes, is ill-equipped to work effectively in such a situation. If the nurse is to be an agent of *change,* a true "helping vehicle" (the beautiful phrase coined by Lucile Matthews of the U. S. Children's Bureau), she must first have some understanding of the poor person and his broad social milieu, of herself, and of her own cultural conditioning.

Rapport. Genuine warmth, interest, friendliness, and kindness grow from the inside out. They cannot be put on from the outside as one would put on a cloak. Rapport is that feeling of relationship between persons which is born of mutual respect, regard, and trust. This sense of relationship gives both helper and helped a deep feeling of working *together.* Its most basic ingredient is concern for people and for persons— a positive orientation toward the human race in general, and a love and concern for individuals in particular.

Acceptance. Acceptance is another way of stating the principle that the nurse must begin where the patient is. To begin to help, the nurse must accept the person as he is in his situation as it exists. She must be concerned with his concerns. She may find it necessary to work with other team specialists through a veritable maze of factors before one individual is ready to accept or even to consider the health practice, or the diet counsel which he needs, or which is desired for him. The nurse may have to spend much time, for example, in coming to understand the meaning of food to this person, before she can begin to explore practical dietary matters with him.

Listening. Here, more than elsewhere, the art of listening—positive, active, creative listening—is vital. The patient must tell his story in his own way. There must be no interruptions with distracting statements or questions; no deflecting of the conversation to someone else's problems. This listening must also be observant. Sequence of statements, subjects introduced, areas of intense feelings, and areas ignored give clues to needs. Throughout, the nurse must sensitively guide, and create a relaxed, nonthreatening atmosphere in a setting where the patient feels free to talk. *And she must listen.* The reason that some frustrated people finally take their problems to the streets may well be that *no one listens to them unless they do.*

Methods. In the light of the factors in the impact of the socioeconomic background, the conditioning that a culture of poverty builds in a person, and the rigid, removed, sterile, antiseptic setting in which most community health agencies operate, it is no wonder that so many of their well-intentioned efforts fail. New methods, approaches, and realistic and creative ideas are needed.

One of the new and exciting approaches to the improvement of the health of low-income families through better food habits is a pilot project conducted in cooperation between the U. S. Federal Extension Service and the extension service of the State of Alabama, in five Alabama counties. Its objectives have been to develop and test

---

TO PROBE FURTHER
Federal food assistance programs*

Two programs administered by the Consumer and Marketing Service of the U. S. Department of Agriculture help to provide more and better food for some 5 million people in the United States.

Donated food. More than half the counties in the United States receive foods that have been acquired by the U. S. Department of Agriculture through its price support and surplus removal operations. Recent reports show that each month nearly 3.5 million people receive staple foods worth about $5 a person. These food items include flour, rice, rolled wheat and oats, bulgur, cornmeal, nonfat dry milk, dried beans, canned chopped meat, peanut butter, shortening, margarine, and raisins. Such foods make an important contribution to the diets of persons in extreme circumstances. For adequate nutrition, however, they need other foods also—fruits, vegetables, meat—and a *person-centered* approach.

Food stamps. A more recently developed program, which is expanding to reach all parts of the country in which it is wanted, is supplementing and supplanting the Food Donation Program in some areas. In June, 1967, some 2 million low-income people in more than 800 cities and counties in 41 states and the District of Columbia improved their diets through the Food Stamps Program. Families participating in the program exchange their small amount of food money for stamps that are worth more than the money given in exchange. On an average, $10 is given in food stamps in exchange for every $6 of money invested. These food stamps can be spent like money at local food stores for any domestic food. Studies show that low-income families are using the food stamps to substantially improve their diets by the addition of more milk, meat, fruits, and vegetables than they could otherwise purchase.

Nutrition education programs. To meet the goals of the Food Donation and Food Stamp programs, nutrition education is essential. The homemakers must be taught to make intelligent food choices, and to plan and prepare nourishing family meals. For this purpose, a number of simple teaching materials have been developed. The core is a series of 21 illustrated pamphlets "Food For Thrifty Families". The leaflets present a wide range of choices in low-cost, nutritious, attractive foods and easily followed recipes, most of which are adapted for top-of-stove cooking. Program aides working closely with low-income families have made effective use of these materials.

---

*Olsen, B. F.: Developing leaflets for use in working with families, J. Amer. Diet. Ass. **50**:481, 1967.

Table 15-10. Economy Family Food Plan—Revised 1964 (designed for temporary use when funds are limited)

Sex-age group*	Milk, cheese, ice cream‡	Meat, poultry, fish§		Eggs	Dry beans, peas, nuts		Flour, cereals, baked goods‖		Citrus fruit, tomatoes		Darkgreen and deep-yellow vegetables		Potatoes		Other vegetables and fruits		Fats, oils		Sugars, sweets	
	Qt.	Lb.	Oz.	No.	Lb.	Oz.	Lb.	Oz.	Lb.	Oz.	Lb.	Oz.	Lb.	Oz.	Lb.	Oz.	Lb.	Oz.	Lb.	Oz.
Children																				
7 months to 1 year	4	1	0	4	0	0	1	0	1	0	0	4	0	0	1	0	0	2	0	2
1 to 3 years	4	1	4	4	0	1	1	12	1	0	0	4	1	0	2	0	0	4	0	4
3 to 6 years	3½	1	8	4	0	4	2	4	1	4	0	4	1	8	2	8	0	6	0	6
6 to 9 years	3½	1	12	5	0	6	3	0	1	8	0	8	2	8	3	0	0	10	0	10
Girls																				
9 to 12 years	5	1	12	5	0	10	2	12	1	12	0	12	2	8	3	4	0	8	0	10
12 to 15 years	6	2	0	6	0	10	3	0	1	12	1	0	3	0	3	8	0	10	0	10
15 to 20 years	6	2	0	6	0	8	2	12	1	12	1	4	2	8	3	4	0	8	0	10
Boys																				
9 to 12 years	5	2	0	5	0	8	3	4	1	8	0	12	2	12	3	4	0	10	0	10
12 to 15 years	6	2	0	5	0	10	4	4	1	12	0	12	3	8	3	8	0	14	0	12
15 to 20 years	6	2	8	5	0	10	5	0	1	12	0	12	4	12	3	8	1	0	0	14
Women																				
20 to 35 years	3	1	12	6	0	10	2	12	1	8	1	8	2	12	3	0	0	8	0	12
35 to 55 years	3	1	12	6	0	10	2	8	1	8	1	8	2	8	2	12	0	6	0	8
55 to 75 years	3	1	8	4	0	6	2	0	1	12	1	0	2	8	2	12	0	6	0	6
75 years and over	3	1	4	4	0	6	1	12	1	12	1	0	2	0	2	4	0	4	0	6
Pregnant¶	5½	2	0	7	0	10	3	0	3	0	2	0	2	8	4	8	0	6	0	6
Lactating¶	8	2	0	6	0	10	4	0	3	0	1	8	3	12	4	8	0	12	0	12
Men																				
20 to 35 years	3	2	0	5	0	8	4	8	1	8	0	12	4	4	3	8	0	14	0	2
35 to 55 years	3	1	12	5	0	8	4	4	1	8	0	12	3	8	3	4	0	12	0	14
55 to 75 years	3	1	8	5	0	6	3	4	1	8	0	12	2	12	3	0	0	12	0	10
75 years and over	3	1	8	5	0	6	3	0	1	8	0	12	2	8	2	12	0	10	0	6

*Age groups include the persons of the first age listed up to but not including those of the second age listed.

†Food as purchased or brought into the kitchen from garden or farm.

‡Fluid whole milk, or its calcium equivalent in cheese, evaporated milk, dry milk, or ice cream.

§Bacon and salt pork should not exceed ⅓ pound for each 5 pounds of meat group.

‖Weight in terms of flour and cereal. Count 1½ pounds bread as 1 pound flour.

¶Three additional quarts of milk are suggested for pregnant and lactating teenagers.

methods for filling three basic needs: (1) reaching and teaching of young families, (2) provision of educational materials related to family financial management, nutrition, housing, and child development, and (3) training of nonprofessional aides to work with poor families under professional guidance and supervision. "Program aides" are being employed.[6] These aides are mature, compassionate women without professional backgrounds, who are being trained and supervised by nutritionists and home economists. They establish contact with low-income, hard-to-reach families, and teach them better ways of simple homemaking. In previous projects with similar goals, trained helpers such as home aides, health aides, or nurses' aides have been used. But they have usually gone into the home to perform a homemaking service while the mother is ill or unable to function. The program aides in the Alabama project are taught by the health professionals of the Extension not to do things *for* the homemaker, but to help the homemaker *help*

herself. The program aides do not decide what will be done, and do not do it for the family. They teach the homemaker how to perform a simple task, prepare a simple food, or make a simple garment—starting with problems that seem important *to the homemaker.* The focus of the program is on education and self-development, rather than on personal help. It is an effort to break the chain of frustration and dependence. Each program aide keeps a working log, which is in effect a diary of her relationships with those persons assigned to her. In some of these logs, the depth of quality in these personal, close-working relationships between aide and homemaker are poignantly revealed.

The early reports of results are encouraging. Some of the families reached through the program live in rural areas, some on the fringes of small towns, and some in urban, low-rent, public housing. Through intensive personal work in the family, and in small discussion groups, the aides have substantially helped 508 young families. Of

Table 15-11. Market basket for lower cost family food plan*

Food group	Food items included
Milk, cheese	Only nonfat dry milk, cheese
Meat, fish, poultry	Stewing beef, ground beef, salt pork, sausage, chicken, fish
Beans, peas, nuts	Dried beans, peanut butter
Flour, cereals, baked goods	Large proportion of flour and cornmeal; only cereals for cooking (no ready-to-eat cereals); rice and macaroni products; bread, crackers, and some sweet crackers
Citrus fruits, tomatoes	Canned orange juice, some fresh oranges, canned tomatoes
Potatoes	Only fresh potatoes (no processed)
Dark green and deep yellow vegetables	Sweet potatoes and carrots
Other vegetables and fruits	Cabbage, onions, bananas, apples; canned apples, corn, fruit juice; dried prunes
Fats, oils	Margarine, lard, and salad dressings
Sugars, sweets	Sugar, syrup, jelly
Accessories	A few seasonings; no soft drinks

*Peterkin, B. B.: Low-cost food plan—choices influence cost, Family Econ. Rev. March, 1967, p. 7-9.

these 508 young homemakers, 40% now use better buying practices than before; 44% have acquired skills in food preparation, and 42% have improved the eating habits of their families. In those families reported to show improvement, the meals are better balanced, better use is made of government-donated foods, or Federal Food Stamps are spent more intelligently. In many instances food storage and kitchen equipment have been improved, the family's consumption of milk has increased, and gardens have been planted.[7]

Economy food plans. The lowest cost family food plan developed by the U. S. Department of Agriculture is the *Economy Family Food Plan* (Table 15-10), designed as a guide for counselors who help homemakers with very low income. The food in this plan, for a family of four for one week, will cost from $20 to $22 (based on December, 1966, food prices in Washington, D. C. area).

Low-cost food plans at still lower cost. In a further attempt to meet the requirements of very low income families, the USDA Low Cost Food Plan (p. 309) has been tested by nutritionists to see if closer buying could reduce its costs still further. Using average selections, the estimated one-week cost of the regular plan for a family of four (parents and 2 school children) was about $26.50 (December, 1966, food prices). When the buying guide shown in Table 15-11, was used, the cost was reduced about 25%, to approximately $19.30 a week.[8]

References
Specific
1. Baker, D., and Beloin, A.: Diets of households in Washington, D. C., Family Econ. Review, June, 1967, pp. 8-11.
2. Cook, F., and Groppe, C.: Saving ways in food buying, Berkeley, California, 1967, University of California Agricultural Extension Service, pamphlet HXT-64, pp. 1-4.
3. Projector, D. S., and Weiss, G. S.: Survey of financial characteristics of consumers, Board of Governors of the Federal Reserve System, 1966. Schoenberg, J. K., and others: Size and composition of consumer savings, Federal Reserve Bulletin, 1967.
4. Family Food Plans, rev. 1964, Hyattsville, Md.,

1964, Agricultural Research Service, Consumer and Food Economics Research Division, U. S. Department of Agriculture.
5. Matthews, L. I.: Principles of interviewing and patient counseling, J. Amer. Diet. Ass. **50**:469, 1967.
6. Spindler, E. B.: Program aides for work in low-income families, J. Amer. Diet. Ass. **50**:478, 1967.
7. Oliver, M.: Pilot study in Alabama, J. Amer. Diet. Ass. **50**:483, 1967.
8. Peterkin, B. B.: Low-cost food plan—choices influence cost, Family Econ. Rev., March, 1967, pp. 7-9.

General
Alexander, M. M., and Stare, F. J.: Your diet: health is in the balance, (Booklet—General Nutrition Education), New York, 1967, Nutrition Foundation.
Beal, V. A.: The nutritional history in longitudinal research, J. Amer. Diet. Ass., **51**:426, 1967.
Collins, P., and Miles, F.: Leaflet Series, Food for family use, University of California Agricultural Extension Service, Berkeley, California, 1965—Use meat in your meals, HXT-70; Bread belongs in every meal, HXT-71; Serve milk and other dairy foods often, HXT-72. Two big steps to good health (vegetables & fruits), HXT-73.
Cook, F., and Groppe, C. C.: Balance food values and cents, University of California Agricultural Extension Service, 1967, HXT-42.
Cook, F., and Groppe, C. C.: Saving ways in food buying, University of California Agricultural Extension Service, 1967, HXT-64.
Family fare: food management and recipes, Home and Garden Bulletin No. 1, Human Nutrition, Consumer and Food Economics Research Divisions, Agricultural Research Service, U. S. Dept. of Agriculture, Washington, D. C., 1966.
Family food plans, rev. 1964, Hyattsville, Maryland, 1964, Agricultural Research Service, Consumer and Food Economics Research Division, U. S. Department of Agriculture.
Food and Nutrition Board, National Research Council, Recommended dietary allowances, ed. 7, 1968, National Academy of Sciences, Washington, D. C., 1968.
Garrett, A. M.: Interviewing—its principles and methods, ed. 25, New York, 1966, Family Service Association of America.
Groppe, C. and Ferree, M.: Leaflet Series, Shopping for . . ., University of California Agricultural Extension Service, Berkeley, California, 1966. Meat, fish, poultry, and eggs, HXT-75; Fruits and vegetables, HXT-76; Milk and dairy products, HXT-77; Bread, cereals, and macaroni, HXT-78.
Hames, P. J., and Robertson, E. C.: Nutritive

value of low income families' diets, J. Amer. Diet. Ass. 30:766, 1954.

Hoff, W.: Why health programs are not reaching the unresponsive in our communities, Public Health Rep. 81:654, 1966.

Irelan, L. M.: Low-income life styles, U. S. Welfare Administration, Pub. No. 14, 1966.

The Interview, Currents in Public Health (Ross Labs.) Vol. 6, No. 4, 1966.

Kaufman, I.: Helping people who cannot manage their lives, Children 13:93, 1966.

Moore, M. C., and others: Using graduated food models in taking dietary histories, J. Amer. Diet. Ass. 51:447, 1967.

Moore, M. L.: When families must eat more for less, Nurs. Outlook 14:66, 1966.

National Live Stock and Meat Board, Lessons on meat, Chicago, 1964.

Reaching 'hard-to reach' families, Currents in Public Health, (Ross Labs.) Vol. 5, No. 7, 1965.

Shopper's guide to U. S. grades of food, Home and Garden Bulletin, No. 58, Washington, D. C., U. S. Department of Agriculture.

Travelbee, J.: What do we mean by rapport, Amer. J. Nurs. 63:70, 1963.

U. S. Department of Agriculture, Agricultural Research Service, Hyattsville, Maryland, Home and garden bulletins for use with "Family food plans," Food for the young couple, 1967, No. 85; Food for the family with young children, 1963, No. 5; Food for families with school children, 1963, No. 13; Food guide for older folks, 1963, No. 17.

U. S. Department of Agriculture, Agri. Res. Serv., Guides for consumers, Home and Garden Bulletins, Washington, D. C. Vegetables in family meals, 1965, No. 105; Eggs in family meals, 1966, No. 103; Poultry in family meals, 1966, No. 110; Beef and veal in family meals, 1967, No. 118.

U. S. Department of Health, Education, and Welfare, Bureau of Family Services, Better health care for people with low incomes, (Leaflet: Summary of the New Title XIX, Medical Assistance Program), Washington, D. C., 1966.

Valante, R. S.: Scavenger hunting, Nurs. Outlook 14:40, 1966.

Zober, M.: Some projective techniques applied to marketing research, J. Marketing 20:265, 1956.

CHAPTER 16

Nutritional deficiency diseases

Out of evident necessity, in its organized beginnings public health work was directed primarily toward the control of communicable disease in man. One of the early manuals, provided a half century ago (1917) for its workers by the American Public Health Association, was oriented to the fulfillment of this need.[1] In the years since that time, communicable disease has come increasingly under control, at least in developed areas of the world. A pronounced shifting of emphasis in public health is now occurring. The primary world health problem today is *malnutrition*. The shift in emphasis to this problem was marked by the Association's publication in 1960 of a companion manual, *Control of Malnutrition in Man.*[2]

World-wide recognition of the public health significance of the nutritional diseases has continued to grow. Observation and experience, however, have also brought deepened awareness of two important interrelated facts: (1) food *alone* is not the answer; (2) a high standard of living does not necessarily solve the problem; even in the midst of plenty malnutrition exists.

As the nutritional deficiency diseases are explored in this chapter, the following questions can be used as a guide. This brief discussion is intended to provide only an initial impetus; it is hoped that the material presented here will stimulate a continued concern and investigation.

First, the general, overall problem should be considered:

1. *The problem.* What is malnutrition? What is its extent and significance in world health today?

2. *Its ecology.* Why does malnutrition exist? What factors combine and interact to cause it?

Second, as each of the basic nutritional deficiency diseases is discussed, these related factors should be considered:

1. *Identification.* What is the nature of the disease? What are its clinical manifestations or associated laboratory findings?

2. *Etiology.* What specific nutritional deficiency is involved? On what type of diet does this disease occur?

3. *Occurrence.* In what inner and outer environment does this disease occur? In persons of what age? Of which sex? Living in what sort of community? In what parts of the world?

4. *Control.* What methods of control are effective in prevention and treatment of this disease?

It will be helpful to look back at the chapters in Unit I in which each of the involved nutrients is discussed in detail, for a review of the nutrient chemistry. In the present chapter, a knowledge of that chemistry will be applied to the clinical disease picture and its public health significance.

MALNUTRITION—WORLD HEALTH PROBLEM
Definitions

Malnutrition. Malnutrition at its fundamental biological level is inadequate supply of nutrients to the cell. A lack of essential nutrients at the cellular level, however, is the result of a complex web of factors: psychological, personal, social, cultural, economic, political, and educational. Each of these factors is a more or less important cause of malnutrition at a given time and place, for a given individual. If these variables are only temporarily adverse, the malnutrition may be acute, and may be alleviated rapidly, leaving no long-standing results or harm to life. But if these variables are continuously adverse and unrelieved, malnutrition becomes chronic. Irreparable harm to life follows, and, eventually, death ensues.

On a biological level, nutritional deficiency diseases may be classified as primary or secondary, according to the availability of the nutrient.

Primary deficiency disease. A primary deficiency disease is a disease that results directly from dietary lack of a specific essential nutrient. For example, scurvy results if the diet is deficient in vitamin C; beriberi results if the diet is deficient in thiamine. The primary deficiency diseases are the subject of this chapter.

Secondary deficiency disease. A secondary deficiency disease is a disease that results from the inability of the body to use a specific nutrient properly. Such inability may result from either of two general types of failure: (1) failure to absorb the nutrient from the alimentary tract into the blood, or (2) failure to metabolize the nutrient normally after it has been absorbed. For example, the malabsorption syndrome is characterized by failure of absorption of fats through the intestinal wall, so that fat is lost in the stool. Phenylketonuria is the inability of the body to metabolize the essential amino acid, phenylalanine, so that phenylalanine is lost in the urine. Secondary deficiency diseases will be discussed in later chapters.

Extent of malnutrition

Human misery and waste of human life from malnutrition, more stark in some regions than in others, occur in both world hemispheres. These effects are more profound and widespread in less developed areas of the world, but are present in the more developed nations also. The course that is already set by a mounting population must collide with the less rapidly growing (and in many areas, diminishing) food supplies. Because of the increasing complexity of society, many persons have only begun to glimpse the magnitude of future needs. The problem is further compounded by the fact that population growth rates often are highest in those countries which can least afford to maintain them. For example, the population of Latin America is the most rapidly growing in the world. Its rate of growth (up to 3.8% a year) is about 1½ times that of the world rate (2% a year). The rapidity of this expansion will lead the Latin America countries to double their population within a generation. In North America the rate of growth is only 1.4% a year.[3]

In many areas, the dangerous race between population growth and the rate of increase in food supply is already being lost. In Latin America, for example, during the last two decades total food production has increased 69%. But the more rapid expansion in population is actually causing a decreasing per capita food supply.[4]

Infant and child mortality and morbidity provide an index to the extent of general malnutrition. In Latin America, in the 1- to 4-year age group, the death rate is twenty to thirty times as high as in the United States and Canada (Fig. 16-1). In some areas the rate is even 50% higher. If the rates of infant and child mortality in Latin America were as low as those in the United States and Canada, 250,000 fewer children in this age group would die each year.[5]

Still more disturbing examples could be cited for other regions in the world, such as parts of Africa, India, the Orient, and the Middle East (Fig. 16-2). The problem is urgent. It is becoming more so.

THE ECOLOGY OF MALNUTRITION

The word "ecology" comes from a Greek word *oikos*, meaning "house." Just as there are many factors and forces within a family's house which interact to influence its

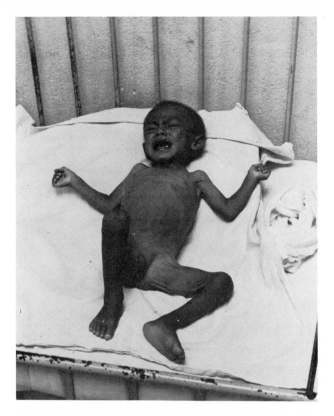

Fig. 16-1. A child in Guatemala suffering from acute malnutrition. Many young children in Latin America die each year from lack of food. (FAO photograph by Y. Nagata.)

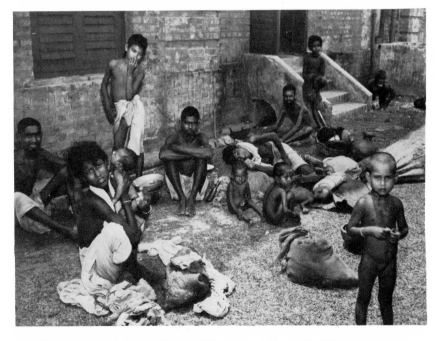

Fig. 16-2. Famine victims in East Pakistan. (FAO photograph by W. Williams.)

members, so there is an even more vast complex of interrelated forces housed in a biological system which produces disease. Many factors work together to produce malnutrition. A disease caused by malnutrition may exist in many varieties, many degrees, and many combinations. It is often complicated by the presence of other diseases, such as tuberculosis, intestinal parasites, or skin sepsis. A synergism is, in fact, known to exist between malnutrition and infection. Each compounds the other, and together they cause more serious illness than either would bring alone. For example, a common infectious disease of childhood such as measles, which would otherwise be mild, in a severely malnourished child may cause death. Infectious diarrhea is a common complication of kwashiorkor, and may be the irreversible factor that causes death.

Some of the many related causes of malnutrition can be classed under the three factors that are classically cited by the epidemiologist as the triad of variables that influences disease: (1) agent, (2) host, and (3) environment.

Agent. The agent that is the fundamental cause of a malnutrition disease is *a lack of food.* Because of this lack, certain nutrients in food which are essential to the sustenance of cellular activity are missing. Various factors may cause or modify this lack of food:

1. *Food quantity.* The total quantity of food ingested may be below the level required to maintain the body tissues. The food deficiency may be partial or complete, seasonal or constant.
2. *Imbalance between community food supply and need.* The amount of food available per person may be reduced by natural disaster (drought, flood), or by man-made disaster (war, overpopulation, poor distribution, poverty).
3. *Food quality.* The food available may be of poor physical quality or biological value.
4. *Food timing.* The food may not be presented (as in infant and child feed-

ing) when needed, in proper balance.

Host. The host is the person—infant, child, adult—who suffers from malnutrition. Various characteristics in the host may influence the disease.

1. *Presence of other disease.* Infections, allergies, metabolic diseases, gastrointestinal diseases, and so on compound the course of malnutrition.
2. *Increased dietary needs.* Any physiologic cause of stress such as growth, pregnancy, lactation, injury, illness, or physical labor increases the demand for nutrients.
3. *Congenital defects.* Premature birth or anatomical defects such as cleft palate influence food intake.
4. *Personal factors.* Ignorance of food needs or food values, carelessness, lack of education, emotional problems, indolence, poor habits, and anorexia influence the kind and amount of food consumed.

Environment. Many environmental factors influence malnutrition. Some are close at hand and may be controlled by the individual. Many more far-reaching ones are too enormous, too powerful, and too remote in their source to be influenced by a single person. Mass action and extensive study are needed to deal with these problems. The following are some of the environmental problems:

1. *Sanitation.* Food contamination causes food loss and produces disease, thus compounding malnutrition.
2. *Culture.* Traditional food habits and customs may hinder nutrition.
3. *Social factors.* Interrelated social problems, such as those created by poverty, racial discrimination, inadequate housing, and family disintegration, may contribute to lack of food and to malnutrition.
4. *Psychological factors.* An example of the many psychological problems that may contribute to malnutrition is maternal deprivation, which may lead to actual or felt rejection of a child, and inadequate feeding.

5. *Economic and political structure.* The economic and political system of a region, which controls the power structure, governs administrative policy and controls channels of food supply and form.

6. *Agriculture.* Geography, climate, food technology, and methods of agriculture influence food supply. What food can and will be produced is determined by the natural resources and their degree of development.

The interaction of some of these factors leading to malnutrition may be visualized in Fig. 16-3.

PROTEIN-CALORIE MALNUTRITION (PCM)

Millions of children throughout the world are exposed to various degrees of protein-calorie malnutrition. It is a health problem of major proportions, which causes a high rate of morbidity and death in children. Its long range effects in those who survive are still incompletely understood. Ritchie Calder,[6] a widely known British writer on science and international affairs, recently voiced the question in the minds of many health workers, "Are the world's malnourished children of today already being maimed in frame and brain as citizens of 1984?" If the suspicions of many investigators are correct, such as those held by Dr. D. B. Jelliffe[7] as a result of his work in Uganda, East Africa, many undernourished populations will prove unable to achieve their full mental, social, and behavioral potential because of a possible long-term effect on brain growth. Should this effect be confirmed, it adds another compelling reason for making an extended effort to combat this widespread public health problem.

In protein-calorie malnutrition a broad clinical spectrum exists between *kwashiorkor* on the one hand and *marasmus* on the other, with many continuous overlapping conditions in between where features of both are found. Although considerable variability is seen, distinctions usually are based upon the nature of the dietary deficiency. In kwashiorkor calories may be sufficient but protein is lacking; in marasmus both calories and protein are deficient.

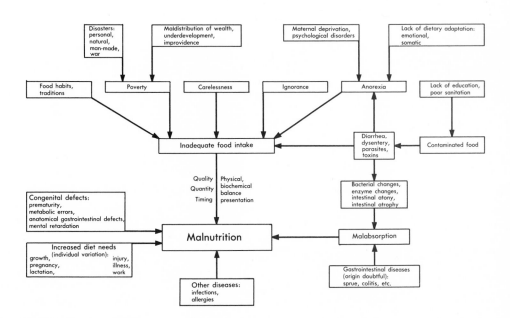

Fig. 16-3. The multiple etiology of malnutrition. (Adapted from Williams, C. D.: Malnutrition, Lancet **2:**342, 1962.)

Kwashiorkor

Identification. The name *kwashiorkor* was first used by Dr. Cecily Williams, in describing her observations and work in the early 1930's with children in Ghana (then known as the Gold Coast). The word comes from the Ghan language and may have several meanings, all usually associated with the mystique of jealousy between siblings, and of physical sickness. It means "the sickness the older child gets when the next baby is born." Sometimes the name "kwashiorkor" is given to the younger child; when his older sibling becomes ill, his sickness is said to be caused by the birth of the second child. Originally, a related meaning of "redness" (derived from the characteristic color of the skin in this disease, which results from depigmentation) was attached to the word, but it is now believed that this interpretation is less correct.

The name is appropriate, for kwashiorkor is the syndrome that develops in a child who, after being weaned from the breast at about the age of one year, on the birth of the next sibling, is given a diet consisting largely of starchy gruels or sugar-water. Such a sequence of events is typical of many cultures in the underdeveloped parts of the world. Before he was weaned, the infant received, in the breast milk, protein and calories adequate for growth. The sharply curtailed diet, based on such starchy foods as tubers (manioc, cassava) or grains (maize), may supply adequate calories as carbohydrate, but its protein content is qualitatively and quantitatively inadequate. Various clinical pictures are determined by local food patterns, involving different degrees of calorie and vitamin deficiencies.

General symptoms. The classical syndrome of kwashiorkor comprises retardation of growth and development with peevish mental apathy (Fig. 16-4), edema, muscular wasting, depigmentation of hair and skin, characteristic scaly changes in skin texture (a "flaky paint" dermatosis, Fig. 16-5), hypoalbuminemia, reversible fatty infiltration of the liver, atrophy of the acini

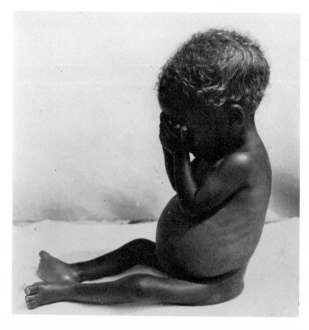

Fig. 16-4. A little African child suffering from kwashiorkor. Note uncurled, graying hair, edema, and skin lesions. (FAO photograph by M. Autret.)

of the pancreas with reduction of the enzymatic activity of the duodenal juice, diarrhea, and moderate anemia (usually normochromic, but occasionally slightly macrocytic). Frequently associated are infections and severe vitamin A deficiency, resulting in permanent blindness. Serious deterioration of patients with kwashiorkor is caused by infections and diarrhea.

Fluid and electrolytes. A consistent characteristic of kwashiorkor is the specific disturbance in water and electrolyte metabolism. Total body water increases and there is marked reduction of total body potassium and retention of sodium. The sodium partially replaces the last of the intracellular potassium, a derangement that critically affects important cell enzyme systems which are normally dependent upon potassium. Factors probably responsible for these fluid and electrolyte disturbances are hypoalbuminemia, endocrine dysfunction, and circulatory failure. A magnesium deficit, similar to that of potassium, has also been described and may also affect cell enzyme function.

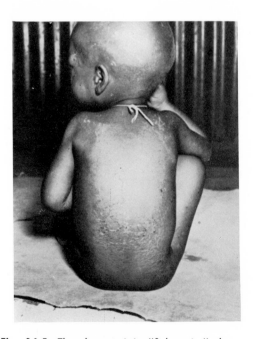

Fig. 16-5. The characteristic "flaky-paint" dermatosis of kwashiorkor.

Fat metabolism. An abnormality of blood lipid transport has also been found in kwashiorkor, which may account for the extremely low levels of vitamin A (the primary fat-soluble vitamin) that characterize the syndrome. There are also alterations in fat synthesis and catabolism. Some studies indicate probable deficiency of essential fatty acids.

Protein metabolism. An extreme protein depletion reaches different degrees in different organs and tissues. Those tissues with faster protein turnover (such as the mucosa and secretory glands in the gastrointestinal system) are affected most. Protein concentrations important to metabolic function, as in enzymes and blood plasma, are greatly disturbed; and there is an extreme decrease in plasma free amino acids.

Vitamins and minerals. Blood levels of vitamins, especially vitamin A, are low. The overall decrease in metabolism, and therefore in the metabolic demand for vitamins, may be so profound that clinical signs of vitamin deficiency may not appear. A similar relationship appears to exist in most cases for iron and copper.

Etiology. Kwashiorkor results from protein malnutrition. Specifically, it results from insufficient quantity or quality of protein (usually both) to meet the demands of growth and cell repair, in the presence of more nearly adequate amounts of calories, usually from starchy foodstuffs. Hunger demands calories, not necessarily protein; and protein foods are more expensive and difficult to produce than starchy foods. Protein deficiency is therefore the lot of a major part of the underprivileged world. Protein *quality* refers to the capacity of a given protein, gram for gram, to promote growth and cell repair. This capacity is usually expressed in terms of biological value (B.V.). The biological value of a given protein is dependent upon the total nitrogen content per 100 calories and the amino acid pattern per gram of nitrogen. Thus, a high quality protein food supplies essential amino acids in the relative amounts required (see Amino Acid Proportionality Pattern p. 000), and supplies in addition sufficient nitrogen for synthesis of the nonessential amino acids which the body needs to build for its own use, and for synthesis of tissue protein and other nitrogen-containing compounds.

Occurrence. Kwashiorkor is usually seen in children in the postweaning years, ages 1 to 4. Particularly in certain areas such as South Africa and Trinidad, where urban mothers practice early weaning so that they may return to paid jobs, it may be seen in younger infants. Kwashiorkor occurs in tropical and subtropical areas, usually in regions where economic, social, and cultural factors combine to make sufficient protein unavailable to the child. It has been shown to be a public health problem in 19 of the 21 countries of the Americas, in all of the countries and territories of Africa south of the Sahara, in India, and in most countries of the Middle and Far East.[8]

Control. Prevention depends upon solution of the socioeconomic factors that underlie the disease. A twofold program adapted to meet individual community needs must include: (1) education concerning improved available sources of dietary protein, (skimmed milk powder, le-

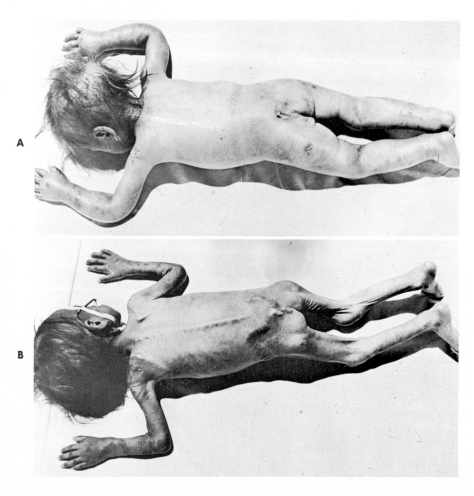

Fig. 16-6. A, Two-year-old child being treated for kwashiorkor. **B,** Two weeks after beginning treatment, edema has disappeared and skin lesions have improved. Note the muscular wasting which had been concealed by the edema. (Courtesy, Pan American Sanitary Bureau, Regional Office of The World Health Organization.)

gumes, fish meal) and (2) motivation to provide adequate food, and means for procuring it.

Treatment. During the first 24 hours of therapy, correction of water and potassium depletion should have priority, especially if diarrhea has been severe. Such correction may prevent sudden death from heart failure. A potassium-containing electrolyte solution such as Darrow's solution is given orally, unless vomiting necessitates intravenous administration. Transfusion of blood and plasma may also be required in severe cases. Beginning on the second day, skimmed milk (usually dry) is given, in a dilution yielding first 10 calories per ounce, then 15. In cases of aggravated digestive disturbance, a formula of lactic acid in fresh skimmed milk (12.5 ml. lactic acid to each ounce of milk) may be used. The size and spacing of feedings are calculated on the basis of individual need. The aim is to provide a protein intake of about 50 grams per day (150 grams of dried skimmed milk). Whole milk should be avoided during the first week because fat is poorly tolerated and may cause diarrhea. Apathetic children usually require hand-feeding. Diuresis, occurring after about seven days of treatment, indicates a favorable response to initial therapy (Fig. 16-6). Thereafter, the caloric content of the diet is increased by the addition of mixed foods suitable to the child's age, which also supply sufficient vitamins and minerals. To give vitamin concentrates during these first two weeks is unnecessary and may even be dangerous.

Marasmus

Identification. The word marasmus comes from a Greek word *marasmos,* which means "wasting." It is applied to the state of chronic total undernutrition in children, which represents a deficiency of both protein and calories in various degrees of severity, and produces a gradual wasting away of body tissue with general emaciation.

General symptoms. Marasmus is characterized by gross underweight. Some children appear almost cadaverous—a living skeleton, skin and bones. There is atrophy of both muscle mass and subcutaneous fat, giving a shrunken, wizened, "old man" appearance to the face (Fig. 16-7), in contrast to the fat, rounded cheeks of children with kwashiorkor. There is little or no dermatosis or depigmentation. Edema is minimal or absent. Diarrhea is common. It may result from infection or from pathogenic microorganisms in the stools, or there may be pre-existing nutritional diarrhea complicated by superimposed infection. Growth rate declines progressively; there are both physical stunting, and mental and emotional impairment. The infant sleeps restlessly, is fretful, apathetic, and withdrawn. Body temperature may be subnormal because of the absence of the insulation that is normally provided by subcutaneous fat, and the child must be kept warm. Metabolic activity is minimal; the heart is weak and urine is scanty; prostration is common.

Fluid and electrolytes. As in kwashiorkor, sodium depletion may occur, especially if diarrhea persists. Little or no water retention is present, in contrast to the gross edema of kwashiorkor.

Fat metabolism. In marasmus, fat absorption, as demonstrated by normal vitamin A absorption, appears to be somewhat less impaired than in kwashiorkor. The enzyme systems for digestion, mechanisms for transport of fat through intestinal wall, and sufficiency of lipid transport protein are conserved for a longer period in this disease.

Protein metabolism. Although serum protein levels are diminished, they are higher than those in kwashiorkor. As general wasting occurs and metabolism approaches basal levels (because amino acids are not provided either endogenously from muscle catabolism or exogenously by the diet), the liver suffers acute and severe protein depletion and loss of its amino acid pool.

Vitamins and minerals. Body stores gradually decline. However, absorption of vitamin A remains normal for some time, in contrast to the depressed absorption in kwashiorkor.

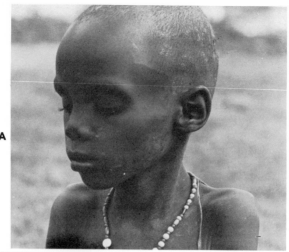

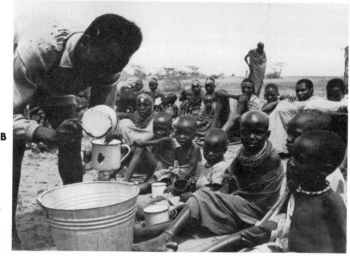

Fig. 16-7. A, African boy suffering from marasmus. His eyesight is poor and his body is emaciated. **B,** The boy's village in Kenya. Victims of famine caused by drought. This soup, brought in twice a week by Red Cross volunteers, is the only nourishing food available. (FAO photographs by Pierre Pittet.)

Hormones. Glucocorticoid secretion remains high in marasmus and is low in kwashiorkor. This important distinction explains many of the differences between the syndromes. When glucocorticoid secretion fails, kwashiorkor develops rapidly, though the exact mechanism of this failure, which follows when caloric intake greatly exceeds that of protein, is unknown.

Etiology. Marasmus is caused by chronic dietary undernutrition, both of calories and of protein; gradual deterioration of body function and atrophy result. Usually deprivation is complete—food, general physical care, and emotional care are all lacking. Such profound deprivation may be found in three basic circumstances. The parents may be poor, and they are often ignorant of food values, so that they do not seek proper food. The parents may have severe mental or emotional problems. This is especially dangerous for the child when the mother is disturbed. She may reject the child and fail to give it care. There may be other disease, such as tuberculosis, chronic gastro-enteritis, dysentery, infectious diarrhea, or parasites, with concomitant lack of proper medical care. All of these conditions thrive in poor socioeconomic settings and the child is caught in these circumstances.

Occurrence. Marasmus is most common in infants 6 to 18 months of age. It occurs in slum conditions in any country where socioeconomic deprivation breeds such diseases. In tropical and subtropical areas, it occurs in much the same pattern in under-developed countries as does kwashiorkor.

Control. Prevention depends upon eradicating the underlying causes of the disease, and thus upon solution of the socioeconomic problems. Treatment follows much the same pattern as that given for kwashiorkor, with initial correction of electrolyte imbalances and a gradual refeeding program. Since rejection and total deprivation are commonly a part of the etiologic picture, treatment also involves gradually holding the infant, as tenderness of his body

allows, keeping the child warm, and the provision of much loving care.

Table 16-1 gives a comparison of the symptoms of kwashiorkor and marasmus.

VITAMIN DEFICIENCY DISEASES
Xerophthalmia

Identification. Xerophthalmia (Gr. *xēros,* dry; *ophthalmos,* eye) is a disease of the eye in which the cornea and conjunctiva become dry. It results from extreme deficiency of vitamin A. The dryness is a consequence of metaplasia of the conjunctiva, causing roughness. Metaplasia of the para-ocular glands leads to a loss of their secretions. Infection usually follows. Early signs are drying, roughness, and wrinkling of the conjunctiva, swelling and redness of the lids, and pain and photophilia. Dry, luster-less patches may be seen on the conjunctiva, and triangular, whitish, foamy spots (Bitot's spots) occur at the limbus conjunctivae. The cornea loses sensitivity, becomes clouded, and ulcers may form. If the disease

Table 16-1. General comparison of symptoms in kwashiorkor and marasmus

Symptom	Kwashiorkor	Marasmus
Growth retardation	x	x
Underweight	x (masked by edema)	x
Apathy, behavioral changes	x	x
Edema	x	—
Muscular wasting	x	x
Depigmentation	x	—
Dermatosis	x	—
Hypoalbuminemia	x	—
Fatty liver	x	—
Diarrhea	x	x
Moderate anemia	x	x
Infection (usual)	x	x
Potassium and electrolyte imbalance (hypokalemia)	x	x
Abnormal fat metabolism	x	—
Low vitamin A absorption	x	—
Protein depletion	x	x
Low body temperature	—	x
Glucocorticoids	—	x

is untreated, the cornea softens (keratomalacia) and perforation may occur, resulting in total blindness.

Night blindness (inability to see in dim light) may also result from lack of vitamin A, and is an early sign of deficiency. Its manifestations vary in degree. A dark-adaptation test is used to determine the rate at which a person's vision is recovered after the visual purple in the retina has been bleached by bright light (see p. 74).

Skin changes also appear in vitamin A deficiency (see Fig. 6-1, p. 75). The skin becomes dry and rough. Papular eruptions occur at the sites of hair follicles, usually on the skin of the thighs and the upper arms, and spread to abdomen and back. The term *phrynoderma* or "toad's skin" has been given to these dermal changes.

Epithelial tissue changes may also occur in prolonged vitamin A deficiency. Degeneration or atrophy of mucous linings in the gastrointestinal and urinary systems become involved and structural changes have been described in the enamel of teeth and in the nervous system. Histologic studies reveal atrophy of glandular tissue and hyperkeratosis.

Etiology. The clinical manifestations are due to a deficiency of preformed vitamin A and its precursor, carotene. Vitamin A is found in animal foods such as liver, dairy fat and eggs, and as carotene in plant foods such as green leafy vegetables, carrots, sweet potatoes, mango, artichokes, and papaya.

The deficiency of vitamin A may be caused by an inadequate diet source (primary deficiency), or a disorder which leads to poor absorption or to poor conversion of carotene (conditional deficiency).

Occurrence. Vitamin A deficiency is one of the commonest nutritional deficiency states. Keratomalacia is typically observed in young children. It is still a major cause of blindness in certain underdeveloped countries. For example, in Indonesia many thousands of cases occur each year and WHO estimates that 5% of all the children in Indonesia have impaired vision or are blind because of vitamin A deficiency.[9] In fact, the entire child population there exists on such a borderline vitamin A level that when a large quantity of free skimmed milk was distributed recently, the increased protein intake caused xerophthalmia and keratomalacia by increasing the attendant requirement for vitamin A. The distribution of the skimmed milk had to be halted until vitamin A capsules could be obtained and given with it.[10] If whole milk had been given, this would not have happened, for natural vitamin A would have been consumed in the cream. Economic factors made the use of skimmed milk necessary.

Control. Prevention is based on education concerning food sources of vitamin A, and the inclusion of more fruits and vegetables in the diet. Treatment is administration of vitamin A, in doses determined by the severity of the clinical condition. Caution should be observed, to avoid hypervitaminosis A from excessive intake. Acute hypervitaminosis A can occur only with a single massive dose (over 1 million I.U.) and is therefore seldom seen. Chronic states have been observed in children who received large amounts (about 100,000 I.U. per day) of vitamin A concentrate over some months. The symptoms of such intoxication are anorexia, growth failure, irritability, skeletal lesions with pain in extremities and periosteal bone thickening, skin itching, fissures at mouth and nose corners, coarsening of hair, and alopecia. The symptoms disappear promptly when the excessive intake is discontinued.

Beriberi

Identification. The clinical picture of beriberi varies according to the age of the patient, and the body tissues primarily affected; but the neuromuscular system is usually involved. The two general types of beriberi are infantile beriberi and adult beriberi.

Infantile beriberi, occurring during the first year of life, is characterized by various symptoms in different cases: convulsive disorders, abrupt onset, respiratory difficulties, and gastrointestinal problems such as constipation and vomiting. Terminal symptoms in severe cases include cyanosis, dyspnea, and tachycardia; sudden death occurs a few hours after onset.[11]

Adult beriberi, usually seen in young adults who are experiencing additional physiological stress such as pregnancy and lactation, may be either a dry or wet form, according to the absence or presence of edema. The symptoms usually result from involvement of the peripheral nerves and related muscle function. First, there may be tingling and numbness of extremities, leg muscle cramps, and later involvement of muscles of the forearms, thighs, and abdominal wall. Paralysis may result. As the heart muscle becomes involved, cardiorespiratory symptoms follow quickly—palpitation, tachycardia, dyspnea, cyanosis, and circulatory collapse. Vomiting and consti-

pation are usually present. The edema in wet beriberi begins in the legs and progresses upward (Fig. 16-8).

Laboratory findings. Since thiamine functions primarily as a coenzyme in glucose metabolism (especially in the conversion of pyruvic acid, see p. 90), laboratory findings in the deficiency disease are related to levels of pyruvic acid and thiamine. There is increased concentration of pyruvic acid in the blood, and decreased levels of body thiamine are noted in urine, circulating blood, and secretions such as breast milk of nursing mothers. Thiamine test loads are used to indicate general body stores.

Etiology. Beriberi is caused by a deficiency of thiamine. Diets based principally on refined cereal grains, such as the polished rice diet found in the Orient, are deficient in thiamine and contribute to development of the disease. A patient may have subsisted on minimal body thiamine stores until additional physiological needs (pregnancy and lactation) increased the requirement for thiamine. When these increased requirements were not met, the disease ensued. Infection and gastrointestinal disturbances affecting absorption may also be precipitating factors.

Occurrence. In children, beriberi occurs mainly during the first year of life. It is seen more often in young adults than in the aged. Persons of both sexes are about equally likely to be affected, except that women are made somewhat more susceptible during the physiological stress of pregnancy and lactation. The disease usually is found among low-income groups, or those ignorant of the need for an adequate diet. Beriberi is endemic in many areas of the worlds such as Japan, Indonesia, China, Malaya, India, Burma, the Philippines, and Brazil. For example, in Thailand, Burma, and Vietnam, it is a major cause of death among infants two to five months of age.[12] Its incidence is actually increasing in some parts of Asia, such as Thailand, where gasoline-driven rice mills have replaced handpounding in small villages. The motordriven rice mills remove more of the hull

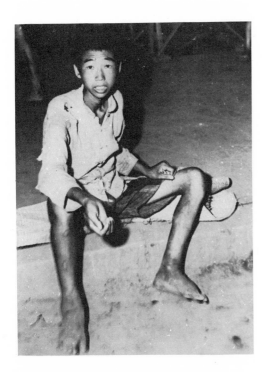

Fig. 16-8. Chinese refugee boy, suffering from multiple nutritional deficiencies. Note the edema in feet and legs, characteristic of wet beriberi. (UNRRA photograph released by FAO.)

and the thiamine-containing germ of the grain; pregnant women therefore eat less thiamine in their food, and mothers secrete less in their milk.[13]

In the Western world, beriberi usually occurs in a milder form and may be associated with other disease. It may occur in poverty-stricken areas, in conjunction with general states of malnutrition, or among persons with alcoholism, in pregnant women with a history of poor diet, in the inmates of some prisons, or in hospitals for the chronically ill geriatric patient or for the mentally ill.

Control. Prevention of beriberi is based upon improvement in economics and education. The aim of such measures is to supply diets adequate in thiamine. General measures of control include laws governing refinement of cereal grains and their enrichment, use of parboiled or converted rice where it is accepted, use of thiamine tablets, brewer's yeast, or extract of rice polishings ("tikitiki") by members of stress groups in the population (expectant and nursing mothers), and education concerning wider food choices and cooking methods to minimize loss of thiamine.

Treatment. In acute infantile beriberi, parenterally administered thiamine is given immediately, 10 to 25 mg. daily. After severe symptoms subside and orally administered thiamine is tolerated, it is continued in oral form at the rate of from 10 to 30 mg. daily until the patient is free of symptoms. Lactating mothers with latent or manifest symptoms should be given 25 to 50 mg. thiamine daily. Both mother and child should continue to receive supplementary thiamine and, in addition, other B-complex vitamins (niacin, pyridoxine, and riboflavin). The diet should be rich in thiamine-containing foods.

Ariboflavinosis

Identification. Ariboflavinosis is the term given to a general group of clinical manifestations that characterize the state of riboflavin deficiency. These characteristic findings include seborrheic dermatitis, cheilosis,

and eye lesions. *Seborrheic dermatitis* is localized to skin folds, as in the groin area, behind the ears, the edges of the nose, and the canthi (angles at either end of the slit between the eyelids). The skin becomes reddened and covered with small, greasy flakes. Hard, sebaceous plugs may develop and project from pores on the nose, cheeks, or forehead. *Cheilosis* is a swelling and reddening of the lips, giving a chapped appearance, with fissures developing at the corners of the mouth. These fissured lesions extend onto the facial skin, rather than into the oral mucosa. Scars of previous lesions are sometimes seen also. *Eye lesions* are less frequently seen. They include photophobia and itching—a feeling of irritation frequently described as "sand in the eyes." The conjunctiva is engorged, there is constant watery secretion (lacrimation: L., *lacrima,* tear), and a capillary overgrowth occurs around the cornea.

Etiology. Diets deficient in riboflavin, one of the B-complex vitamins, induce these symptoms. Such diets are lacking in animal protein foods such as milk, meat, or fish; and in leafy vegetables and legumes—all sources of riboflavin. Riboflavin deficiency frequently develops in association with deficiencies of other B-vitamins such as niacin and thiamine, in situations of poverty, ignorance, chronic alcoholism, or illness such as prolonged diarrhea.

Occurrence. Riboflavin deficiency occurs in many underdeveloped areas, such as parts of Africa, Asia, India, Indonesia, the Caribbean, and Newfoundland. It is rarely seen in the United States, although it was formerly a public health problem in the southern states.

Methods of control. A supply of foods containing adequate amounts of riboflavin is basic to prevention. Riboflavin is easily destroyed by exposure to light. Such good sources as milk must be protected from excessive exposure to light in order to ensure retention of their riboflavin content. Other sources that may be incorporated into the diet in any of various forms include cheese, meats, whole grain or enriched cereals, eggs, legumes, nuts, and most vegetables. Foods used as staples in a given country (wheat flour, cornmeal, rice, bread) may be the focus of an enrichment program. In the United States, such basic foods are usually enriched with riboflavin.

Acute ariboflavinosis is treated by the oral administration of 10 to 20 mg. of riboflavin daily, divided into several doses, replacement of attendant vitamin deficiencies by the administration of other vitamins, and a generally well-balanced diet containing from 3,000 to 3,500 calories.

Pellagra

Identification. Clinical manifestations of pellagra, a disease resulting from niacin deficiency, are of four types. *Gastrointestinal disturbances* include anorexia, general indigestion, weight loss, and diarrhea (which is often severe). *Stomatitis* is a swelling and reddening of the tongue, with hypertrophy, then atrophy, of the papillae. The entire buccal mucosa becomes involved with reddening, a burning sensation, and tissue erosion. *Dermatitis* is a highly characteristic sign of pellagra. The lesions resemble burned areas, and become much more painful upon exposure to sunlight. The dermatitis occurs most often on exposed portion of the skin (hands, forearms, feet, lower legs, neck, and face), but may also be seen in skin folds, where the surface is subject to irritation, as around the scrotum, vulvae, and anus. Infection often occurs as the lesions rupture. Healing leaves darkly pigmented areas. *Neurological change* includes mental apathy, depression, and anxiety of various degrees. In extreme cases, serious disorientation, confusion, and dementia may occur.

Etiology. Pellagra is caused by a deficiency of niacin (a B-complex vitamin) and the amino acid tryptophan, a precursor of niacin. Upon its conversion in the body, about 60 gm. of tryptophan yields 1 mg. of niacin; hence, 60 gm. of tryptophan is called a "niacin equivalent." The incidence of pellagra is especially high in populations whose staple food is corn, because corn is low in both tryptophan and niacin. Pellagra may also be a conditioned response complicating other chronic disease involving diarrhea or poor food intake, or in chronic alcoholism with associated general malnutrition.

Occurrence. In the southern United States, especially in rural areas, pellagra was formerly widespread. However, since wheat flour, cornmeal, and other grains have been enriched, and since the general diet has been improved, pellagra is seen only occasionally in areas of poverty or in association with other disease affecting food intake or food utilization. Pellagra still occurs in parts of Egypt, Romania, and southern Yugoslavia, mostly in rural areas and villages where the diet tends to be little varied.

Control. Pellagra is prevented by a diet adequate in tryptophan and niacin. The dietary recommendation is stated in terms of niacin equivalents (17 to 21 mg. equivalents daily) to include tryptophan sources as well as preformed niacin. Nutrition education should focus on available food sources, enrichment possibilities (especially for cornmeal, because it is often the staple food of patients with this disease), and dietary variety. Agricultural improvements to extend livestock production and crop diversification are fundamental to maintenance of adequate dietary resources.

Patients with acute pellagra require large amounts of niacin, usually as much as 300 to 500 or more mg. of niacinamide daily. Usually a multivitamin preparation is given also, and a balanced diet furnishing about 3,000 calories, adequate amounts of good quality protein, and foods rich in niacin.

Pyridoxine (vitamin B₆) deficiency

Identification. A deficiency of pyridoxine has been reported to cause convulsions and hypochromic anemia in infants. Adults with multiple vitamin deficiency states characterized by muscle weakness and fatigue have responded to pyridoxine therapy. Additional proof of the effects of pyridoxine deficiency on the nervous system is the fact that an antagonist of pyridoxine, isonicotinic acid hydrazide (isoniazid), which is used in the treatment of pulmonary tuberculosis, causes peripheral neuritis and occasional convulsions. The hypochromic anemia occurring with these neurological symptoms is thought to be caused by alteration of cellular metabolism of vitamin B_6.

When the diet is deficient in pyridoxine, or when the metabolism of vitamin B_6 is obstructed by an antagonist such as isoniazid, products of abnormal metabolism of the amino acid tryptophan (such as xanthurenic acid) appear in the urine. A tryptophan-load test (giving 10 gm. of the amino acid in water or fruit juice, then measuring the urinary output of xanthurenic acid) may therefore be used to determine the presence of pyridoxine deficiency. Women in the latter half of pregnancy may evidence vitamin B_6 deficiencies in response to such tests, yet give no clinical evidence of deficiency.

Etiology. Since vitamin B_6 occurs in many natural foods, a deficiency is unlikely to occur in persons taking a well-balanced diet. The only instances of deficiency that have been reported occurred in infants fed a prepared formula in which the pyridoxine content had been destroyed by autoclaving. The convulsions that followed were quickly controlled by administration of vitamin B_6.

Control. The best prevention of pyridoxine deficiency is a mixed diet made up of a wide variety of foods. About 2 mg. of the vitamin a day is adequate for body needs. Additional pyridoxine (5 to 10 mg.) may be required during pregnancy to counteract the altered tryptophan metabolism, and 50 to 100 mg. is needed for protection against the neuritis experienced during treatment with pyridoxine antagonists for other diseases.

Folic acid deficiency
(megaloblastic anemia)

Identification. A deficiency of folic acid in human beings produces a macrocytic anemia associated with megaloblastic arrest in red blood cell production. Production of white blood cells and platelets

is also hindered. Clinical manifestations include: (1) the weakness and pallor usually associated with anemias, and (2) degeneration of surface mucosal tissue, resulting in ulceration and secondary infections, sore tongue, and gastrointestinal disturbances such as diarrhea and poor fat absorption. A similar type of megaloblastic anemia occurs with the deficiency of vitamin B_{12} that is secondary to pernicious anemia. Folic acid deficiency anemia may be distinguished by trial therapy. If the anemia is due to a deficiency of folic acid, a reticulocyte response will be evident within 7 to 10 days after administration of folic acid, and blood values will return to normal.

Etiology. Folic acid deficiency may be due to one of several causes: (1) a primary dietary lack, (2) poor intestinal absorption of the vitamin, or (3) increased metabolic demands, as during late pregnancy and the rapid growth of early infancy, and in concurrent ascorbic acid deficiency.

The diets of persons evidencing nutritional folic acid deficiency are particularly lacking in animal protein foods and green vegetables. These should be supplied from adequate and varied food sources.

Occurrence. Folic acid deficiency occurs usually in conjunction with general malnutrition. The pregnant woman is especially susceptible. The infant also is at risk because of the increased physiological stress of growth, because of infections, or because of ascorbic acid deficiency resulting from a poor diet.

Control. Generally, diets that supply adequate amounts of the other B-complex vitamins will be adequate in folic acid also. Doses of 5 to 20 mg. of folic acid may be given in cases of deficiency. The most intelligent approach to protection against the anemia of folic acid deficiency is the use of a well-balanced, varied diet providing optimum overall nutrition.

Vitamin B_{12} deficiency
(pernicious anemia)

Identification. Clinical manifestations of pernicious anemia are anorexia, nausea, vomiting, diarrhea, abdominal pain, and weight loss. General signs of anemia are present—weakness, dyspnea, and palpitation. There may be a characteristic lemon-yellow tinge to the skin, and the liver and spleen may enlarge. Some patients may experience spinal cord degeneration which produces difficulty in walking, in sense of position, and in vibratory sense in the legs. Characteristic changes in the development of red blood cells result in a wide variety of abnormal sizes and shapes. The normal free gastric hydrochloric acid is absent.

Etiology. The vitamin B_{12} deficiency of pernicious anemia is secondary to an inherent lack of intrinsic factor in the gastric juice. The cause of this defect is not known; heredity is thought to be a factor.

Occurrence. Pernicious anemia occurs most often in middle-aged persons. Seldom is it seen in those under thirty years of age. The rates of occurrence in the two sexes do not differ. It seems to be more common in persons having type A blood than in those having type O blood, and to be more common in white-skinned than in dark-skinned persons.

Control. No means of preventing pernicious anemia is known; however, it may be treated effectively by injecting doses of vitamin B_{12} to bypass the absorption defect. The anemia may also be relieved by the administration of folic acid, but this form of therapy is contraindicated because it fails to control the degenerative changes in the central nervous system.

Iron medication or giving blood by transfusion is usually unnecessary. Rest and a high-protein diet supplemented with a multivitamin preparation provide supportive care.

Scurvy

Identification. Scurvy is a nutritional deficiency disease directly associated with a lack of vitamin C (ascorbic acid). The antiscorbutic activity of the vitamin has been well established.[14-16] Scurvy develops after the body tissue stores of ascorbic acid have been exhausted.

Clinical manifestations. Since ascorbic acid performs many vital physiologic functions, related especially to formation of connective tissue, collagen, and the integrity of capillary walls (see p. 110), the clinical manifestations of scurvy involve tissue deterioration and changes of hemorrhagic origin.

SKIN. The skin becomes dry, rough, and often has a dingy brown color. Scaly, raised areas, called perifollicular hyperkeratotic papules, develop around the hair follicles in the skin. The follicular hemorrhages develop around these papules (see Fig. 7-4, p. 111). These skin changes usually occur on the arms and legs, the buttocks, and the back. Purpura (L., "purple"), hemorrhaging into the skin which produces a reddish-purple discoloration with the appearance of a bruise, appears first on the lower extremities and then spreads upward. Pinpoint hemorrhages produce small red spots called petechiae, which may coalesce into areas of purpura and finally, if large enough, into even larger areas called ecchymoses (G. *ek,* out; *chymos,* juice). Sometimes a whole extremity may be involved with extravasated blood.

MUSCLES. Deep hemorrhages in the muscle tissue may produce brawny areas of induration, resulting from hardening and thickening of the tissue. Phlebothrombosis (clotting in a vein) may follow.

JOINTS. Scurvy may also be manifested by hemorrhages into the cavities of joints, which cause local heat, painful swelling, and immobility. This condition is called *hemarthrosis.* The joint pain causes scorbutic infants to lie in a characteristic position, supine with the knees partially flexed and the thighs externally rotated—the only position of comfort. This position is sometimes called the scorbutic pose.

GUMS. The gums are spongy, friable, grossly swollen, and bleed easily at the slightest touch. As tissue hemorrhaging continues, thromboses form in the blood vessels and infarcts occur, producing blue-red discoloration. The teeth become loosened and may fall out. Infection is frequent.

FAILURE OF WOUND HEALING. Any trauma, even small, produces ulcerated areas. New wounds fail to heal, or if they are apparently healed, they break open again under the slightest stress.

ANEMIA. Anemia usually accompanies scurvy. It is due partially to hemorrhagic blood loss, but also to the erroneous metabolic interrelationships of vitamin C with folic acid and with iron. Concurrent deficiency of other nutrients also contributes to the anemia.

Age variance. Since the clinical picture of scurvy is modified by growth, the manifestations vary with the patient's age.

Adult scurvy is characterized by general weakness, lassitude, irritability, and vague, dull, aching pains in the muscles and joints of the lower extremities. There may be weight loss and dyspnea. The classic hemorrhagic changes occur in skin, muscles, and gums. The levels of vitamin C in the blood and urine are below normal.

Infantile scurvy differs from that found in adults because the reaction to vitamin C deficiency in the growing bones of children differs from that in the mature bones of adults. The growing ends of long bones in infants and children are particularly affected by insufficiency of vitamin C. Microscopic fractures, small defects or cracks, occur, associated with bleeding into the subperiosteal space. These defects progress to separation of the epiphyses and malformation of the bone, as calcified cartilage which has not been destroyed or withdrawn as in the normal process, piles up in the zone of provisional calcification. This gives the long bone the shape of a club. Characteristic changes occur also in the growing ribs. Because of the pull of the respiratory muscles, the costochondral junctions are deformed. The central part of the chest is sunken and there is a sharp prominence of the bony ends of the ribs (costochondral beading).

Etiology. Scurvy results directly from a dietary lack of vitamin C. The most concentrated food sources of this vitamin are citrus fruits, tomatoes, and odd plants such as the acerola, a cherry-like fruit grown in tropical regions. Additional sources include other fruits and vegetables such as berries

and potato. Human milk has an appreciable vitamin C content (4 to 8 mg. per 100 ml.). Commercially prepared cows' milk, however, has almost none, as this vitamin is destroyed by pasteurization and other processing. Breast-fed infants, therefore, secure a sufficient supply of vitamin C, whereas bottle-fed infants require vitamin C supplementation.

Scurvy is most likely to occur in persons subsisting on limited, monotonous diets. Three groups are most at risk: (1) infants fed processed cows' milk and little else, with no vitamin supplementation, (2) men living alone, preparing their own meals, subsisting on little more than cereals, bread, and milk, and (3) psychoneurotic individuals eating bizarre diets. For example, a case of advanced scurvy was recently reported in a thirty-six-year-old woman who had been following a ritualistic Zen macrobiotic diet.[17]

Occurrence. Normally, infants are born with vitamin C adequate for several months, so that infantile scurvy rarely occurs before the age of 4 months. Peak incidence is at about nine months of age, with some cases occurring at about two years of age. Under normal conditions, after age 2, children usually eat enough of the adult diet to prevent the clinical disease. However, certain groups of children are at greater risk, for example, institutionalized or defective children. Among adults, scurvy occurs more frequently in the aged because diets are more likely to be insufficient.

As the American public has become better informed about food values, ascorbic acid supplementation, and available food sources, the incidence of scurvy has greatly decreased in the United States. However, as recently as 1955, a rise in the incidence of scurvy in Canada led the American Academy of Pediatrics to conduct a survey in the United States, which revealed 713 pediatric cases of scurvy, and a hospital admission rate of about one patient with scurvy in every 3,300 admissions.[18]

Control. Scurvy can be prevented by a well-balanced diet which includes some primary sources of vitamin C, such as citrus fruits, or a wide variety of secondary sources in fruits and vegetables (leafy greens, potatoes). Cases of frank scurvy respond quickly and dramatically to therapeutic doses of vitamin C of about 200 mg. or more daily. For example, all bleeding ceases in twenty-four hours, gums heal in three or four days, and a leg that has been ecchymotic from hip to heel becomes normal in three weeks on such a regimen.

Rickets

Identification. Rickets, a disease directly related to impaired metabolism of calcium and phosphorus, is manifested in defective bone growth and changes in the body musculature. The impaired mineral metabolism in rickets may have many causes, but by far the commonest cause is a deficiency of vitamin D. The vitamin D may be preformed in food, or formed in the body (the skin) through the action of short ultraviolet radiations such as those in sunlight. Vitamin D is necessary for the absorption of calcium and phosphorus, and for their deposit in bone tissue.

Clinical manifestations. Characteristic clinical manifestations of rickets result from failure of calcification of the growing portions of bones. The resultant rarefaction of bone tissue may be observed by comparing x-rays of rachitic bones with x-rays of corresponding normal bones. The involved bones are deformed by the stress of weight-bearing, or even by the normal pull of attached muscles. Characteristic musculoskeletal and metabolic changes in rickets include the following.

HEAD. The head appears large, due to the development of thickened areas in the temporal and parietal regions of the skull. The top of the skull appears flat, and is often depressed toward the middle. These skull deformities result from lying supine: the continued weight of the brain pressing upon the back of the skull causes thinning of the bones and flattening of the back of the head. Such areas of softening in cranial bones are called areas of *craniotabes*.

LEGS AND ARMS. When the child begins to sit erect, the effect of gravity upon the legs in the sitting position is to pull the epiphyses out of position. Bizarre deformities then develop in several different planes. The result is a combination of bowed thighs and knock-knees. In addition, a deformity called "saber skin" (anterior curving just above the ankle) may occur in the lower end of the tibia as it is tilted backward by the weight of the foot while the child is lying or sitting. Because of his muscular weakness, when the child is sitting he attempts to support his trunk with his outstretched, pronated hands. This pressure causes a knobbing deformity at the wrists and a bowing of the arms. Later, when standing or walking is attempted, the weight of the child's body causes further bowing of the legs (see Fig. 6-2, p. 79).

RIBS. The costochondral junctions become enlarged and knobs form. These appear as rows resembling strings of beads, which run parallel to the sternum and curve outward toward the lower end of the thorax. This beaded effect is the characteristic "rachitic rosary." With time, bending of the ribs and cartilage occurs, which interferes with normal expansion of the chest during respiration. A funnel-shaped depression develops in the lower end of the sternum, in addition to the overall "pigeon-breasted" effect produced by the rickets.

SPINE. Because his muscles are lax and hypotonic, the infant tends to slump when he tries to sit up. Gradual curving of the spine may follow, leading to kyphosis (Gr., "humpback").

ABDOMEN. The lax muscles of the abdomen and intestines may bring about protuberance of the abdomen (Fig. 16-9). Constipation often results from the intestinal atony.

TEETH. Infantile rickets does not affect the first temporary teeth, because these are fairly well-developed at birth; but the dentition of permanent teeth, which are forming during this period, may be affected with resultant alteration in the tooth structure.

TETANY. The impaired balance of calcium

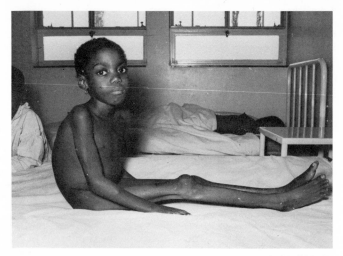

Fig. 16-9. African girl suffering from malnutrition. Note skeletal deformities of spine (kyphosis) and protuberant abdomen, often seen in rickets. (FAO photograph by Pierre Pittet.)

and phosphorus in the body fluids—lowering of the blood calcium, or decrease in the availability of calcium—may produce tetany in the rachitic patient. During the healing period, as calcium is withdrawn from the blood for bone mineralization, the blood calcium may be diminished and may remain low. This lowered level alone may not be sufficient to produce overt tetany; but the stress of a superimposed febrile illness may cause the latent tetany to become manifest in convulsions.

Etiology. In full-term infants, rickets is most commonly produced by a deficiency of vitamin D. In premature infants, deficiencies of calcium and phosphorus contribute to the development of the disease. Since a large amount of the fetal skeleton is mineralized during the last trimester of pregnancy, the body of a baby born four weeks prematurely contains only a little more than half the total calcium present in the normal full-term infant. In addition, the premature infant is smaller than the full-term infant, and so has a more limited food capacity. Finally, human milk rarely can supply his demands for calcium. In these combined circumstances, his rapid growth and slow rate of calcification may cause early, severe rickets. His milk should be fortified both with dried skimmed milk,

to provide sufficient usable mineral to prevent rickets, and with supplementary vitamin D, necessary for utilization of these minerals.

Refractory forms of rickets have been observed, some of which are genetically acquired. A variety of signs appear in different members of the same family.[19] The clinical picture is similar; there are retarded growth and skeletal deformities. However, these unusual forms may be differentiated by their great resistance to vitamin D therapy. For example, a case has been reported in which the serum vitamin D levels were about twenty times greater than normal, and 1 million units of vitamin D daily were required for healing, with a necessary maintenance dose thereafter of 440,000 units daily.[20]

Occurrence. Vitamin D-deficiency rickets is observed most frequently in infants between the ages of six and eighteen months. Rarely does it have its onset after the first two to three years of life. Other forms of rickets are usually first observed after this early period. In all forms, however, disturbance of calcium-phosphorus metabolism is the direct cause of the disease. In the north temperate zone, vitamin D-deficiency rickets has its onset most frequently in the spring. It is unusual in the tropics, where the body is exposed to more sunlight. It occurs more often in dark-skinned races, whose skin pigmentation inhibits the passage of ultraviolet rays. The customary diet of natives in the frigid zone is protective against rickets, as it contains fish oils and animal fat sources of vitamin D. In regions where breast-feeding is practiced the incidence is also reduced, chiefly because the ratio of calcium to phosphorus in human milk is lower than in cows' milk, not because there is a significant difference between the vitamin D content (or lack of vitamin D) in the two milks.

Control. Supplementation of the diet with vitamin D effectively controls rickets. Exposure to sunlight is also effective, but in many areas this is seasonal and limited, thus uncertain as a source of the vitamin. Calcium and phosphorus adequate for human infants are supplied by either human milk or a diluted cows' milk formula. The milk enrichment program presently followed in the United States, in which each quart of milk is fortified with 400 I.U. of vitamin D, has greatly reduced the incidence of vitamin D-deficiency rickets; nevertheless, the disease is still seen despite these preventive measures.

Recovery from rickets follows the usual therapeutic dose of 2,000 to 4,000 units of vitamin D. Extreme skeletal deformities are occasionally corrected surgically, although certain deformities are not amenable to treatment. Many of these decrease with time, however.

Hemorrhagic disease of the newborn (vitamin K deficiency)

Identification. Since vitamin K is fairly widespread in nature, especially in green leaves of various kinds (spinach, cabbage, cauliflower), and is also synthesized by intestinal bacteria, a deficiency is relatively uncommon in adults. Exceptions may exist in patients who lack bile (necessary for the absorption of vitamin K) or in those with intestinal diseases (sprue or chronic diarrhea) which hinder its absorption. However, newborn infants lack stores of vitamin

K at birth, have a sterile gastrointestinal tract and hence no bacterial synthesis, and do not obtain an adequate dietary supply in milk. Therefore, there is a fall in prothrombin activity in the blood during the first few days of life and life-endangering hemorrhages may result.

Etiology. Vitamin K is necessary to the synthesis of prothrombin by the liver (p. 83). If this first stage in the blood clotting mechanism does not proceed, hemorrhaging may result.

Occurrence. Some authorities have estimated that possibly one in every 1,000 newborn infants dies from hemorrhage preventable by treatment with vitamin K. Milder hemorrhage, preventable by treatment, is believed to have a much higher incidence.

Control. Hemorrhagic disease of the newborn can be prevented by giving parenterally small doses of water-soluble vitamin K analogues to newborn infants. Excess amounts of vitamin K may be toxic, even lethal. The Council on Drugs of the American Medical Association has recommended single doses of the water-soluble analogues equivalent to 1 mg. of synthetic vitamin K for prophylaxis and treatment.[21]

MINERAL DEFICIENCY DISEASES
Tetany

Identification. Tetany, first described by Trousseau in 1885, is characterized by neuromuscular irritability which manifests itself in various degrees of intermittent tonic muscle spasm, usually paroxysmal in nature and involving the extremities. Convulsive seizures may follow. The three major manifestations of tetany are:

1. *Carpopedal spasm* (Gr. *karpos*, L. *carpus*, wrist; L. *pedalis*, foot). Tonic contracture of the hands and feet is the most characteristic sign of tetany. In carpal spasm, the thumb is drawn into the cupped palm, the wrist is flexed, and the hands are abducted. The fingers are flexed at the metacarpophalangeal joints, but are extended at the more distal joints. This posture of the hand may be produced in patients with latent tetany by maintaining a firm, con-

stricting grip on the patient's upper arm for two or three minutes. The appearance of carpal spasm (Trousseau's sign) is evidence of latent tetany. In manifest tetany, such spasms occur spontaneously; they may be transitory or may continue for days at a time. In the pedal spasm, the sole of the foot is cupped and the toes are flexed inward. Both the arms and legs may be abducted and rigidly flexed.

2. *Laryngospasm.* The abductor muscles of the larynx spasmodically contract, producing *inspiratory stridor* (L. *stridor,* harsh sound), usually a high-pitched, crowing sound, heard as the patient breathes in. In extreme cases this spasmodic impedance of breathing may cause deep cyanosis; on rare occasions death has occurred during an attack.

3. *Convulsions.* Generalized convulsions may occur at long or short intervals. The patient (usually an infant) becomes unconscious. The body is in a rigidly tonic state with intermittent clonic jerkings. The hands are tightly clenched and held in the carpospasmodic position.

Etiology (serum calcium to phosphorus ratio). Any condition that lowers the blood calcium, or decreases the availability of the calcium that is present in the blood, or produces alkalosis may cause tetany. Ionized calcium, phosphate, carbon dioxide, and the acidity of the blood serum exist together in a relationship which may be expressed as follows:

$$\frac{Ca \times HPO_4 \times HCO_3}{pH} = K$$

K is constant. This indicates that if the carbon dioxide and the pH remain constant, the product of the calcium content (normally 10 to 11 mg. per 100 ml.) and of the phosphate content (normally 3.0 to 3.5 mg. per 100 ml.) of the serum must be constant between 30 and 40. In tetany, the calcium content drops to 6 mg. per 100 ml. and the phosphate rises to 5 or 6 mg. per 100 ml. to maintain the constant product. (See Calcium to Phosphorus Ratio, p. 120.)

Clinical forms of tetany may be classified according to these blood ratios.

Hypocalcemic tetany is produced by a decrease in the serum calcium. Tetany of the newborn may be due to temporary hypofunction of the parathyroid glands; initial feedings of whole cows' milk, with its relatively high phosphate content, give too heavy a phosphate load for renal clearance. In response to the increased serum phosphate, serum calcium falls in order to maintain the constant calcium to phosphorus product. This state is sometimes called milk tetany of the newborn. A number of rare disorders, such as vitamin D-resistant rickets and renal tubular lesions may produce hypocalcemia and therefore potential tetany.

Hyperventilation tetany is produced by over-breathing, which results in respiratory alkalosis (see p. 173). The pH of the blood and the relationships between blood carbon dioxide, calcium, and phosphorus are upset, thus disturbing the balance that is necessary to maintenance of the constant product.

Gastric tetany results from loss of chloride ions. Such loss may occur in excess vomiting, in repeated gastric lavage, in pyloric stenosis, or in high intestinal obstruction. As a result of the chloride loss, the serum chloride is reduced and the bicarbonate elevated, increasing the blood pH, and its carbon dioxide content (see Metabolic Alkalosis, pp. 131, 174).

Bicarbonate tetany occasionally results from excess oral or intravenous intake of sodium bicarbonate, which elevates both the blood pH and the blood carbon dioxide content. Administering bicarbonate in the presence of vomiting or renal insufficiency is extremely dangerous.

Control. The control of tetany depends upon control of the causative circumstance or condition. Primary attention is given to removing the cause or resolving the underlying disturbance. Calcium or ammonium chloride may be given orally if vomiting has subsided. The orally administered dose usually does not take adequate effect in less than twenty-four hours. For immediate control, an injection of magnesium sulfate, (10%

solution, 1 ml. per kg. body weight), may be given intramuscularly. Any respiratory depressant effects may be counteracted by parenteral injection of a soluble calcium salt such as calcium lactate or calcium gluconate. The latter may also be given intramuscularly.

Osteomalacia and osteoporosis

Identification and etiology. Both osteomalacia and osteoporosis are diseases of impaired calcium and phosphorus metabolism with resulting changes in bone formation. They may be distinguished according to cause and result.

Osteomalacia is the adult form of rickets. It is caused by a deficiency of vitamin D, calcium, or phosphorus in the diet; or by a deficiency of the vitamin D that is produced by exposure to sunlight, especially during periods of increased physiologic need as in pregnancy and lactation; or by factors that hinder the proper metabolism of vitamin D, calcium, and phosphorus. Such a hindering factor may be a defect in renal tubular reabsorption, resulting in imbalances in serum calcium or phosphorus; a malabsorption syndrome such as sprue or steatorrhea, which makes calcium unavailable to the body, and allows it to be lost in the feces; or resistance to vitamin D. The most common contributing factors are: (1) failure to absorb calcium, in prolonged steatorrhea or uremia, with excess fecal excretion of calcium phosphate, and (2) general malnutrition, and dietary deficiency of calcium and vitamin D during the stress demands of pregnancy and lactation. The resulting osteomalacia is a softening of the bones due to their demineralization, accompanied by general weakness and aching.

Osteoporosis is a metabolic disorder that usually occurs in persons older than 50 years, especially women after the menopause. The latter is called involutional or postmenopausal osteoporosis. It is believed to be due to the age-related decline in secretions of anabolic hormones by the sex glands and pituitary glands. No doubt other factors also contribute, such as lack of stim-ulating exercise and malnutrition, especially protein malnutrition. The result is a decrease in bone-forming activity (ossification) with a consequent reduction in the amount of bone, although the composition of the bone remains normal. Hypercalcinuria may occur, especially when prolonged immobilization is a factor; and renal calculi frequently develop. Manifestations include weakness, anorexia, hip and back pain, muscle tenderness and cramping, stooped posture, decreased height due to shrinkage of the spine, and a tendency of the bones to fracture easily.

Occurrence. In addition to its frequency in postmenopausal women, osteomalacia occurs in adults during periods of extreme malnutrition and semistarvation, such as in war or famine. Pregnant women are a high-risk group because of their increased needs, especially those who have undergone several pregnancies while taking an inadequate diet. Osteomalacia of pregnancy and lactation is endemic in India and the Middle East because the practice of purdah confines women indoors which gives them very little exposure to sunlight.

Control. Prevention of osteomalacia is based on adequate dietary provision of calcium, phosphorus, and vitamin D, and treatment for any disease or other factor that prevents the proper utilization of these nutrients. The intake of these nutrients must be increased during pregnancy and lactation. Immediate treatment with therapeutic doses of vitamin D, as in rickets, is indicated. Establishment of overall dietary improvement should follow.

Osteoporosis is combated by the administration of combined male and female hormones. Dietary intake of vitamin D, calcium, and protein should be increased.

Iron deficiency anemia

Identification. The general clinical manifestations of iron deficiency anemia are similar to those of all types of anemia: weakness, pallor, fatigability (a sense of being "dead-tired"), headache, and palpitation. If the anemia becomes more severe there may be increased shortness of breath and some degree of cardiac enlargement. In time, some persons with chronic iron deficiency anemia adapt their level of work to their hematologic status, and live at this reduced level of activity.

Clinical manifestations. Distinctive signs of iron-deficiency anemia include the following.

Nails. The fingernails of many patients become brittle and flat, and develop longitudinal ridges. In some cases the changes are so marked that the nails are concave instead of normally convex, so that they appear spoon-shaped—a condition called *koilonychia,* (Gr. *koilos,* hollow; *onyx, onych,* nail). The nail beds are pale.

Tongue and mouth. A papillary atrophy of the tongue is seen in about half the patients, and some have fissures at the corners of the mouth. The mouth is sore and in severe cases there may occasionally be some difficulty in swallowing (the Plummer-Vinson syndrome).

Gastrointestinal. Gastritis, achlorhydria, and gastric atrophy are common. Other complaints include anorexia, flatulence, epigastric distress, and constipation. The liver and spleen may be enlarged.

Hands and feet. Some patients experience numbness and tingling of the hands and feet, but these symptoms are less pronounced than in pernicious anemia.

Laboratory findings. In iron-deficiency anemia, the red blood cells contain less than the normal amount of hemoglobin; they are small and pale (microcytic hypochromic anemia). The total hemoglobin level is always below normal, and is more strikingly reduced than is the red blood cell count. The erythrocyte count may even be about normal (4.5 to 5.5 million per mm.) while the hemoglobin value is as low as 5 gm. per 100 ml. (normal range, 14 ± 2 gm. per 100 ml. for women; 16 ± 2 gm. per 100 ml. for men). The serum iron level is low, and the total iron-binding protein level is above normal.

Etiology. Since iron performs important physiologic functions in oxygen transport and cellular respiration, the body guards its small supply, using it over and over again. In conditions of physiologic stress such as growth, menstruation, pregnancy, or hemorrhage (often compounded by poor diet and impaired absorption), a negative iron balance may develop. Anemia is the result.

Infants and children. The body of a newborn infant contains about 500 mg. of iron. When the normal person has reached maturity, this amount has increased by 2.5 to 4.5 gm. This represents an average increase of 0.35 to 0.60 mg. per day! The infant is vulnerable to iron deficiency because milk is a poor source of iron. The premature infant, especially if born to a malnourished mother, is in even greater jeopardy, as he lacks the normal quantity of iron stores present at birth in tissues, particularly in the liver and blood.

Women in their reproductive years. During normal menstruation, a woman loses from 35 to 70 ml. of blood per period, representing a total loss of iron in hemoglobin of 15 to 25 mg. Over the span of her reproductive years, the normal woman has a continuous average iron loss of 0.5 of 1.0 mg. per day. Without adequate replacement in her diet, she is obviously in a precarious state of iron balance. Pregnancy deprives her of still further iron. The net iron demand of a full-term pregnancy has been conservatively estimated to be from 500 to 700 mg. It is evident that frequent, multiple pregnancies take their toll and must lead to iron deficiency if precautionary iron therapy is not given.

Blood loss. Acute hemorrhage is an evident emergency, for which the patient usually receives immediate blood replacement. Chronic blood loss, especially gradual, occult gastrointestinal bleeding, may go unnoticed and drain the body reserves. Parasitic infections of the intestines may also cause a continuous blood loss.

Poor absorption. Diseases such as chronic diarrhea, infection, sprue, steatorrhea, or celiac disease hinder absorption of iron. These often compound such stress situations as growth and pregnancy, and increase the iron need.

Poor diet. A diet high in cereal content, and low in animal protein and green vegetables is usually low in iron. Unfortunately, this is the common dietary pattern of many people who lack the money, means, or knowledge necessary to improve their diets. During such periods the iron-deficiency is compensated in some degree by increased efficiency of iron absorption (p. 133).

Occurrence. Iron deficiency anemia is a world health problem. It occurs in all countries, but is particularly prevalent (affecting in some areas as many as 20% of the population) in the Middle East, northern Africa, and Asia. The high-risk groups in any population are children, women in their reproductive years, and those suffering from chronic illness and infection.

Control. Where it can be achieved, correction of the factors that increase the requirement for iron (numerous pregnancies, parasitic infections and so on) makes a significant contribution to the control of iron-deficiency anemia. The enrichment of cereals by iron should be considered, especially where cereals are the staple food. Optimum diet and supplementation of the diet with iron are important during periods of stress such as growth and pregnancy.

Treatment of iron deficiency anemia consists of giving a simple ferrous salt, such as ferrous sulfate or ferrous gluconate. The gastrointestinal difficulties that attend the ingestion of iron salts may be minimized by taking it after meals so that it is mixed with the food in the stomach. Abnormal blood loss should also be sought and, if it is occurring, must be corrected.

Goiter

Identification. Goiter (L. *guttur*, throat) is enlargement of the thyroid gland. The normal thyroid gland is about the size and shape of a lima bean. In states of iodine deficiency the gland undergoes compensatory enlargement and may reach many times its normal size, until it becomes plainly visible at a distance of several feet (Fig. 16-10).

Simple goiter. In simple goiter, compensatory mechanisms may suffice to produce adequate amounts of thyroxine (the thyroid hormone), so that hypothyroidism may not cause general symptoms and signs resulting from metabolic imbalance. The goiter is then manifest only in mechanical

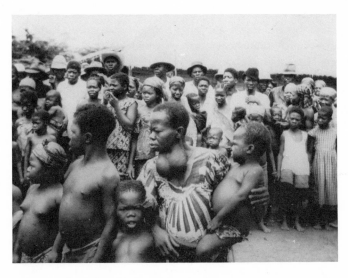

Fig. 16-10. Goiter and hyperthyroidism among children and adults in central Africa. (FAO photograph by Marcel Ganzin.)

problems, such as the local disfigurement, compression of the trachea with consequent hoarseness of the voice, chronic nonproductive cough, possible difficulty or discomfort in swallowing, or congestion of the face.

Cretinism. In areas where the soil is poor in iodine and goiter has affected a number of generations, severe iodine deficiency in mothers produces an endemic form of cretinism in the offspring, characterized by stunted growth, dwarfism, and various degrees of mental retardation. This profound result of continued iodine deficiency was recognized as long ago as 1871 by C. H. Flagge, an English physician. "Goiter is the earlier effect of the endemic influence; cretinism shows itself when the action of that influence is intensified by operating on more than one generation."[22]

Etiology. Simple goiter is the result of failure of the thyroid gland to receive sufficient iodine to maintain its normal structure and function. Thyroxine is 65% iodine. When adequate iodine is not present, the gland's compensatory effort to produce the needed hormone results in its enlargement.

The dietary lack of iodine may be due to environmental factors—a deficiency of the mineral in soil and water. The deficiency may also be caused by factors that make the dietary iodine unavailable by interfering with its absorption or metabolism. Such goitrogenic substances are found in cabbage, Brussels sprouts, soybeans, peanuts, turnips, and rutabagas. Further causes of deficiency are conditions such as chronic infection that increase the iodine requirement.

Occurrence. Goiter may occur in persons of any age. After puberty, the incidence is somewhat greater in girls. In areas where examination of school children reveals a 5 to 10% incidence, goiter is a significant public health problem. In countries where the use of iodized salt has become an accepted public health practice, the incidence of goiter has been greatly reduced.

Control. Goiter may be prevented by a sufficient supply of iodine in the diet. The most practical means of ensuring adequate intake is the iodization of table salt. A content of 1 part iodine to 10,000 to 20,000 parts of salt is recommended in the Western Hemisphere; lower levels are used in Europe. Prevention is more effective than treatment, for in longstanding goiter, treatment has little effect; the chronic fibrosis is not reversible. Iodine may be administered to vulnerable groups (children, pregnant and lactating women), but is only a temporary measure.

METHODS OF COMBATING MALNUTRITION

Malnutrition is the world's primary health problem. How shall it be solved? It is evident that the problem is complex, and that it has no simple answer. The discussion must end as it began with a restatement of the two-fold premise: (1) supplying food alone is not the answer, and (2) the problem is not confined to economically deprived populations.

Requirements for solution of the problem of malnutrition

An approach to the problem of malnutrition must embrace three basic factors—medical care, health education, and responsibility of the persons involved.

Medical care. A direct attack involving case-finding, clinical diagnosis, and treatment is a primary concern. All the resources of the medical team are needed for this aspect of the approach. But treating malnutrition and then sending the patient back into the environment that produced it is like putting a strip of adhesive bandage over a cancer.

Long-range control and prevention must focus on education and responsibility.

Health education. In addition to medical treatment, a balanced program must include nutritional rehabilitation and health education. This education must begin with the health personnel. At times it seems that a few members of the health professions, whether working in the United States or in a foreign country, become encased in a

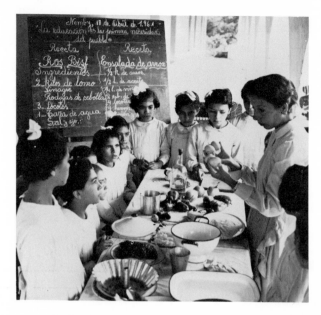

Fig. 16-11. In many underdeveloped countries the school provides the way to health. Here, children in Paraguay are being taught cooking and hygiene. In turn, they pass on to their parents the elementary knowledge of health and nutrition. (WHO photograph by Paul Almasy.)

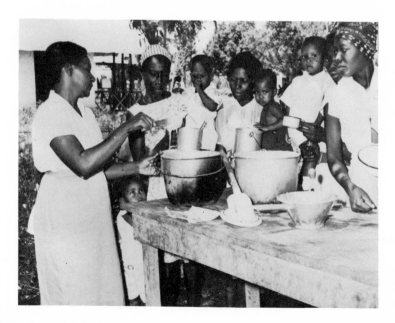

Fig. 16-12. Practical help for mothers in Haiti. Recuperation of malnourished children is aided not only by giving badly needed food, but also by teaching mothers the rudiments of nutrition and proper food preparation.

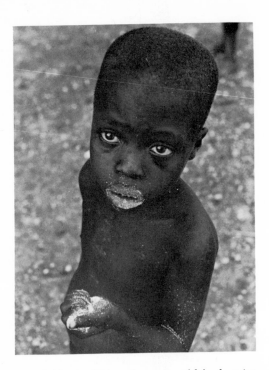

Fig. 16-13. A child eating a mouthful of maize flour at a FAO food distribution center in Northern Dahomey. Recent drought in Dahomey and Togo brought famine to the area and necessitated aid from world health groups. (FAO photograph by C. Bavagnoli.)

crystallized rigidity, unable to learn from what meets the eye. Education must also reach the patients themselves, their parents and families, and the public (Fig. 16-11). It must constantly develop, in order to accommodate the constant changes in people, in the circumstances of their lives, in food products, and in scientific knowledge. It must be person-centered and practical (Fig. 16-12). The principles discussed in the previous chapter apply here. Often the most significant nursing care in such situations is personal teaching and supportive encouragement.

Responsibility. Ultimately, the success of any efforts to combat malnutrition in a community must rest upon a developed sense of responsibility in the people involved. The responsibility for providing sound, relevant health care rests with members of the health professions. The responsibility for helping to provide a safe and adequate food supply, to explore food enrichment laws, agricultural methods, marketing practices, consolidation of control programs, supporting research, education, and technical development rests with the persons who form and administer the economic and po-

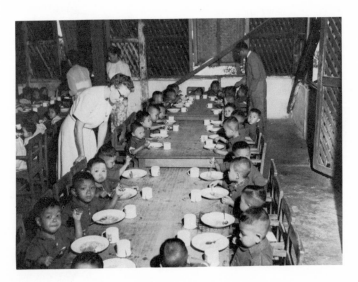

Fig. 16-14. Fish flour preparation served to children in Rangoon day nursery to combat protein deficiency. FAO nutritionist helps the Burmese nutrition staff with this program. (FAO photograph by S. Bunnag.)

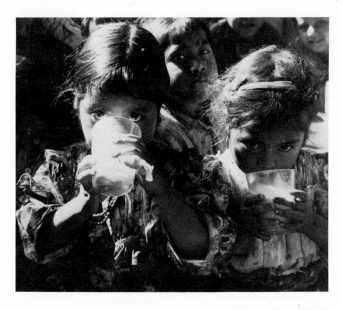

Fig. 16-15. Guatemalan children drinking Incaparina at school. After much experimentation, the Institute of Nutrition of Central America and Panama (INCAP) has succeeded in developing Incaparina, an inexpensive protein product of high nutritive value. It is now well liked and widely used in Central America. (WHO photograph by Todd Webb.)

litical structure of the country. Responsibility for meeting health needs in daily life at the local level rests with community leaders. Responsibility for meeting personal and family health needs, for maintaining interest in good nutrition, for making certain that information is correct and clearly understood, and for carrying out the discipline that is required for the development of sound food habits rests with individuals and with the heads of families.

World health groups such as the World Health Organization, the Food and Agriculture Organization, UNICEF, and others are actively and earnestly engaged in the mammoth task of combating malnutrition (Figs. 16-13 and 16-14). Many other national and local groups in the United States and other countries are working toward the same goals. Food supplements such as the protein substance "Incaparina," which was developed by the Institute of Nutrition for Central America and Panama (INCAP) in Guatemala City are being studied and used to add needed nutrients to inadequate regional diets (Fig. 16-15). Research and

education programs are helping to provide knowledge and tools.

Ultimately, the welfare of a nation rests upon the health of its people. George Herbert, an English poet who lived from 1593 to 1633 wrote, "Whatsoever was the father of a disease, an ill diet was the mother." He was far wiser than even he knew!

References
Specific

1. Emerson, H., editor: Control of communicable diseases in man, ed. 1, New York, 1917, The American Public Health Association.
2. Nordseik, F. W., editor: Control of malnutrition in man, New York, 1960, The American Public Health Association.
3. Statistical bulletin, Vol. 45, 1964, Metropolitan Life Insurance Company.
4. The State of food and agriculture, 1965, Review of second postwar decade, 1965, Food and Agriculture Organization.
5. Health Conditions in the Americas (1961-62), Pub. No. 104, 1964, Prepared for the Meeting of the Directing Council, Pan American Health Organization/World Health Organization.
6. Calder, R.: Proceedings of meeting on nutrition of the preschool child, Washington D. C., 1965, National Academy of Sciences.

7. Jelliffe, D. B.: Effect of malnutrition on behavioral and social development, Proceedings Western Hemisphere Nutrition Congress, Chicago, 1965, American Medical Association.

8. Scrimshaw, N. S., and Béhar, M.: World-wide occurrence protein malnutrition, Fed. Proc. **18**:82 (Suppl. 3, Pt. 2), 1959.

9. Joint FAO/WHO Expert Committee on Nutrition, Fourth Report, WHO Tech. Rep. Ser. 97, 1955.

10. Oamen, H. A. P. C.: Clinical experience on hypovitaminosis A, nutritional disease. In Kinny, T. D., and Follis, R. H., Jr., editors: Proceedings of Conference on Beriberi, Endemic Goiter and Hypovitaminosis A, Fed. Proc. **17**:162 (Suppl. 2, Pt. 2), 1958.

11. Burgess, R. C.: Beriberi, 6. Special problems concerning beriberi, B. Infantile beriberi, Fed. Proc. **17**:39 (Suppl. 2, Pt. 2), 1958.

12. Schaefer, A. E.: Nutritional deficiencies in developing countries, J. Amer. Diet. Ass. **42**: 295, 1963.

13. Scrimshaw, N. S.: Malnutrition and the health of children, J. Amer. Diet. Ass. **42**:203, 1963.

14. Burns, J. J., editor: Vitamin C, Ann. N. Y. Acad. Sci. **92**:1, 1961.

15. Tolbert, B. M.: Report on the second year of research on ascorbic acid, biological function and chemistry, Contract No. DA-49-193-MD-2611. Office of the Surgeon General, U. S. Army, 1966.

16. Wagner, A. F., and Folkers, K.: Vitamins and coenzymes, New York, Interscience, 1961, p. 208.

17. Sherlock, P., and Rothschild, E. O.: Scurvy produced by a Zen macrobiotic diet, J.A.M.A. **199**:794, 1967.

18. Fraser, D.: Nutritional problems in North America, Proceedings, Western Hemisphere Nutrition Congress—1965, Council on Foods and Nutrition, Chicago, Ill., 1966, American Medical Association.

19. Fraser, D.: Clinical manifestations of genetic aberrations of calcium and phosphorus metabolism, J.A.M.A. **176**:281, 1961.

20. Bakwin, H., and others: Refractory rickets, Amer. J. Dis. Child **59**:560, 1940.

21. Council on Drugs, Doses of water-soluble vitamin A analogues in hemorrhagic disease of the newborn, J.A.M.A. **164**:1331, 1957.

22. Flagge, C. H.: On sporadic cretinism occurring in England, Medico-Chirurgical Transactions **54**:155, 1871.

General

Akbarian, M., Yankopoulos, N. A., and Abelmann, W. H.: Hemodynamic studies in beriberi heart disease, Amer. J. of Med. **41**:197, 1966.

Béhar, M., and others: Treatment of severe protein deficiency in children (kwashiorkor), Amer. J. Clin. Nutr. **5**:506, 1957.

Burgess, R. C.: Beriberi, 6. Special problems concerning beriberi, B. Infantile beriberi, Fed. Proc. **17**:39(Suppl. 2, Pt. 2), 1958.

Clinical nutritional problems in the United States today, Nutr. Rev. **23**:1, 1965.

Follis, R. H.: Deficiency disease, Springfield, Illinois, 1958, Charles C Thomas, Publisher.

Follis, R. H.: Some unsolved problems concerning the pathogenesis of human deficiency disease syndromes, Amer. J. Clin. Nutr. **6**:459, 1958.

Frenk, S., and others: Fatty liver in children—kwashiorkor, Amer. J. Clin. Nutr. **6**:298, 1958.

Goiter and iodine deficiency, Nutr. Rev. **22**:169, 1964.

Goldsmith, G.: Niacin—tryptophan relationships in man and niacin requirement, Amer. J. Clin. Nutr. **6**:479, 1958.

Gordon, J. E.: Chairman, Subcommittee on Communicable Disease, Control of communicable disease in man, ed. 9, New York, 1960, American Public Health Association.

Gubbay, E. R.: Beri-beri heart disease, Canad. Med. Ass. J., **95**:21, 1966.

Joliffe, N., editor: Clinical nutrition, New York, 1962, Harper and Row, Publishers.

King, C. G.: Trends in international nutrition programs, J. Amer. Diet. Ass. **48**:297, 1966.

McConnell, J. F.: The deposed one, Amer. J. Nurs. **61**:78, 1961.

McCullough, F. S.: Vitamin A deficiency in African children in Northern Rhodesia, J. Pediat. **60**:114, 1962.

McLaren, D. S.: Xerophthalmia: a neglected problem, Nutr. Rev. **22**:289, 1964.

Nordin, B. E. C.: Calcium balance and calcium requirement in spinal osteoporosis, Amer. J. Clin. Nutr. **10**:384, 1962.

Nordsick, F. W., editor: Control of malnutrition in man, New York, 1960, American Public Health Association.

Nutritional rickets and parathyroid function, Nutr. Rev. **21**:271, 1963.

Patwardhan, V. N.: Nutritional anemias—WHO research program: early developments and progress deport of collaborative studies, Amer. J. Clin. Nutr. **19**:63, 1966.

Progress in meeting protein needs of infants and preschool children, Washington, D. C., 1961, National Academy of Sciences, National Research Council, Pub. No. 843.

Schaefer, A. E.: Nutritional deficiencies in developing countries, J. Amer. Diet. Ass. **42**:295, 1963.

Scrimshaw, N. S.: Malnutrition and the health of children, J. Amer. Diet. Ass. **42**:203, 1963.

Scrimshaw, N. S., and others: Kwashiorkor in children and its response to protein therapy, J.A.M.A. **164**:555, 1957.

Sebrell, W. H.: Changing concept of malnutrition, Amer. J. Clin. Nutr. **20**:653, 1967.

Shaw, J. H.: Nutrition and dental caries, J.A.M.A. **166**:633, 1958.

Stiebeling, H. K.: Our share in better world nutrition, J. Amer. Diet. Ass. **45**:315, 1964.

Sydenstricker, V. P.: The history of pellagra, its recognition as a disorder of nutrition and its conquest, Amer. J. Clin. Nutr. **6**:409, 1958.

Walker, A. R. P.: Osteoporosis and calcium deficiency, Amer. J. Clin. Nutr. **16**:327, 1965.

Weaver, J. C.: The food crisis of humanity, J. Amer. Diet. Ass., **32**:795, 1956.

Williams, C. D.: Malnutrition, Lancet **2**:342, 1962.

Williams, C. D.: Maternal and child health services in developing countries, Lancet **1**:345, 1964.

Williams, C. D.: Self-help and nutrition—real needs of underdeveloped countries, Lancet **146** (6807):323, 1954.

Williams, C. D.: What is health education?, Lancet **1**:1205, 1966.

Williams, R. R.: Can we eradicate the classical deficiency diseases?, J. Amer. Diet. Ass. **36**:31, 1960.

NUTRITION IN
THE NURSING SPECIALTY

Not only in public health nursing, but also in the other nursing specialties, the nurse-clinician will seek to identify the nutritional needs of her patients and to explore with them ways of meeting these needs. In Unit III, five of the nursing specialties will be considered, and in respect to each area ways will be discussed in which concern for significant nutritional needs can be integrated into total patient care.

The first three chapters of this unit are concerned with the principles of nutrition as applied to the physiologic stress periods of gestation, lactation, and normal growth and development—to the well-being of mothers and children. In obstetric nursing the first concern is antepartum care, the nutritional demands of pregnancy; then, in postpartum care, the nurse is concerned with helping the new mother sustain lactation and initiate the first feedings of her newborn infant. In the chapter on "Nutrition during Pregnancy and Lactation" these needs are explored, the difficulties in setting nutritional standards are discussed, and some realistic guidelines for patient care are established.

In pediatric nursing, the nurse is con-cerned with providing for the needs of children during each stage of growth from infancy through adolescence. In the chapter on "Nutrition for Growth and Development: Infancy, Childhood, and Adolescence" these needs are traced through each stage of development, and it is stressed that food and feeding are not only essential to physical growth but also are an intimate part of the total human developmental process. The following chapter, "Nutritional Therapy in Childhood Diseases," reviews general therapeutic nutritional needs in diseases such as those of the gastrointestinal system that affect digestion and absorption and genetic diseases that affect metabolism of key nutrients.

The remaining three chapters of this unit identify nutritional components of patient care in geriatric nursing, rehabilitation nursing, and psychiatric nursing. In each instance, the emphasis is upon the patient, his unique experience and needs, and the nurse's discovery, together with the patient, of how basic principles of nutrition, the meanings of food and feeding, may be applied in ways that will help him move toward health and fulfillment.

CHAPTER 17

Nutrition during pregnancy and lactation

Human reproduction involves complex processes of rapid, specialized growth. Both mother and child possess tremendous powers of adaptation that enable them to meet the demands of this growth. Gestation has well been called "the epitome of purposeful growth."

Because the maintenance of the health of body tissues is dependent upon certain essential chemical nutrients in food, it is evident that the development of the infant is directly related to the diet of the mother. However, experience has shown that widely differing diets have sustained individual mothers through successful pregnancies, and the medical literature has reported conflicting and controversial observations concerning the nutritional requirements during pregnancy. Thus, the thoughtful student might well ask, what reasonable basis is there for establishing nutritional recommendations for my prenatal patient? What metabolic stress does the process of gestation place on the mother? How does this stress compare with that of lactation? What effects do complications of pregnancy have on the nutritional needs of the mother? As a guide in the nurse's search for answers that she may apply realistically to patients under her care, it will be well to consider some of the background studies in the physiology of gestation and lactation as they relate to nutritional needs. The following questions should be used to guide further study:

1. What influence does maternal nutrition have on the outcome of pregnancy?
2. How does the physiology of gestation relate to antepartum nutritional needs? How may these needs be met through food choices?
3. How may general dietary problems associated with pregnancy (for example, gastrointestional difficulties and weight control) best be met?
4. How should the diet be managed in complications of pregnancy?
5. What are the nutritional needs of the lactating mother?
6. What place does nutrition education have in maternity nursing?

THE RELATION OF NUTRITION AND PREGNANCY
Background

For centuries, in all cultures, a great body of folklore has surrounded pregnancy. Many traditional practices and diets have been followed, which have had little basis in fact; and much clinical advice was based only on supposition. It was not until the 1920's that articles in the medical literature began to outgrow baseless assumptions and dogmatic statements, and to reflect scientific experiment and careful observation. For example, Paddock[1] advanced the idea that the pregnant woman should be advised to eat a mixed diet including a variety of foods, and that excessive weight gain was to be avoided. Soon thereafter, Toverud[2] of Norway first expressed his working hypothesis that "a child is nutritionally nine months old at birth." This biologic axiom gained enthusiastic acceptance; however, sound research was needed to undergird his appeal.

In 1943, *Nutrition Reviews* pointed out the need to study prenatal nutrition. The editors contended that, "No period in the development and growth of the child has been more neglected than the prenatal period."[3] In the same year, the recommended dietary allowances of the National Research Council were published for the first time. They have undergone continuous revisions. From their initial appearance, they have provided guidelines widely used by scientific and lay groups.

The controversy surrounding diet in pregnancy, which began in the 1920's and 1930's, continued to grow in scope during the 1940's and 1950's. Many investigators brought forth seemingly conflicting evidence concerning the influence of maternal diet on the outcome of pregnancy. Several widely-known studies may be cited as examples, two as evidence for, and two as evidence against its importance.

Positive evidence

The Toronto study. In a large prenatal clinic in Toronto, Canada, during World War II, Ebbs and his co-workers[4] conducted a study of the diet of pregnant women and its effects, based on the women's records of food intake during one week. Half of the women were judged by their records to have "poor diets; below the recommended standards." Within this group of women with "poor diets," a subgroup received, from the fourth month until term, a food supplement that raised their nutritional level to optimum standards. Without knowing to which group or subgroup each woman belonged, the clinic's obstetrician and pediatrician rated the pregnancies, labors, postpartum periods, and babies as good, fair, poor, or bad—depending upon minor complaints or major

complications. The results revealed that 36% of the women on "poor diet" had poor or bad prenatal ratings; whereas only 9% of the women who received the supplement that raised the nutritional intake to the optimum level had poor or bad ratings.

The Boston study. The studies of Burke and her co-workers[5] at the Boston Lying-in Hospital during the early 1940's have often been used to support the contention that the quality of the prenatal diet has a high correlation with reproductive performance. Using a detailed dietary questionnaire, Dr. Burke interviewed a number of pregnant women and rated their diets according to the recommended dietary allowances of the National Research Council, and then compared these ratings to the outcome of their pregnancies. She reported that most of the superior infants were born to mothers with good to excellent diets. All stillborn, all premature, all "functionally immature," all but one of the infants who died within a few days of birth, and a majority of those born with morbid congenital defects were delivered by women whose diet had been inadequate during gestation.

Negative evidence

The Vanderbilt study. Over several years during the 1950's one of the largest and most extensive studies of prenatal nutrition that has been reported was conducted at Vanderbilt University in Tennessee, by McGanity and Darby and their co-workers.[6,7] For the total population served by an obstetric clinic (2,338 women) all of whom were in a relatively low income bracket, these investigators compared average daily nutrient intakes, blood and urine nutrient levels, and the incidence of obstetric complications. Although the average nutrient intake was not in all cases equal to the recommended allowances of the National Research Council, the intakes were not particularly low, nor were dietary supplements routinely ordered for women of the studied group. Their diets were varied and revealed no consistent pattern of food prejudice or fad associated with pregnancy. Their daily caloric intake, especially during the second and third trimesters, decreased on the average about 200 calories, probably partially reflecting response to their physicians' advice, and partially reflecting lessened activity. To the question of whether there was evidence that improved nutrition could be expected to prevent the occurrence of gestational complication, Dr. McGanity's answer was no. These observations led him to three general conclusions. (1) Dietary intakes greater than the recommended dietary allowances of the Food and Nutrition Board do not bestow additional protective benefits during pregnancy. (2) The recommended standards for caloric intake may be too high for the expectant mother of today. (3) A diet that will provide the essential nutrients is usually readily obtainable. He therefore expressed the opinion that the need for broad-spectrum nutritional supplementation during pregnancy, at that time routinely advised by many obstetricians (and the doses usually given) were questionable. He indicated that, to be effective, the use of supplements should be based on an understanding of the normal physiologic changes associated with the reproductive process.

The Aberdeen study. The strictly controlled, more recent (1958-1959) study by Thomson[8] in Aberdeen, Scotland, was of 713 primiparas, comprising a sample of all pregnant women in the city, grouped according to the registrar general's official designations of social class. For one week during the seventh month of pregnancy, each of these women weighed all nutrients before consuming them, and recorded these weights. A subsample, resurveyed six weeks later, showed close agreement in recorded intake. Nutrient intake varied directly with social class, but even the lowest values were higher than those of the poor diet group in the Toronto study. These dietary ratings were compared with outcome of the pregnancies. The results varied over a broad range. No statistically significant correlations could be found. Thomson concluded that, "The correlations between food intake during pregnancy and the outcome of pregnancy are so elusive that they are far from easy to demonstrate, even by ad hoc survey methods."

Difficulties and limitations in determining needs

It is evident from these studies and from the wide experience of many clinicians, that a number of difficulties and limitations impede the determination of specific nutritional requirements during pregnancy. Several reasons may be given.

Age and parity of the mother. The teenage mother adds her own needs presented by her continuing growth to those introduced by her pregnancy. At the other end of the reproductive span, hazards increase with age. The number of pregnancies and the intervals between them influence the needs of the mother and the outcome of pregnancy.

Pre-conception nutrition. The mother brings to gestation all of her previous life experiences, including her diet. Her general health and fitness, and her state of nutrition at the time of her infant's conception are products of her lifelong dietary habits and possibly of generations before her own conception. The woman is the product of the growth that has preceded.

Complex metabolic interactions of gestation. Three distinct biological entities are involved in pregnancy—the mother, the fetus, and the placenta. Constant metabolic interactions go on among them. Their functions, while being unique, are at the same time interdependent. Any number of variables, therefore, may combine in ways that make the determination of general needs difficult.

Individual needs and adaptations. Individual nutritional needs vary with time and circumstance; but homeostatic mechanisms appear to operate with special efficiency during pregnancy. Even when nutritional limitations are extreme, as has been demonstrated for example in deprived populations during war time,[9] the pregnant female organism possesses great metabolic capacities for adapting to suboptimal intakes of essential nutrients.

The answer to the problem

Is there then a dilemma and a nutritional paradox? What reasonable inference can be drawn from these complexities and apparent contradictions?

Parts of the answer may be drawn from three sources.

The perinatal concept. The prefix "peri" comes from the Greek root meaning "around, about, or surrounding." As knowledge and understanding increase, it is realized the whole of the individual's life experiences surrounding the pregnancy must be considered. The nutritional status developed over previous years of living, and the establishment of reserves for possible future pregnancies are both important. All things considered, in the light of life needs, to focus only upon the brief nine-month period of gestation is far too narrow an approach.

The life continuum concept. The concept of the life continuum naturally follows the perinatal concept. Each child becomes a part of the ongoing continuum of life. Through the food she eats, each mother gives to her unborn child the nourishment required to initiate and sustain fetal growth; but she carries over the same nutritional principles in her feeding and teaching of the growing child—principles which he, in turn, internalizes and passes on to his child. Perhaps it should be said, which *she* in turn passes on to *her* child, for it is the nutritional development of the girl child that is of particular concern in this case; she is the potential mother of future generations.

Adequate, not excessive, diet. From the studies cited, it is clear that the excessive diet has no foundation for use. Obesity is a deterrent to a successful pregnancy. Excessive food is to be avoided. The *quality* of the diet, not its quantity, is the important consideration. A good diet that supplies the needs of this individual mother and the essential nutrients required for reproduction is basic.

NUTRITION IN PREGNANCY
The physiology of gestation
Fetal development

The development of the fetus undergoes three distinct morphologic phases: implantation, differentiation of major organs and tissues, and the intensive growth period.

Implantation (first two weeks). Prior to conception, the endometrium, the membrane that lines the uterus, is prepared for the reception of the ovum by thickening and developing an increased blood supply. The fertilized ovum develops into a sphere called the *blastocyst*, which has an inner and an outer layer of cells. The outer layer of cells will later contribute to the formation of the placenta, which will carry nutrients from the mother to the fetus, and waste products from the fetus into the maternal circulation for disposal. Because they are related to nourishment, these cells are called "trophoblasts" (Gr. *trophe*, nourishment; *blastos*, germ or cell). They develop within nine to ten days of fertilization of the ovum. The blastocyst imbeds itself in the endometrium, which invaginates to receive it. Here it is anchored by the trophoblasts. The trophoblasts also differentiate into two layers. One layer, in intimate relationship with the uterus, maintains important nutrient relationships with the mother. The ovum rapidly increases in size, largely as a result of the growth of the second layer, the *syncytium* (Gr. *syn*, with; *kytos*, cell), so named because it consists of cells whose protoplasm is continuous with that of the contiguous cells. The syncytium develops from the trophoblast; the syncytial trophoblast is that layer of the trophoblast which is in closest relation to the uterus. It is a highly structured, highly complex tissue, which becomes an important part of the placenta, where it helps to provide nourishment to the growing fetus. An idea of its complexity can be gained from the fact that this tissue is similar to the visceral epithelium in Bowman's capsule (surrounding the renal glomerulus) and in the convoluted tubules. This complex development represents an adaptation to the need for rapid transport of fluid and solute nutrients.

By the completion of seven to ten days' development, the cell mass (now the embryonic disc) is ready to differentiate into a thick plate of primitive ectoderm and an underlying layer of endoderm.

Differentiation of major organs and tissues (two to eight weeks). During the second phase of fetal development, rapid, dramatic changes take place in the developing embryo. The three basic layers of tissue (the "germ layers") are formed—ectoderm, mesoderm, and endoderm (Gr., *ektos,* outside; *mesos,* middle; *endon,* within; *derma,* skin). These three germ layers give rise to the various organs and tissues of the body in very specific ways. From the ectoderm come the entire nervous system and the epidermis. From the endoderm develop the lining of the gastrointestinal tract and such derivative organs as the liver, pancreas, and thyroid. From the mesoderm come the skeleton, connective tissues, the vascular and urogenital systems, the dermis, and most of the skeletal and smooth muscles. By the seventh week, the body has begun to take form. Although the head remains large relative to the size of the body during the embryonic period, the body has begun to grow rapidly also. By now the neck can be recognized, the tail filament has disappeared, and by the end of the seventh or eighth week, the embryo can be identified as human. It is evident that with such rapid development of specialized cells, the nutritional status which the mother brings to conception and to these crucial early weeks is significant in the successful outcome of the pregnancy.

Intensive growth period (eight weeks to term). From the eighth week on the changes are less dramatic but equally vital to the entire future life of the developing human being. The specialized tissues continue to develop and grow during this period of most rapid fetal growth. There is also intensive *maternal* physiologic growth during this period; the mother's body undergoes nutritional reconditioning, and reserves are laid down to meet the demands of approaching labor, the period immediately following labor, and lactation.

The placenta

Definition and function. The placenta (L. "a flat cake") is an oval, spongy structure which at term is six to seven inches in diameter and weighs about one pound. It is expelled following parturition and is then commonly called the afterbirth. The placenta is a complex, highly specialized organ. Its primary function is to transport and store oxygen and nutrients from the mother to the developing fetus and to return the end products of fetal metabolism to the maternal blood. The fetus, in a highly selective manner, draws its nutrients for growth and development from the placental stores supplied by the mother. From the time the fertilized egg is implanted in the uterus to full maturation and birth, the fetus depends for these functions entirely upon this specialized placental structure. The placenta consists of physiologic divisions, specialized in function, and particularly adapted to serve each of these essential purposes.

Specialized functional parts. The specialized functional parts of the placenta are the fetal portion, the maternal portion, and the intervillous spaces.

Fetal portion (chorion frondosum). The essential parenchyma (functional part of an organ as distinguished from its purely structural parts) of the placenta is its trophoblast. Soon after implantation of the fertilized ovum, the highly invasive trophoblast penetrates the endometrium. It develops a functional outer shell or layer of cells called the syncytium. From the syncytium develop small villous protrusions; the surface of the villi are covered with even finer projections called microvilli. A similar structure in the small intestine provides maximum absorbing surface. This placental network of villi is adapted to serve the same purpose. The fetal portion of the placenta is called the *chorion,* and the projections are called the chorionic villi. Some villi extend to the endometrium as anchoring villi, but the majority end freely and continue to divide as the placenta develops, thus increasing the total absorbing surface.

Maternal portion (decidua basalis). The

name comes from the Latin word *decidua,* "falling off" (a tissue that will fall off after parturition) and the Latin and Greek root *basis,* the "base or lowest part." As the invasion of the endometrium continues, maternal blood vessels are tapped, and vacuoles in the cytoplasm coalesce to form larger *lacunae* (L. *lacuna,* a pit). The lacunae are hollow spaces that soon fill with blood from the endometrial arteries and veins. These spaces join and form a labyrinth of channels and columns lined with the highly selective, functional, trophoblast cells. These cells, the major agents for nutrition and homeostasis, are the survival links for the fetus.

Intervillous spaces. As Ramsey's[10] beautiful radiographic work clearly shows, like so many minute springs or fountains, vertical maternal arteries push blood, in funnel shaped spurts, up from the floor of the decidua basalis. The blood flows around the chorionic villi that lie free in the intervillous spaces, bathing their surfaces and exchanging metabolic material. Then, as maternal blood pressure dissipates, the blood is dispersed laterally into endometrial veins. The intervillous spaces serve as the depot of transfer, and the chorionic villi serve as the agents of transfer. Through highly selective transport mechanisms similar to those operating in the small intestine and in the kidney, essential metabolic substances move across the trophoblast membrane by three basic mechanisms. Most of the small molecules (water, oxygen, electrolytes) move across membranes in this manner according to need and are guided, by osmotic pressures (passive diffusion). Somewhat larger molecules (nutrients such as dextrose, amino acids, vitamins), primarily for nutrition, move across the membrane by specialized carrier systems of active transport. Some of the larger molecules such as proteins are absorbed by means of the invaginating process called pinocytosis (see p. 158). In view of this highly selective transport activity provided by the placental membrane, perhaps the common term "placental barrier" is mislead-ing. A better term may be "placental membrane."

Maternal nutrient needs

What nutrients must the mother take to supply the fetus and her own changing body optimally for this critical gestation period?

During the first trimester (the first three months), the fetus is small and undergoes differentiation, so the mother's relative nutrient requirements are not increased from normal adult needs. These nutrients are, however, essential during this vital period; only the *quantitative* need for them is not increased. The importance of a diet that contains balanced portions of essential nutrients in normal individual quantity continues into the second trimester.

The last three months of pregnancy is the period during which a greater *amount* of key nutrients is required by the fetus, as it lays down stores for growth. This need for increased amounts of certain nutrients is indicated by the recommended daily allowances outlined by the National Research Council (Table 17-1). It should be remembered that the recommended allowances provide a margin of safety above minimal requirements to allow for wide variations of need among individuals. For example, the reference woman in the table is age eighteen to thirty-five years, weighs 128 pounds, is 64 inches tall, lives in a temperate climate, and is a normally active, healthy woman. Obviously, variations from this state would need to be considered as the nurse counsels with individual expectant mothers. The increased quantitative need for nourishment by pregnant adolescents should be noted. The need for individual counseling and for correct use of these recommendations as guidelines is clearly stated by the Council: "They are not called 'requirements' because they are not intended to represent merely literal (minimal) requirements of average individuals, but [the levels are sufficiently high] to cover substantially the individual variations in the requirements of normal people." In

Table 17-1. Recommended daily dietary allowances for pregnancy and lactation (National Research Council, 1968 revision)

Nutrients	Nonpregnant girl 12-14 yrs. 47 kg. 103 lbs.	Nonpregnant girl 14-18 yrs. 53 kg. 117 lbs.	Nonpregnant woman 25 yrs. 58 kg. 128 lbs.	Pregnancy (last half) Added need	Pregnancy Girl 12 to 14 yrs.	Pregnancy Girl 14 to 18 yrs.	Pregnancy Woman 25 yrs.	Lactation (850 ml. daily) Added need	Lactation Girl 12 to 14 yrs.	Lactation Girl 14 to 18 yrs.	Lactation Woman 25 yrs.
Calories	2,300	2,300	2,000	200	2,500	2,500	2,200	1,000	3,300	3,300	3,000
Protein (gm.)	50	55	55	10	65	65	65	20	75	75	75
Calcium (gm.)	1.3	1.3	0.8	0.4	1.7	1.7	1.2	0.5	1.8	1.8	1.3
Iron (mg.)	18	18	18	—	18	18	18	—	18	18	18
Vitamin A (I.U)	5,000	5,000	5,000	1,000	6,000	6,000	6,000	3,000	8,000	8,000	8,000
Thiamine (mg.)	1.2	1.2	1.0	0.1	1.3	1.3	1.1	0.5	1.7	1.7	1.5
Riboflavin (mg.)	1.4	1.5	1.5	0.3	1.7	1.8	1.8	0.5	2.0	2.0	2.0
Niacin equivalent and tryptophan (mg.)	15	15	13	—	15	15	15	5	20	20	20
Ascorbic acid (mg.)	45	50	55	10	60	60	60	10	60	60	60
Vitamin D (I.U.)	400	400	—	—	400	400	400	—	400	400	400

considering the needs of the normal pregnant woman, therefore, the nutrient elements should be reviewed in terms of the general amount of increased intake indicated, why this increase is recommended, and how it may be obtained in basic foods.

Protein. An additional daily allowance of 10 gm. of protein is recommended during the second half of pregnancy, raising the 55 gm. required by the average normal nonpregnant woman to 65 gm. daily. This represents an increase of about 20%, or one-fifth.

Protein, with its essential constituent, nitrogen, is the nutritional element that is basic to growth. Nitrogen balance studies give some indication of the large amounts of nitrogen used by the mother and child during pregnancy. A study of fetal tissue composition revealed that during the last half of gestation the amount of nitrogen stored by the embryo rose from 0.9 to 55.9 gm. The mature placenta at term has stored about 17 gm. of nitrogen; the amniotic fluid contains 1 gm. An estimated 17 gm. of nitrogen is incorporated in the developing maternal breast tissue; nearly 40 gm. in the increased uterine tissue. In addition, a maternal reserve of 200 to 350 gm. is stored for the approaching losses during labor and parturition (from 300 to 500 ml. or more of blood may be lost during delivery) and in preparation for the physiologic demand of lactation.

In summary, to meet the demands posed by the rapid growth of the fetus, by enlargement of the uterus, mammary glands, and placenta, by the increase in maternal circulating blood volume, and by the formation of amniotic fluid and storage reserves for labor, delivery, and lactation, more protein is essential.

Milk, meat, egg, and cheese are complete protein foods of high biologic value. Protein-rich foods also contribute other nutrients such as calcium, iron, and B vitamins. The amounts of these foods that would supply the quantities of protein needed are indicated in the recommended daily food plan (Table 17-2).

Calories. Contrary to popular notion, calories should not be appreciably increased during pregnancy. The common contention, "But I have to eat for two, so I need twice as much!" could well be countered with the reply, "But certainly not for two of the *same size!*" The increases in the latter half of pregnancy are *qualitative.* They are increases in specific essential nutrients; only in limited degree are they quantitative (increases in total amounts). Only 200 calories additional to the amount ingested by the nonpregnant woman is recommended; this represents only about a 10% increase over the usual previous intake.

Usually, the pregnant woman becomes less active as she nears term. Excessive weight gain increases the hazards to her health and should be avoided.

A few extra calories may be taken in any foods that the expectant mother may desire, provided that the basic food needed for nutrient increases is included in the total diet.

Minerals. The need for calcium and iron should be particularly emphasized during the last half of pregnancy.

Calcium. It is recommended that the woman in the last half of gestation increase her daily calcium intake by 0.4 gm. Since the suggested intake for the nonpregnant woman is 0.8 gm., the total daily intake during the last half of pregnancy should be 1.2 gm. This is about a 50% increase.

The importance of calcium to the mother and fetus is suggested by the size of the increase that is recommended. Calcium is the essential element for the construction and maintenance of bones and teeth. It is also an important constituent of the blood clotting mechanism (p. 83), and is used in normal muscle action and other essential metabolic activities. Balance studies indicate that the calcium used by the maternal organism increases from about 4 gm. at the middle of pregnancy to about 30 gm. at term. Fetal tissue studies reveal an increase in the quantity of calcium stored, from about 1 gm. at the middle of gestation to about 23 gm. at term. For the rapid mineralization of skeletal tissue during this final period of growth, more calcium is essential.

Dairy products are a primary source of calcium. Therefore, some increase in milk or equivalent milk foods (cheese, ice cream, skimmed milk powder used in cooking) is recommended. Additional calcium is obtained in whole or enriched cereal grain and in green or leafy vegetables. Because an occasional woman in the latter part of pregnancy experiences cramping of the muscles of the legs (induced, perhaps, by a transitory imbalance in the serum calcium to phosphorus ratio and the relatively high phosphorus content of milk), some health workers routinely advise pregnant women to drink no milk. If she eliminates milk altogether from her diet, the woman deletes an excellent source of other important nutrients, including protein, riboflavin, and vitamin A. To control the minor complaint of muscular cramping, would it not be more reasonable to simply indicate to her the amount of milk (3 to 4 cups) or *equivalent milk foods* that will supply her needs? Perhaps this patient likes milk or wants to use it in cooking. To take her calcium in this form would satisfy both the patient and her adviser.

Iron. A woman should maintain a daily intake of 18 mg. of iron throughout her childbearing years. This amount would replenish menstrual losses and restore tissue and liver reserves after each pregnancy. It is probable that iron supplements to dietary sources will be needed.

The increase in maternal circulating blood volume during pregnancy has been estimated to be from 20 to 40%. Iron is essential to the formation of hemoglobin; an adequate supply of this mineral is therefore important to maintain the mother's hemoglobin level. If low preconception stores are suspected, if there is a history of anemia, or if there is doubt concerning adequate dietary iron sources, iron supplementation may be indicated. Iron is also needed for fetal development, especially for storage of reserve in the liver. About a three to four months' supply of iron is stored in the de-

veloping fetal liver to supply the infant's need after birth; this is necessary because his first food, milk, lacks iron. Adequate maternal iron stores also fortify the mother against the blood losses at delivery.

Liver contains far more iron than any other food. Patients who dislike liver may be encouraged to use it more frequently by suggestions concerning appetizing ways of serving it. Other meat, dried beans, dried fruit, green vegetables, eggs, and enriched cereals, are additional sources of iron.

Vitamins. Increased amounts of vitamins A, B, C, and D are recommended during pregnancy.

Vitamin A. A daily increase of 1,000 I.U. is recommended for the latter half of pregnancy (about a 20% increase over the usual adult intake). Vitamin A is an essential factor in cell development, maintenance of the integrity of epithelial tissue, tooth formation (p. 76), normal bone growth, and vision. Liver, egg yolk, butter or fortified margarine, dark green and yellow vegetables, and fruits are good food sources.

B vitamins. There is an especially increased need for B vitamins during pregnancy. These are usually supplied by a well-balanced diet. When the physician doubts that the pregnant woman is taking an adequate diet, he may find it necessary to prescribe supplements. The B vitamins are important as coenzyme factors in a number of metabolic activities, energy production, function of muscle and nerve tissue, and therefore play key roles in the increased metabolic activities of pregnancy.

Vitamin C. Special emphasis must be laid on the pregnant woman's need for ascorbic acid. A daily increase of 5 to 10 mg. is recommended. Added to the adult recommendation of 55 mg. this makes a recommended daily total of 60 mg. during the latter half of pregnancy, or nearly a 20% increase. Ascorbic acid is exceedingly important to the growing organism. It is essential to the formation of intercellular cement substance in developing connective tissue and vascular systems. It also increases the absorption of the iron that is needed for the increasing quantities of hemoglobin. The expectant mother should be encouraged to eat additional quantities of foods that are common sources of vitamin C, such as citrus fruit, berries, melon, and cabbage.

Vitamin D. Adults who lead active lives entailing adequate exposure to sunlight, probably need no additional source of vitamin D. However, during pregnancy, the increased need for calcium and phosphorus presented by the developing fetal skeletal tissue necessitates additional vitamin D to promote the absorption and utilization of these minerals. Four hundred I.U. of vitamin D is recommended for the latter half of pregnancy. Frequently supplementary vitamin D is ordered by the physician. Food sources include fortified milk, but-

ter, liver, egg yolk, and fortified margarine.

Daily food pattern. A diet consisting of a variety of foods can supply needed nutrients and can make eating a pleasure. Adequate amounts of the nutrients during the early part of pregnancy, and the increased quantities of certain substances needed during the latter half may be met by intelligently planning around a daily food plan, using the key foods suggested. Such a daily food pattern is suggested in Table 17-2 and may be used as a helpful guide.

GENERAL DIETARY PROBLEMS
Gastrointestinal problems

During pregnancy, several gastrointestinal difficulties may be encountered. These are highly individual in form and extent and will require individual counseling or

Table 17-2. Daily food plan for pregnancy and lactation

Food	Nonpregnant woman or during first half of pregnancy	Second half of pregnancy	Lactation
Milk, cheese, ice cream, skimmed or buttermilk (food made with milk can supply part of requirement)	2 cups	3 to 4 cups	4 to 5 cups
Meat (lean meat, fish, poultry, cheese, occasional dried beans or peas)	1 serving (3 to 4 ounces)	2 servings (6 to 8 oz.); include liver frequently	2½ servings (8 oz.)
Eggs	1	1 to 2	1 to 2
Vegetable* (dark green or deep yellow)	1 serving	1 serving	1 to 2 servings
Vitamin C-rich food* Good source—citrus fruit, berries, cantaloupe Fair source—tomatoes, cabbage, greens, potatoes in skin	1 good source or 2 fair sources	1 good source and 1 fair source or 2 good sources	1 good source and 1 fair source or 2 good sources
Other vegetables and fruits	1 serving	2 servings	2 servings
Bread† and cereals (enriched or whole grain)	3 servings	4 to 5 servings	5 servings
Butter or fortified margarine	As desired or needed for calories	As desired or needed for calories	As desired or needed for calories

*Use some raw daily.
†One slice of bread equals one serving.

control. Usually, the complaints are relatively minor; but if they persist or become extreme, they will need attention from the physician. These problems include:

Nausea and vomiting. This complaint is usually mild and transitory, and limited to early pregnancy. It is commonly called "morning sickness," because it occurs more often upon rising than later in the day. A number of factors may contribute to this condition. Some are physiologic; they are traceable to the hormonal changes that occur in early pregnancy. These changes are probably accentuated in some patients by psychologic factors, various situational tensions, or anxieties concerning the pregnancy itself. Simple treatment usually suffices to improve food toleration. Small, frequent meals, fairly dry, and consisting chiefly of easily digested energy foods such as carbohydrates are most readily tolerated. Liquids are best taken between meals instead of with the food. If the condition develops to *hyperemesis* (severe, prolonged, persistent vomiting), the physician will probably hospitalize the patient and feed her intravenously to avoid complications.

Constipation. This complaint is seldom more than minor. The pressure of the enlarging uterus upon the lower portion of the intestine may make elimination somewhat difficult. Increased fluid intake and use of naturally laxative foods such as whole grains with added bran, dried fruits (especially prunes and figs), other fruits, and juices usually induce regularity. Laxatives should be avoided; they should not be used except under the physician's supervision.

Weight control

Optimum weight of the mother at conception appears to make an important contribution to a successful pregnancy. In most studies concerning the relation of nutrition to pregnancy, both underweight and overweight conditions have been shown to be asociated with problems during gestation or labor, or with unfavorable conditions of the infant at birth. Women who are underweight at conception and fail to gain adequately during the first two trimesters have a higher risk of premature labor or of giving birth to small babies. Overweight women, especially those whose general diet is inadequate in nutritional quality, are at a higher risk of developing toxemia or producing stillborn infants.

In addition to obstetrical hazards, excessive weight gain is to be avoided for other general health reasons. Strain on the muscles of the legs and back is a common cause of discomfort, fatigue, and pain in the back and legs. The excess weight tends to remain after the pregnancy, so that each successful pregnancy begins with the mother at a higher weight level. This accumulation can lead to added health problems as the woman grows older.

Total weight gain during pregnancy. In a broad study of weight gain in normal and toxic pregnancies, Chesley[11] found that the total weight gain averaged 24 lbs. In those patients the average gain in the first trimester was only 2 lbs.; whereas approximately 11 lbs. were accumulated during each of the last two trimesters. There was a wide variance in the individual rates of weight gain; during the third trimester and toward term, the variability was even more marked.

The average weight of the products of a normal pregnancy are given in the following list:

Products	Weight (lbs.)
Fetus	7.5
Placenta	1
Amniotic fluid	2
Uterus (weight increase)	2.5
Breast tissue (weight increase)	3
Blood volume (weight increase)	4 (1,500 ml.)
	20

Most obstetricians recommend a weight gain of about 16 to 24 lbs. with an average of 20 lbs. This represents the sum of the products of pregnancy indicated in the preceding list. Additional weight usually remains with the mother after delivery.

Rate of weight gain. Chesley's study indicated that far more rapid gain occurred during the latter part of pregnancy. Most physicians consider the increment satisfactory if it is about 2 lbs. during the first trimester and averages no more than 3 lbs. monthly during the second and third trimesters. Wide fluctuations in weight will be observed carefully by the physician.

Dietary management. Control of excess calories should be focused upon foods that are less essential to the fetus and mother—excess fats, sugar, and starches—not upon curtailment of the essential nutrients in the daily food pattern (see Table 17-2). A diet of 1,500 calories usually meets the

need for weight control and, with wise planning, can assure the needed nutrients. Such a general pattern is shown in Table 17-3.

Sodium restriction. Although views are conflicting concerning sodium restriction in pregnancy, there seems to be evidence that some control is warranted. Usually, strict control at the lower level of 500 to 1,000 mg. is unnecessary except in cases of therapeutic need, when it will be individually prescribed by the physician. Moderate curtailment, however, to about 2 to 3 gm. of sodium daily, is probably helpful. This level

Table 17-3. Diets for pregnancy varying in caloric content

	2,400 calories	1,800 calories	1,500 calories
Milk	3 to 4 cups	3 to 4 cups	3 to 4 cups skimmed
Meat, fish, poultry	2 servings	2 servings, lean	2 servings, lean
Eggs	1 to 2	1 to 2	1 to 2
Fruit	2 servings citrus, 1 other	2 servings citrus, 1 other	2 servings citrus, 1 other
Vegetables	4 servings, including potato and dark green leafy or yellow vegetable	4 servings, including potato and dark green leafy or yellow vegetable	4 servings, including potato and dark green leafy or yellow vegetable
Bread and cereals	4 servings whole grain or enriched	4 servings whole grain or enriched	4 servings whole grain or enriched
Butter or margarine	3 teaspoons	3 teaspoons	3 teaspoons
Other foods	Sugar, desserts, fat for cooking; other foods to meet caloric needs	None (sugar substitute may be used for sweetening)	None (sugar substitute may be used for sweetening)

Typical meal pattern

Breakfast	**Lunch**	**Dinner**
Fruit or juice (citrus)	Meat or meat substitute (egg, cheese)	Meat, lean (seafood, poultry)
Egg	Vegetable (green or yellow)	Potato
Cereal and/or bread— 1 tsp. butter	1 bread (or 2)	Cooked vegetable (green or yellow)
Milk	1 tsp. butter (or margarine)	Raw vegetable—salad
Coffee	Fruit (citrus)	1 bread—1 tsp. butter
	Milk (skimmed)	Fruit
		Milk (skimmed)

can be achieved by following two simple rules. *No salt should be added to foods.* Moderate or small amounts may be used in cooking, but no salt may be added at the table. *No obviously salty foods should be eaten.* This includes all such foods as meat and other foods preserved in salt such as ham, bacon, pickles, olives, potato chips, and cheese.

If a more specifically outlined diet is desired, the exchange system (p. 479) may be used with the pattern given below.

COMPLICATIONS OF PREGNANCY
Anemia

Anemia is common during pregnancy. Clinicians report that about 10% of the pa-tients in large prenatal clinics in the United States have hemoglobin concentrations of less than 10 gm. per 100 ml., and a hema-tocrit reading below 32. Anemia is, of course, more prevalent among the poor, many of whom live on diets barely ade-quate for subsistence; but anemia is by no means restricted to the lower economic groups. Disregarding some of the heredi-tary anemias, some of the more common acquired types encountered in pregnancy are categorized here according to their cause.

Iron deficiency anemia. A deficiency of iron is by far the most common cause of anemia in pregnancy. The cost of a single normal pregnancy in iron stores is large

---

Diet of 1,500 calories for weight control in pregnancy using the exchange system of dietary control (see Food Exchange Groups, pp. 483 and 484)

Total day's exchanges

4 milk exchanges (skimmed)
Vegetable A (as desired, 2 to 4 servings)
1 vegetable B exchange
4 fruit exchanges (2 citrus)
4 bread exchanges
8 meat exchanges (2 eggs; 6 oz. meat)
4 fat exchanges

Suggested meal pattern

Breakfast

1 fruit exchange
1 meat exchange (1 egg)
1 bread exchange
1 milk exchange
Coffee or tea

Lunch or supper

Meat exchange (3 oz. lean meat or exchange)
Vegetable A (any)
1 bread exchange
1 fat exchange
1 fruit exchange
1 milk exchange
Coffee or tea

Dinner

Meat exchange (3 oz. lean meat)
Vegetable A (any)
1 vegetable B
1 bread exchange
2 fat exchanges
1 fruit exchange
1 milk exchange
Coffee or tea

Snacks

1 bread exchange
1 fruit exchange
1 milk exchange

(about 700 to 800 mg.). Of this amount, nearly 300 mg. is used by the fetus; the remainder is utilized in the expansion of maternal red cell volume and hemoglobin mass. This total iron requirement exceeds the available reserves in the average woman. Studies have indicated that most women in the United States have low stores of iron.[12] The additional amount of iron needed during pregnancy may be made up in some women by increased dietary intake and increased efficiency of absorption; but in other women the iron level is borderline prior to pregnancy and insufficient to meet the augmented requirement. Anemia results. Usually, the requirements of the fetus, which increase during the last trimester, will continue to be met by transfer of the iron across the placenta; it is the mother who will suffer the iron deficiency. Doses of iron compound given orally, supplying about 200 mg. of iron daily, are usually adequate for treatment. This oral therapy should be continued for three to six months after the anemia has been corrected in order to replenish the depleted stores. Meanwhile, ways of including more iron-rich foods in her diet should be explored with the patient.

Hemorrhagic anemia. Anemia due to blood loss is more likely to occur during the puerperium than during gestation. Blood loss may occur earlier, however, as a result of abortion or ruptured tubal pregnancy. Most patients undergoing these physiologic disasters receive blood by transfusion, but iron therapy may be indicated in addition to support the formation of hemoglobin needed for adequate replacement.

Megaloblastic anemia. Megaloblastic anemia of pregnancy almost always results from folic acid deficiency. An analysis of the diet of these women usually reveals that they eat few if any vegetables (especially green leafy ones) and seldom take animal protein. Manifestations include intensification of nausea, vomiting, and anorexia. As the anemia progresses, the anorexia is more marked, thus further com-

pounding the nutritional deficiency. The folic acid requirement of the adult woman, estimated by Herbert[13] to be from 50 to 100 μg. per day, is considerably increased by pregnancy. Both the trophoblast and the fetus are sensitive to folic acid inhibitors, and therefore probably have high metabolic requirements for folic acid and its derivatives. The placenta and the fetus appear to concentrate folic acid efficiently, since the fetus may have an adequate store while the mother is severely deficient in this compound. Pritchard[14] has reported one case in which the hemoglobin levels of the newborn infant were 18 gm. or more per 100 ml. while the maternal levels were as low as 3.6 gm. per 100 ml.

Toxemia

Where man lacks precise knowledge he often must proceed on the basis of inference; but the human tendency to allow assumption to become dogma sometimes impedes the discovery of fact. In their development over the years, medicine, nursing, and nutrition have not been free from such errors. Certain assumptions about "the enigma of obstetrics"—toxemia—probably afford an example. Toxemia of pregnancy has been aptly called "the disease of theories." The literature abounds with conflicting views and open controversy concerning its etiology and treatment. Eastman and Helman[15] recently reviewed thirteen separate theories of the etiology of toxemia. Perhaps the most soundly based of these theories is that toxemia results from uterine ischemia (impaired blood flow); but this concept, like the others, is founded on assumption and has not been proved. Brewer[16,17,18] and a number of other clinicians[19,20] have presented clinical and laboratory evidence that toxemia is a disease of malnutrition, and that the malnutrition affects the liver and its metabolic activities. Certainly, as Mengert and Tweedy[21] have stressed, toxemia is classically associated with poverty; it has been encountered most often in women subsisting on inadequate diets who have little or no medical care.

It is evident that much more knowledge must be gained through research before this problem can be solved. Its urgency is evident from a few statistics. Toxemia occurs in 6 to 7% of all pregnancies. It accounts for the majority of all maternal deaths (about 1,000 deaths annually in the United States), and for the majority of all deaths of newborn infants (some 30,000 stillbirths and neonatal deaths per year). Most of these deaths could be prevented by good prenatal care, which inherently includes attention to sound nutrition. Many studies such as those discussed in the beginning of this chapter indicate that a general state of good nutrition, which a woman *brings to her pregnancy and maintains throughout it,* provides her with optimum resources for adapting to the physiologic stress of gestation. Her fitness during pregnancy is a direct function of her past nutrition.

Classification and clinical manifestations. Toxemia is generally classified and defined according to its manifestations. It is usually seen in the third trimester, toward term. Among its clinical manifestations are hypertension, edema, albuminuria, and in severe cases, convulsions and coma.

The broad descriptive classification of toxemia outlined by the American Committee on Maternal Welfare (revised 1952) is widely used:

I. Acute toxemia of pregnancy (onset after the twenty-fourth week)
  A. Pre-eclampsia
    1. Mild
    2. Severe
  B. Eclampsia (convulsions or coma; usually both when associated with hypertension, proteinuria, edema)
II. Chronic hypertensive (vascular) disease with pregnancy
  A. Without superimposed acute tox- or edema)
    1. Hypertension known to exist before beginning of the pregnancy
    2. Hypertension discovered during the pregnancy (earlier than the twenty-fourth week and persisting into the postpartum period)
  B. With superimposed acute toxemia

Treatment. Specific treatment varies according to the patient's symptoms and needs. Optimum nutrition is a fundamental aspect of therapy. Emphasis is laid on protein foods of high biologic value, and sources of vitamins and minerals for correction and maintenance of metabolic balance.

Pre-existing chronic conditions

Pre-existing conditions such as diabetes and heart disease are managed during pregnancy according to the general principles of care related to pregnancy and to the particular disease (pp. 487 and 523). With the physiologic stress of pregnancy added to that of disease, closer medical supervision is required. The pregnancy and the pre-existing disease affect each other, and enhance the difficulty of control. The therapeutic responsibility is frequently shared by internist and obstetrician. With their close observation of mother and child, cooperation by the patient, and good nutritional and nursing care, complications are minimized.

NUTRITION DURING LACTATION

The physiologic stress of lactation is even greater than that of pregnancy. The lactating mother consequently requires more dietary additions than does the pregnant woman. A comparison between the nutritional needs and daily food pattern of women in these two states may be made in Tables 17-1 and 17-2.

Nutritional needs

The basic nutritional requirements during pregnancy persist throughout lactation, with the following additions.

Protein. An increase of 10 gm. over the quantity recommended for the pregnant woman (20 gm. more than the usual adult allowance) is recommended during lactation, making a total daily protein allowance of about 75 gm.

Calories. The greatest recommended increase is in calories. Eight hundred calories daily more than in the prenatal diet (1,000 calories more than the usual adult allowance) is needed for lactation, making a daily total of about 3,000 calories.

This additional requirement of 1,000 calories for the overall total lactation process (about 120 calories per 100 ml.) represents two factors.

1. *Milk content.* An average daily milk production for lactating women is 850 ml. (30 ounces). Human milk has a caloric value of about 20 calories per ounce. Thus, these 30 ounces of milk have a value of 600 calories.
2. *Milk production.* The metabolic work involved in producing this amount of milk utilizes from 400 to 420 calories.

In view of these two amounts (600 for milk content plus 400 for milk production) the nurse is clearly justified in assuring the young mother who desires to breast-feed her baby that these calories do indeed go into milk production—not into her own figure!

Minerals. The quantities of calcium and iron required by the lactating mother are not greater than those needed during pregnancy. The increased amount of calcium that was required during gestation for mineralization of the fetal skeleton is now diverted into the mother's milk. Iron, since it is not a principal mineral component of milk, need not be increased for milk production per se.

Vitamins. The increased quantity of vitamin C recommended for the pregnant women is also recommended for the lactating mother. No further augmentation is needed, since milk contains little vitamin C. Increases over the mother's prepartum intake are recommended, however, in vitamin A (2,000 I.U. more) and the B-complex vitamins, riboflavin and niacin (about a one-third increase over the quantities taken during pregnancy). These vitamins are important coenzyme factors in cell respiration, glucose oxidation, and energy metabolism; the quantities needed therefore invariably increase as caloric intake increases.

Fluids. A practice sometimes neglected, because fluids may not be considered a nutrient, but which is highly significant to adequate milk production, is the increased intake of fluids. Water, beverages such as juices, tea, coffee, and milk, all add to the fluid necessary to produce milk, a fluid tissue.

Rest and relaxation. In addition to the augmented diet, the mother who would breast-feed her baby requires rest, moderate exercise, and relaxation. Often the nurse may help the mother by counseling with her about her new family situation; together they may develop plans to accommodate these needs.

Summary concept. Throughout the experience of pregnancy and lactation, intelligent care is based on general nutritional fitness and attention to individual needs. And these are but a continuation of a women's lifetime nutritional experience.

References
Specific
1. Paddock, C. E.: Diet in pregnancy, Surg. Gynec. Obstet. **31**:71, 1920.
2. Toverud, G.: The influence of nutrition on the course of pregnancy, Milbank Mem. Fund. Quart. **28**:7, 1950.
3. Nutrition in pregnancy, Nutr. Rev. **1**:81, 1943.
4. Ebbs, J., Tisdall, E. F., and Scott, W. A.: The influence of prenatal diet on the mother and the child, J. Nutr. **22**:515, 1941.
5. Burke, B. S., and others: Nutrition studies during pregnancy, Amer. J. Obstet. Gynec. **46**:38, 1943.
6. McGanity, W. J., and others: The Vanderbilt Cooperative Study of Maternal and Infant Nutrition. VIII. Some nutritional implications, J. Amer. Diet. Ass. **31**:582, 1955.
7. McGanity, W. J., and others: Vanderbilt Cooperative Study of Maternal and Infant Nutrition. XII. Effect of reproductive cycle on nutritional status and requirements, J.A.M.A. **168**:2138, 1958.
8. Thomson, A.: Diet in pregnancy, Brit. J. Nutr. **1**(12):446, 1958; **2**(13):190, 1959; **3**(13): 509, 1959.
9. Smith, C.: Effects of maternal undernutrition upon the newborn infant in Holland (1944-1945), J. Pediat. **30**:229, 1947.

10. Ramsey, E., Corner, G. W., and Donner, M. W.: Serial and cineradiographic visualization of maternal circulation in the primate (hemochorial) placenta, Amer. J. Obstet. Gynec. **86**:213, 1963.
11. Chesley, L. C.: Weight changes and water balance in normal and toxic pregnancy, Amer. J. Obst. Gynec. **48**:565, 1944.
12. Pritchard, J. A., and Mason, R. A.: Iron stores of normal adults and replenishment with oral iron therapy, J.A.M.A. **190**:897, 1964.
13. Herbert, V., and others: Minimal daily adult folate requirement, Arch. Int. Med. **110**:649, 1962.
14. Pritchard, J. A.: Megaloblastic anemia during pregnancy and the puerperium, Amer. J. Obst. Gynec. **83**:1004, 1962.
15. Eastman, N. J., and Hellman, L. M.: Williams' obstetrics, ed. 13, New York, 1966, Appleton-Century-Crofts.
16. Brewer, T. H.: Metabolic toxemia of late pregnancy, Springfield, Illinois, 1966, Charles C Thomas, Publisher.
17. Brewer, T. H.: Limitations of diuretic therapy in the management of severe toxemia: the significance of hypoalbuminemia, Amer. J. Obstet. Gynec. **83**:1352, 1962.
18. Brewer, T. H.: Role of malnutrition, hepatic dysfunction and gastrointestinal bacteria in the pathogenesis of acute toxemia of pregnancy, Amer. J. Obstet. Gynec. **84**:1253, 1962.
19. Call, M., and Lorentzen, D.: Rupture of the liver associated with toxemia, Obstet. Gynec. **25**:466, 1965.
20. Maqueo, M., Ayala, L., and Cervantes, L.: Nutritional status and liver function in toxemia of pregnancy, Obstet. Gynec. **23**:222, 1964.
21. Mengert, W. F., and Tweedie, J. A.: Acute vasospastic toxemia: therapeutic nihilism, Obstet. Gynec. **24**:662, 1964.

General

Anderson, E. H., and Lesser, A. J.: Maternity care in the United States, Amer. J. Nurs. **66**:1539, 1966.
Benjamin, F., and others: Serum levels of folic acid, B_{12}, and Fe in anemia of pregnancy, Amer. J. Obstet. Gynec. **96**:310, 1966.
Brown, M. W.: Prenatal care, (Children's Bureau, U. S. Dept. of Health, Education, and Welfare), Bronxville, New York, 1967, Child Care Publishers, Inc.
Chopra, J. G., and others: Anemia in pregnancy, Amer. J. Public Health **57**:857, 1967.
Davis, M. E., and Rubin, R.: Obstetrics for nurses, Philadelphia, 1966, W. B. Saunders Company.
Eastman, N. J.: Expectant motherhood, Boston, 1957, Little, Brown and Company.

Editorial: Weight gain and pregnancy, J.A.M.A. **164**:877, 1957.
Edwards, C. H., and others: Odd dietary practices of women, J. Amer. Diet. Ass. **30**:976, 1954.
Fitzpatrick, E., Eastman, N. J., and Reeder, S. R.: Maternity nursing, ed. 11, Philadelphia, 1966, J. B. Lippincott Co.
Hagbord, L.: Pregnancy and diabetes mellitus, Springfield, Illinois, 1961, Charles C Thomas, Publisher.
Iron deficiency anemia, Tech. Rep. Series No. 182, Geneva, 1959, World Health Organization.
Jeans, P. C., Smith, M. B., and Stearns, G.: Incidence of prematurity in relation to maternal nutrition, J. Amer. Diet. Ass. **31**:576, 1955.
Josey, W. E.: The role of nutrition in the management of pregnancy: a review of recent studies, Amer. J. Clin. Nutr. **2**:303, 1954.
Lowenberg, M. E.: Philosophy of nutrition and application in maternal health services, Amer. J. Clin. Nutr. **16**:370, 1965.
Lutwak, L.: Osteoporosis—a mineral deficiency disease?, J. Amer. Diet. Ass. **44**:173, 1964.
Macy, I. G., and Kelly, H. J.: Food for expectant and nursing mothers. In Stefferud, A., editor: Food, the yearbook of agriculture, 1959, Washington, D. C., 1959, U. S. Dept. of Agriculture.
Mayer, J.: Nutrition and lactation, Postgrad. Med. **33**:380, 1963.
Mayer, J.: Some aspects of the relation of nutrition and pregnancy, Postgrad. Med. **33**:277, 1963.
Mayer, J.: Treatment of obesity in adults, Postgrad. Med. **38**:A133, 1965.
McGanity, W. J.: Obesity and the obstetrician, J.A.M.A. **186**:39, 1963.
Mullins, H.: Overweight in pregnancy, Lancet **1**:146, 1960.
Nutrition in pregnancy, Sym. IV, Council on Foods and Nutrition, Chicago, Illinois, 1958, American Medical Association.
Nutrition in pregnancy and lactation, Tech. Rep. Series No. 302, Geneva, 1965, World Health Organization.
Page, E. W., and Page, E. P.: Leg cramps in pregnancy, Obstet. Gynec. **1**:94, 1953.
Pike, R. L.: Sodium intake during pregnancy, J. Amer. Diet. Ass. **44**:176, 1964.
Reis, R. A., DeCosta, E. J., and Allweiss, M. D.: Diabetes and pregnancy, Springfield, Illinois, 1952, Charles C Thomas, Publisher.
Rust, H.: A survey of food habits of pregnant women, Amer. J. Nurs. **60**:1636, 1960.
Sand, R. X.: Obesity and pregnancy, Amer. J. Obstet. Gynec. **83**:1617, 1962.
Scrimshaw, N. S.: Nutrition functions of maternal and child health programs in technically underdeveloped areas, Nutr. Rev. **20**:33, 1962.
Seifrit, E.: Changes in beliefs and food practices in pregnancy, J. Amer. Diet. Ass. **39**:455, 1961.

Semmens, J. P., and McGlamory, J. C.: Teen-age pregnancies, Obstet. Gynec. **16**:31, 1960.

Sisson, T. R. C., and Lund, C. J.: The influence of maternal iron deficiency on the newborn, Amer. J. Clin. Nutr. **6**:376, 1958.

Smith, C. A.: Effect of maternal nutrition upon pregnancy and the newborn, J. Amer. Diet. Ass. **25**:665, 1949.

Smith, C. A.: Prenatal and neonatal nutrition, Pediatrics **30**:145, 1962.

Sodium intake in pregnancy: two views, J.A.M.A. **200**:42, 1967.

Stearns, G.: Nutritional state of the mother prior to conception, J.A.M.A. **168**:1655, 1958.

Stearns, G.: Prenatal nutrition and infant health, Children **5**:145, 1958.

Streiff, R. R., and Little, A. B.: Folic acid deficiency in pregnancy, New Eng. J. Med. **276**:776, 1967.

Taylor, R. G.: Some significant developments in maternal and child health nursing, Nurs. Outlook **8**:442, 1960.

Tompkins, W. T., and Wiehl, D. G.: Nutritional deficiencies as a causal factor in toxemia and premature labor, Amer. J. Obstet. Gynec. **62**:898, 1951.

Tompkins, W. T., and others: The underweight patient as an increased obstetric hazard, Amer. J. Obstet Gynec. **69**:114, 1955.

Thaxton, A.: Teaching expectant parents what they want to know, Amer. J. Nurs. **62**:112, 1962.

Ullery, J. C., Hollenbeck, Z. J. R., and Meiling, R. L.: Textbook of obstetrics, St. Louis, 1965, The C. V. Mosby Co.

Wallace, H.: Teen-age pregnancy, Amer. J. Obstet. Gynec. **92**:1125, 1965.

Wayler, T. J., and Klein, R. S.: Applied nutrition, New York, 1965, The Macmillan Company.

Wellin, E.: Maternal and infant feeding practices in a Peruvian village, J. Amer. Diet. Ass. **31**:889, 1955.

Woody, N. C., and Woody, H. B.: Management of breast feeding, J. Pediat. **68**:344, 1966.

Yankauer, A., and others: What mothers say about childbearing and parents' classes, Nurs. Outlook **8**:563, 1960.

CHAPTER 18

Nutrition for growth and development: infancy, childhood, and adolescence

Growth may be defined, essentially, as an increase in size. Biologic growth of an organism takes place through cell multiplication. Development is the associated process in which growing tissues and organs take on increased complexity of function. Thus, since both processes are part of one whole, the combined terms *growth and development* form a unitary concept which indicates the magnitude and quality of maturational changes.

At birth, the newborn infant displays evidence in form and function of the tremendous growth and development that has already taken place during his fetal life. He brings to the beginning of his life cycle the heritage of generations before him and the physical resources provided him by the maternal organism. It is upon this heritage and these resources that his total life experience will make indelible imprint. Therefore, the molding of growth and development factors in these early impressionistic years is of vital import.

Physiologic growth is dependent upon special chemical nutrients in the food a person eats and the biochemical processes of metabolism which supply the right elements in the right place, at the right time, for the formation and maintenance of body tissues. However, human growth and development involves far more than the physical process alone. It encompasses social and psychologic influences and relationships, the whole of the environment and culture which nurtures the individual growth potential. Food and feeding during these highly significant years do not, indeed cannot, exist apart from this broader, overall concept of growth and development. The *whole* process produces the *whole* person. This study, therefore, will use this approach. Within this framework food and feeding will be considered as a part of the whole development of the child. Age group nutritional needs and the food which supplies them will be adapted to the general psychosocial as well as physical maturation normally achieved at that age. These related questions may be helpful guides for study:

1. What is the normal physical growth pattern for children?
2. In what ways may growth of children be determined? What general nutritional problems do United States surveys reveal?
3. What psychosocial problems face the growing child? What related developmental tasks does he learn in each age period? How are these related to food and feeding?
4. What are the basic nutritional needs for normal growth and development of children?
5. How may these combined physical and psychosocial needs in each age group be met in food choices and feeding practices?

Throughout the study it should be remembered that although the discussion is in terms of general needs at a given

369

age level, wide individual variations exist within normal ranges. Thus, in the care of children the nurse should never lose sight of the individual child and his own unique needs and growth potentials.

GROWTH AND DEVELOPMENT
Physical growth

Normal life cycle growth pattern. The normal human life cycle follows four general phases of overall growth.

Infancy. During the first year the infant grows rapidly, the rate tapering off somewhat in the latter half of the year. At age six months, he will probably have doubled his birth weight and at one year may have tripled it. Thus, a baby weighing 7 lbs. at birth will weigh approximately 14 lbs. at six months and about 21 lbs. at one year of age.

Latent period of childhood. During the years between infancy and adolescence, the rate of growth slows and becomes erratic. At some periods there are plateaus; at others, small spurts of growth. The overall rate, being erratic, affects appetite accordingly; at times a child will have little or no appetite, and at others he will eat voraciously.

Adolescence. The second rapid growth spurt occurs during adolescence in association with the manifold physical changes of puberty. Due to the hormonal influences, multiple body changes occur including development of long bones, sex characteristics, and fat and muscle mass development.

Adult. In the final phase of the normal life cycle, growth levels off in the adult plateau and gradually declines during senescence.

Parameters of growth in children

Physical growth. There is a wide variance in the physical growth of children. Several basic measures are used to determine this growth.

Weight and height. Weight and height are the common general measures of physical growth. They form, however, a crude index without giving finer details of individual variations. Generally, as the child's growth is supervised, his weight and height are compared with the "average" measures of weight and height for his age.

Body measurements. In addition to general weight and height, several body measurements are helpful indicators of growth. These include the recumbent length of the infant and small child as compared with the standing height as he grows older. Also, head circumference is a valuable measure in infants but is seldom taken routinely after three years of age. Other circumference measures are those of the chest, the abdomen, and the leg at its maximal girth of the calf. An additional measure is that of pelvic breadth which is taken with a broad sliding caliper. Other measurements made with calipers may include skin fold thicknesses. Longitudinal growth studies in research centers employ many measures of development (Fig. 18-1).

Clinical signs. Various clinical signs of optimum growth may be observed as measures. These include general vitality, a sense of well-being, posture, the condition of gums and teeth, of the skin, the hair, the eyes, the development of muscles, and nervous control. A number of these clinical signs and observations of nutritional status are summarized in Table 18-1.

Laboratory data. In addition, finer measures are obtained by various laboratory tests. These include studies of blood and urine to determine levels of vitamins, hemoglobin, and so on. X-rays of the bones in the hand and wrists may also be taken to indicate degree of ossification.

Nutritional analysis. A measure of the growth of a child may be based upon a nutritional analysis of his general eating habits. A diet history form and an analysis chart such as those suggested for use in family diet counseling (pp. 292 and 294) may be used.

Mental growth. Measures of mental growth usually involve abilities in communication and the development in ability to handle abstract and symbolic material in thinking. The child originally thinks very

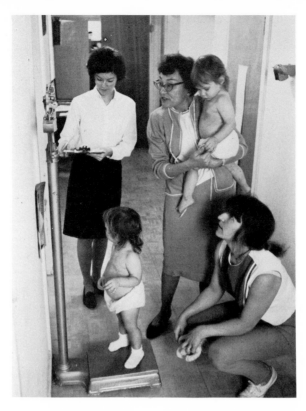

Fig. 18-1. Growth and development study being conducted at University of California in Berkeley. Here weight of twins in the study is being recorded. Many other measures are taken, some using calipers.

literally. As he develops in mental capacity, he increasingly can handle more than single ideas and develop constructive concepts.

Emotional growth. Emotional growth is measured in the capacity for love and affection, the ability to handle frustration and its anxieties, to control aggressive impulses, and to channel hostility from destructive to constructive activities.

Social and cultural growth. Social development of a child is measured in terms of his ability to relate to others and to participate in group living in his culture. These social and cultural behaviors he learns first through his relationships with his parents, then with his family. As his horizon broadens, he develops relationships with those outside the family, with friends, and with those in the community. For this reason a child's play in his early years is a highly purposeful activity.

NUTRITIONAL REQUIREMENTS

Calories—total energy needs. During childhood, the demand for calories is relatively large. However, there is a great variation in need with age and condition. For example, approximately 50% of the five-year-old's calories are needed for basal metabolic requirements. Another 5% is involved in the specific dynamic action of food, which includes the various metabolic processes involved in the digestion, absorption, and metabolism of food substances. Therefore, 55% of his calories are involved in the metabolic activities of basal metabolism and food digestion. Physical activity requires 25% of his calories, growth needs 12%, and 8% is represented in fecal loss. In recent revisions of the National Research Council (1963 and 1968) for nutrient recommendations, the caloric allowances were reduced for children. The reduced general

Table 18-1. Clinical signs of nutritional status

	Good	Poor
General appearance	Alert, responsive	Listless, apathetic, cachexic
Hair	Shiny, lustrous; healthy scalp	Stringy, dull, brittle, dry, depigmented
Neck (glands)	No enlargement	Thyroid enlarged
Skin (face and neck)	Smooth, slightly moist; good color, reddish-pink mucous membranes	Greasy, discolored, scaly
Eyes	Bright, clear; no fatigue circles beneath	Dryness, signs of infection, increased vascularity, glassiness, thickened conjunctiva
Lips	Good color, moist	Dry, scaly, swollen; angular lesions (stomatitis)
Tongue	Good pink color, surface papillae present, no lesions	Papillary atrophy, smooth appearance; swollen, red, beefy (glassitis)
Gums	Good pink color; no swelling or bleeding, firm	Marginal redness or swelling, receding, spongy
Teeth	Straight, no crowding, well-shaped jaw, clean, no discoloration	Unfilled caries, absent teeth, worn surfaces, mottled, malposition
Skin (general)	Smooth, slightly moist, good color	Rough, dry, scaly, pale, pigmented, irritated, petechia, bruises
Abdomen	Flat	Swollen
Legs, feet	No tenderness, weakness, or swelling; good color	Edema, tender calf, tingling, weakness
Skeleton	No malformations	Bowlegs, knock-knees, chest deformity at diaphragm, beaded ribs, prominent scapulae
Weight	Normal for height, age, body build	Overweight or underweight
Posture	Erect, arms and legs straight, abdomen in, chest out	Sagging shoulders, sunken chest, humped back
Muscles	Well developed, firm	Flaccid, poor tone; undeveloped, tender
Nervous control	Good attention span for age; does not cry easily, not irritable or restless	Inattentive, irritable
Gastrointestinal function	Good appetite and digestion; normal, regular elimination	Anorexia, indigestion, constipation or diarrhea
General vitality	Endurance, energetic, sleeps well at night; vigorous	Easily fatigued, no energy, falls asleep in school, looks tired, apathetic

activity of children in an industrialized society requires fewer calories. Of these calories, carbohydrate is the main energy source. It is important also as a protein-sparer to ensure that protein vital for growth will not be diverted for energy needs. Fat calories are important, although caution should be exercised against an excess. Certain fatty acids are essential, especially linoleic acid. A characteristic eczema has been observed in infants whose diets were deficient in linoleic acid.

Protein. Protein is the *growth element* of the body. It supplies the essential amino acids which are necessary for formation and maintenance of muscle and nerve tissue, and of bone matrix. Protein also serves as an integral part of most body fluids and secretions such as enzymes, hormones, lymph, and plasma. As stated in the chapter on protein, these essential amino acids have to be supplied in proper amounts and proportion and timing for tissue protein to be synthesized (p. 51).

The final determinant for the protein requirement of a child is his overall growth pattern. His requirements per unit of body weight gradually decrease. For example, during the first six months of life he requires about 2.0 gm. of protein per kilogram body weight. This amount relative to body weight gradually decreases until adulthood, when his protein need is about 1 gm. per kilogram body weight. By and large, the healthy, active, growing child will consume his needed amount of calories and proteins in the variety of food provided him.

Water—body content and consumption. Water is essential to life second only to oxygen. The human need for water is well established. The infant need, however, is even greater than that of the adult. The infant's body content of water, for example, is from 70 to 75% of his body weight, whereas in the adult, water comprises only from 60 to 65% of the total body weight. Also, in the infant a relatively large amount of the total water is outside the cell, and thus is more easily lost.

The infant's requirement for water is

related to the caloric intake and the specific gravity of the urine. Generally, an infant consumes daily an amount of water equivalent to 10 to 15% of his body weight. The adult consumes daily an amount of water equivalent to 2 to 4% of his body weight. The approximate daily requirements of children for water, calories, and protein are outlined in Table 18-2.

Minerals. A number of minerals relate to special body function and are essential in body metabolism. Two minerals particularly vital to the growing child are calcium and iron.

Calcium. Calcium is necessary for the rapid bone mineralization that takes place during growth. In the newborn infant only the central sections of large bones are mineralized. An x-ray taken at this time would give the appearance of a collection of disconnected, separate bones. Calcium is also needed for the developing teeth, for muscle contraction, nerve irritability, blood coagulation, and the action of the heart muscle.

Iron. Iron is necessary for the formation of hemoglobin. Iron is also used as a component of several oxidative enzymes. Since the infant's fetal store is diminshed in about three to four months, and his basic food, milk, lacks iron, the infant soon needs solid food additions to supply iron. Such foods as meat, enriched cereal, and egg yolk, accomplish this purpose.

Vitamins. In the chapters on vitamins it was learned that a large number are essential for growth and maintenance. In fact, the word vitamin refers to their essential character. They were so named because they are necessary to life and play many key roles in body metabolism. There are several vitamins for which growth requirements have been set.

Vitamin A. Vitamin A is a necessary constituent of the substance in the eye, visual purple, which regulates adaptations to light and dark. It is also used in bone and tooth development, and in the formation and maturation of epithelial tissue such as in the skin, the eye, and in the digestive, res-

Table 18-2. Approximate daily requirements of children for calories, protein, and water*

Age in years	Calories†		Protein	Water†	
	per kg.	per lb.	gm. per kg.‡	ml. per kg.	oz. per lb.
Infancy§	110	50	2.0 to 3.5	150	2¼
1 to 3	100	45	2.0 to 2.5	125	2.0−
4 to 6	90	41	3.0	100	1½
7 to 9	80	36	2.8	75	1.0+
10 to 12	70	32	2.0	75	1.0+
13 to 15	60	27	1.7	50	¾
16 to 19	50	23	1.5+	50	¾
Adult	40	18	1.0	50	¾

*Nelson, W. E., editor: Textbook of pediatrics, ed. 8, Philadelphia, 1964, W. B. Saunders Company, p. 109.
†At least 10% variation.
‡To convert gm. per kg. to gm. per lb., divide by 2 and subtract 10% of the quotient. Thus 4 gm. per kg. is equivalent to 1.8 gm. per lb.
§Needs during the first weeks are lower; during the first 6 months they are relatively higher than during the last 6 months.

piratory, urinary, and reproductive tracts.

B-complex vitamins. The main B-complex vitamins include thiamine, niacin, and riboflavin.

THIAMINE. Thiamine is directly related to carbohydrate metabolism; hence, to caloric intake. As caloric needs increase, thiamine needs increase. It is evident then that thiamine needs accompany the caloric demands for energy. Thiamine functions as an important coenzyme factor, especially in the oxidation of pyruvic acid and therefore is important to energy production for use in body activity and metabolic work. In growth, there is increased anabolic activity and increased physical activity, both of which increase energy demands.

NIACIN. Niacin is also an important coenzyme factor in metabolic activities. It is required for cellular oxidation.

RIBOFLAVIN. Riboflavin also acts as a coenzyme factor in metabolism, in reactions involving amino acids and fatty acids as well as carbohydrates. Table 18-3 shows that beginning with the preadolescent period, there is a difference in requirements of riboflavin for boys as compared with those for girls. Usually the requirements for boys are larger due to their increasing

size and change in muscle mass and body weight.

Other B vitamins. Several B vitamins are associated with the proper formation of red blood cells and therefore are important during growth. These include cobalamin, pyridoxine, and folic acid.

COBALAMIN (vitamin B_{12}). A deficiency of vitamin B_{12} is associated with juvenile pernicious anemia due to a defect in the absorption of the vitamin because of an absence of the necessary intrinsic factor in the gastric juice.

PYRIDOXINE (vitamin B_6). A deficiency of pyridoxine is associated with nerve and muscle irritability and a hypochromic anemia.

FOLIC ACID (folacin). A deficiency of folic acid is associated with megaloblastic anemia, especially in infancy.

Vitamin C. Vitamin C plays an important role in the growth period in several ways:

1. It participates in the formation of intercellular cement substance in all tissues. In this role, vitamin C is especially needed in the rapidly growing tissue of a child.

2. It facilitates the absorption of essential iron.

3. It participates actively in a number of other general metabolic activities including mineralization and enzyme systems. For example, ascorbic acid is probably a coenzyme in the metabolism of phenylalanine and tyrosine, both of which are important amino acids for growth.

Vitamin D. Vitamin D is essential during growth for the absorption and utilization of calcium and phosphorus needed for bone development. It regulates the absorption of these minerals, probably by affecting the permeability of intestinal membranes. It also aids in the anchoring of the minerals in the bone by regulating the level of serum alkaline phosphatase.

Vitamin K. Vitamin K is essential in the formation of prothrombin by the liver (p. 83), an initial element in the blood-clotting mechanism. A lack of vitamin K is not usually a dietary problem, because it is synthesized by intestinal microorganisms. However, since the newborn lacks these microorganisms at birth, he is usually given vitamin K to avoid any hemorrhagic tendencies.

Vitamin E. Although no definitive mechanisms are as yet determined, current research indicates possible growth-associated functions of vitamin E, perhaps in relation to muscle metabolism and to erythrocyte fragility (pp. 81 and 82).

Hypervitaminoses A and D. Hypervitaminoses A and D (pp. 77 and 80) are possibilities when for prolonged periods excess amounts of the vitamins are given, because of a misunderstanding, ignorance, or carelessness. Parents should be counseled to use only the amount directed and no more. Symptoms of toxicity from excess vitamin A include anorexia, slow growth, drying and cracking of the skin, enlargement of the liver and the spleen, swelling and pain of long bones, and bone fragility. Symptoms of toxicity from excess vitamin D include nausea, diarrhea, weight loss, polyuria, nocturia, and eventually calcification of soft tissues, including that of renal tubules, blood vessels, bronchi, stomach, and heart.

Summary of nutritional needs

A summary of the nutritional needs for growth is presented in Table 18-3, as recommended by the National Research Council in their 1968 revisions. Since the original publication of these recommendations in 1943, the Council has made six revisions as new knowledge has been gained from research. In Table 18-3 a summary of the new 1968 dietary allowances is given for comparative study. In the allowances of protein the reduced recommendations are based on basal calorie requirements, the generally good quality of protein in an average American diet, with appropriate increments for growth on the basis that gain in body weight is 18% protein. Some allowance is then added to cover individual variability within a large population. There were also general reductions in calorie allowances.

The allowances for vitamin C were significantly reduced based on indications that the previous ample safety margin was excessive and produced no added beneficial effects. The allowances for iron during late childhood and adolescence were raised. These increases were deemed wise to cover losses in normal iron exchange, needs for iron retention during growth, and additional menstrual losses in adolescent girls.

These overall allowances include safety margins to cover individual variations in healthy, normal children. As such they are *guidelines* for needed amounts of nutrients which can be attained with a variety of common foods.

AGE GROUP NEEDS

Throughout the human life cycle, food and feeding not only serve to meet nutritional requirements for growth and physical maintenance, but they also relate intimately to personal psychosocial development. The nutritional age group needs of children cannot be understood apart from the child's overall maturation as a person. Erik Erikson,[1-3] professor of Human Development at Harvard University, has contributed much

Table 18-3. Recommended daily dietary allowances for growth (National Research Council 1964 and 1968 reviews)*

	Age (yrs.)	Wt. (lbs.)	Calories	Protein gm.	Calcium gm.	Iron mg.	Vitamin A I.U.	Vitamin B complex Thiamine mg.	Riboflavin mg.	Niacin mg.	Vitamin C mg.	Vitamin D I.U.
Infants:	0 to 1/6	9	(495) 480	(14) 9	(.6) .4	(5) 6	1,500	(.4)	(.5) .2	(6) 5	(30) 35	400
	1/6 to 1/2	15	(825) 770	(24) 14	(.6) .5	(5) 10	1,500	.4	.5	(6) 7	(30) 35	400
	1/2 to 1	20	900	(28) 16	(.8) .6	(7) 15	1,500	.5	(.8) .6	(7) 8	(30) 35	400
Children:	1 to 2	26	(1,200) 1,100	(32) 25	(.8) .7	(8) 15	2,000	(.5) .6	(.8) .6	(9) 8	40	400
	2 to 3	31	1,250	(32) 25	.8	(8) 15	2,000	(.5) .6	(.8) .7	(9) 8	40	400
	3 to 4	35	(1,600) 1,400	(40) 30	.8	10	2,500	(.6) .7	(1.0) .8	(11) 9	(50) 40	400
	4 to 6	42	1,600	(40) 30	.8	10	2,500	(.6) .8	(1.0) .9	11	(50) 40	400
	6 to 8	51	(2,100) 2,000	(52) 35	(.8) .9	(12) 10	3,500	(.8) 1.0	(1.3) 1.1	(14) 13	(60) 40	400
	8 to 10	62	2,200	(52) 40	(.8) 1.0	(12) 10	3,500	(.8) 1.1	(1.3) 1.2	(14) 15	(60) 40	400
Boys:	10 to 12	77	(2,400) 2,500	(60) 45	(1.1) 1.2	(15) 10	4,500	(1.0) 1.2	(1.4) 1.3	(16) 17	(70) 40	400
	12 to 14	95	(3,000) 2,700	(75) 50	1.4	(15) 18	5,000	(1.2) 1.4	(1.2) 1.4	(20) 18	(80) 45	400
	14 to 18	130	(3,400) 3,000	(85) 60	1.4	(15) 18	5,000	1.4	(2.0) 1.5	(22) 20	(80) 55	400
Girls:	10 to 12	77	(2,200) 2,250	(55) 50	(1.1) 1.2	(15) 18	4,500	(.9) 1.1	1.3	15	(80) 40	400
	12 to 14	97	(2,500) 2,300	(62) 50	1.3	(15) 18	5,000	(1.0) 1.2	(1.5) 1.4	(17) 15	(80) 45	400
	14 to 16	114	(2,300) 2,400	(58) 55	1.3	(15) 18	5,000	(.9) 1.2	(1.3) 1.4	(15) 16	(70) 50	400
	16 to 18	119	2,300	(58) 55	1.3	(15) 18	5,000	(.9) 1.2	(1.3) 1.5	15	(70) 50	400

*The 1964 recommendations appear in parentheses before the new 1968 recommendations in those places where changes have been made. If no figure precedes a given nutrient listing, no change was made by the Council in its allowance for that nutrient.

insight to an understanding of this pattern of human growth and its critical periods of development. Dr. Erikson has identified eight stages in man's growth, and a basic psychosocial problem or crisis with which one struggles at each stage. The developmental problem at each stage has a positive ego value and a conflicting negative counterpart:

Infancy—trust versus distrust
Toddler—autonomy versus shame and doubt
Preschooler—initiative versus guilt
School-aged child—industry versus inferiority
Adolescent—identity versus role confusion
Young adult—intimacy versus isolation
Adult—generativity versus stagnation
Old age—ego integrity versus despair

Given favorable circumstances, a growing child develops the positive aspect of his developmental problem at each life stage, and therefore builds increasing strength to meet the next crisis. However, the struggle at any age is not forever won at that point. A residue of the negative remains and in periods of stress, such as those encountered in illness, regression in some degree usually occurs. But as the child gains mastery at each stage of development, assisted by significant relationships of a positive nature surrounding him, integration of self-controls takes place. Various related developmental tasks surround each of these stages and its core problem. These are learnings that, when accomplished, contribute to successful resolution of the core problem. Therefore, these developmental tasks are integrated and associated with the normal physical maturation at that point. In each of these stages of childhood, food choices and feeding practices are related to the general age group characteristics.

Infancy (birth to 1 year)
The premature infant

Characteristics. Although premature infants vary in weight and development, a child is usually considered premature if he is born at fewer than 270 days of gestation or if he weighs less than 5.5 pounds. The premature infant lacks the nutritional and developmental resources provided in the final weeks of normal gestation. Thus, he faces survival hazards. He is a fragile, unfinished product. He has much more water and less protein and minerals per pound of body weight than the full-term baby. There is little subcutaneous fat and his bones are poorly calcified. The neuromuscular system is incompletely developed, making normal sucking reflexes weak or absent. The digestive ability and renal function may be limited. The immature liver lacks adequate iron stores and developed metabolic enzyme systems.

Food and feeding. Despite these handicaps, however, relatively simple feeding routines are usually effective, and good growth results may be expected, if the child is also kept warm[4] and free from infection.

Type of milk. Breast milk alone is seldom adequate because it lacks sufficient protein for the rapid growth of the premature infant. Fat is poorly tolerated due to the immature digestive apparatus. Therefore, the usual milk of choice is skimmed or partially skimmed diluted cow's milk with added carbohydrate as needed. This may be supplemented by breast milk should the mother desire. Until the infant is strong enough to nurse at the mother's breast, the milk may be expressed manually or with a common hand breast pump. Feedings are usually delayed twenty-four to thirty-six hours following birth. The comparative inactivity and low heat production of the infant, plus his relatively large body water content reduce his immediate need for calories. Also, his weakness and the danger of aspiration make some feeding delay advisable. The first feedings are usually sterile 5 to 10% solutions of glucose in water. A few milliliters are given at frequent intervals gradually building up the amount, and adding small amounts of milk formula.

Generally, one needs to proceed more slowly with smaller infants and never to hurry with any. Usually by the time an infant is a week old, he should be receiving about 50 to 60 calories per pound (approximately 2½ oz. of formula per pound per day). There is increased need for supplement of vitamins C and D; approximately 35 to 50 mg. of ascorbic acid and 500 to 1,000 I.U. of vitamin D are usually given during the second and third weeks respectively, depending on individual need. Ascorbic acid is needed for the intermediate metabolism of phenylalanine, an amino acid essential to growth. Vitamin D is needed for the rapid mineralization of bones.

Methods of feeding will vary with the infant's strength and the nurse's experience. The feedings may be given by medicine dropper, by bottle with a soft nipple having larger than usual holes, or by gavage. Care must be taken in all methods to avoid aspiration. This is especially true with the gavage method. For use in gavage feeding, the tube is a small soft plastic one with a rounded tip to avoid tissue trauma, and there are two holes on either side of the tip. The tube is passed through the nose until one inch of the lower end is in the stomach. Proper depth placement in the stomach is guided by markings on the tube made according to the measure of the individual infant. Correct anatomic placement is tested by placing the free end in water. If bubbles appear in the water, the tube is in the trachea. It should be withdrawn immediately and reinserted. Careful control of amount of feeding and rate of flow is necessary.

The full-term infant

Physical characteristics. The growth rate during infancy is rapid. Consequently, energy requirements are high. The full-term infant has the ability to digest and absorb proteins, a moderate amount of fat, and simple carbohydrates. He has some difficulty with starch since amylase, the starch-splitting enzyme, is not being produced. However, as starch is introduced, this enzyme functions. His renal system functions well but he needs more water relative to his size than an adult does to manage renal excretion. Teeth do not erupt until about the fourth month so his initial food is liquid or semiliquid. He has limited nutritional stores from gestation, especially in iron, so he needs supplements of vitamins and minerals, first in concentrate and later in solid food additions to his milk. *The newborn's rooting reflex* and his somewhat recessed lower jaw are natural adaptations for feeding at the breast.

Psychosocial development. The core psychosocial problem in infancy is the development of *trust versus distrust.* Feeding is his main means of establishing human relationships. The close mother-infant relationship in the feeding process fills his basic need to build trust. The need for sucking and the development of oral organs, lips and mouth, as sensory organs, represent adaptations to ensure an adequate early food intake. As a result, food becomes the infant's general means of exploring his environment. As muscular coordination involving the tongue and the swallowing reflex develop, he will accept solid foods beginning at about the second month.[5] As he grows he will begin to evidence a desire to help feed himself. If his needs for food and love are fulfilled in this early relationship with the mother, and in broadening relationships with other family members, trust is developed. He evidences this trust by an increasing capacity to wait for his feedings while they are being prepared.

Breast-feeding. The female breasts, or mammary glands, are highly specialized secretory organs. They are composed of glandular tissue, fat, and connective tissue. The glandular tissue is composed of fifteen to twenty lobes, each containing many smaller units called *lobules.* In the lobules, secretory cells called *alveoli* or *acini* form milk from the materials supplied to them by a rich capillary system in the connective tissue. During pregnancy, the breast is prepared for lactation. The alveoli enlarge and multiply, and toward the end of the prenatal period, secrete a thin yellowish fluid called *colostrum.* After delivery, the breast secretion is colostrum for two to four days (10 to 40 ml. a day) until milk production begins about the third day. This colostrum provides some initial nutrition for the infant. It contains more protein and minerals than breast milk but less carbohydrate and fat. It is also thought to impart helpful antibodies to the newborn.

The first milk is a transition form from colostrum; it gradually assumes the composition and form of mature breast milk by the third or fourth week. Milk is produced under the stimulation of a hormone, *prolactin,* produced by the anterior pituitary gland. After the milk is formed in the mammary lobules by the clusters of secretory cells (the acini or alveoli), it is carried through converging branches of the lactiferous ducts to reservoir spaces under the *areola,* the pigmented area of the skin surrounding the nipple. These reservoir spaces for the milk are called *ampullae.* From fifteen to twenty excretory lactiferous ducts carry the milk from the ampullae out the surface of the nipple. Other pituitary

hormones, principally *oxytocin* and to a lesser extent *vasopressin,* stimulate the ejections of the milk from the alveoli to the ducts, releasing it so the baby can obtain it. This is commonly called the let down reflex. It causes a tingling sensation in the breast and the flow of milk. The initial sucking of the baby stimulates this reflex.

Feeding techniques. The rooting reflex of the newborn, his oral needs for sucking, and his basic hunger drive usually make breast-feeding simple for the healthy relaxed mother who is nutritionally sustained by an adequate diet for milk production. Several suggestions to the mother who chooses to nurse her baby may be helpful.

1. She should assume the position which is most relaxing. It may be reclining in bed initially (Fig. 18-2). Later a rocker or other comfortable chair with arm support and a low foot stool usually provide support.

2. The baby should be cradled in her arms in a semireclining position against the breast. The warm touch of the breast on his

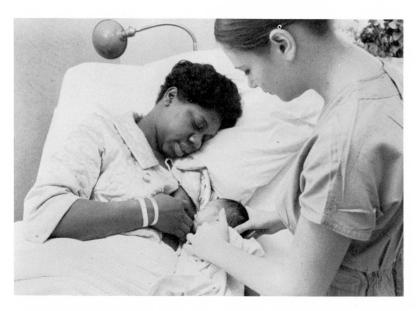

Fig. 18-2. Breast feeding the newborn infant. Note that the nurse, in assisting the mother, avoids touching the infant's outer cheek so as not to counteract his natural rooting reflex at the touch of the breast.

cheek will stimulate the natural rooting reflex causing him to turn his head *toward* the direction of the touch and to begin sucking motions with his mouth. Therefore his outer cheek should not be touched with the hand in an effort to turn his head toward the breast. This only confuses him; the reflex causes him to turn his head away from the breast toward the hand.

3. The baby should grasp most of the areola in his mouth, not merely the outer tip of the nipple. This wider grasp compresses the ampullae underneath the areola

and expresses the milk. If he grasps only the tip of the nipple, his mouth will clamp off the milk flow instead and may cause nipple irritation.

4. In the beginning, both breasts may be used at one feeding. After lactation is established, probably alternate breasts will be used for each feeding.

5. Usually, a hungry infant will get his fill of milk in about the first five minutes of nursing or he may continue for some twenty minutes. He has had a sufficient amount and is obviously satisfied when he

Table 18-4. Comparison of human milk and cow's milk*

	Human milk			Whole cow's milk		
Water (%)	87	to	88	83	to	88
Protein (%)	1.0	to	1.5	3.2	to	4.1
Lactalbumin	.7	to	.8	.5		
Casein	.4	to	.5	3.0		
Sugar (lactose) (%)	6.5	to	7.5	4.5	to	5.0
Fat (%)	3.5	to	4.0 (more oleic acid and fewer of the volatile fatty acids)	3.5	to	5.2
Minerals (%)	.15	to	.25	.7	to	.75
Calcium	.034	to	.045	.222	to	.179
Phosphorus	.015	to	.04	.09	to	.196
Magnesium	.005	to	.006	.013	to	.019
Sodium	.011	to	.019	.05	to	.06
Potassium	.048	to	.065	.138	to	.172
Iron	.0001			.00004		
Vitamins (per 100 ml.)						
A (I.U.)	60	to	500	80	to	220†
D (I.U.)	.4	to	10.0	.3	to	4.4† (+400 per qt.)
C (I.U.)	1.2	to	10.8	.9	to	1.4†
Thiamine (mg.)	.002	to	.036	.03	to	.04†
Riboflavin (mg.)	.015	to	.080	.10	to	.26†
Niacin (mg.)	.10	to	.20	.10		
Digestion				Occurs less rapidly		
Emptying of stomach				Occurs less rapidly		
Curd	Soft, flacculent			Hard, large		
Calories per fluid oz.	20			20		

*Adapted from Nelson, W. E., editor: Textbook of pediatrics, ed. 8, Philadelphia, 1964, W. B. Saunders Company, p. 135. (Data assembled from a number of sources.)
†Pasteurized.

stops nursing and is disinterested in more.

6. Feedings may be given according to the hunger needs of the baby. Usually these will be at closer intervals for the newborn, perhaps every two to three hours. About three to four hour intervals will suffice as he develops.

7. After each feeding, the baby should be held erect on the mother's shoulder to allow him to expel swallowed air. Sometimes this is necessary during the feeding or also after he has been back in his crib.

8. After lactation is established, an occasional bottle feeding may replace the breast feeding if the mother desires or has need to be away.

9. No particular food per se in the mother's diet influences milk production or disturbs the infant. The mother's basic needs are for specific nutrients and fluids as outlined in the lactation diet on pp. 365 and 366.

Care of the breasts. A properly fitting brassiere should be worn day and night to provide adequate support. It should be changed daily to a clean one. A folded clean white cloth (for example, a man's handkerchief) placed inside the bassiere will absorb any milk that may leak between feedings. Plastic brassiere liners should be avoided as they curtail air circulation and prevent adequate drying of the nipple area.

Plain water is best for cleansing. Soap and alcohol are too drying; boric acid should not be used. The nipples should be dried well.

If difficulty with nipples should occur (cracking or infection), the milk may be expressed with a hand breast pump and fed to the baby in bottles for a few days until the nipples heal. A nipple shield is sometimes satisfactorily used while healing occurs.

Bottle-feeding. Artificial feeding of cow's milk formula by bottle may be preferred by the mother. A comparison of the composition of human milk and cow's milk gives the basis for the formula ingredients, since the objective is to modify the cow's milk to make its nutrient proportions similar to those in human milk. The basic differences in protein, carbohydrate and minerals are shown in Table 18-4.

Cow's milk contains about twice as much protein and about six times as much mineral matter as does human milk. This is not surprising because the growth rate of the calf, for whom cow's milk was intended, is much greater than that of the infant. The calf is running about shortly after birth and reaches maturity in a matter of months, whereas it takes a year to get a human offspring on its feet and years more for him to reach full physical growth. Human milk, on the other hand, has more carbohydrate than cow's milk. Therefore, for use in infant feeding, the cow's milk is modified in two ways. It is diluted with water to reduce the protein and mineral salts, and it is mixed with a simple sugar to increase the carbohydrate content. The sugar may be in the form of corn syrup,

Table 18-5. Basic twenty-four-hour formula

Age	Ounces of whole milk per pound body weight per day	Sugar*	Water
First 2 weeks	1½ (¾ oz. evap.)	½ oz. (1 tbsp.)†	Add amount necessary
2 weeks to 2 months	1½ to 2 (1 oz. evap.)	¾ to 1 oz. (2 tbsp.)†	to bring total solution
After 2 months	2 (1 oz. evap.)	1 oz. (2 tbsp.)†	to amount required

*May be granulated, corn syrup, or malt-dextrin preparation.
†2 tablespoons granulated sugar or corn syrup = 1 oz.; 4 tablespoons Dextrimaltose = 1 oz.

granulated sugar, or a special sugar for infants such as Dextrimaltose. A basic 24-hour formula pattern is given in Table 18-5.

Formula preparation and sterilization. Keeping the area of preparation, the utensils, and the hands clean is simple initial sanitation. The clean utensils and the ingredients should be assembled. Canned evaporated milk is commonly used with a simple sugar such as corn syrup. Tap water in the indicated amount is added to the correct amount of sugar and milk. After the formula has been measured and mixed, it is poured into clean bottles in the amount needed for each feeding. The bottles are capped and sterilized according to direction. The terminal method of sterilization is usually preferred because it is simpler than the aseptic technique and is less likely to permit contamination in handling. In the so-called aseptic technique, the equipment is sterilized first. The formula is made in a sterile container with boiled water, then poured into sterile bottles. It is highly doubtful that in the average kitchen this technique would actually be aseptic.

Pictured steps in the preparation of the formula and use of the terminal sterilization process are available in most hospitals for use in teaching mothers (Fig. 18-3). Several points are important to stress when the nurse is discussing or demonstrating the method with new mothers.

1. Simple cleanliness should be observed in the preparation area, the utensils, and the mother's hands. This is no more than good hygiene in any family food preparation.
2. An accurate ingredient measures should be made according to the pediatrician's directions.
3. After capping, the cap assemblies should be *loose* on the bottle to allow for steam circulation during sterilization.
4. After water in the sterilizing container comes to a boil, a full *twenty-five minutes* of boiling should be allowed to adequately protect the formula.
5. When the container has cooled and bottles are removed, the cap assemblies should be screwed down

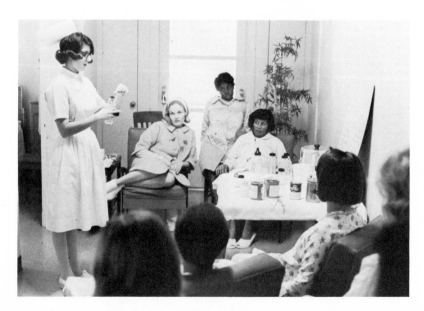

Fig. 18-3. Student nurse giving a demonstration in formula preparation to mothers of newborn infants.

firmly to seal the bottles. The bottles should be refrigerated until use.

6. After each feeding, any unused formula should be disposed of. It should not be recapped for later use.

Feeding techniques. The child should be cradled in the arm as in breast feeding (Fig. 18-4). The close human touch and warmth are important to him. The bottle should be inclined to keep the nipple filled with milk to minimize the swallowing of air.

When the infant is obviously satisfied, he should not be forced to accept more milk, regardless of what is remaining in the bottle. A healthy infant will take what he needs; he should be the guide. A suggested schedule of feedings is given in Table 18-6.

After the infant has been fed, he should be held erect against the mother's shoulder to expel any swallowed air.

Breast feeding versus bottle feeding. The question always arises of whether breast feeding or bottle feeding is better. That question may be countered by asking, better for whom, better in what circumstance, and better in what way. An *unqualified* yes or no to either method does not answer the question.

It is a human tendency, it seems, to react to situations in extremes, basing one's acts or attitudes on personal bias of which there are some forms in everyone. Perhaps *complete* objectivity is really an impossible state. Traditionally, for years, health workers have responded to this question with unequivocable support of breast feeding. Yet the fact remains, as surveys indicate, that

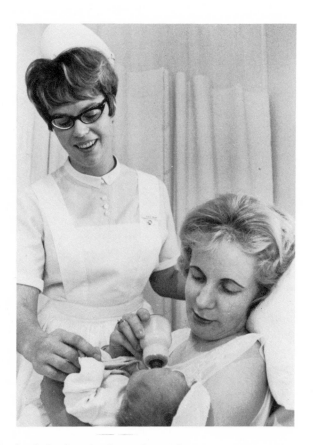

Fig. 18-4. Initiating bottle feedings for the newborn infant.

Table 18-6. Suggested schedule on an approximate four hour basis

Age	Oz. per feeding	Number of feedings	Time of feedings
First week	2 to 3	6	6, 10, 2, 6, 10, 2
Two to four weeks	3 to 5	6	6, 10, 2, 6, 10, 2
Second to third months	4 to 6	5	6, 10, 2, 6, 10
Fourth and fifth months	5 to 7	5	6, 10, 2, 6, 10
Sixth and seventh months	7 to 8	4	6, 10, 2, 6
Eighth to twelfth months	8*	3	7, 12, 6

*4 oz. milk may be given midafternoon.

today in the United States nearly 80% of all infants are bottle-fed. Perhaps this changing pattern in Western culture is due in part to the evolving view of the female breast less as a source of food for babies and more as a stimulating sex symbol, or in part, to the increasing industrialization in Western society and employment of women outside the home. For whatever the reason, more babies in modern American culture are being bottle-fed, and still children are growing up to be healthy adults. With better present-day knowledge of milk processing and food chemistry, a general high standard of living and of community food and water supply, objective studies of the nutritional state of growing infants and children show little difference between infants fed human milk and those fed a wide variety of cow's milk formulas. Thus, from a purely physical and nutritional standpoint, in a technically developed culture where reasonably high standards of environmental sanitation prevail and safe community food and water supplies are maintained, either feeding method suffices. Even routine sterilization of formula is unnecessary in United States cities as the unsterile city water supply is bacteriologically safe for infants to use.[6] Even the traditional warming of the bottle does not seem to be necessary.[7]

Therefore, to the degree that any one of these overall qualifying states is altered in any one particular situation, to that degree and in that situation, the individual answer must be found. For example, on this basis a health worker in an urban slum situation or a nurse on a medical team in an undeveloped area of the world, where the health of the environment and safe sources of alternative food were questionable, would encourage breast feeding. In these situations, it may be life-saving to the infant.

But where these questions of environmental sanitation do not apply, a factor to be considered is the psychosocial aspect. An interesting recent study by Dr. Martin Heinstein[8] indicates that in some instances, under certain emotional conditions involving the sex of the child, the emotional character of the mother (warm or cold) and the quality of the interaction between the two, from a psychological point of view, breast feeding may actually be contraindicated. In former years, before the development of adequate formula feeding methods and elevation of the standard of living, concern for the infant's physical health was uppermost in recommending breast feeding. Heinstein's study seems to indicate that there is now more than the physical health of the infant to consider as in former years. The mother and the infant are a feeding *couple* and the needs of both are involved.

In American society, reasonable counseling with expectant mothers and fathers, seems to be based on two main factors.

(1) If the *environmental sanitation and food supply* factors are positive, either method of feeding will meet the physical need. (2) If *the emotional and psychological character of the mother and the mother-child relationship* factors are negative, breast feeding may be contraindicated. In the last analysis, therefore, given a healthy environment and an emotionally mature mother and father, whether the mother chooses breast feeding or bottle feeding, she should be supported in her own decision. This decision should be made early in pregnancy so that wise ways and means of implementing her choice may be explored with her. Sometimes the pitfall is the physician's or the nurse's or the nutritionist's inadequacy in handling a mother who really does desire to breast-feed her infant, but because of the health worker's own ignorance and lack of training in this regard, he advises her to switch to a formula.

Solid food additions. Apparently there is no one sequence to the addition of solid foods to the infant's diet. Whatever solid food is offered first or at what time seems to be largely a matter of individual preference of the mother or of the pediatrician. It is far less often based on the individual infant's needs. Observation and experience have led many investigators to the conclusion that the infant's digestion and assimilation are much more adaptable than was once thought.[9] A number of studies indicate varying ages at which solid foods are accepted by the infant. Beal[5] found that the average age of willing acceptance for cereals was from 2½ to 3½ months, for vegetables from four to 4½ months, for meat and meat soup from 5½ to six months (Fig. 18-5). Fruits were accepted at progressive early ages, often as early as 2½ to three months. Other investigators[10] indicate that there are certain critical or sensitive periods in the development of children in which their maturation brings them to a readiness for an activity. For example, at six to seven months, the child is developmentally ready to chew solids (as distinguished from thickened feedings), and if he is not given solids when he is able to chew feeding problems may occur later.

Two factors seem to be guiding principles. *Necessary nutrients* are the needs, not any one food per se. The general direction of a physician to a mother that she give her child "table foods" without any exploration of what "table food" at home is, may be giving an unwise prescription, depending upon the level of the household hygiene or the family food pattern. *Food is a basis of learning.* Theoretically, if additional nutrients in concentrated form were given to the child, he could get along well only on milk during his infancy. However, food serves not only for physical sustenance but also supplies other personal and cultural needs. The addition of foods characteristic of a culture is a basis of teaching a cultural pattern of eating. On this foundation the child will continue to base his food habits. Good food habits begin early in life and may be continued as the child grows older.

A guideline for the addition of solid foods to the infant's diet is given in Table 18-7. Individual practices will vary widely around this sequence. By the time a child is approximately eight or nine months old, he should have attained a fairly good ability to eat so-called family foods, chopped, cooked foods, simply seasoned, without recourse to a large number of special infant foods.

Childhood
Toddler (one to three years)

Physical characteristics and growth. Following the first year, the child's growth rate slows. Although his rate of gain is less, the pattern of growth produces significant changes in his body form. His legs become longer. He begins losing his baby fat. There is less body water and more water in the cells. He begins to look and feel less like a baby and more like a child. There are fewer energy demands because of the slackened growth. However, important muscle development takes place. Muscle

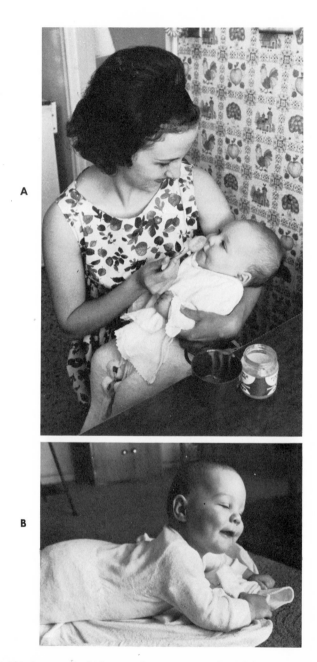

Fig. 18-5. A, This five month old boy is taking a variety of solid food additions and is developing wide tastes. Here feeding has become a bond of relationship between mother and child, and is serving not only as a source of physical growth but also of psychosocial development. **B,** Optimum physical development and security are evident, the result of sound nutrition and loving care.

mass development accounts for about one-half of the total gain during this period. As the child begins to walk and stand erect, more muscle is needed to strengthen the body. There is special need, for example, for big muscles of the back, the buttocks, and the thighs. The overall rate of skeletal growth slows, but there is more deposit of mineral rather than great lengthening of bones. The increased mineralization strengthens the bones to support the in-

creasing weight. The child has about six or eight teeth at the beginning of the toddler period. Most of his deciduous teeth have erupted by the time he is three years of age.

Psychosocial development. The toddler's psychosocial development is pronounced. The core problem with which he struggles is the conflict between *autonomy and shame*. He has an increasing sense of self —of "I"—of being a person, distinct and in-

Table 18-7. Guideline for addition of solid foods to infant's diet during the first year*

When to start	Foods added	Feeding
First month	Vitamins A, D and C in multi-vitamin preparation (according to prescription)	Once daily at a feeding time.
Second to third month	Cereal and strained cooked fruit; Egg yolk (at first, hard boiled and seived, soft boiled or poached later)	10:00 A.M. and 6:00 P.M.
Third to fourth month	Strained cooked vegetable and strained meat	2:00 p.m.
Fifth to seventh month	Zweiback or hard toast	At any feeding
Seventh to ninth month	Meat: beef, lamb, or liver, (broiled or baked and finely chopped) Potato: baked or boiled and mashed or sieved.	10:00 or 6:00 P.M.

Suggested meal plan for age eight months to one year or older		
7:00 A.M.	Milk	8 oz.
	Cereal	2 to 3 tbsp.
	Strained fruit	2 to 3 tbsp.
	Zweiback or dry toast	
12:00 NOON	Milk	8 oz.
	Vegetables	2 to 3 tbsp.
	Chopped meat or one whole egg	
	Puddings or cooked fruit	2 to 3 tbsp.
3:00 P.M.	Milk	4 oz.
	Toast, zweiback or crackers	
6:00 P.M.	Milk	8 oz.
	Whole egg or chopped meat	
	Potato, baked or mashed	2 tbsp.
	Pudding or cooked fruit	2 to 3 tbsp.
	Zweiback or toast	

*Semisolid foods should be given immediately after breast or bottle feeding. One to two teaspoons should be given at first. If food is accepted and tolerated well, the amount should be increased to one to two tablespoons per feeding.
Note: Banana or cottage cheese may be used as substitution for any meal.

dividual, apart from his mother, not just an extension of her. As his physical mobility increases, he has an increasing sense of independence. His growing curiosity leads to much exploration of his environment. Increasingly his mouth is his means of exploring. Touch is important to him. It is his means of learning what objects are like. Often his constant use of "no" is not perverse negativism as much as it is his struggle with his ego needs in conflict with his mother's efforts to control him. He wants to do more and more for himself, and his attention span is fairly short because of his increasing diversion of interest to other things around him.

Food and feeding. Calorie needs are not high during the toddler age. They increase very slowly; an increase of only 300 to 500 calories is required over the two year span. At about one year of age he needs approximately 1,000 calories, and only 1,300 to 1,500 calories by the time he is three years old. From ages one to two, some children do not eat as many calories as they did in the second half of infancy. Knowledge of the child's decreased need for calories and of his struggle for autonomy which often involves refusal of food will help the mother avoid conflict with the toddler about his eating.

Protein needs are relatively large in comparison to caloric needs. The child requires about 1.0 gm. of protein per pound of body weight. There is rapid growth of muscle and other body tissues. At least half of this protein should be of animal origin, since animal protein has high biologic value. Calcium and phosphorus are also needed for the bone mineralization. The bones are strengthening to keep pace with the muscle development and increasing activity. Two to three cups of milk are sufficient for the child's needs. Sometimes excess milk intake, a habit carried over from infancy, may exclude some solid foods from the diet. As a result the child may be lacking iron and develop a "milk anemia." On the other hand, a child may dislike milk, and milk solids may be used in soups, cus-

tards, or puddings, and dry milk can be used in cereals, mashed potatoes, meat loaf, and so on. A variety of food should be offered the child, avoiding an emphasis on refined sweets. These should be reserved for special occasions, not for constant habitual use or bribe mechanisms to get a child to eat.

In summary, two factors are important for the mother to know, understand, and practice during this period. (1) The child needs fewer calories but more protein and mineral matter for growth. Hence, a variety of foods should be offered in smaller amounts to provide key nutrients. (2) The child is struggling for autonomy. This struggle often takes the form of refusal of food and a desire to do things for himself before he is fully able to do them completely. If the mother offers a variety of foods in small amounts, supports and encourages some degree of food choice and self-feeding in the child's own ceremonial manner, eating can be a pleasant, positive means of development. It can help satisfy his growing need for independence and his desire for ritual. The mother needs to maintain a calm, relaxed attitude of sympathetic interest, to understand his struggle and give help where needed, but to avoid both over-protection and excessive rigidity.

Preschool child (three to six years)

Physical characteristics and growth. Physical growth continues in spurts. On occasion the child bounds with energy; his play is hard play—running, jumping, testing new physical resources. At other times he will sit for increasing periods of time engrossed in passive types of activities. His mental capacities are developing. He is doing more thinking, and is exploring his environment. Specific nutrients need emphasis.

Protein requirements continue to be relatively high. The preschool child needs daily about 40 gm. of good quality protein, such as is found in milk, meat, egg, and cheese. He continues to need calcium and iron for storage. Since United States surveys indicate that vitamins A and C are likely to be lacking in the diets of preschool and growing children, a variety of fruits and vegetables should be provided.

Psychosocial development. Each age period builds upon the previous one. The toddler who has been provided the physical and psychosocial resources by understanding and able parents has a foundation on which the preschool period builds. The child is continuing to form life patterns in attitudes and basic eating habits as a result of his social and emotional experiences. The twofold guiding principle for parents remains the same—to provide the right food to meet physical needs and the right climate to promote and support social and emotional growth.

The core problem with which the preschool child struggles during these ages is essentially that of *initiative versus guilt.* He is beginning to develop the superego (the conscience). As his locomotion and his powers of locomotion increase, he has increasing imagination and curiosity. This very capacity often leads him into troubled feelings about his changing attitudes, especially toward his parents. This is a period of increasing imitation and of sex identification. The little boy will imitate the father. The little girl will imitate the mother. In their play, much of this becomes evident in the use of grown-up clothes and role-playing in domestic situations. Eating assumes, therefore, greater social aspects. The family meal time is an important means of this socialization and sex identification. The children imitate their parents and others at the table. Depending upon the example of the parents and other family members, this may be negative rather than positive training.

Food and feeding. Of all the food groups, vegetables usually are less well liked by most children, yet they contain vitamins and minerals needed for growth. Consideration given to the way they are prepared and served is valuable. Children like crisp raw vegetables better than cooked ones. They have a keen sense of taste. Flavor and texture are important.

They usually dislike strong vegetables such as cabbage and onions. Tough strings cause problems. Tough parts are hard to manage and should be removed. For example, it is easy to break a crisp piece of celery and remove the strings before giving it to the child. Children also react to consistency of vegetables. Because they prefer their foods luke-warm, some foods may remain on their plates and become dry and gummy and hence are refused. Children usually prefer single foods to combination dishes such as casseroles or stews. In such combinations the foods lose their identity and flavors are intermingled. The child prefers a single food that he can identify and that has retained its characteristic texture, color, and form. He likes food he can eat with his fingers. Frequently, when appetites lag, fruit may be substituted for vegetables. Often a variety of raw fruit and raw vegetables cut in finger-sized pieces and offered to a child for his own selection, provides a resource of needed nutrition. Fruit in a gelatin base is usually liked and if a child has a choice in selecting the color of the gelatin, often it is accepted more readily.

Because of his developing social and emotional needs, the preschool child frequently follows food jags that may last for several days. However, this is usually short lived and of no major concern.

It is helpful when the child can set his own goals in quantity of foods. His portions need to be relatively small. Often, if he can pour his own milk from a small pitcher into a small glass, he consumes a greater amount. The quantity of milk needed usually declines during these years. The child will consume two to three, rarely four, cups of milk during the day. Smaller children like their milk more luke-warm, not icy cold. Also, they prefer it in small glasses which hold about ½ to ¾ of a cup, rather than in large adult size glasses. Meat should be tender, easy to chew or cut; hence, ground meat is popular.

The preschool period is one of increasing growth for the child. Life-time food habits are forming. Food continues to play an important part in developing his personality. Group eating becomes significant as a means of socialization. The child learns to control strong dislikes at the family table or in group situations away from home. He may be involved in nursery or play-school situations in which he eats with other children. Here he learns a widening variety of food habits, and forms new social relationships.

School-age child (six to twelve years)

Physical characteristics and growth. The school-age period has been called the latent period of growth. The rate of growth slows and body changes occur very gradually. Resources, however, are being laid down for the growth needs to come in the adolescent period, and it has been called sometimes the lull before the storm. By now, the body type is established. Growth rates will vary widely within this period. Girls usually outdistance boys by the latter part of the period.

Psychosocial development. The core problem with which the child struggles during these years is the tension between *industry and inferiority.* There is increasing mental development and ability to work out problems. With widening horizons, new school experiences, and challenging learning opportunities, the child is involved in activities that develop his sense of adequacy and accomplishment. He develops his ability to cooperate in group activities. He begins moving from a dependence on parental standards toward standards of his peers in preparation for his own coming maturity. Pressures are generated for self-control of his changing body. These pressures produce changes in previously learned habits, and the negative attitudes that are sometimes asserted are but evidence of these struggles for growing independence. There is a temporary disorganization of previous learning and developed personality, a sort of loosening up of the personality pattern for the inevitable changes ahead in adolescence. A number of years ago an insightful observer[11] called the latter part of this period the "soaking the beans before you cook them." It is a diffuse period of gangs, of cliques, of hero-worship, of pensive day-dreaming, of emotional stresses, of learning to get along with other children.

Food and feeding. The slowed rate of growth during this latent period results in a gradual decline in the food requirement per unit of body weight. This decline continues up to the latter part of the period when there is a gradual increase in need during the preadolescent period because reserves are being laid down for the demands of the adolescent period to come. Likes and dislikes are a product of earlier years and continue in patterns set before. Family attitudes are imitated. There is an increasing interest and participation in other activities which compete with mealtimes. The breakfast meal may be an inadequate one for the young child whose growth and development maturation lead a working mother to give the child more responsibility, often leaving him alone to prepare food for himself. In such situations, meals are make-shift or nonexistent. The school lunch program provides a nourishing noon meal for many children who would not otherwise have one. Midafternoon snacking is common. The snack may be sweets of empty calories, or it may be an opportunity for additional needed nourishment.

Food behavior reflects the child's developmental changes. Manners and punctuality at meals sometimes are a family problem. The source of conflict usually comes from unrealistic parental expectations, expecting adult manners from a child. Too often parents may seek to train children by constant correction at the table, rather than setting the example in their own behavior. In these years of imitation, children learn more from a good example lived before them daily than from a constant negative fault-finding or correction. Such a negative approach is hurtful in the child's struggle against inferiority feelings, especially when it occurs before people who are significant to the child—his teacher or his peers. Often, however, the school-age child has increasing exposure to positive learning opportunities in the classroom, where nutrition is integrated in other activities. Also, he can observe many food attitudes and taste new foods in a group school lunch program that he may not accept otherwise.

Adolescence (twelve to eighteen years)

Physical characteristics and growth. During the adolescent period, with the onset of puberty, the final growth spurt of childhood occurs. Maturation during this period varies so widely that chronological age as a reference point for discussing growth ceases to

be useful, if indeed it ever was. *Physiologic age* becomes more important in dealing with individual boys and girls. It accounts for wide fluctuations in metabolic rates, in food requirements, in scholastic capacity, and even in illness. These capacities can be more realistically viewed only in physiologic growth terms.

The body changes in the adolescent period result from hormonal influences regulating the development of the sex characteristics. The rate at which these changes occur varies widely and is particularly distinct in growth patterns that emerge

Table 18-8. Tool for summarizing growth and development needs of children

Age group	Core psychosocial problem	Growth and development characteristics	Food and feeding
Infant (Birth to 1 year)	Trust vs. distrust		
Toddler (1 to 3 years)	Autonomy vs. shame and doubt		
Preschool child (3 to 6 years)	Initiative vs. guilt		
School-age child (6 to 12 years)	Industry vs. inferiority		
Adolescent (12 to 18 years)	Identity vs. diffusion		

Table 18-9. Food intake for good nutrition according to food groups and the average size of servings at different age levels*

Food group	Servings per day	1 year	2 to 3 years	4 to 5 years	6 to 9 years	10 to 12 years	13 to 15 years
					Average size of servings at each age level		
Milk and cheese (1.5 oz. cheese = 1 cup milk)	4	½ cup	½ to ¾ cups	¾ cup	¾ to 1 cup	1 cup	1 cup
Meat group (protein foods)	At least 3						
Egg		1 egg	1 egg	1 egg	1 egg	1 egg	1 or more
Lean meat, fish, poultry (liver once a week)		2 tbsp.	2 tbsp.	4 tbsp.	2-3 oz. (4-6 tbsp.)	3-4 oz.	4 oz. or more
Peanut butter			1 tbsp.	2 tbsp.	2-3 tbsp.	3 tbsp.	3 tbsp.
Fruits and vegetables	At least 4, including:						
Vitamin C source (citrus fruit, berries, tomato, cabbage, cantaloupe)	1 or more (twice as much tomato to as citrus)	⅓ cup citrus	½ cup	½ cup	1 med. orange	1 med. orange	1 med. orange
Vitamin A source (gree or yellow fruits and vegetables)	1 or more	2 tbsp.	3 tbsp.	4 tbsp. (¼ cup)	¼ cup	⅓ cup	¾ cup
Other vegetables (potato, legumes)	2 or more	2 tbsp.	3 tbsp.	4 tbsp. (¼ cup)	⅓ cup	½ cup	¾ cup
or							
Other fruits (apple, banana)		¼ cup	⅓ cup	½ cup	1 medium	1 medium	1 medium
Cereals (whole grain or enriched)	At least 4						
Bread		½ slice	1 slice	1½ slices	1-2 slices	2 slices	2 slices
Ready-to-eat cereals		½ oz.	¾ oz.	1 oz.	1 oz.	1 oz.	1 oz.
Cooked cereal (including pastes, rice, etc.)		¼ cup	⅓ cup	½ cup	½ cup	¾ cup	1 cup or more
Fats and carbohydrates	To meet caloric needs						
Butter, margarine, mayonnaise, oils: 1 tbsp. = 100 calories		1 tbsp.	1 tbsp.	1 tbsp.	2 tbsp.	2 tbsp.	2-4 tbsp.
Desserts and sweets 100 calorie portions: ⅓ cup pudding or ice cream 2 3" cookies, 1 oz. cake, ⅓ oz. pie, 2 tbsp. jelly, jam, honey, sugar		1 portion	1½ portions	1½ portions	3 portions	3 portions	3 to 6 portions

*Bennett, M., and Hansen, A.: Nutritional requirements. In Nelson, W., editor: Textbook of pediatrics, ed. 8, Philadelphia, 1964, W. B. Saunders Company, p. 123.

between the sexes. A thirteen-year-old girl, for example, who is past puberty, is about 2 years ahead of a boy the same age in development—sometimes she feels as if it were five.

Other physical growth differences emerge between the sexes. In the girl there is an increasing amount of subcutaneous fat deposit, particularly in the abdominal area. The hip breadth increases and the bony pelvis widens in preparation for reproduction. A pelvic girdle of subcutaneous fat results. This is often a source of anxiety to many figure-conscious young girls. In the boy, physical growth is manifest more in an increased muscle mass and in long bone growth. His growth spurt is slower than that of the girl, but he soon passes her in weight and height, and at age eighteen weighs about 140 pounds.

Reaction to disease. During this transitional period of rapid growth, the physical resistance of the adolescent to infectious disease seems lessened. For example, the incidence of tuberculosis during the adolescent period, especially in girls, is a matter of concern to public health offiicials.[12] Usually the incidence of such disease and the individual reaction to it is related to the physical nutritional resources the adolescent brings to the metabolic demands of the pubertal growth period. Also, increased activity of sweat glands and lack of good skin care make acne of face and back a common and vexing problem.

Psychosocial development. Adolescence is an ambivalent period full of stresses and strains. On the one hand the child looks back to the securities of earlier childhood. On the other hand, he reaches for the maturity of adulthood. The core problem with which the adolescent struggles is that of *identity versus diffusion.* The search for self begun in early childhood reaches a climax in the identity crisis of the teen years. The profound body changes associated with sexual development cause changes in body image and resulting tensions in maturing boys and girls. Individual variance is great in response to these ten-

sions, depending upon the resources that have been provided for them in their earlier developmental years. In American society, adolescent children continue to have problems in a rigid school system which groups them only by an arbitrary chronological age rather than by a plan which considers their physiologic and mental ages. Frustrations are often generated during this period in many adolescents, and, no doubt, have an effect upon their adult lives.

The identity crisis of the teen years, largely revolving around sexual development and preparation for an adult role in a complex society, produces many psychologic, emotional, and social tensions. The period of rapid physical growth is relatively short, only two to three years. However, the attendant psychosocial development continues over a longer period. The pressure for peer group acceptance is strong, and fads in dress and food habits are common. Also, in a technically developed society such as in the United States, where high values are placed on education and achievement, prolonged preparation for careers often delays marriage and establishment of the new family far beyond the initiation of the reproductive years. Social tensions and family conflicts are created. These conflicts may have nutritional consequences as the teen-ager eats away from home more often, and develops a snacking pattern of his own food choices.

Food and feeding. Caloric needs increase with the metabolic demands of growth and energy expenditure. Although individual needs vary, girls consume fewer calories than boys (from 2,000 to 2,500 a day; boys need 2,500 to 3,000 a day). Sometimes the large appetite characteristic of this growth period leads an adolescent to satisfy his hunger with carbohydrate foods and to slight essential protein foods.

Protein needs for adolescent growth are large, especially during the pubertal changes in both sexes, and for the developing muscle mass in boys. From 50 to 60 gm. of protein sustain daily needs and maintain nitrogen reserves.

Minerals particularly needed are calcium and iron. Bone growth demands calcium. Menstrual iron losses in the adolescent girl predispose her to simple iron deficiency anemia. In some areas where iodized salt use does not ensure sufficient iodine for the increased thyroid activity associated with growth, a deficiency state may result.

Vitamins are necessary regulators of metabolic activity. The B vitamins are needed in increased amounts, especially by boys, to meet the extra demands of energy metabolism and muscle tissue development. Intakes of needed vitamin C and vitamin A may be low because of erratic food intake.

Eating habits. Physical and psychosocial pressures influence eating habits. By and large, the adolescent boy fares better than the girl. His large appetite and the sheer volume of food it leads him to consume usually assure his intake of adequate nutrients. The adolescent girl, however, is less fortunate. Most United States surveys show her to be most vulnerable to nutritional deficiencies in comparison to other age-sex groups in the general population. Two factors combine to help produce this result. (1) Because of her physiologic sex differences associated with fat deposits during this period and her comparative lack of physical activity, she gains excess weight easily. (2) Social pressures and personal tensions concerning figure control will sometimes cause her to follow unwise self-imposed crash diets for weight loss. As a result, she may be malnourished at the very time in her life when her body is laying down reserves for coming reproduction. The hazards of such eating habits to her future course during potential pregnancies is clearly indicated in the studies relating preconception nutritional status to the outcome of gestation (pp. 351-353).

SUMMARY OF NEEDS FOR GROWTH

Throughout human growth, therefore, it is apparent that nutritional resources to meet physical growth are conditioned by the food habits and feeding practices which are psychosocially and culturally derived. Large numbers of growing children have these resources and arrive at adulthood vigorous and happy. Unfortunately, many others do not.

A helpful tool to use in reviewing these developmental needs for growth is given in Table 18-8. A brief summary of each age group should be filled in, relating the core psychosocial problem and its related developmental characteristics and physical maturation to food and feeding needs for each stage of growth. As a result of this study, the student should have a more realistic, sound *working knowledge* of normal growth and development needs, which will enable her to help young children who are struggling to grow up, and their parents who are trying to guide them.

References
Specific
1. Erikson, E.: Youth and the life cycle, Children **7**:43, 1960.
2. Erikson, E.: Childhood and society, ed. 2, New York, 1963, W. W. Norton and Company, Inc., pp. 247-274.
3. Duvall, E. V.: Family development, ed. 2, Philadelphia, 1962, J. B. Lippincott Co.
4. Silverman, W. A., and Parke, P.: Keep him warm, Amer. J. Nurs. **65**:81, 1965.
5. Beal, V. A.: On the acceptance of solid foods and other food patterns of infants and children, Pediatrics **20**:448, 1957.
6. Gibson, J. P.: Is formula sterilization necessary? J. Pediat. **55**:119, 1959.
7. Holt, L. E., and others: A study of premature infants fed cold formulas, J. Pediat. **61**:556, 1962.
8. Heinstein, M.: Behavioral correlates of breast-bottle regimes under varying parent-infant relationships, Monograph, Society for Research in Child Development, No. 88, Vol. 28, No. 4, 1963.
9. Smith, C. A.: Current trends in the feeding of infants and children, J.A.M.A. **161**:728, 1956.
10. Illingworth, R. S., and Lister, J.: The critical or sensitive period, with special reference to certain feeding problems in infants and children, J. Pediat. **65**:839, 1964.
11. Redl, F.: Preadolescents: what makes them tick? Child Study **21**:44, 1933-1934.
12. Johnson, J. A.: Nutritional studies in adolescent girls and their relation to tuberculosis, Springfield, Illinois, 1953, Charles C Thomas, Publisher.

General

General nutrition

Beeuwkes, A. M., and Wallin, B. D.: From this day forward . . . (White House Conferences on Children), J. Amer. Diet. Ass. **49**:289, 1966.

Food and Nutrition Board, Recommended dietary allowances, ed. 7, Pub. No. 1694, National Academy of Sciences, National Research Council, Washington, D. C., 1968.

Lesser, A. J.: The significance of the 1965 Social Security amendments for child health programs (1965 Martha May Eliot Award Address), Columbus, Ohio, 1965, Ross Laboratories.

Martin, E.: Robert's nutrition work with children, Chicago, 1954, University of Chicago Press.

Nelson, W. E., editor: Textbook of pediatrics, ed. 8, Philadelphia, 1964, W. B. Saunders Company.

Ohlson, M. A.: The calcium controversy, J. Amer. Diet. Ass. **31**:333, 1955.

Scrimshaw, N. S.: Ecological factors in nutritional disease, Amer. J. Clin. Nutr. **14**:112, 1964.

Scrimshaw, N. S.: Malnutrition and the health of children, J. Amer. Diet. Ass. **42**:203, 1963.

Stefferud, A., editor: Food, the yearbook of agriculture, 1959, Washington, D. C., 1959, The U. S. Dept. of Agriculture.

Infancy

Food and Nutrition Board: Meeting protein needs of infants and children, Pub. No. 843, 1961, National Academy of Sciences, National Research Council.

Food and Nutrition Board: The composition of milks, a compilation of the comparative composition and properties of human, cow, and goat milk, colostrum, and transitional milk, Bull. No. 254, 1953, National Academy of Sciences, National Research Council.

Guthrie, H. A.: Nutritional intake of infants, J. Amer. Diet. Ass. **43**:120, 1963.

György, P.: Trends and advances in infant nutrition, Nurs. Outlook **6**:516, 1958.

Heseltine, M., and Pitts, J. (Co-chairmen): Joint Committee Maternal and Child Health and Food and Nutrition Sections, American Public Health Association, Economy in nutrition and feeding of infants, Amer. J. Public Health **56**:1756, 1966.

Hill, L. F., and others: On the feeding of solid foods to infants, Pediatrics **21**:685, 1958.

Lathrop, D. B.: Bacteriological counts on infant formulas mixed in the home, Arch. Pediat. **73**:451, 1956.

Legady, C.: A failure to thrive, Nurs. Forum **1**:56, 1965.

Lubchenko, L. O.: Formulas and nutrition, Amer. J. Nurs. **61**:73, 1961.

McClure, M. H.: When she chooses breast feeding, Amer. J. Nurs. **57**:1002, 1957.

O'Keefe, M.: Advice from a nurse-mother (breast feeding), Amer. J. Nurs. **63**:61, 1963.

Richmond, J. B., and Pollack, G. H.: Psychological aspects of infant feeding, J. Amer. Diet. Ass. **29**:656, 1953.

Sarto, J., Sr.: Breast feeding: preparation, practice, and professional help, Amer. J. Nurs. **63**:58, 1963.

Silver, H. K.: Sterilization and preservation of formulas for infants, Pediatrics **20**:993, 1957.

Smith, C. A.: Overuse of milk in the diets of infants and children, J.A.M.A. **172**:567, 1960.

Stilb, G., and others: Some practical considerations of economy and efficiency in infant feeding, Amer. J. Public Health **52**:125, 1962.

Vaughn, V. C., and others: A study of preparation of formulas for infant feeding, J. Pediat. **61**:547, 1962.

Wood, A. L.: The history of artificial feeding of infants, J. Amer. Diet. Ass. **31**:474, 1955.

Childhood

Bernstein, N.: Rehabilitating a child with a severe feeding problem, J. Amer. Diet. Ass. **36**:131, 1960.

Breckenridge, M. E.: Food attitudes of 5-12 year old children, J. Amer. Diet. Ass. **35**:704, 1959.

Cady, E., and Carrington, E.: Retraining a child to eat, J. Am. Diet. Ass. **33**:605, 1957.

Dierks, E. C., and Morse, L. M.: Food habits and nutrient intakes of preschool children, J. Amer. Diet. Ass. **47**:292, 1965.

Poehler, H. R.: Dealing in a habit clinic with eating problems of children, J. Amer. Diet. Ass. **25**:696, 1949.

Pre-school child malnutrition, primary deterrent to human progress, Pub. No. 1282, Washington, D. C., 1966, National Academy of Sciences, National Research Council.

Teply, L. J.: Nutritional needs of the pre-school child, Nutr. Rev. **22**:65, 1964.

Weng, L.: A bookshelf on nutrition and the pre-school child, J. Amer. Diet. Ass. **30**:570, 1954.

Weng, L.: Nutrition and the preschool child, Amer. J. Clin. Nutr. **3**:150, 1955.

Adolescence

Coleman, J. S.: The adolescent society, the social life of the teenager and its impact on education, New York, 1961, The Free Press.

Edwards, C. H., and others: Nutrition survey of 6,200 teen-age youth, J. Amer. Diet. Ass. **45**:543, 1964.

Everson, G. J.: Bases for concern about teenagers' diets, J. Amer. Diet. Ass. **36**:17, 1960.

Gallagher, J. R.: Some aspects of adolescents' medical care, Postgrad. Med. **31**:190, 1962.

Gallagher, J. R.: Weight control in adolescence, J. Amer. Diet. Ass. **40**:519, 1962.

Hammar, S. L.: The role of the nutritionist in an adolescent clinic, Children **13**:217, 1966.

Hinton, M. A., and others: Eating behavior and

dietary intake of girls 12 to 14 years old, J. Am. Dietet. A., **43**:223, 1963.

Huenemann, R., and others: A longitudinal study of gross body composition and body conformation and their association with food and activity in a teen-age population: view of teen-age subjects on body conformation, food, and activity, Amer. J. Clin. Nutr. **18**:325, 1966.

Huenemann, R., and others: Teen-agers' activities and attitudes toward activity, J. Amer. Diet. Ass. **51**:433, 1967.

Peckos, P. S., and Heald, F. P.: Nutrition of adolescents, Children, Vol. 11, No. 1, 1964.

Roth, A.: The teenage clinic, J. Amer. Diet. Ass. **36**:27, 1960.

Semmens, J. P.: 14,000 teenage pregnancies, Amer. J. Nurs. **66**:308, 1966.

Semmens, J. P., and McGlamory, J. C.: Teen-age pregnancies, Obstet. Gynec. **16**:31, 1960.

Spindler, E. B., and Acker, G.: Teen-agers tell us about their nutrition, J. Amer. Diet. Ass. **43**:228, 1963.

CHAPTER 19

Nutritional therapy in childhood diseases

The child's reaction to illness is conditioned by his past experiences and the common growth and development patterns of childhood. Sick or well, all children struggle to accomplish indispensable tasks of physical and psychosocial development. As Erikson[1] points out, however, during illness some degree of regression occurs. Therefore, in exploring patient needs and planning relevant nursing care, not only must the particular age group needs of the child be considered, but also his individual responses to the experience of illness according to his own unique resources.

Nutritional therapy will play an important role in the nursing care of a child. The basic normal nutritional needs of his particular growth period, as outlined in the previous chapter, will take on added significance as a foundational resource for meeting the physiologic stress of disease. These food factors need to be assured in his diet. In some instances, dietary modifications will need to be made to accommodate a particular disease condition. The alert, observant, and sensitive nurse will find many opportunities throughout her pediatric nursing to provide learning experiences for children and their parents in the principles of health care. A fundamental part of this health care is good nutrition.

Therefore, the general needs of the hospitalized child will be looked at first, and in the light of these basic needs, the factors involved in planning his nutritional care will be considered. With this background,

a few of the diseases involving nutritional consideration will be used as examples of adjusting normal nutritional needs for therapeutic care.

This study will revolve around the following questions:

1. What role does nutritional therapy play in meeting the needs of ill children?
2. What nutritional therapy is used in the management of gastrointestinal problems of infants and children?
3. What are genetic diseases? How are they related to nutrients?
4. What is the basic genetic defect in phenylketonuria and galactosemia? How are the results of these defects managed in the child's diet? What are the public health implications?
5. What are the principles of care in juvenile diabetes?
6. What is the wise approach in childhood to nutritional care of common public health problems such as obesity and dental caries?

THE HOSPITALIZED CHILD

Good nursing care essentially centers upon two factors: (1) determining the needs of the patient, and (2) planning wise nursing action to meet these needs. Many authorities have emphasized that nursing practices considered helpful of themselves are not necessarily helpful to a particular patient in a particular situation. This is especially true in the care of children. But

397

here the nurse has an added responsibility. She must be able to communicate with children. This ability comes from knowing children and caring about their concerns. It is based upon an indefinable quality of feeling for them which enables her to establish contact with a child who is often very inarticulate, emotionally disoriented, and physically ill. A consideration of the basic needs of the ill, hospitalized child is an essential first step. Then plans for nutritional care will be an integral part of total nursing care.

Basic needs of ill children

Physical care. Quality medical care and supervision is of primary consideration. The child is hospitalized at the direction of his

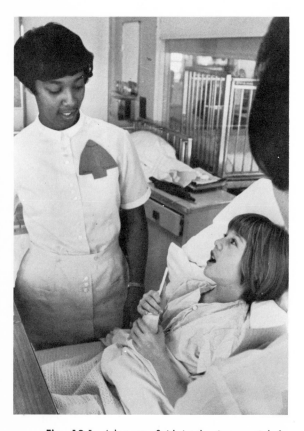

Fig. 19-1. Adequate fluid intake is essential for children, especially during illness. Here student nurses encourage a child to drink some orange juice.

physician who carries the medical responsibility for the child's health. He relies heavily, however, upon other members of the health team in the total care of the child, particularly upon the nurse for supportive nursing care. Often it is the high quality of this nursing care by a sensitive, skilled, attuned nurse, that makes the difference in the child's illness and helps him to recovery of health again. A major aspect of her nursing care will be close observation of the child's food attitudes and intake, and his fluid intake keeping both the doctor and the dietitian informed of these attitudes and needs (Fig. 19-1; see also Table 18-2).

Emotional support. The hospitalized child usually has anxieties and fears. These anxieties may stem from separation from his family, especially his mother, and from his fears concerning his illness and its treatment. A number of factors influence a child's adjustment to hospitalization. These include his age, how ill he is, the kind of care he receives, and the inner personal resources he may have developed thus far from all his past experiences which enable him to cope with his present situation. His particular life experiences may have given him few resources to meet this added crisis. He may be malnourished or lack emotional strength and control. Because she is closest to him and in more constant attendance, the child's nurse is in a key position to help provide support for his emotional needs. To do this, however, she must have an understanding of his emotional needs and provide wise ways of meeting them.

Optimum nutrition. Food is an essential principle in physical and emotional recovery from illness. It is a fundamental means of metabolic return to health, even in this age of miracle drugs. Sometimes this simple fact is forgotten. The biochemical base of health functions at the cellular level through the media of innumerable chemicals and their metabolic interactions. These chemicals or their precursors must be obtained in food. The problem in nutritional care of children, therefore, is twofold. The necessary food must be provided, and the food must be eaten by the child. Usually in a qualified hospital there is adequate administration and trained personnel equipped to accomplish the first aim. The crux of the problem is more often the second need— the acceptance of the food by the child. This aspect of the problem becomes the responsibility of the nurse.

Plans for nutritional care

In planning for the nutritional care of the child, the nurse must consider his general age group needs, any necessary diet modifications, the individual child, and his family.

Age group needs. What age is the child and in what stage of growth? What related developmental age group needs is he struggling with just now? How are these in any way related to feeding, to food, and to fluid intake?

Diet modifications. What is his illness? Is it long or short term? Does it hinder his eating ability in any way? Does it require any dietary modifications? If so, what changes and why? Have these needs been discussed with the dietitian or nutritionist?

The child's acceptance of food. Up to this point in her exploration of the child's needs the nurse may find his food well planned and prepared. But if the child does not eat it, it does him no good. Upon the child's acceptance of the food hinges the success of his nutritional care. Granted that hospital food is usually not exactly like mother's home cooking, it still can be made appetizing and interesting to stimulate lagging appetites.[2] Exploration of the child's reason or reasons for not eating and ingenuity in ways of presenting the food to him will pay great dividends.

Reasons for food rejection. A number of things may contribute to the child's poor appetite and his refusal of food.

Illness. The child may be too ill or weak to eat. He may have some physical intolerance for the food. He may require liquid or soft food, food substitutions, or gentle help in feeding.

Anxiety. The child may be tense and frightened because he is separated from his family, especially his mother. The strange and unfamiliar surroundings may frighten him. He may be concerned about his illness and its outcome. Involving his parents in plans for his care, or helping to make arrangements for his mother to be with him, usually provide needed security and support.[3] Also, helping him to talk about his fears, understanding and accepting him and his fears, or providing simple brief explanations of his care and his treatment as needed all help to reduce his anxiety, to gain his confidence, and give him added resources with which to cope.

Presentation of food. Often the child rejects food because of the way in which it is presented to him. For example, an ill two-year-old is confronted with a tray full of wan food and man-sized utensils unceremoniously planted before him by a large, forbidding, strange adult with the command, "Now eat!" and is overwhelmed. Worse yet, force-feeding a child with inner conflicts only adds more trauma. Some children already wear battle scars of home combat with an adult over food!

Ways of achieving food acceptance. Nurses, dietitians, and physicians experienced in caring for children have devised numerous ways of presenting food. Basically, these ways of helping a child to eat revolve around two related factors—self-selection and a warm mealtime atmosphere.

Self-selection. Allowing a child to have some degree of choice in his food is helpful. Following the early classic experience of Davis[4] with children's self-selection of foods, the staff of the same Chicago hospital in which those experiments took place brought food in sufficient variety to the pediatric ward in a heated conveyor. The children were allowed to select their food from the items displayed.[5] Another hospital in Colorado recently capitalized upon its western heritage and converted their pediatric food cart into a "chuck wagon" outfitted with all the covered wagon trimmings. Periodically the "chuck wagon" travels to the pediatric ward and the adolescent areas of the hospital for evening "chow time." A "cowboy," assisted by nurses and a dietitian, dispenses food selected by the young patients.[6] Several other children's hospitals have planned cafeteria service and group eating for all their ambulatory patients. Although such activities may not be possible in all hospitals, a selective menu from which the child, with guidance, may help select his own food, is a step in that direction. Some consideration of a child's likes and dislikes, with encouragement in convalescence to try new tastes in foods, also helps to achieve food acceptance.

Warm mealtime atmosphere. The manner in which the food is served and a warm atmosphere at mealtime are major influences on the child's reaction. The following factors may help to build this atmosphere:

1. *Personnel.* The warm, supportive manner of the personnel serving the food is of inestimable value. They must know the children and have a feeling for them. Food is served attractively in proper-sized, small portions and in correct, child-sized utensils. Bed patients are made as comfortable as possible and assisted as needed (Figure 19-2).

2. *Group eating.* Often ambulatory patients may eat at small tables in family style. Interest is heightened if the children are involved in the preparation; for example, setting the table, serving as host and hostess, passing the food, and refilling serving dishes as needed. Nurses may eat with the children occasionally and find in sharing food not only a means of observing and learning more about their patients, but also an important vehicle of establishing feeling relationships with them.

3. *Festive days.* Observance of holidays and birthdays with special food or favors or

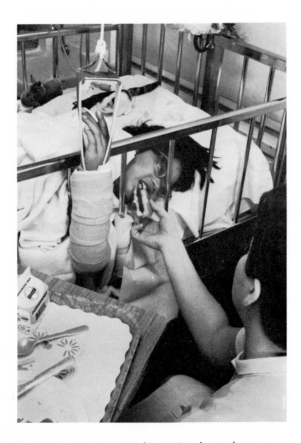

Fig. 19-2. Child with fractured arm is assisted in eating by student nurse.

decorations will help to interest children and give support.

4. *Familiar food.* Consideration should be given to ethnic food habits. Sometimes a familiar food or dish from home that is not contraindicated by the child's illness will stimulate his appetite and interest in eating, and secure for him needed nourishment. Preparing food and ethnic dishes to which the child is accustomed, or flavoring food according to his familiar tastes, are helpful to a child, especially one confined to bed for an extended period.

Family involvement. Exploration of the child's home eating habits with his mother and of the ways she prepares and serves his food, will give helpful background for planning the child's nutritional care while he is in the hospital. Also, such discussions provide opportunity for parents to express their own anxieties about the child, and lead to mutual learning concerning normal growth and developmental needs of children. If the child requires any special diet modifications, these needs may also be discussed with the parents, helping them to explore ways the child's needs may be fitted in with family eating habits.

GASTROINTESTINAL PROBLEMS OF INFANTS AND CHILDREN
General disturbances

Infantile colic. Infantile colic is the name given to paroxysmal intermittent periods of loud, continuous crying. It is not uncommon in newborns and lasts no longer than the third month. It is usually seen only in firstborn infants and seldom in their subsequent siblings. Because it occurs rather routinely in the evening hours between five or six o'clock and midnight, medical and nursing care is usually better directed toward the ragged nerves of the new, inexperienced parents than to the infant himself. It is a self-limiting difficulty ending spontaneously during the first three months. However, to young, tense parents this brief interval of time may seem an eternity.

Treatment usually involves careful history-taking, discovering attitudes and feeding practices. The child may be underfed and simply screaming because he is hungry, or he may be overfed by a zealous young mother and have abdominal discomforts. In other cases his formula may be rapidly changed from day to day by an experimenting mother. (One young mother changed her baby's formula seven times in as many days.) Also, the common pacifier is much more in current vogue, with the blessing of most pediatricians.[7,8] At least, the pacifier has the value of closing the opening from which the cacophony emanates. Mostly, however, treatment involves explanation and moral support to the parents, with reassurance that their child is growing normally. They may take courage from the knowledge that such an active, energetic child with high neuromotor function often develops faster than his more passive peers. He may hold up his head, walk, sit, and talk sooner. He has excellent energy potential for becoming a vigorous and vocal adult. One tongue-in-cheek reviewer has called such a baby "one having the pent-up energy of a born protester and a larnyx of unquestioned competence."[9]

Simple functional vomiting. Regurgitation, or "spitting up," is common in most young infants. Its cause is usually gastric distention from overfeeding or from air-swallowing during feeding or crying. Related factors may be ineffective burping and leaving the baby in a supine (on his back) position rather than a prone (on his stomach) position after feeding. Also, overactivity and semiacrobatics at the hands of doting fathers and grandparents soon after he has been fed may stimulate regurgitation. Temperature of the feeding may be a factor, as feedings that are too hot may induce vomiting. Milk at room temperature is better tolerated, and even cold feedings have evoked no difficulty in a number of infants.[10] Again, simple attention to possible causative factors and reassurance to the young mother will provide adequate care.

Constipation. The old adage, "It is not what he eats, but what eats him!" is correctly applied to constipation. Dietary manipulation is often not a fundamental cure but simply a helpful adjunct. *Psychogenic* constipation may occur during the ages one to two while the child is being toilet trained. Sometimes a compulsive anal-fixated mother, who believes in an arbitrary timetable of elimination ("a daily bowel movement is absolutely essential to health") imposes stringent toilet disciplines on the child, scolding him for failure and rewarding him for perfect performance. The child soon learns that he can suppress the natural impulse to defecate, and he uses this power as a weapon in his conflict with his mother. In time, the habit weakens normal peristalsis. Stools become dry and difficult to pass. Correction of the problem involves adjustment of the parent-child relationship and a resulting easing of the conflict and tensions. The mother needs to learn two simple physiologic facts—toxins are not absorbed from fecal material, and, therefore, a *daily* stool is not essential to the child's health.

Occasional simple physiologic constipation is usually transient. It is aided by moderately reducing the milk intake, increasing the carbohydrate intake (for example, increasing the sugar somewhat in the formula), increasing fruits and vegetables, and increasing the water intake.

Diarrhea

Fluid and electrolytes. Diarrhea in infants may be a more serious problem, especially if it is prolonged and associated with infection. Because of his relatively high water content and his large area of intestinal mucosa in proportion to body surface area, the infant's fluid and electrolye reserves may be rapidly depleted. The sequence of steps leading to dehydration in Chapter 9 on Water and Electrolytes should be reviewed. Common mild diarrhea usually responds to simple treatment. This consists of reducing the food intake, especially of carbohydrate and fat in the formula, and increasing the water intake, sometimes including in it oral electrolyte replacements. More serious forms involving

infection and producing marked dehydration and acidosis are medical emergencies calling for immediate parenteral fluid and electrolyte therapy. The loss of potassium can be dangerous, as hypokalemia affects action of the heart muscle.

Oral feedings. After initial essential replacement of fluid and electrolytes, and when the infant is able to take oral feedings more readily, they are resumed. Water, glucose, and balanced salt solutions may be used, followed by milk mixtures, breast milk, or substitutes such as Probana (a high-protein formula with banana powder), or Nutramigen (a casein hydrolysate free of galactose) as stool volume decreases. Calories are increased to normal requirements as soon as possible. Such agents as pectin and kaolin may thicken the stools, but most authorities agree they have little or no therapeutic usefulness in severe infant diarrhea. Although views differ, pediatricians generally discount the previous practice of completely starving patients with acute diarrhea, a practice which was based on the erroneous belief that avoidance of oral intake put the bowels at rest.[11] Also, tea should not be given to the child. The xanthines in tea stimulate and excite children, and in some cases cause diuresis, which in turn only aggravates the fluid imbalance.

The celiac (malabsorption) syndrome

Identification. In 1889 a London physician named Gee observed a number of malnourished patients having a diarrheal disease and distended abdomens. He gave the name *celiac* to the general clinical syndrome, from the Greek word *kolia*, meaning "belly" or "abdomen." For several decades thereafter, confusion existed among a number of conditions with the same four basic symptoms, all of which were clinical manifestations of intestinal malabsorption: (1) general malnutrition, (2) multiple, foul, bulky, foamy, greasy stools, (3) distended abdomen, due to an accumulation of improperly digested and inadequately absorbed material and to abnormal gas accumulations, and (4) secondary vitamin deficiencies.

Etiologic classification. Beginning in the 1930's, with advances in new knowledge, it became clear that the term *celiac* covered not one but a group of entities, each distinguished by its etiology, but having the same general clinical manifestations of intestinal malabsorption and hence steatorrhea. Three basic contributions of knowledge have helped to clarify these disease entities. In the late 1930's Anderson and others[12,13] distinguished *cystic fibrosis of the pancreas* as a separate disease entity, by the absence of pancreatic enzymes in the duodenal juice. A group of Dutch workers[14] in the early 1950's identified a separate *gluten-induced enteropathy* as a leading cause of the syndrome in children. In the mid-1950's Shiner[15,16] developed a peroral biopsy technique. Using a flexible tube with a suction-guillotine tip, small tissue samples of the intestinal mucosa could be obtained for microscopic study. Electron micrographs of these tissues have consistently shown an eroded mucosal surface without the number or form of villi normally seen, and with sparce microvilli. This erosion effectively reduces the absorbing surface areas as much as 95%. As a result of these and other studies, the various diseases of the malabsorption syndrome have been grouped according to etiology. The general causes of steatorrhea are given in the following outline: [*]

A. Impaired digestion of fat
  1. Inadequate lipolysis due to absence of pancreatic lipase
     a. Cystic fibrosis of pancreas
     b. Congenital hypoplasia of exocrine pancreas
     c. Dietary protein deficiency
  2. Inadequate emulsification of fat due to exclusion of bile from intestine
     a. Atresia of bile ducts
     b. Obstructive jaundice (e.g. viral hepatitis)

B. Impaired absorption of fat
  1. Inadequate length of small bowel or increased transport time
     a. Extensive surgical resection
     b. Intestinal fistulas
     c. Increased intestinal motility due to diarrhea
  2. Obstruction of intestinal lymphatics
     a. Exudative enteropathy due to lymphatic anomalies
     b. Tuberculosis
     c. Hodgkin's disease
     d. Lymphosarcoma
  3. Inflammatory disease or involvement of intestinal mucosa in systemic diseases
     a. Intestinal infections and infestations
     b. Regional enteritis
     c. Ulcerative colitis
     d. Gaucher's disease
     e. Niemann-Pick disease
     f. Scleroderma
  4. Biochemical dysfunction of mucosal cells
     a. Gluten-induced enteropathy
     b. Parenteral diarrhea (in infancy)
     c. Severe starvation

C. Basic mechanism obscure[†]
     a. Incomplete obstruction of intestinal tract (malrotation, stenosis, blind-loop syndrome, etc.)
     b. Idiopathic steatorrhea
     c. Gastrointestinal allergy
     d. Acanthocytosis
     e. Hypoparathyroidism
     f. Sugar-splitting enzyme deficiencies

The principal causes of the celiac syndrome are cystic fibrosis of the pancreas, gluten-induced celiac disease, idiopathic celiac disease or steatorrhea, and exudative enteropathy. These conditions are characterized by excessive intestinal loss of serum protein, often with abnormalities of the intestinal lymphatics. An excellent summary of these disease entities has been outlined

---

[*]Nelson, W. E., editor, Textbook of pediatrics, ed. 8, Philadelphia, 1964, W. B. Saunders Company, p. 723.

[†]Familial dysautonomia (Riley-Day syndrome) and ganglioneuroma may be responsible for diarrhea, but it has not been established whether steatorrhea occurs.

recently by di Sant'Agnese and Jones.[17] The two entities most commonly encountered in children are (1) gluten-induced entropathy, usually called celiac disease, and (2) cystic fibrosis of the pancreas.

Gluten-induced enteropathy (celiac disease)

Etiology. The celiac syndrome seen in children is apparently caused by an enzymatic defect or metabolic error in the intestinal mucosal cells, brought out by wheat or rye gluten. It is thought to be a genetic defect, although the mechanism is unknown. In adults, the condition is known as nontropical sprue. In the process of the disease, the villi of the intestinal mucosa atrophy, greatly reducing the absorptive and secretory surface. Tissue changes occur in the mucosal cells, which brings on pathologic lesions of varying sorts. Whether these mucosal changes are reversible or not is controversial. Efforts of some investigators to return patients to regular diets after initial improvement on a low-gluten regimen have been successful in a few cases with children, but the majority (mostly adults) have not responded. Most of the children seem to recover from the overt disease by school age. Apparently, however, the disease process is in remission, as it may appear again in adult years. Most adults with sprue give a history of having had celiac disease in childhood.

The protein *gluten* is found mainly in wheat and rye. It is composed of two fractions, *glutenin* and *gliadin*. The gliadin fraction is mainly responsible for the malabsorption in gluten-induced enteropathy. About 47% of the weight of the wheat gliadin has been identified as the amino acid *glutamine*. Studies of this amino acid seem to implicate it in the biochemical defect. It is now apparent that the steatorrhea is a secondary manifestation caused by the primary biochemical reaction to gliadin in sensitive patients.

Clinical symptoms. In children who develop gluten-induced celiac disease, the onset usually occurs between the ages of six months to eighteen months, with symptoms appearing later in those who were breast-fed babies. It usually begins with a chronic course, which may suddenly be worsened by a celiac crisis, usually triggered by an infection. This is a severe episode of dehydration and acidosis in which there are large, watery stools and copious vomiting. It is an acute medical emergency. There is chronic diarrhea with passage of characteristic foul, foamy, bulky, greasy stools. About 80% of the ingested fat appears in the stools, usually in the form of soaps and fatty acids. There is progressive malnutrition with signs of deficiency states secondary to the malabsorption—anemia, rickets, and an increased bleeding tendency. The abdomen is grossly distended. There is loss of subcutaneous fat tissue, leaving the buttocks flattened and wrinkled with folds of skin. The child takes on the emaciated, apathetic, and fretful appearance of malnutrition.

Idiopathic steatorrhea is the term given to the disease clinically identical to gluten-induced enteropathy. It is sometimes called idiopathic celiac disease, a source of frequent confusion. The only distinction is in etiology. Idiopathic steatorrhea is *not* induced by gluten and hence does not respond to a clinical trial with a low gluten regimen.

Dietary management of gluten-induced enteropathy would be better defined as *low-gluten* rather than *gluten-free*, because it is impossible to remove all the gluten completely and there is evidence that a small amount of gluten is tolerated by most patients.[18] Wheat and rye are the main sources of gluten, and gluten is also present in oats and barley. Therefore, these four grains (wheat, rye, oats and barley) are eliminated from the diet. Corn and rice are the substitute grains used. The offending grains are obvious in cereal form, but they are also used as ingredients (thickeners or fillers) in many commercial products. Therefore, specific instructions must be outlined to the child's parents, giving the principal omissions in each main food group and

General clinical dietary management during acute and follow-up phases of celiac disease in infants and young children

Stage I

    Celiac crisis—1 to 3 days

        Intravenous replacement therapy of fluid and electrolytes

Stage II

    Initial oral feedings—1 to 6 months (depending on patient's initial condition and individual response)

        High protein, low fat, starch-free feedings (until diagnosis of gluten-induced enteropathy is clearly established, all types of starch are omitted)

            Formulas

            1. Protein milk with glucose and banana powder

            2. Skimmed milk (Probana or Hi Pro)

    According to age of child, add simple carbohydrate foods for additional caloric requirements—fruit juice, *ripe* banana, cooked or canned fruit in syrup (pureed), such as applesauce; protein—strained meat, beginning with beef and liver

Stage III

    Gradual liberalization of diet—indefinite period depending on individual clinical course; form of food will remain soft or pureed

        Meats—lean (no fat); add seafood with caution

        Eggs

        Vegetables, pureed

        Fruits, pureed—fruit ices, fruit whips

        Cereal—corn and rice (small amounts)

        Miscellaneous—gelatin desserts, honey, sugar

    General meal pattern

        Breakfast

            Fruit juice (citrus or apple)

            Fruit (ripe banana or other pureed or soft fruit)

            Egg (no added fat)

            Low-fat cottage cheese or meat (strained or finely ground), if desired

            Formula

        Lunch

            Lean meat (strained or finely ground)

            Vegetable—cooked (strained, or chopped, depending on age)

            Fruit—cooked, stewed or soft

            (Starch: 1 small serving—corn or rice cereal)

            Formula

        Dinner

            Meat, strained (may substitute cottage cheese or egg)

            Vegetable (strained or chopped, depending on age)

            Dessert—gelatin desserts or fruit

            Formula

        Evening

            Formula

        Between meal feedings—depending on appetite

a basic meal pattern. Commercial products involving gluten and careful label-reading habits should also be discussed.

Good dietary management varies according to the age of the child, his clinical status, and pathologic conditions. Generally, however, the course of treatment will follow the stages outlined on p. 405 during the acute and follow-up phases with infants and young children. For continuing use, a dietary program such as the guideline below may be followed. An excellent summary of the practical details of dietary management of patients with the celiac syndrome has been outlined by E. M. Mike.[19]

Cystic fibrosis of the pancreas

Identification and clinical manifestations. Cystic fibrosis is a generalized hereditary disease of children that involves the exocrine glands and affects many tissues and organs. In past years its prognosis was poor. Few children with early disease survived past ten years of age. However, with better knowledge of the disease and improved diagnostic tests, clinical treatment and antibiotic therapy, prognosis has improved. Cystic fibrosis usually produces characteristic clinical manifestations:

1. Pancreatic deficiency with greatly diminished digestion of food caused by the absence of pancreatic enzymes

2. Malfunction of mucus-producing glands with accumulation of thick, viscid secretions and subsequent respiratory difficulty and chronic pulmonary disease
3. Abnormal secretions of the sweat glands containing high electrolyte levels
4. Possible cirrhosis of the liver arising from bilary obstruction and increased by malnutrition or infection

Treatment, therefore, is based on three factors: (1) control of respiratory infection, (2) relief from the effects of extremely viscid bronchial secretions, and (3) maintenance of nutrition. The digestive deficiency and malabsorption character of cystic fibrosis is evident in the nature of the child's stools. They are similar to those in celiac disease (typically bulky, mushy, greasy, foul, foamy), but they also contain more undigested food. Only about half (50% to 60%) of the child's food is absorbed. Thus the child with cystic fibrosis has a much more voracious appetite.

Dietary management. The basic objective of nutritional therapy is to compensate for the large loss of nutrient material resulting from the insufficiency of pancreatic enzymes. Apparently protein hydrolysates, split fats (emulsified, simple fats), and simple sugars are assimilated readily.[20]

Low gluten diet for patients with celiac disease

Diet principles
1. Calories—high, usually about 20% above normal requirement, to compensate for fecal loss
2. Protein—high, usually 6 to 8 gms. per kg. body weight
3. Fat—low, but not fat-free, due to impaired absorption
4. Carbohydrate—simple, easily digested sugars (fruits, vegetables) should provide about one half of the calories.
5. Feedings—small, frequent feedings during ill periods; afternoon snack for older children
6. Texture—smooth, soft, avoiding irritating roughage initially, using strained foods longer than usual for age, adding whole foods as tolerated and according to age of child
7. Vitamins—supplements of B vitamins, vitamins A and B in water-miscible forms, and vitamin C
8. Minerals—iron supplements if anemia present

Continued.

Low gluten diet for patients with celiac disease—cont'd

Food groups	Foods to use	Foods to avoid
Milk	Milk (plain or flavored with chocolate or cocoa) Buttermilk	Malted milk; preparations such as Cocomalt, Hemo, Postum, Nestle's chocolate
Meat or substitute	Lean meat, trimmed well of fat Eggs, cheese Poultry, fish Creamy peanut butter (if tolerated)	Fat meats (sausage, pork) Luncheon meats, corned beef, frankfurters, all common prepared meat products with any possible wheat filler. Duck, goose Smoked salmon Meat prepared with bread, crackers, or flour
Fruits and juices	All cooked and canned fruits and juices Frozen or fresh fruits as tolerated, avoiding skins and seeds	Prunes, plums (unless tolerated)
Vegetables	All cooked, frozen, canned as tolerated (prepared *without* wheat, rye, oat, or barley products); raw as tolerated	Any causing individual discomfort All prepared with wheat, rye, oat, or barley products
Cereals	Corn or rice	Wheat, rye, oat, barley; any product containing these cereals.
Breads, flours, cereal products	Breads, pancakes, or waffles made with suggested flours (cornmeal, cornstarch; rice, soybean, lima, potato, buckwheat)	All bread or cracker products made with gluten, wheat, rye, oat, barley, macaroni, noodles, spaghetti, any sauces, soups, or gravies, prepared with gluten flour, wheat, rye, oat, or barley
Soups	Broth, bouillon (no fat, cream; no thickening with wheat, rye, oat, or barley products); soups and sauces may be thickened with cornstarch	All soups containing wheat, rye, oat, or barley products
Desserts	Cornstarch, rice, or tapioca puddings; custard, fruit ice, plain ice milk, sherbet, gelatin desserts, fruit whips; special cakes or cookies made with allowed flours only	Pies, cookies, cakes, doughnuts, ice cream, prepared mixes
Fats and oils	Cottonseed, corn, soybean, or olive oil Olives French dressing; true mayonnaise or other dressing made with cornstarch Limited amounts of butter, margarine	Meat fat, bacon, lard Salad dressings or mayonnaise thickened with flour (check label) Coconut or oil Excessive chocolate Nuts
Sugars and sweets	All sugars, syrups, honey, molasses, jellies Marshmallows or sauce	Candies containing wheat, rye, oat, or barley products Avoid excessive use of high fat candy (most candy bars)
Seasonings	As desired, soy sauce	Fat seasonings or gluten products not allowed
Vitamins	Aqueous multivitamins; B complex	

Table 19-1. Principles of dietary management for patients with cystc fibrosis

Principle	Reason
High calorie	Energy demands of growth and compensation for fecal losses; large appetite usually ensures acceptance of increased amounts of food
High protein	Usually tolerated in large amounts; excess above normal growth needs required to compensate for losses
Moderate carbohydrate	Starch less well tolerated, simple sugars easily assimilated
Low to moderate fat, as tolerated	Fat poorly absorbed, but tolerance varies widely
Generous salt	Food generously salted to replace sweat losses; salt supplements in hot weather
Vitamins	Double doses of multivitamins in water-soluble form (vitamin E supplements sometimes used as low blood levels of the vitamin have been observed); vitamin K supplements with prolonged antibiotic therapy
Pancreatic enzymes	Large amounts given by mouth with each meal (may be mixed with cereal or applesauce for infants) to compensate for pancreatic deficiency—powdered pancreas containing steapsin, trypsin, and amylapsin (Pancreatin, or other pancreatic extracts such as Cotazyme or Viokase).

There is a wide variation, however, in tolerance for fat, and the amount of fat intake is usually prescribed according to the character of the stools. Large increases of protein seem to be well tolerated and are needed for replacement of losses and for growth.

Dietary programs for cystic fibrosis are similar to those outlined for celiac disease, the food used varying in form according to the age of the child. The diet differs, however, in that gluten sources need not be restricted, and, of course, there is greater emphasis on quantity of food. The important principles of dietary management for patients with cystic fibrosis are summarized in Table 19-1.

Cleft palate

Feeding difficulties in infants and young children may result from abnormalities in the structure of the mouth. When the parts of the upper jaw and of the palate separating the mouth and nasal cavity do not fuse properly during fetal development, the anatomic abnormality creates difficult feeding problems. The premaxillary and maxillary processes normally fuse early in gesta-

tion (between the fifth and eighth week of intrauterine life) and fusion of the palate is completed about one month later. If this fusion fails to occur, cleft lip (harelip) or cleft palate results. Since the infant is unable to suck adequately, early feedings are tiring and lengthy. A softened nipple with enlarged opening, through which the infant can obtain milk by a chewing motion, is helpful. In some instances a medicine dropper or gavage feedings may be used initially. The infant should be held in an upright position and fed slowly, in small amounts, to avoid aspiration. There should be brief rest periods and frequent burping to expel the large amount of air swallowed. If acid foods such as orange juice are irritating, ascorbic acid supplement is usually prescribed. As solid foods are added they may be mixed with milk in the bottle and given in gruel or thickened form through a large nipple opening.

Surgical repair of a cleft palate is usually carried out over the growth years, depending upon the extent of the deformity and the growth of the child. During this period the child may be cared for by a group of specialists to handle his overall development. This group may be found in larger medical centers and is called the cleft palate team. Preparation for surgery demands good nutritional status. Following surgery, special nursing care is essential. The infant or child is usually fed a fluid or semifluid diet using a medicine dropper or a spoon. Great care must be exercised to protect the suture line and avoid any strain.

GENETIC DISEASES
Genetic inheritance concept

The concept of "inborn errors of metabolism" was first postulated by Sir Archibald Garrod in 1908. Though he probably had no clear conception of enzyme action, he pointed the way to a large number of conditions known today as genetic diseases that result from an inherited autosomal recessive mutant gene.

Definitions. The following is a review of the meanings of some key terms involved in the basic concept of genetic disease:

1. A *chromosome* is a rod-shaped body developed in the cell nucleus. Each human cell contains 46 chromosomes arranged in

23 pairs. One pair forms the sex chromosomes carrying the sex trait, and the remaining 22 pairs control the other various characteristics of the cell and of the individual.

2. *Autosomes* are any of the chromosomes other than the sex characteristics.

3. *Genes* (Gr. *gennan*, to produce) are self-reproducing particles in the cells, located at definite individual points (loci) on chromosomes. Each gene is a long, double-stranded molecule (helix) of DNA *(deoxyribonucleic acid)*, with a special arrangement of its components—its so-called genetic code (see p. 52).

A *mutant gene* (L. *mutare*, to change) is an altered form of a gene which can be transmitted to the offspring. Why genes mutate is not known. Probably temperature, irradiation, or infection are involved. A mutant gene is an abnormal gene that keeps on reproducing itself in successive generations.

4. The genes on the respective pairs of chromosomes are almost identical with each other, so they, too, form pairs, or so-called

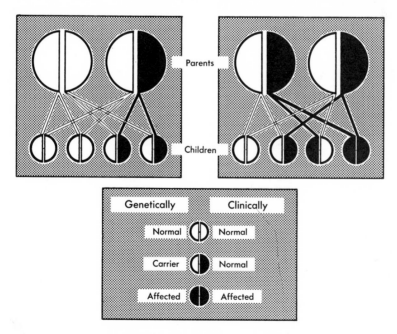

Fig. 19-3. Pattern of genetic disease. Transmission of recessive traits follows Mendel's law. If two carriers marry, one child will be normal, one child will manifest the trait, and two children will be carriers.

links of genes. A gene trait is *recessive,* (does not manifest itself) if it does not match its partner. The recessive gene must be carried by both parents to cause a defect.

5. *Heterozygote* is an individual in which the members of one or more gene pairs are unlike. Such a person is called a "carrier" of the trait, but he does not manifest its symptoms. Transmission of recessive traits to successive generations follows the pattern established by Mendel (Fig. 19-3). If two carriers marry, the risk for each birth is 25% manifest trait, 50% carriers, 25% normal (neither carrier nor manifesting the trait).

Genetic control of heredity and cell function

Control of heredity. When the human ovum (female sex cell) is fertilized by the sperm (male sex cell) the fertilized ovum from which the new individual develops contains 46 chromosomes, 23 contributed by the sperm cell from the father and 23 contributed by the ovum from the mother.

These 46 chromosomes align themselves in 23 pairs in the fertilized ovum, and with each successive cell division (mitosis) by which growth occurs in the new life, these same pairs of chromosomes are duplicated in the nucleus and become a part of the new cell. Thus, the gene pattern of the original chromosomes received at conception from the parents remains to determine the offspring's inherited traits of sex, physical appearance, eye color, and so on.

Control of cell function. The genes not only control common hereditary characteristics in this manner, but they also control the metabolic function of the cell by their control of the synthesis of specific metabolic enzymes. There are one thousand or more protein enzymes which control essentially all the chemical reactions which take place in cells. Each one of these enzymes is a *specific* protein synthesized by a *specific* DNA pattern in a *specific* gene (see p. 65). Therefore, when a specific gene is abnormal (mutant) the enzyme whose synthesis it controls cannot be made. And, in turn, the metabolic reaction controlled by

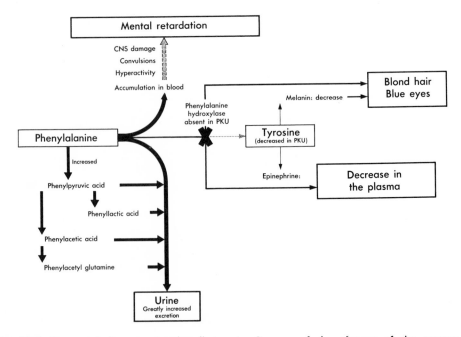

Fig. 19-4. The metabolic error in phenylketonuria. Because of the absence of the enzyme phenylalanine hydroxylase, the essential amino acid phenylalanine cannot be converted to tyrosine.

that enzyme cannot take place. The result is a genetic disease manifesting symptoms relative to those reaction products. Two such diseases are *phenylketonuria* and *galactosemia*.

Phenylketonuria (PKU)

Metabolic defect. Phenylketonuria was first observed in 1934 by a Norwegian biochemist and physician, Asbjorn Fölling. It is a genetic disease resulting from a mutant autosomal recessive gene. The normal gene controls the synthesis of the liver enzyme, *phenylalanine hydroxylase*, which oxidizes *phenylalanine*, an essential amino acid, to *tyrosine*, another amino acid. Since the gene is defective, the enzyme cannot be produced, and the reaction does not proceed normally (Fig. 19-4). Phenylalanine accumulates in the blood and its alternate metabolites, the phenyl acids, are excreted in the urine. One of these acids, *phenylpyruvic acid*, is a phenylketone; hence the name, phenylketonuria. This acid gives the characteristic green color reaction with ferric chloride (the basis for the "diaper test" of the infant's urine to detect the presence of phenylketonuria).

Clinical symptoms. The most profound effect which may occur in untreated phenylketonuria is mental retardation. The I.Q. is usually below 50, and most frequently under 20. The damage to the central nervous system probably occurs within the first two years. The patient may learn to walk, but few learn to talk. There is increased motor irritability, hyperactivity, convulsive seizures, and biazarre behavior—disorientation, failure to respond to strong stimuli, catatonic-like positions, fright reactions, and screaming episodes.

Because tyrosine is used in the production of the pigment material *melanin*, phenylketonuric children usually have blond or light brown hair and blue eyes. The skin is fair and susceptible to eczema. Tyrosine also is involved in the production of epinephrine by the adrenal gland, accounting for the low blood level of epinephrine in the child.

The urine frequently has a strong musty odor from the presence of large amounts of phenylacetic acid (Fig. 19-4). Sometimes this is the first thing the mother notices, leading her to seek a physician's care. This was the case in the initial discovery of the

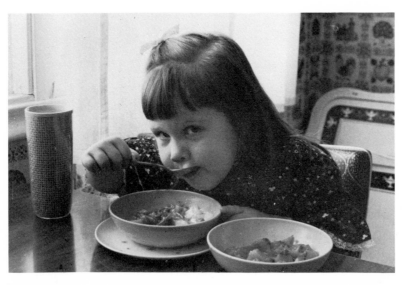

Fig. 19-5. PKU. This child is a delightful, perfectly developed 2-year-old. Screened and diagnosed at birth, she has eaten a carefully controlled low phenylalanine diet and is growing normally.

disease when a mother of two mentally retarded children complained of this unusual odor in the children's urine and called it to Dr. Fölling's attention, thus stimulating his active interest and study of the disease.

Dietary management. Treatment of phenylketonuria is dietary. A low phenylalanine diet is used to reduce the serum phenylalanine and prevent the high levels that cause the clinical symptoms, especially the central nervous system damage. Since phenylalanine is an essential amino acid necessary for growth, it cannot be totally removed from the diet. Blood levels of phenylalanine are constantly checked and the diet is calculated to allow the limited amount of phenylalanine, usually between 10 and 20 mg. per kg. body weight (the diet of a normal child contains 100 to 200 mg. of phenylalanine per kg. body weight). This amount will maintain the blood levels within acceptable ranges (2 to 6 mg. per 100 ml.) to prevent symptoms. Normal phenylalanine blood levels range from 1 to 3 mg. per 100 ml. of blood. In the untreated

phenylketonuric child they may run as high as sixty times this amount.

Milk substitute formula. Milk has a relatively high phenylalanine content, so the first need for the infant is a milk substitute. The formula is usually made from Lofenalac, a special casein hydrolysate balanced with fats, carbohydrates, vitamins, and minerals. One measure of Lofenalac powder in 2 oz. of water makes a formula of twenty calories per ounce and is well accepted by the infant. A small designated measure of milk may be added to the Lofenalac formula to adjust the phenylalanine content.

Low phenylalanine diet. As the child grows (Fig. 19-5), solid foods are added to the diet as calculated according to their phenylalanine content. These food additions are selected from a list of phenylalanine food exchange groups or equivalents. The diet is prescribed by the physician according to the child's blood phenylalanine test, and calculated by the nutritionist in terms of numbers of food choices

Table 19-2. Food lists for use with low phenylalanine diet*

Food	Amount	Phenylalanine (mg.)	Protein (gm.)	Calories
Vegetables (Each serving listed contains approximately 15 mg. phenylalanine)				
Baby and Junior				
Beets	7 tbsp.	15	1.1	35
Carrots	7 tbsp.	15	0.7	28
Creamed spinach	1 tbsp.	16	0.4	6
Green beans	2 tbsp.	15	0.3	7
Squash	4 tbsp.	14	0.4	14
Table vegetables				
Asparagus, cooked	1 stalk	12	0.6	4
Beans, green, cooked	4 tbsp. (¼ cup)	14	0.6	9
Beans, yellow, wax, cooked	4 tbsp. (¼ cup)	15	0.6	9
Bean sprouts, mung, cooked	2 tbsp.	18	0.6	5
Beets, cooked	8 tbsp. (½ cup)	14	0.8	34
Beet greens, cooked	1 tbsp.	14	0.2	3
Broccoli, cooked	1 tbsp.	11	0.3	3
Brussels sprouts, cooked	1 medium	16	0.6	5
Cabbage, raw, shredded	8 tbsp. (½ cup)	15	0.7	12

*Bureau of Public Health Nutrition of the California State Department of Public Health, 1961 revision, PKU, a diet guide for parents of children with phenylketonuria, Berkeley, California, pp. 7-11.

Table 19-2. Food lists for use with low phenylalanine diet—*cont'd*

Food	Amount	Phenylalanine (mg.)	Protein (gm.)	Calories
	Vegetables—*cont'd*			
Table vegetables—*cont'd*				
Cabbage, cooked	5 tbsp. (⅓ cup)	16	0.8	12
Carrots, raw	⅙ large (¼ cup)	16	0.5	16
Carrots, cooked	8 tbsp. (½ cup)	17	0.5	23
Cauliflower, cooked	3 tbsp.	18	0.6	6
Celery, cooked, diced†	4 tbsp. (¼ cup)	15	0.4	6
Celery, raw†	1 8-inch stalk	16	0.5	7
Chard leaves, cooked	2 tbsp.	19	0.6	6
Collards, cooked	1 tbsp.	16	0.5	5
Cucumber slices, raw	8 slices, ⅛ inch thick	16	0.7	12
Eggplant, diced, raw	3 tbsp.	18	0.4	9
Kale, cooked	2 tbsp.	20	0.5	5
Lettuce†	3 small leaves	13	0.4	5
Mushrooms, cooked†	2 tbsp.	14	0.4	35
Mushrooms, fresh†	2 small	16	0.5	3
Mustard greens, cooked	2 tbsp.	18	0.6	6
Okra, cooked†	2 3-inch pods	13	0.4	7
Onion, raw, chopped	5 tbsp. (⅓ cup)	14	0.5	20
Onion, cooked	4 tbsp. (¼ cup)	14	0.5	19
Onion, young scallion	5 5-inch long	14	0.5	23
Parsley, raw, chopped†	3 tbsp.	13	0.4	5
Parsnips, cooked, diced†	3 tbsp.	13	0.3	18
Peppers, raw, chopped†	4 tbsp.	13	0.4	12
Pickles, dill	8 slices, ⅛ inch thick	16	0.7	12
Pumpkin, cooked	4 tbsp. (¼ cup)	14	0.5	16
Radishes, red, small†	4	13	0.4	8
Rutabagas, cooked	2 tbsp.	16	0.3	10
Spinach, cooked	1 tbsp.	15	0.4	3
Squash, summer, cooked	8 tbsp. (½ cup)	16	0.6	16
Squash, winter, cooked	3 tbsp.	16	0.6	14
Tomato, raw	½ small	14	0.5	10
Tomato, cooked	4 tbsp. (¼ cup)	15	0.6	10
Tomato juice	4 tbsp. (¼ cup)	17	0.6	12
Tomato catsup	2 tbsp.	17	0.6	34
Turnip greens, cooked	1 tbsp.	18	0.4	4
Turnips, diced, cooked	5 tbsp. (⅓ cup)	16	0.4	12
Soups (condensed)				
Beef broth	1 tbsp.	14	0.5	3
Celery	2 tbsp.	18	0.4	19
Minestrone	1 tbsp.	17	1.5	25
Mushroom	1 tbsp.	11	0.2	17
Onion	1 tbsp.	14	0.6	8
Tomato	1 tbsp.	11	0.2	11
Vegetarian vegetable	1½ tbsp.	17	0.4	14

†Phenylalanine calculated as 3.3% of total protein.   Continued.

Table 19-2. Food lists for use with low phenylalanine diet—*cont'd*

Food	Amount	Phenylal- anine (mg.)	Protein (gm.)	Calories
Fruits (Each serving listed contains approximately 15 mg. phenylalanine)				
Baby and Junior				
Applesauce and apricots	16 tbsp. (1 cup)	15	0.6	205
Applesauce and pineapple	16 tbsp. (1 cup)	11	0.5	176
Apricots with tapioca	16 tbsp. (1 cup)	16	0.6	187
Bananas	8 tbsp. (½ cup)	14	0.6	97
Bananas and pineapple	16 tbsp. (1 cup)	18	0.6	187
Peaches	10 tbsp.	15	0.7	124
Pears	12 tbsp. (¾ cup)	16	0.5	106
Pears and pineapple	16 tbsp. (1 cup)	17	1.0	166
Plums with tapioca	12 tbsp. (¾ cup)	16	0.5	163
Prunes with tapioca	12 tbsp. (¾ cup)	16	0.5	152
Fruit juices				
Apricot nectar	6 oz. (¾ cup)	14	0.6	102
Cranberry juice	12 oz. (1½ cup)	15	0.6	39
Grape juice	4 oz. (½ cup)	14	0.5	80
Grapefruit juice	8 oz. (1 cup)	16	1.2	104
Orange juice	6 oz. (¾ cup)	16	1.2	84
Peach nectar	5 oz. (⅔ cup)	15	0.5	75
Pineapple juice	6 oz. (¾ cup)	16	0.6	90
Prune juice	4 oz. (½ cup)	16	0.5	84
Table fruits				
Apple, raw	4 small 2½-inch diam.	16	0.8	176
Applesauce	16 tbsp. (1 cup)	12	0.6	192
Apricots, raw	1 medium	12	0.5	25
Apricots, canned	2 med. 2 tbsp. syrup	14	0.6	80
Avocado, cubed or mashed‡	5 tbsp. (⅓ cup)	16	0.6	80
Banana, raw, sliced	4 tbsp. (¼ cup)	15	0.4	32
Blackberries, raw‡	5 tbsp. (⅓ cup)	14	0.6	25
Blackberries, canned in syrup‡	5 tbsp. (⅓ cup)	13	0.5	55
Blueberries, raw or frozen‡	12 tbsp. (¾ cup)	16	0.6	60
Blueberries, canned in syrup‡	10 tbsp.	16	0.6	140
Boysenberries, frozen, sw.‡	8 tbsp. (½ cup)	16	0.6	72
Cantaloupe	5 tbsp. (⅓ cup)	16	0.4	15
Cherries, sweet, canned in syrup‡	8 tbsp. (½ cup)	16	0.6	104
Dates, pitted, chopped	3 tbsp.	18	0.7	96
Figs, raw‡	1 large	18	0.7	40
Figs, canned in syrup‡	2 figs in 4 tsp. syrup	16	0.6	90
Figs, dried‡	1 small	16	0.6	40
Fruit cocktail‡	12 tbsp. (¾ cup)	16	0.6	120
Grapes, American type	8 grapes	14	0.5	24
Grapes, American slipskin	5 tbsp. (⅓ cup)	16	0.6	25
Grapes, Thompson seedless	8 tbsp. (½ cup)	13	0.8	64
Guava, raw‡	½ medium	13	0.5	35
Honeydew melon‡	¼ small 5-inch melon	13	0.5	32

‡Phenylalanine calculated as 2.6% of total protein.

Table 19-2. Food lists for use with low phenylalanine diet—*cont'd*

Food	Amount	Phenylal-anine (mg.)	Protein (gm.)	Calories
	Fruits—cont'd			
Table fruits—cont'd				
Mango, raw‡	1 small	18	0.7	66
Nectarines, raw	1-2 inches high, 2 inches diam.	15	0.4	45
Oranges, raw	1 medium 3 inches diam. or ⅔ cup sections	15	1.1	60
Papayas, raw‡	¼ med. or ½ cup	14	0.6	36
Peaches, raw	1 medium	15	0.5	46
Peaches, canned in syrup	2 medium halves	18	0.6	88
Pears, raw	1 3 x 2½ inches	14	1.3	100
Pears, canned in syrup	2 med. halves 2 tbsp. syrup	14	1.3	78
Pineapple, raw‡	16 tbsp. (1 cup)	16	0.6	80
Pineapple canned in syrup‡	2 small slices	13	0.5	93
Plums, raw	½ 2-inch plum	12	0.3	15
Plums canned in syrup	3–2 tbsp. syrup	16	0.5	91
Prunes, dried	2 large	14	0.4	54
Raisins, dried seedless	2 tbsp.	14	0.5	54
Raspberries, raw‡	5 tbsp. (⅓ cup)	13	0.5	25
Raspberries, canned in syrup‡	6 tbsp.	14	0.5	78
Strawberries, raw‡	8 large	16	0.6	32
Strawberries, frozen‡	6 tbsp.	14	0.5	108
Tangerines	1½ large	15	1.2	66
Watermelon‡	½ cup cubes	13	0.5	28
	Breads and cereals (Each serving listed contains approximately 30 mg. phenylalanine)			
Baby and Junior				
Cereals, ready to serve				
Barley	3 tbsp.	32	0.8	24
Oatmeal	2 tbsp.	34	0.8	16
Rice	5 tbsp. (⅓ cup)	30	0.6	40
Wheat	2 tbsp.	30	0.6	17
Creamed corn	3 tbsp.	30	0.5	27
Sweet potatoes (Gerber's)	3 tbsp.	32	0.5	31
Table foods				
Cereals, cooked				
Cornmeal	4 tbsp. (¼ cup)	29	0.6	29
Cream of rice	4 tbsp. (¼ cup)	35	0.7	34
Cream of Wheat	2 tbsp.	27	0.6	16
Farina	2 tbsp.	25	0.5	18
Malt-o-Meal	2 tbsp.	27	0.5	17
Oatmeal	2 tbsp.	32	0.7	18
Pettijohns	2 tbsp.	24	0.5	19

‡Phenylalanine calculated as 2.6% of total protein.
§Low phenylalanine recipes in Phenylalanine-restricted diet recipe book, 1966, Berkeley, State of California Department of Public Health.

Continued.

Table 19-2. Food lists for use with low phenylalanine diet—*cont'd*

Food	Amount	Phenylal-anine (mg.)	Protein (gm.)	Calories
Breads and cereals—cont'd				
Table foods—cont'd				
Ralston	2 tbsp.	34	0.7	18
Rice, brown or white	4 tbsp. (¼ cup)	35	0.7	34
Wheatena	2 tbsp.	27	0.5	19
Cereals, ready to serve				
Alpha Bits	4 tbsp. (¼ cup)	32	0.6	28
Cheerios	3 tbsp.	32	0.6	20
Corn Chex	4 tbsp. (¼ cup)	29	0.6	32
Cornfetti	5 tbsp. (⅓ cup)	31	0.6	46
Cornflakes	5 tbsp. (⅓ cup)	29	0.6	30
Crispy Critters	4 tbsp. (¼ cup)	30	0.6	28
Kix	5 tbsp. (⅓ cup)	31	0.6	31
Krumbles	3 tbsp.	32	0.7	26
Rice Chex	6 tbsp.	32	0.7	49
Rice flakes	5 tbsp. (⅓ cup)	33	0.6	32
Rice Krispies	6 tbsp.	30	0.6	40
Rice, puffed	12 tbsp. (¾ cup)	30	0.6	38
Sugar Crisp, puffed wheat	4 tbsp. (¼ cup)	30	0.6	46
Sugar Frosted Flakes	5 tbsp. (⅓ cup)	29	0.6	55
Wheat Chex	10 biscuits	30	0.6	22
Wheaties	3 tbsp.	26	0.5	20
Wheat, puffed	6 tbsp.	30	0.6	16
Crackers				
Barnum Animal	5	30	0.6	45
Graham (65 per lb.)	1	26	0.5	30
Ritz (no cheese)	2	24	0.5	34
Saltines (140 per lb.)	2	29	0.6	28
Soda (63 per lb.)	1	36	0.7	30
Wheat Thins (248 per lb.)	5	30	0.6	45
Corn, cooked	2 tbsp.	32	0.7	17
Hominy	2 tbsp.	32	0.7	17
Macaroni, cooked	1 ½ tbsp.	31	0.7	20
Noodles, cooked	3 tbsp.	32	0.7	20
Popcorn, popped	5 tbsp. (⅓ cup)	31	0.6	17
Potato chips	4 2-inch diameter	30	0.6	44
Potato, Irish, cooked	3 tbsp.	33	0.8	31
Spaghetti, cooked	1 tbsp.	24	0.5	14
Sweet potato, cooked	2 tbsp.	25	0.4	31
Tortilla, corn	1½ 6-inch diameter	30	0.8	31
Fats				
(Each serving listed contains approximately 5 mg. phenylalanine)				
Butter	1 tbsp.	5	0.1	100
French dressing, commercial	1 tbsp.	5	0.1	59
Margarine	1 tbsp.	5	0.1	100
Mayonnaise, commercial	½ tbsp.	5	0.1	30
Olives, green or ripe	1 medium	5	0.1	12

Table 19-2. Food lists for use with low phenylalanine diet—*cont'd*

Food	Amount	Phenylal-anine (mg.)	Protein (gm.)	Calories
Desserts				
(Each serving listed contains approximately 30 mg. phenylalanine)				
Cake§	¹⁄₁₂ of cake			
Cookies Rice flour§	2			
Corn starch§	2			
Cookies, Arrowroot	1½			
Ice cream				
Chocolate§	⅔ cup			
Pineapple§	⅔ cup			
Strawberry§	⅔ cup			
Jello	⅓ cup			
Puddings§	½ cup			
Sauce, Hershey	2 tbsp.			
Wafers, sugar, Nabisco	5			

Free foods

Apple juice
Beverages, carbonated
Gingerbread§
Guava butter
Candy
    Butterscotch
    Cream mints
    Fondant
    Gum drops
    Hard
    Jelly beans
    Lollipops
Cherries, Maraschino
Fruit ices (if no more than ½ cup used daily)
Cornstarch
Jell-Quik
Jellies
Kool-Aid
Lemonade
Molasses
Oil
Pepper, black, ground
Popsicles, with artificial fruit flavor
Rich's Topping
Salt
Shortening, vegetable
Soy sauce
Sugar, brown, white, or confectioner's
Syrups, corn or maple
Tang
Tapioca

§Low phenylalanine recipes in Phenylalanine-restricted diet recipe book, 1966, Berkeley, State of California Department of Public Health.

allowed daily from each food group. Then a meal pattern of feedings is made out for the mother to follow. The phenylalanine food exchange groups forming the basis of the low phenylalanine diet are outlined in Table 19-2. It is not known yet how long such a diet must be continued. One clinician has suggested it may be possible to relax the dietary controls as early as age 4,[21] but at present, it is probably wise to continue the diet at least until the child is six to eight years old.

Family counseling. The parents charged with the care of a phenylketonuric child face physical, emotional, and financial tension. Depending upon their personal resources and strength in all three areas, the course may be stormy or relatively stable. They must understand and accept the absolute necessity of following the diet carefully, so patient and understanding teaching must be done. Frequent home visits by the public health nurse or nutritionist may be a source of guidance and support as the child grows older (Fig. 19-6). Other family members and any subsequent siblings should be

tested for phenylketonuria also. Supervised by a competent physician, whose medical care is supported by the nurse and nutritionist and mature and wise parents, the phenylketonuric child will grow and develop normally. Such a child, diagnosed at birth by widespread screening programs, has a healthy and happy adulthood ahead, instead of the profound disease consequences he would probably have experienced so few years ago.

Public health implications. Phenylketonuria screening surveys have shown it to occur more frequently than originally estimated. These surveys indicate an incidence of about one in every ten thousand births. The possibilities of severe mental retardation from undiagnosed and untreated phenylketonuria make public health implications obvious. A number of tests have been developed to detect the disease. They are listed on p. 419.

The more recent, sensitive tests of blood samples have been the basis of new laws in several states making mandatory the screening of all newborns for phenylketonuria.

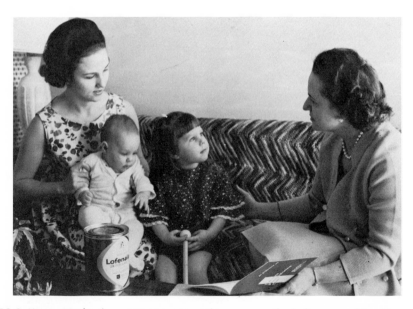

Fig. 19-6. Home visits by the nutritionist support this young mother's fine care of her two-year-old daughter, a phenylketonuric child screened at birth. Careful, understanding diet control has enabled this child to develop normally in all respects. Here she sits between her mother and the nutritionist, interested and alert. The young child, a boy, is normal.

TO PROBE FURTHER
Tests used in phenylketonuria

Test	Method	Use
Urine tests		
Diaper test	10% ferric chloride dropped on freshly wet diaper. Green spot is positive, indicates probable PKU.	Cheap. Useful in screening large groups of infants, but not of value until the infant is at least 6 weeks of age.
Phenistix* test	Prepared test stick pressed against wet diaper or dipped in urine. Green color reaction indicates probable PKU.	Simple; more accurate than diaper test. Useful in screening large groups of infants, but not of value until after infant is 6 weeks of age.
Dinitrophenyl-hydrazine (DNPH) test†	0.5 to 1 ml. of urine placed in test tube, and equal amount of DNPH solution added. Immediate pale yellow-orange color reaction is negative. A gradual change to opaque bright yellow is positive and indicates probable PKU.	Cheap, accurate, but more complicated than diaper test or Phenistix; most useful in clinical setting to confirm these tests.
Blood serum phenylalanine tests		
Guthrie inhibition assay method‡	Drops of blood placed on filter paper. Lab uses a bacterial growth inhibition test. Level above 8 mg. phenylalanine per 100 ml. blood diagnostic of PKU.	Effective in newborn period. Used also to monitor PKU diet. Blood easily obtained by heal or finger puncture. Inexpensive; used for wide-scale screening.
LaDu-Michael method§	5 ml. of blood; serum separated and tested for phenylalanine. Level above 8 mg. per 100 ml. blood indicates PKU. In PKU patients, level above 8 to 12 mg. phenylalanine per 100 ml. blood indicates loss of dietary control.	Useful diagnostic tool, and to monitor PKU diet. Requires blood drawn from patient, and the lab method is difficult (test not available in many labs).

*Manufactured by Ames Company, Elkhart, Indiana.
†Centerwall, W., and Centerwall, S.: Phenylketonuria, U. S. Children's Bureau, Pub. No. 338, Washington, D. C., 1961, Government Printing Office.
‡Guthrie, R.: Blood screening for phenylketonuria, J.A.M.A., 178:863, 1961.
§LaDu, B., and Michael, P.: An enzymatic spectriphotometric method for the determination of phenylalanine in blood, J. Lab. Clin. Med., 55:491, 1960.

Continued.

Tests used in phenylketonuria—cont'd

Test	Method	Use
McCaman and Robins fluorimetric method‖	5 ml. of blood; serum separated and tested for phenylalanine. Level above 8 mg. indicates PKU or loss of dietary control.	Diagnostic and diet monitoring tool. Lab procedure more simple than LaDu-Michael method. Test not available in many labs.

‖McCaman, M., and Robins, E.: Fluorimetric method for the determination of phenylalanine in the serum, J. Lab. Clin. Med., 59:885, 1962.

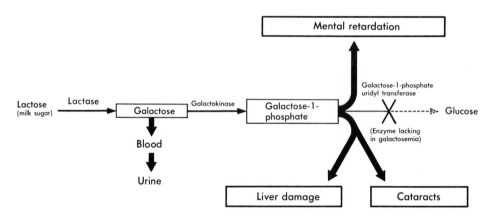

Fig. 19-7. Metabolic error in galactosemia. Because of the absence of the enzyme galactose-1-phosphate uridyl transferase galactose cannot be converted to glucose.

The inhibition assay test, developed by Dr. Robert Guthrie[22-24] of the University of Buffalo, is a highly specific blood test, sensitive as early as the third day of life. A simple heel puncture is made and the blood is absorbed on specially treated absorbing paper. Another definitive blood test is the fluorimetric procedure developed by McCaman and Robins.[25] In California both of these tests are approved for use under the regulations which are now part of the State Administrative Code, Title 17. These new amendments, which make phenylketonuria screening mandatory throughout the state for all newborns, were signed into law by the 1965 legislature and became effective January 1, 1966.

Galactosemia

Metabolic defect. Galactosemia is also a genetic disease caused by a missing enzyme. The metabolic defect, transmitted by a single autosomal recessive gene, is illustrated in Fig. 19-7. The incidence of galactosemia is lower than that of phenylketonuria; it occurs about once in 25,000 to 50,000 births.

The missing enzyme, *galactose-1-phosphate uridyl transferase,* is one of three enzymes that control steps in the conversion of galactose to glucose. Milk, the infant's first food, contains a large amount of the disaccharide lactose (milk sugar) which is acted upon by the intestinal digestive enzyme *lactase* (see p. 16) to produce the

Foods which may be included or should be excluded in a galactose-free diet*

Food categories	Foods included	Foods excluded†
Milk and milk products	None; Nutramigen and soybean milks used as milk substitutes	All milk of any species and all products containing milk, as skim, dried, evaporated, condensed; yogurt; cheese; ice cream; sherbet; malted milk
Legumes	All may be included if facilities are available for monitoring erythrocyte galactose-1-phosphate	
Meat, fish, and fowl	Plain beef, chicken, fish, turkey, lamb, veal, pork, and ham	Creamed or breaded meat, fish or fowl; sausage products, such as weiners, liver sausage, cold cuts containing milk; organ meats, such as liver, pancreas and brain
Eggs	All	None
Vegetables	Artichokes, asparagus, beets, broccoli, cabbage, carrots, cauliflower, celery, chard, corn, cucumber, eggplant, green beans, kale, lettuce, mustard, okra, onions, parsley, parsnips, pumpkin, rutabagas, spinach, squash, tomatoes	Sugar beets, peas, lima beans; creamed, breaded or buttered vegetables; canned or frozen vegetables; corn curls (if lactose is added during processing)
Potatoes and substitutes	White and sweet potatoes, yams, macaroni, noodles, spaghetti, rice	Any creamed, breaded, or buttered; French fried or instant potatoes if lactose is added during processing
Breads and cereals	Any that do not contain milk or milk products‡	Prepared mixes, such as muffins, biscuits, waffles, pancakes; some dry cereals; Instant Cream of Wheat. *Read labels carefully.*
Fats	Margarines and dressings which do not contain milk or milk products; oils, shortenings; bacon	Margarines and dressings containing milk or milk products; butter; cream; cream cheese
Soups	Clear soups; vegetable soups which do not contain peas or lima beans; consommés	Cream soups, chowders, commercially prepared soups containing lactose
Desserts	Water and fruit ices; gelatin; angel food cake; homemade cakes, pies, cookies made from acceptable ingredients	Commercial cakes and cookies and mixes; custard, puddings, ice cream made with milk; any containing chocolate
Fruits	All fresh; canned or frozen that are not processed with lactose	Any canned or frozen processed with lactose
Miscellaneous	Nuts and nut butters, unsalted popcorn, olives, pure sugar candy, jelly or marmalade, sugar, corn syrup	Gravy, white sauce; chocolate, cocoa, toffee, peppermints, butterscotch, caramels, molasses; instant coffee, powdered soft drinks, monosodium glutamate, some spice blends, chewing gum

*Koch, R., M.D., and others: Nutrition in the treatment of galactosemia, J. Amer. Diet. Ass. 43:220, 1963.
†In all instances, labels should be read carefully and any product which contains milk, lactose, casein, whey, dry milk solids, or curds should be omitted.
‡In each area, bakeries should be contacted and a list of acceptable products made available.

monosaccharides glucose and galactose. After galactose is initially combined with phosphate to begin the metabolic conversion to glucose, it cannot proceed further in the galactosemic infant. Galactose-1-phosphate and galactose rapidly accumulate in the blood and in various body tissues.

Clinical symptoms. The excess tissue accumulations of galactose cause rapid damage to the untreated infant. The child fails to thrive, and clinical evidences are apparent soon after birth. Liver damage brings jaundice, hepatomegly with cirrhosis, enlargement of the spleen, and ascites. Death usually results from hepatic failure. If the infant survives, the continuing tissue damage and accompanying hypoglycemia in the optic lens and the brain cause cataracts and mental retardation.

Dietary management. The main indirect source of dietary galactose is milk. Therefore, *all* forms of milk and lactose must be removed from the diet. In this instance, a galactose-*free* diet can be used. Although galactose is part of certain body structures, the needed amounts can be synthesized by the body. The milk substitute usually used for infant feeding is Nutramigen, a complete protein hydrolysate that is free of galactose. Careful attention must be given to avoid lactose from other food sources as solid foods are added to the infant's diet. An outline of foods to use and to avoid is given on p. 421. Parents must be carefully instructed to check labels on all commercial products. Table 19-3 gives products which normally contain lactose. Even drugs contain lactose occasionally as an ingredient.

Public health implications. Although original estimates place the incidence of galactosemia at one in every 25,000 to 50,000 births, there is evidence that it may not be so rare. Asymptomatic carriers have been detected in families of galactosemic

Table 19-3. Typical uses of lactose*

Ascorbic acid and citric acid mixtures	Monosodium glutamate extender
Buttermilk	
Cakes and sweet rolls	Party dips
Canned and frozen fruits and vegetables	Penicillin and other antibiotics
Caramels, fudge, and tableted candies	Pharmaceutical bulking agents, fillers, and excipients
Cheese foods and spreads	Pie crusts and fillings
Cookies and cookie sandwich fillings	Powdered coffee cream
Cordials and liqueurs	Powdered soft drinks
Cottage cheese and cottage cheese dressings	Puddings
Dietetic and diabetic preparations	
Dried soups	Salad dressings
Easter egg dyes and dye carrier	Sherbets, frozen desserts, and ices
	Simulated mother's milk; infant food formulas
Fireworks, flares, and pyrotechnics	Sour cream
French fries and corn curls	Spice blends
Frozen cultures	Starter cultures
Health and geriatric foods	Sweetened condensed milk
High-solids ice cream	Sweetness reducers in icings, candies, preserves, and fruit pie fillings
Instant coffee	
Instant potatoes	Tablets (food and pharmaceutical)
Meat products	Tinctures
Modified skimmed milk	Vitamin and mineral mixtures

*Koch, R., and others: Nutrition in the treatment of galactosemia, J. of Amer. Diet. Ass. 43:221, 1963.

children and in other individuals. Also, continuing reports give increasing incidence. The severe and rapid effects of the disease and the profound effects on body organs and tissues, especially on the brain, make attention to early diagnosis at birth and subsequent careful treatment with a galactose-free diet mandatory. Tests have been developed for such immediate screening. Cord blood may be used immediately after birth to establish a diagnosis, using a simple test for galactose-1-phosphate activity in erythrocytes. Children detected may be carefully followed with continuing blood tests every two to three months to monitor the diet.[26] Since a carrier can also be identified by a lowered enzyme level in the red cells, it may be advisable to eliminate lactose from the prenatal diet of a mother detected as a carrier.

Juvenile diabetes
Dietary management

Diabetes and its management is discussed in Chapter 25. Several principles, however, of the care of diabetes occurring in children are important to emphasize here.

Pediatricians usually hold one of three opinions concerning a philosophy of diet management for diabetic children. These are rigid diet control, the "free" diet, and the moderate approach.

Rigid diet control. This approach perhaps arises from experience in previous years, before development of more sensitive and varied types of insulin to meet individual needs, and from the more severe nature of the disease in children. A rigid, calculated and weighed diet (weighed on a gram scale) is prescribed and followed in some clinics. Pediatricians who still follow this approach apparently feel that the more brittle, labile form of diabetes in children, as compared with its more stable form in adults, requires this rigid supervision. In such programs, urine sugars are carefully checked frequently, with a sugar-free urine the criterion as a measure for control.

"Free" diet. Quotation marks are needed around the word "free," because most pedi-

atricians who use this term really do not mean *absolutely* free. However, they do seem to feel that a somewhat unlimited approach to diet (food as the child desires or has appetite for) should be followed. Insulin is usually adjusted to cover the food intake, and some sugar spillage in the urine is allowed. The rationale given for such an approach is the psychological benefit it has for the child.

Moderate approach. The more moderate approach, avoiding the tension of extreme rigidity on the one hand and the inconsistencies of a purely "free" regimen on the other, is followed by the majority of pediatricians. This approach is based on two realistic principles: (1) the normal physical and psychosocial growth development needs of the child, and (2) the nature of diabetes in children and the needs it imposes for balance and consistent habits.

Normal nutritional needs for growth and development. During the formative growth years, an optimum nutritional base is essential to health. These physiological needs for growth and the psychosocial developmental paths that accompany each stage of normal development have been outlined in the previous chapter. The normal nutritional needs of the child are fundamental.

Accommodations to diabetes. The insulin-sensitive type of diabetes in children appears different from diabetes that occurs in adults in their middle or older years of life. The child developing diabetes is likely to be undernourished when the disease is first discovered. It usually runs a more labile course and requires closer consideration and consistent, sound, self-care by the patient. Also, the erratic pattern of physical activity in children and the emotional struggles of obtaining maturity impose additional needs for sympathetic guidance, balance, and control.

Nutrient ratio. A balanced diet for children includes adequate quantities of protein, carbohydrate, and fat to meet growth and energy demands.

PROTEIN. Optimum levels for growth are about 1.5 gm. per kilogram body weight for children under three years of age, and 1 gm. per kilogram body weight for older children.

CALORIES. Calories should be sufficient for activity and growth. Carbohydrates should contribute 40% to 50% of the total calories, to supply the major source of energy. Fat should be sufficient but not excessive, *moderation* being the key. As the child grows older, weight control will be an important part of general care, and dietary habits of moderation in the use of fat will be helpful to that end. Also, because carbohydrate and fat metabolism is so intimately associated and interrelated, both factors are well considered together in the management of diabetes.

VITAMINS AND MINERALS. Optimal intake of vitamins and minerals should be assured for the metabolic requirements of growth. A well-planned and consistently followed balanced diet should supply these needs. Occasionally, however, where adequate diet may be questionable, or a greater margin of safety is desirable, the physician may prescribe supplements.

Distribution of meals. The distribution of food through the day should be based on the absorption rate and activity of the insulin used and on the general family meal pattern. Usually these needs are met with three fairly equal meals at breakfast, lunch, and dinner, with an added afternoon and evening snack. A midmorning snack may also be required by a younger child.

Regularity and portion sizes. The establishment of regular habits and a routine schedule are important factors in early and continuing stabilization of the diabetes. Day-to-day needs and activities will influence the schedule, but these may be accommodated in the day's balanced plan. The three balance factors are always food, insulin, and exercise, with additional considerations during periods of infection.

Exchange system of dietary control. For some two decades a system of dietary control based on food equivalents has been in common use throughout the United States for planning diabetic diets.[27] This plan is based on the concept that if foods are of fairly equal composition, it does not matter which of them is used. Thus, foods commonly used are grouped according to like composition, and these groups are called "exchange groups." The diet plan outlines for the mother and the child a meal pattern based on the number of choices from each of the food groups for each meal. With such a plan, flexibility and freedom of choice within the food groups is possible. A listing of these exchange food groups is given on pp. 483 and 484.

Teaching program for juvenile diabetes. The keystone of treatment and the basis of continuing care should be an early, thorough, and understanding teaching program for the child and his family. There should be no discounting of the fact that the child has diabetes, but at the same time it should not be used as a crutch or excuse to deprive the child from developing normal responsibility and maturity along with his peers. That he is essentially a "normal" healthy person, given the wise control of his diabetes, is an important concept to grasp. He is not primarily a diabetic child—he is a normally growing and developing child who has diabetes. There is a great difference in the two perspectives.

Time of instruction. Many later problems in control may be avoided by careful and thorough instruction at the initial development of the diabetes. Time spent in the beginning often saves time and tears later. Parents and child need time and opportunity to accept their new situation and make adequate psychological adjustment to it. By and large, mature adjustment to any problem is aided by sound knowledge of its nature. This is especially true in the care of juvenile diabetes, for the essential aim is to build in the patient as he grows an independence from the physician for ordinary day-to-day care of the diabetes, and the development of a mature sense of responsibility and self-direction. In the last analysis, the welfare of the person with diabetes—as with almost all persons—is in his own hands.

Content of instruction. The instructions

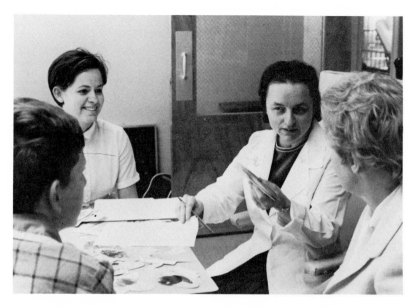

Fig. 19-8. Initial diet counseling with a 13-year-old boy having newly diagnosed juvenile diabetes mellitus. The dietitian discusses basic nutritional needs with the patient and his mother, assisted by the student nurse working with the patient on the ward.

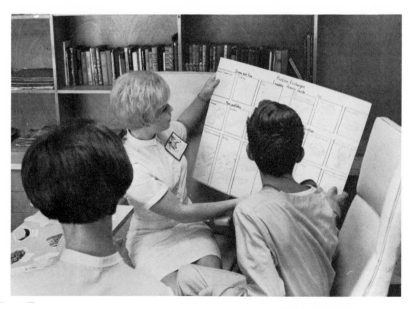

Fig. 19-9. Student nurses have numerous follow-up conferences with the patient as part of a planned teaching program (see Table 19-5). They prepare learning materials and use them to involve the patient in self-care activities.

Table 19-4. Teaching plan and record for diabetic child and parents

Patient's name_____

	Discussion	Return Explanation	Demonstration	Return Demonstration	Date	P = Parents C = Child Remarks
Conference with physician						
Hand out illustrated booklet on diabetes						
Diabetes						
Acidosis						
Insulin shock						
Collecting and testing urine						
Method used at home						
Hand out "The Child with Diabetes"*						
Giving insulin injections						
Type of insulin						
Site of injection						
Hand out "Watch these Injection Sites"†						
Rotation of injection						
Procedure						
Mixing insulin						
Equipment for insulin (same as home)						
List of equipment to buy						
Cost and where purchased (Review comparison costs of all equipment)						

*Reprint: *ADA Forecast,* The child with diabetes, Vol. 1, No. 3, May-June, 1953.
†Reprint: *ADA Forecast,* Watch these injection sites, Vol. 4, No. 1, Jan., 1951.

Table 19-4. Teaching plan and record for diabetic child and parents—*cont'd*

Patient's name_____

	Discussion	Return Explanation	Demonstration	Return Demonstration	Date	P = Parents C = Child Remarks
Diet						
Diet history						
School						
Amount						
Conference with dietitian						
Exercise						
Gym and sports						
Hygiene						
Feet						
Skin						
Girls—avoid panty girdles						
Time schedule arranged with family						
Home routine						
Weekends						
Diabetic camp (purpose, costs, application, procedure)						
"Forecast"						
Medic Alert (purpose, application, procedure)						
School						
Conference with school nurse						
Testing urine						
Giving insulin						
Reference materials						

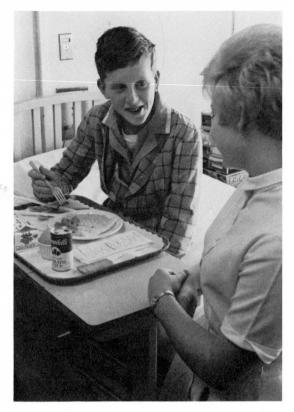

Fig. 19-10. As a result of knowledge and understanding of needs, given in a supportive manner at the very beginning signs of diabetes, his disease is controlled. He is a normal young boy, enjoying his food, secure in his own knowledge and in the care of the health team and his family.

should include basic needs for routine care: (1) an understanding of diabetes, (2) a realistic diet plan to meet normal needs, provide a basis for balance of the diabetes, and fit in with family food patterns, (3) techniques of insulin administration and minor adjustment, (4) urine testing for sugar, (5) the keeping of reasonable daily records according to need, (6) personal cleanliness and skin care, (7) recognition of early signs of insulin shock and how to treat it, and (8) recognition of early signs of acidosis and the need for immediate medical care.

A check list for planning such a teaching program as is followed in many clinics is given in Table 19-4. Active involvement of the patient and his family in practice ses-

sions and feedback discussion is essential (Figs. 19-8 to 19-10).

FOOD ALLERGIES IN INFANTS AND CHILDREN

The care of the allergic child is often frustrating and formidable, both for the child and for his parents. A wide variety of environmental, emotional, and physical factors influence the child's reaction, and a suitable regimen is sometimes difficult to find. Since sensitivity to protein substances is a common basis of the allergy, the early foods of infants and children are frequent offenders. Children tend to become less allergic to food sources as they grow older and respond more to inhalent allergens.

Milk. Cows' milk has long been and continues to be the most common cause of allergic disease in young infants. Park's classic case, nearly a half century ago (1920), of an infant with violent vomiting reactions to minute amounts of milk, is well known. The child's severe response was only overcome by a long, gradual, desensitizing program, beginning at six weeks of age with a single drop of diluted cows' milk and bringing the child to a tolerance for one pint of milk a day by the time he was three years old. Other such reports of violent reactions are found in the literature. Current observation indicates that milk allergy occurs in about 1 to 2% of all infants and accounts for some 30% of the cases among allergic infants.[28]

The allergy to milk usually causes gastrointestinal difficulties such as vomiting, diarrhea, and colic. The problem is generally identified by clinical symptoms, family history, and a trial on a milk-free diet, using a substitute formula such as a soybean preparation (for example, Sobee) or a meat formula. However, pediatricians agree generally that there may be a tendency among some clinicians to over-diagnose milk allergy in infants and children with diarrhea, colic, irritability, and skin rash. Thus, a remission of symptoms on a milk-free diet should always be followed by a trial on milk again to determine if it does indeed

Rowe Elimination Diets*—straight lines enclose foods in the cereal-free elimination diets 1, 2, and 3, a commonly used combination

Diet 1	Diet 2	Diet 3	Diet 4
Rice	Corn	Tapioca	Milk†
Tapioca	Rye	White potato	Tapioca
Rice biscuit	Corn pone	Breads made of any	Cane sugar
Rice bread	Corn-rye muffin	combination of soy,	
	Rye bread	lima and potato	
	Ry-Krisp	starch and tapioca	
		flours	
Lettuce	Beets	Tomato	
Chard	Squash	Carrot	
Spinach	Artichoke	Lima beans	
Carrot	Asparagus	String beans	
Sweet potato or yam			
		Peas	
Lamb	Chicken (no hens)	Beef	
	Bacon	Bacon	
Lemon	Pineapple	Lemon	
Grapefruit	Peach	Grapefruit	
Pears	Apricot	Peach	
	Prune	Apricot	
Cane sugar	Cane or beet sugar	Cane sugar	
Sesame oil	Mazola oil	Sesame oil	
Olive oil‡	Sesame oil	Soy bean oil	
Salt	Salt	Salt	
Gelatin, plain or	Gelatin, plain or	Gelatin, plain or	
flavored with lime	flavored with	flavored with lime	
or lemon	pineapple	or lemon	
Maple syrup or syrup	Karo corn syrup	Maple syrup or syrup	
made with cane sugar	White vinegar	made with cane sugar	
flavored with maple		flavored with maple	
Royal baking powder	Royal baking powder	Royal baking powder	
Baking soda	Baking soda	Baking soda	
Cream of tartar	Cream of tartar	Cream of tartar	
Vanilla extract	Vanilla extract	Vanilla extract	
Lemon extract		Lemon extract	

*Rowe, A. H.: Elimination diets and the patient's allergies, ed. 2, Philadelphia, 1944, Lea & Febiger.
†Milk should be taken up to two or three quarts a day. Plain cottage cheese and cream may be used. Tapicoa cooked with milk and milk sugar may be taken.
‡Allergy to it may occur with or without allergy to olive pollen. Mazola oil may be used if corn allergy is not present.

cause the symptoms to reappear. Only then should the child be labeled as allergic.[29]

Other frequent responses among infants allergic to milk are skin problems such as rashes, eczema, and respiratory difficulties such as wheezing or runny nose. Often these symptoms appear and disappear spontaneously, regardless of dietary changes. But they tend to be more often caused by food if gastrointestinal problems are also present with them.

Egg, wheat, and other foods. The albumin in egg white is a potential allergen, and hence is usually added to the infant's diet following earlier use of egg yolk. Wheat is also a fairly common food allergen among allergic children. The specific biochemical sensitivity to gluten (a protein found in wheat) in the child with gluten-induced celiac disease (p. 404) may be considered an example, although the biochemical defects in the mucosal cell in celiac disease probably represent a different sensitivity mechanism.

Dietary management. In an allergic child's diet, foods are usually added slowly, common offenders being excluded in early feedings. In some cases a series of diagnostic diets, such as the Rowe Elimination Diets (p. 429), may be used to identify the offending food. Each of the four basic diets is used for a trial period. If no change occurs in the allergic condition, the patient is given the next diet. If, however, on a given diet the patient's symptoms improve, it is assumed that the offending food is not in that diet list. Then foods are added one at a time to test the patient's response. If a given food causes return of the allergy, the food is then identified as an offending allergen and is eliminated from use. Guidance in the substitution of special food products and in the use of special recipes should be provided for the child's mother by the nutritionist and the nurse.

The following is a general hypoallergy diet list of foods that should be avoided:

Egg
Fish
Wheat
Strawberries
Tomatoes
Pork
Bacon
Citrus fruit
Nuts
Peanut butter
Chocolate
Pineapple
Milk* or milk products

Family education. The education of the parents and family of an allergic child should include a knowledge and understanding of the allergic state and the many

*Use soybean milk substitute.

factors that influence it. If specific foods have been definitely identified as offenders, careful guidance to the mother to eliminate these from the child's diet will follow. Discussion of the food's common use in daily meal patterns, and its occurrence in a number of commercial products and other hidden sources will make label reading and attention to recipes of prime consideration. As the child grows older, the allergic reaction to the given food may wane, and it may be gradually readded to the diet.

OBESITY IN CHILDREN

Great variations in weight and height occur among normal, healthy children. Therefore, a criteria for establishing a definition of obesity in children is somewhat difficult. Moreover, the important contribution of Bruch[30] states that in some cases the state of obesity may be an important resolution in the child's personality of deep-seated psychiatric problems. Nonetheless, reports continue to indicate that approximately 10% of the children in the United States are obese.[31] Later reports confirm these findings. Also, from a preventive medicine point of view, the development of obesity in childhood is a significant factor in avoiding problems in adulthood associated with the overweight state. The problem of obesity in children is complex. An increased understanding may be gained by clarification of words used in discussing obesity, by considering some of the causes for its development, and by comparing the basic types of obesity.

Associated definitions. In view of the controversy and divergent opinion concerning exact terminology, the Committee on Nutrition of the American Academy of Pediatrics recently gave these definitions for terms used:

Hunger—a biologic phenomenon predominantly learned and unconditioned
Appetite—a learned response usually in intimate association with the memory of past food experiences
Anorexia—absence of desire for food in

circumstances where one might ordinarily anticipate such a desire

Satiety—the lack of desire to eat which ensues after eating, predominantly determined by postingestion factors

Palatability—related to preingestion factors such as taste, aroma, texture, appearance, color, temperature and association with past experiences

Causes of obesity

Cultural factors. Many cultural factors condition food intake. There is much seasonal emphasis, such as the Christmas and Thanksgiving feasts, and emphasis upon eating certain foods at certain times, all of which habits are culturally derived. Also, meal patterns are different in different cultures. The three-meals-a-day pattern is a cultural one, not a biological necessity. Some indication exists that less food more often may be better to control weight than larger meals less frequently. However, there needs to be some consideration of the type and frequency of the snacks. Too often among growing children these foods tend to be rich in carbohydrate and relatively low in content of other nutrients and only serve to give excess calorie intake.

Body needs and food habits. Sometimes the classic experiments of Davis[4,5] are called upon to support the contention that children will eat what they need. However, some difficulty exists in interpretation of these studies. Apparently the children in her group were only offered "good" foods and they had no opportunity to select an imbalanced diet. Also, these children seem to have spent some time in tasting the food before settling down to more restricted use of their preferred foods, which suggests that *learning* rather than *instinct* guided their choice. Observation and research indicate that new habits do form in accordance with body needs, but that old established habits persist as regulators of food selection, even after the need for those habits is no longer present.

Excessive parental concern with poor appetite during latent growth period. The normal growth pattern follows a rapid period of growth during the first year with a slump in food intake during the latent childhood years as a result of the normal slowed and erratic growth pattern. Frequently during this period mothers express dissatisfaction with the amount of food their children eat. As a result they tend to overfeed them, pushing food at periods of time when such an intake is not needed for growth.

Decreased physical activity. There is also evidence from research and observation that in the age of automation there is a decreasing amount of physical activity among growing children. The California study of Huenemann's group[32] emphasizes this aspect of developing obesity in children. Her results showed that American teen-agers today have less activity and frequently evidence little interest in securing more.

Types of obesity

The pattern of the growth years and the study of developing obesity during these years points to two types of obesity.

Developmental obesity. Studies indicate that at birth fat accounts for about 12% of the infant's body weight.[33] During the middle of the first year there is usually more fat in males than in females. By the time the infant is one year old, fat accounts for about 24% of the body weight. As the child continues to grow through the childhood years, this general percent of fat remains essentially constant, relative to the desired weight for height and age. Heald[34] indicates that the peak for onset of juvenile obesity occurs during the first four years of the child's life and that it is established by the time the child is eleven years old. About the twelfth year the percent of body fat increases in girls and the development of lean body mass begins to rise sharply in boys.

The developmental form of obesity begins early in life. The cells become supersaturated with fat and additional cells are recruited from connective tissue for fat deposit. With the increasing weight, additional bone and muscle cells must also increase to help carry the load. As a result, these children are usually taller, have an advanced bone age, and have been consistently obese since infancy. Their percentage of lean body mass is high, and so also is the fat deposit.

Reactive obesity. The reactive type of obesity usually results from intense and oft-repeated episodes of emotional stress. As a result of the stress period, the child overeats and his weight often assumes an up-and-down type of weight pattern. His body composition is high in fat, but not in the lean body mass observed in the developmental type of obesity.

Implications for food practices during the growth years

Several implications of these studies and observations appear reasonable in considering feeding patterns of the early growth years.

Fat content of infant formulas and quantity fed. With the knowledge regarding the rapid growth of the first year and the normal laying down of fat during that period, questions can be raised concerning the fat content of infant diets and formulas. The attitude of mothers who insist on the emptying of the bottle with every feeding of formula beyond the infant's obvious desire for food can also be questioned.

Sex differences in early years. If the sex differences at the early age of two or three years in calorie expenditure all considered, it should be realized that all toddlers are not going to eat the same amount of food. The basal metabolic rate is higher in the male than in the female during the second and third year of life. Therefore, parents should be prepared for very early differences among young boys and young girls.

Overfeeding in the preschool years. Overfeeding during the years of slow growth can make a large contribution to the development of continuing obesity. The peak onset of developmental types of obesity is during these early years. Mothers of young children would be well advised to offer them the enjoyment of a wide variety of food in realistic portion sizes.

Decreased activity of elementary school years. Prior to the beginning of the school years the child engages in much strenuous physical play, testing his developing strength and motor capacity. Usually this is more independent spontaneous activity and there is not yet a set schedule for the day. With the continuing experiences of school, the child becomes more sedentary in his recreational pattern as well as his school activities. This great change in energy expenditure during ages seven to eleven calls for guidance from mothers concerning food intake habits.

Adolescent sex differences in body composition. The increasing tendency for fat deposit in the teen-age girl, in comparison to greater increase in lean body mass in the teenage boy, makes weight control a greater problem for the girl. Guidance from parents in a supportive, accepting manner, especially for young girls, is needed.

DENTAL CARIES

Incidence. Dental decay is a prevalent disease among young children. Almost no one escapes it. According to surveys, over 99% of the children in the United States at one time or another are affected by it, and there seems to be little pattern to its incidence. It is found in well-fed and in undernourished children. Perhaps because it is so common and seldom causes grave problems, it is often dismissed with indifference or ignored. Yet it remains and continues to disfigure, cause pain, and cost money.

Etiology. Three factors combine to produce tooth decay, the susceptible host, oral bacteria, and the diet.

The susceptible host. Inherent differences in caries susceptibility vary widely among individual children. Some of these are hereditary differences in the anatomical characteristics of the tooth, but the ultimate form is influenced by interrelationships between these inherited characteristics and the environment that sustains its development during its formative period. Since teeth once formed are stable structures, it is evident that this positive nutritional influence can only have effect during growth and development of the enamel-forming organ and the tooth bud. Certain vitamins and minerals, especially vitamins A and D, calcium, and phosphorus, do play a part during this period (see p. 76). Studies indicate that fluoride ingestion during this period may have a direct influence on tooth formation.[35]

Oral bacteria. In humans, streptococci comprise the highest number of bacteria in the dental plaque, the gelatinous coating of the teeth.[36] They seem to have a particular affinity for carbohydrates and act upon them rapidly. It has been shown in controlled tests that only thirteen minutes after carbohydrate was present as a substrate, streptococci alone lowered the pH of the dental plaque from 6.0 to 5.0.[36] However, the oral flora is complex, and bacterial effects can vary from symbiosis between two or more microorganisms. It is their substrate that is mandatory for the metabolism of caries-producing organisms. This substrate is carbohydrate.

The diet. As *carbohydrate* food accumulates in the mouth, it provides the necessary media for the normal growth of acidogenic microorganisms which cause tooth decay. In sites of greatest food particle retention around the teeth, and on food textures that adhere and remain more readily (sticky, gummy), the bacterial activity is greatest. Persistent and continuous eating of adhesive carbohydrates, therefore, is a prime factor in tooth decay. The most convincing proof of this fact comes from a five year study in Sweden[37,38] in which a steady, controlled diet situation at a constant caloric level was maintained with a group of institutionalized patients. Over the years, different variables were added at different times. Supplementation of vitamins and minerals produced no difference. But the addition of carbohydrates brought about marked changes. One group eating bread containing 50 gm. of sugar one time a day

had no caries increase, but this same amount was distributed through the day at four different times, and definite increase in caries did occur. Also, a large amount of carbohydrate (300 gm.) taken in liquid form with meals produced no change, but when this same amount was given as milk chocolate four times a day between meals, the incidence of caries was greater and increased even more when caramels were used. During every period when the candy was withdrawn, the caries attack rate decreased.

The other dietary element which has a large influence on dental caries is *fluoride.* Repeated studies consistently confirm about 60% reduction in the incidence of dental caries in children, both in pre- and postnatal exposure to fluoridated water. A significant extensive project on the dental caries activity in children from eleven areas in five western states (Oregon, Idaho, Montana, Utah, and Washington) found the one most significant factor was the fluorides in the water supplies. Dental caries rates in the children consuming the fluoridated water were less than half those in the children whose water was fluoride-free.[39,40]

Dietary implication. While the problem of dental caries is by no means solved, recent advances in the knowledge of nutrition and its relationship to caries provide helpful steps in that direction. Two nutritional factors seem apparent. *Adhesive carbohydrates* (sweets, candy bars, caramels) consumed at frequent intervals *do* increase dental caries. Also, carbohydrates in liquid form are less cariogenic than those in solid form. *Fluoridated public water supplies do decrease dental caries rates.*

References
Specific

1. Erikson, E.: Childhood and society, ed. 2, New York, 1963, W. W. Norton and Company, Inc., pp. 247-274.
2. Weng, L., Heseltine, M., and Bain, K.: Children will eat hospital food, Hospitals **30:**64, 1956; **30:**74, 1956.
3. Fagin, C. M.: Why not involve parents when children are hospitalized?, Amer. J. Nurs. **62:**78, 1962.

4. Davis, C. M.: Self-selection of diet by newly weaned infants, Amer. J. Dis. Child 36:651, 1928.
5. Davis, C. M.: A practical application of some lessons of the self-selection of diet study to the feeding of children in hospitals, Amer. J. Dis. Child 46:743, 1933.
6. Chuck wagon for the pediatric floor, J. Amer. Diet. Ass. 51:432, 1967.
7. Spock, B.: Baby and child care, New York, 1957, Pocket Books, Inc.
8. Meyer, H. F.: A clinical interpretation of the "colicky" infant, Postgrad. Med. 24:627, 1958.
9. Current aspects of infant nutrition in daily practice. 1. Evansville, Indiana, 1962, Mead Johnson & Co., p. 1.
10. Holt, L. E., and others: A study of premature infants fed cold formulas, J. Pediat. 61:556, 1962.
11. Keitel, H. G., editor: The pediatric clinics of North America, pitfalls in clinical practice. I. Vol. 12, No. 1, 1965.
12. Andersen, D. H.: Cystic fibrosis of the pancreas and its elation to celiac disease, Amer. J. Dis. Child 56:344, 1938.
13. Andersen, D. H.: History of celiac disease, J. Amer. Diet. Ass. 35:1158, 1959.
14. Dicke, W. K., Weijer, H. A., and Van de Kamer, J. H.: Caeliac disease. 2. The presence in wheat of a factor having a deleterious effect in cases of caeliac disease, Acta Paediat. 42:34, 1953.
15. Shiner, M.: Duodenal biopsy, Lancet 1:17, 1956.
16. Rubin, C. E., and others: Studies of celiac disease. I. The apparent identical and specific nature of the duodenal and proximal jejunal lesion in celiac disease and idiopathic sprue, Gastroenterology 38:28, 1960.
17. Di Sant' Agnese, P. A., and Jones, W. O.: The celiac syndrome in pediatrics, J.A.M.A. 180:308, 1962.
18. Weijers, H. A., Van de Kamer, J. H., and Dicke, W. K.: Celiac disease. In Advances in pediatrics, Vol. 9, Chicago, 1957, Year Book Publishers.
19. Mike, E. M.: Practical dietary management of patients with the celiac syndrome, Amer. J. Clin. Nutr. 7:463, 1959.
20. Holt, L. E., Jr., McIntosh, R., and Barnett, H. L.: Pediatrics, ed. 13, New York, 1962, Appleton-Century-Crofts, p. 464.
21. Horner, F. A., and others: Termination of dietary treatment of phenylketonuria, New Eng. J. Med. 266:79, 1962.
22. Guthrie, R.: Letters to the Journal—Blood screening for phenylketonuria, J.A.M.A. 178:863, 1961.
23. Guthrie, R., and Susi, A.: A simple phenylalanine method for detecting phenylketonuria in large populations of newborn infants, Pediatrics 32:338, 1963.
24. Guthrie, R., and Whitney, S.: Phenylketonuria: detection in the newborn infant as a routine hospital procedure, Children's Bureau, U. S. Dept. Health, Education, and Welfare, Washington D. C., 1965, Government Printing Office.
25. McCaman, M. W., and Robins, E.: Fluorimetric method for the determination of phenylalanine in serum, J. Lab. Clin. Med. 59:885, 1962.
26. Kirkman, H. N., and Maxwell, E. S.: Enzymatic estimation of erythrocytic galactose-1-phosphate, J. Lab. Clin. Med. 56:161, 1960.
27. Caso, E. K., and Stare, F. J.: Simplified method for calculating diabetic diets, J.A.M.A. 133:169, 1947.
28. Bachmann, K., and Dees, S. C.: Milk allergy. II. Observations on incidence and symptoms of allergy and milk in allergic children, Pediatrics 20:400, 1957.
29. Keitel, H. G., editor: The pediatric clinics of North America, pitfalls in clinical practice. I. Vol. 12, No. 1, 1965, p. 27.
30. Bruch, H.: The importance of overweight, New York, 1957, W. W. Norton and Company, Inc.
31. Johnson, M. L. Burke, B. S., and Mayer, J.: The prevalence and incidence of obesity in a cross-section of elementary and secondary school children, Amer. J. Clin. Nutr. 4:231, 1956.
32. Huenemann, R., and others: Teen-agers' activities and attitudes toward activity, J. Amer. Diet. Ass. 51:433, 1967.
33. Wallace, W. M.: Why and how are children fat?, Pediatrics 34:303, 1964.
34. Heald, F. P., and Hollander, R. J.: The relationship between obesity in adolescence and early growth, J. Pediat. 67:35, 1965.
35. Brudevold, F.: Chemical composition of the teeth in relation to caries. In Sognnaes, R. F., editor: Chemistry and prevention of dental caries, Springfield, Illinois, 1962, Charles C Thomas, Publisher, pp. 32-88.
36. Gibbons, R. J., and others: Studies of the predominant cultivable microbiota of dental plaque, Arch. Oral Biol. 9:365, 1964.
37. Stralfors, A.: Investigations into the bacterial chemistry of dental plaques, Odon. T. 58:151, 1950.
38. Gustafsson, B. E.: Vipeholm dental caries study; effects of different levels of carbohydrate intake on caries activity of 436 individuals observed for 5 years, Acta Odont. Scand. 11:232, 1954.
39. Tank, G., and Starvick, C. A.: Dental caries experience of school children in Corvallis,

Oregon, after 7 years of fluoridation of water, J. Pediat. **58**:528, 1961.

40. Tank, G., and Starvick, C. A.: Caries experience of children one to six years old in two Oregon communities (Corvallis and Albany). I. Effect of fluoride on caries experience and eruption of teeth, J.A.D.A. **69**:749, 1964.

General
The hospitalized child

Hoble, B. M.: We admit parents, too, Amer. J. Nurs. **57**:865, 1957.

Nelson, W. E., editor: Textbook of pediatrics, ed. 8, Philadelphia, 1964, W. B. Saunders Company.

Nutrition, Growth and illness in children, Nutr. Rev. **20**:101, 1962.

Rose, M. H.: Communicating with children, Nurs. Outlook **9**:428, 1961.

Wallace, M. V.: Feeding the hospitalized child, J. Amer. Diet. Ass. **29**:449, 1953.

General gastrointestinal problems and celiac disease, cystic fibrosis, cleft lip and palate

Andersen, D. H., and Mike, E. M.: Diet therapy in the celiac syndrome, J. Amer. Diet. Ass. **31**:340, 1955.

Anderson, C. M., and others: Caeliac disease, gastrointestinal studies and effect of dietary wheat flour, Lancet **1**:836, 1952.

Feeding cleft palate children, Dover, Delaware, 1958, Delaware State Board of Health, Division of Crippled Children and Nutrition Services.

MacCollum, D. W., and Richardson, S. O.: Care of the child with cleft lip and cleft palate, Amer. J. Nurs. **58**:211, 1958.

Meyer, H. F.: Infant foods and feeding practice, Springfield, Illinois, 1960, Charles C Thomas, Publisher.

Miles, M.: Family centered care for cystic fibrosis, Nurs. Outlook **11**:718, 1963.

Review: The celiac syndrome (malabsorption) in pediatrics, Nutr. Rev. **21**:195, 1963.

Schwab, L., Callison, C., and Frank, M.: Cystic fibrosis, Amer. J. Nurs. **63**:62, 1963.

Weijers, H. A., and van de Kamer, J. H.: Some considerations of celiac disease, Amer. J. Clin. Nutr. **17**:51, 1965.

Zickefoose, M.: Feeding the child with a cleft palate, J. Amer. Diet. Ass. **36**:129, 1960.

Phenylketonuria and galactosemia

Acosta, P. B., and Centerwall, W. R.: Phenylketonuria: dietary management, J. Amer. Diet. Ass. **36**:206, 1960.

Bureau of Public Health Nutrition of the Calif. State Dept. of Public Health, The phenylalanine-restricted diet; A diet guide for parents of children with phenylalanine (booklets), 1966, Berkeley, State of California Department of Public Health.

Centerwall, W. R.: Phenylketonuria, J. Amer. Diet. Ass. **36**:201, 1960.

Fincke, M. L.: Inborn errors of metabolism, J. Amer. Diet. Ass. **46**:280, 1965.

Groves, R., and Schloesser, P.: A state program to control phenylketonuria, Amer. J. Nurs. **64**:74, 1964.

Guest, G. M.: Hereditary galactose disease, J.A.M.A., **168**:2015, 1958.

Harrison, H. E., and Harrison, H. C.: Aminoaciduria in relation to deficiency diseases and kidney function, J.A.M.A. **164**:1571, 1957.

Horner, F. A., and others: Termination of dietary treatment of phenylketonuria, N. Eng. J. Med. **266**:79, 1962.

Hsiu, D. Y.: Phenylketonuria: a study of human biochemical genetics, Pediatrics **38**:173, 1966.

Koch, R., and others: Nutrition in the treatment of galactosemia, J. Amer. Diet. Ass. **43**:216, 1963.

Koch, R., and others: Nutrition in the treatment of phenylketonuria, J. Amer. Diet. Ass. **43**:212, 1963.

O'Flynn, M. E.: Diet therapy in phenylketonuria, how long should it continue?, Amer. J. Nurs. **67**:1658, 1967.

Ragsdale, N., and Koch, R.: Phenylketonuria: detection and therapy, Amer. J. Nurs. **64**:90, 1964.

Shaw, K. N. F., and others: The clinical team looks at phenylketonuria, Children's Bureau, U. S. Department of Health, Educational, and Welfare, Washington, D. C., 1965.

Solomons, G.: Evaluation of the effects of terminating the diet in phenylketonuria, J. Pediat. **69**:596, 1966.

Stacey, H.: Coordination of long-term care of PKU children, J. Amer. Diet. Ass. **42**:311, 1963.

Umbarger, B.: Phenylketonuria: dietary treatment, Amer. J. Nurs. **64**:96, 1964.

Wright, S. W.: Phenylketonuria, J.A.M.A. **165**:2079, 1957.

Juvenile diabetes

Etzwiler, D., and Sines, L.: Juvenile Diabetes and its management, J.A.M.A. **181**:304, 1962.

Hooker, A. D.: Camping and the diabetic child, J. Amer. Diet. Ass. **37**:143, 1960.

Jackson, R. L.: Nutritional management of children with diabetes mellitus, J.A.M.A. **168**:42, 1958.

Marble, A.: The future of the child with diabetes, J. Amer. Diet. Ass. **33**:569, 1957.

Owen, G. M., editor: Juvenile diabetes mellitus, Proceedings of Ross Conference on Pediatric Research, Columbus, Ohio, 1965, Ross Laboratories.

Obesity

Forbes, G. B.: Lean body mass and fat in obese children, Pediatrics **34**:308, 1964.

Hathaway, M., and Sargent, D.: Overweight in children, J. Amer. Diet. Ass. **40**:511, 1962.

Norman, J. M.: Treating obesity in children, J. Amer. Diet. Ass. **30:**695, 1954.

Wright, F. H.: Preventing obesity in childhood, J. Amer. Diet. Ass. **40:**516, 1962.

Dental caries in children

Bibby, B. G.: Carogenicity of foods, J.A.M.A. **177:**316, 1961.

Control of tooth decay, Committee on Dental Health, Food and Nutrition Board, Washington, D. C., 1953, National Academy of Sciences, National Research Council.

Dunning, J.: Biased criticism of fluoridation, Nutr. Rev. **18:**6, 1960.

Fluoridation is here to stay, J. Amer. Diet. Ass. **65:**578, 1962.

Johansen, E.: Nutrition, diet, and calcium metabolism in dental health, Amer. J. Public Health **50:**1089, 1960.

Miller, C. D.: Effect of restricting hours of feeding on dental decay, J. Nutr. **76:**278, 1962.

Nutrition in tooth formation and dental caries, Symposium 8, Council on Foods and Nutrition, American Medical Association, Chicago, Illinois, 1960.

Shaw, J.: Nutrition and dental caries, J.A.M.A. **160:**633, 1958.

Tank, G.: Recent advances in nutrition and dental caries, J. Amer. Diet. Ass. **46:**293, 1965.

Weiss, R., and Trithart, A.: Between-meal eating habits and dental caries experience in preschool children, Amer. J. Public Health **50:**1097, 1960.

CHAPTER 20

Nutrition for the aging
and the aged

The previous three chapters have formed a unit on maternal-child health. In these chapters the human life cycle has been reviewed from the point of conception through the prenatal period to birth, and continuing through the growth and development years of childhood to maturity. In the nursing care of individuals in each of these stages of growth, these basic human developmental needs have been related to optimum nutritional care. This chapter views the middle and latter years of the life span in the same way—as part of the whole growth pattern. Each phase of development along the way has meaning only in relation to the whole.

Following the tumultuous adolescent years from age thirteen to eighteen, when youth in American society is struggling with the core problem of identity versus identity diffusion, of learning who he is and where he is going, three more basic stages in man's life span, as identified by Erikson (see p. 377), complete his development.

Young adulthood (ages 18 to 40). In the years of young adulthood, the individual, now launched on his own, must resolve the core problem of *intimacy versus isolation.* If he achieves this goal, he is able to build an intimate relationship leading to marriage or self-fulfillment in other personal relationships. But if he fails to do so, he becomes increasingly isolated from others. These are the years of career beginnings, of establishing one's own home, of parenthood, of starting young children on their way

through the same life stages, and of early struggles to make one's way in the world.

Adulthood (ages 40 to 60). In the years of adulthood, the core problem the individual faces is *generativity versus self-absorption.* The children have now grown and gone to make their own lives in turn. These are the years of the "empty nest," the coming-to-terms with what life has offered, and of finding expression for stored learning in passing on life's teachings. It is a regeneration of one life in the lives of young persons following the same way. To the degree that these inner struggles are not won, there is increasing self-absorption, a turning-in upon one's self, and a withering rather than a regenerating.

Senescence (ages 60 to 80+). In the last stage of life (old age, senescence) the final core problem is resolved between *integrity versus despair.* Depending on one's resources at this point, there is either a predominant sense of wholeness and completeness, or a sense of distaste, of bitterness, of revulsion, and of wondering what life was all about. If the outcome of life's basic experiences and problems has been positive, the individual arrives at old age a rich person—rich in wisdom of the years. Building on each previous level, his psychosocial growth has reached its positive human resolution.

Not all of the elderly patients for whom the nurse cares will be able to say with Browning at this point that this is the "best of life for which the first was made." Some of them will not have resolved the core psychosocial conflicts and struggles with which they wrestled in previous stages. They arrive at middle and later years poorly equipped to deal with the adjustments and health problems that may face them. Many others, however, for whom the nurse cares will have been enriched by life's experiences in their maturing process. They will bring enrichment to the nurse's life in turn, and the nurse-patient relationship will be mutually rewarding.

As the developmental needs of individuals in these middle and later years are studied, and integration of nutrition into nursing care is sought, the following questions should be considered:

1. What social and economic problems does the aging person face in American society?
2. What is the biological nature of the aging process? Is it the same in all aging persons?
3. What is the role of nutrition in the aging process? Are needs for specific nutrients changed in any way?
4. What clinical problems may aging individuals encounter? How is nutrition related to these problems?
5. What practical daily living problems might the aged patient have related to eating?
6. Are there community resources available to help meet the aged person's needs?

Two important concepts should develop, therefore, as a result of this study: (1) aging is an *individual* process, and (2) aging is a part of a *total life* process. These two basic concepts will govern all other aspects of need during these years—biologic, nutritional, socioeconomic, psychosocial, and spiritual.

GERONTOLOGY AND GERIATRICS—APPROACH TO THE STUDY OF AGING

Several terms are used in discussing the middle and later years of life. A clarification in meaning will be helpful.

Gerontology and geriatrics. The word *gerontology* comes from two Greek words, *geron* meaning "old man," and *logos* meaning "study of." It is the study of the process of aging and its phenomena. The word *geriatrics* comes also from the Greek word *geron,* and from *iatrike,* meaning "medical treatment." It is the study and treatment of diseases of old age. Geriatrics, therefore, is a fairly narrow medical term. For purposes of this study the idea behind the much broader term "gerontology" will be used.

Aging and the aged. The two terms aging and aged have comparative yet distinct meanings. *Aging* is a life process. The age of a person or an object is from the point of its beginning existence to the present time. Thus, human aging is the total life process. It begins at conception and ends at death. It may be somewhat startling to think that even now every person is aging, and has been since the moment he was conceived. But it is a biologic truth. *Aged* refers to one who is old. He has arrived near the end of the aging process and bears visible physical signs of the gradual process of decline. Sometimes people are spoken of as young-old (those in the ages 60 to 75) and of old-old (those over 75) because marked distinctions may exist among persons in these two age brackets.

Senescence and senile. Senescence comes from a Latin verb *senescere* which means "to grow old." It refers to the process of growing old, or more specifically, to the latter period of life, old age. It is similar to the Latin root for adolescence, for example, which means "to grow up," or the latter period of attaining physical maturity. The word *senile* is from the Latin word *senilis* which simply means "old." However, common usage has given it a negative clinical connotation, a meaning which should not be attached to *normal* old age.

The pattern emerges of a life continuum. Aging is a positive concept. It encompasses the whole of life and each period has its own unique potentials and fulfillments. The period of middle and later years is no exception. Its own particular capacities can be lived to the fullest. These are attitudes the nurse may have opportunity to help support in her patients.

SOCIOECONOMIC AND PSYCHOLOGIC FACTORS

The increasing industrialization and urbanization of American society, the complexity of the culture it is building, and the changes in age distribtuion in the population have all brought about changes in the life of the aging person in the United States today.

Population changes. Not only has the general population been increasing rapidly, but significant shifts have also occurred in the age distribution. Increasing longevity has produced a larger number of persons in the older age group. More people are living longer. By 1975, 12%, or over 22 million, of the American population will be 65 years of age or over. However, biostatisticians such as Yerushalmy[1] point out that there is need for more knowledge of *qualitative* longevity, how the interdependence of biologic and environmental factors affects the quality of the lengthened life. Quantitative statistics alone do not reveal the many subtle individual differences. He raises significant questions such as: Do stressful experiences at one period of life have a measurable effect on subsequent survival? Do repeated exposures to physical and mental stresses in early life leave their mark on the individual?

In general, this increased longevity is influenced by two factors, medical care and improved living standards.

Medical care. The great progress in care of infants and children has reduced infant mortality, controlled communicable diseases, and improved child care. The increased availability and quality of medical care during adult years is also a factor in health during the maturing years. But there has been relatively little progress in control of chronic disease in old age.

Improved general living standards. With an increasing national economy and affluence, the general United States living standards are high. For many, this factor has led to increased education, better housing, and improved nutrition during the growth and early adult years. In older age, however, problems in socioeconomic status

increase for many. The factors which have contributed to the increased number of older persons in the population have medical, social, and economic implications.

Social and economic factors. America's increasing industrialization and subsequent changing social attitudes have affected the position of the older person in American society. Economic insecurity often creates pressures. An increasing policy of early retirement in industry and employment difficulties with advancing age create financial pressures. Changing social attitudes toward the elderly person and his capacities have increased institutional care and segregation in living situations. The older person is oftened removed from the stimulus of involvement in the activities of society.

Psychologic factors. Financial pressures and a decreasing sense of acceptance and accomplishment have developed in many old persons anxieties and a loss of personal values. Many feel inadequate. They do not have a sense of belonging, of self esteem, or of achievement. They are often lonely, restless, unhappy, and uncertain. The experiences of visiting nurses working with elderly persons in the community have led them to identify basic common personal needs. Austin[2] has summarized these well:

1. An income and economic security through socially useful and personally satisfying means
2. A sense of *maximum* personal effectiveness
3. A suitable place in which to live
4. The spending of leisure time constructively
5. A sense of positive and well-integrated social relationships within the family and the community
6. A sense of achieving and maintaining spiritual values and goals

THE BIOLOGIC NATURE OF THE AGING PROCESS

Biologic changes. From a biologic standpoint there is limited knowledge of the process of aging. The general biologic process extends over the entire life span and is conditioned by experiences that have gone on before. In the later ages, however, there is a cell loss and reduced cell metabolism. Studies[3] have shown that during the ages 30 to 90 there is gradual reduction in the performance capacity of most organ systems. For example, the speed of conducting a nerve impulse diminishes by 15%, the rate of blood flow through the kidney is reduced 65%, and the resting cardiac output is reduced by 30%. The pulmonary function (the maximum voluntary ventilatory capacity) is reduced 60%, and there is a reduced recovery rate following a displacing stimulus. For example, in a glucose tolerance test the blood sugar level takes longer to return to normal, and the pulse rate and respiration after exercise take longer to return to normal.

There seems to be an overall, gradual reduction in the body's reserve capacities, an important cause of which is the gradual reduction of cellular units (for example, nephrons are lost from the kidney as functioning units; there is a loss of pulmonary functional tissue). Some resulting physiological factors may affect food patterns. For example, there may be a diminished secretion of digestive juices, a decreased motility of the gastrointestinal tract, and a decreased absorption and utilization of nutrients.

Individuality of the process. The biologic changes are general. The persons in the advancing years of life will display a wide variety of individual reaction. Each person bears the imprint of his individual trauma and accumulation of disease experience. This has a direct effect upon his individual aging process. Therefore, specific needs of individuals must always be remembered and considered when discussing general aging and general nutritional needs. It seems, therefore, that the greatest influence of nutrition on the aging process takes place in earlier years. Nutrition's most effective role is in the growth and middle years, which prepare the individual to meet the gradually declining metabolic processes of old age.

NUTRITIONAL REQUIREMENTS
Calories

Standard allowances. The reduced basal energy requirement, caused by losses in functioning protoplasm, and the reduced physical activity combine to create less demand for calories in advancing age. The statement of the Food and Agriculture Organization indicates a reduction in calories of approximately 7.5% for each decade past age twenty-five. The standard allowances of the National Research Council are based on estimates of a decrease in metabolic activity of about 5%. The average estimate is an approximate caloric requirement of 1,800 calories. Men will require more—about 2,200 calories.

These standards seem to be borne out by various studies of the food intake patterns of older people. For example, in the San Mateo County study in California there was a reported caloric intake for men aged fifty to seventy of 2,165 to 2,618 calories, and an intake for women the same ages of 1,586 to 1,780 calories.[4] Other reports indicate the caloric intake of aged women living at home to be approximately 1,500 calories. However, there is need for much more information on the daily life activities of older people and the degree of energy that they may be capable of expending. The calorie requirements are highly individual, according to activity. Primary consideration must also be given to the living status of the individual and the degree of his or her activity in various phases of life. Perhaps the simplest criterion for judging adequacy of caloric intake is the maintenance of *normal* weight.

Carbohydrates. At least 70 to 75% of the total calories should be provided in the form of carbohydrate or fat. Otherwise, part of the protein will be diverted for use as energy rather than tissue maintenance. The label "nonprotective" or "empty" that is frequently put on carbohydrate and fat foods is not entirely correct. They perform important functions in providing energy and protecting protein for tissue metabolic activities. The actual optimum amount of carbohydrate intake is unknown, but it is usually recommended that about 50% of the calories come from carbohydrate foods. Easily absorbable sugars are not contraindicated and there is usually no disturbance in carbohydrate metabolism. The fasting blood sugar level has been found to be essentially normal in the aged.[5] There should be a fairly free choice of carbohydrate foods according to individual digestion or metabolism situations.

Fats. Fats usually contribute about 20% of the total calories. They provide a source of energy, important fat-soluble vitamins, and essential fatty acids. A reasonable objective is the avoidance of large quantities of fat with more emphasis upon the quality of fat consumed. The digestion and absorption of fats may be delayed in the elderly person but they are not greatly disturbed with age. There is no need to be unduly restrictive. Enough fat for meal palatability aids appetite. Fat loads, however, should be avoided because of the delayed absorption capacity in elderly persons.

Protein

Standard allowances. The National Research Council recommends a continuation of the daily protein intake for the aging individual at the same adult allowance given for age twenty-five—0.9 gm. per kg. body weight. Even this amount provides an allowance for a wide variation in individual needs. Also, although there may be increased need for protein during illness or convalescence or after a wasting disease, the overall mass of actively metabolizing tissue decreases with age. There usually is no increased requirement for protein per se under normal circumstances. The difficulty in establishing precise protein requirements is evidenced by the conflicting reports of studies. Some of the data obtained from population groups in institutions may have some questionable applications to relatively healthy persons living a fairly active life at home, engaged in business, professional, and social interests.

Most investigators agree, however, that age itself does not alter adult protein needs.

Protein value. Needs are influenced by (1) the biologic value of the protein (the quantity and ratio of its amino acids), and (2) adequate caloric value of the diet. It is estimated that one-fourth to one-half of the protein intake should come from animal sources with the remainder from plant protein sources. If animal and plant protein foods are consumed at the same meal, there is better utilization of the incomplete plant protein for tissue synthesis, as the lacking amino acids may be supplied by the animal protein foods. It is estimated that protein should supply from 15% to 20% of the day's total calories. There is usually no need for supplemental amino acid preparations as some food faddists may claim. They are expensive, unpalatable, irritating, impractical, and an inefficient source of available nitrogen.

Vitamins

The sale of so-called geriatric vitamin preparations, especially of the B complex, implies that the requirement for them increases with age. There may be gradually decreasing tissue stores with normal aging but long-term studies show no difference in requirement from that for normal adults. The problem in some individual cases may stem from inadequate normal intake rather than from an increased need. A well-selected mixed diet should supply all the essential vitamins in normally needed quantities. Increased therapeutic needs in illness should be evaluated on an individual basis.

Minerals

There is also no need for increased minerals in normal aging. The same adult allowances are sufficient on a continuing basis and are supplied by a well-balanced diet. Two essential minerals which may be lacking in poor diets, however, are iron and calcium. Encouragement may need to be given to some individuals to ensure adequate dietary sources among their daily food choices.

Water

The need for water varies with environment. A liberal intake should be assured, with thirst as the general guide.

CLINICAL NEEDS

Chronic illness such as heart disease often creates additional problems for aging persons. Also, although physiologic needs for nutrients do not increase with age, other environmental factors may contribute to illness and produce clinical needs.

Malnutrition

By and large, poor dietary habits in young adulthood, as with any other personal habits, tend to be set and accentuated in older age. Although surveys show on the average adequate total calorie intakes, there is frequent evidence of inadequate distribution of these calories in food choices. For example, there may be fewer animal proteins (meat, egg, cheese, milk), more use of grain and other starch in breads and cereals, fewer vegetables and fruits, and more sweets and desserts (even to the extent of about 20% of the day's calories). Also, older persons are frequent prey to claims of food faddists concerning restorative food products, tonics, regulators, and so on.

Causes of malnutrition. Numerous factors may contribute to developing malnutrition in an elderly person.

Oral problems. Poor teeth or poorly fitting dentures may make chewing difficult. Poor appetite and limited financial means for adequate dental care may discourage efforts to seek improvement of the situation. Also buccal mucosa changes in the mouth, and decrease or change of quality in salivary secretions may cause difficulty in eating.

Gastrointestinal problems. Numerous gastrointestinal complaints, from vague indigestion to specific disease (peptic ulcer, diverticulitis), sometimes effectively reduce food intake and curtail the needed nutrients. A variety of other acute or chronic illnesses may limit food intake or utilization.

Personal factors. Financial resources may be limited with little money available to purchase needed food. There may be a lack of knowledge of the food needed for a well-balanced diet. Boredom, loneliness, anxiety, insecurity, and apathy compound the problem. Especially if an older person lives alone, the social value of eating is gone. Also, he may lack adequate cooking, refrigeration, or storage facilities and have no means for transportation to obtain food and bring it back to his home. Often a vicious cycle ensues—his funds are low, he hesitates to spend, goes without, builds increasing weakness and lethargy, which leads to still less interest and incentive. Finally, he is ill.

Implications for nursing care. Such a patient needs much understanding care and support to build improved eating habits (Fig. 20-1). Helpful nursing attitudes and actions are based on an understanding and realistic approach.

Food habits should be analyzed carefully. The nurse must listen well to learn the patient's attitudes and precise situation and its limiting factors. Nutritional needs can be met with a variety of foods, and suggestions can be adapted to fit his particular needs and personal situation, as well as his desires. Suggestions should be administered in a practical and realistic manner.

The nurse should not moralize. "Eat this because it is good for you" should be struck from every nurse's and nutritionist's vocabulary. It has little possible value for any patient, much less one who is struggling to maintain his personal integrity and self-esteem.

Interest should be encouraged in food variety and seasoning. A bland and unattractive diet is presumed by many to be necessary for all elderly persons. It is not. A variety of food, and adventure with new foods, tastes and seasonings, often prove to be the needed stimulae for poor appetite and lack of interest in eating. Sometimes

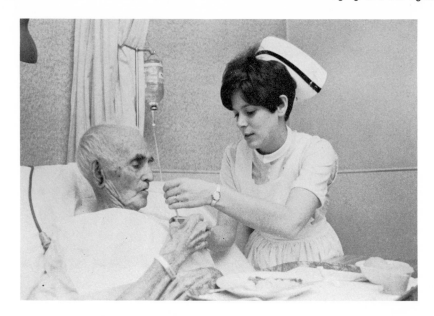

Fig. 20-1. Care and support in feeding an elderly patient. Assistance is given by the student nurse as needed to ensure optimum nutrition.

smaller amounts of these foods and more frequent meals are helpful.

Obesity

In a different sense, obesity may be considered a form of malnutrition. It is a potential health hazard, indicated in a number of degenerative diseases. In fact, Mayer[6] indicates that the prevention of obesity in earlier growth years may be the major nutritional measure one may take in preparation for old age.

Causes of obesity. Many of the same living situations and emotional factors may cause obesity by contributing to compensatory overeating or poor food choices. Also, there is usually decreased physical activity, and the maintenance calorie requirement is lessened.

Individual approach. Discouraging reports come from clinicians attempting weight reduction programs with older persons. It is difficult indeed to change long-standing habits or long-standing obesity. Certainly, in most cases, a reasonable approach should be followed with no drastic measures or diet, planning only for a slow,

gradual loss. Because individual calorie requirements vary widely and individual personalities and problems are unique, personal and realistic planning with the individual patient, followed by supportive guidance and encouragement, usually pays the greatest dividends.

COMMUNITY RESOURCES
Professional organizations

The American Geriatrics Society. The American Geriatrics Society was organized in 1942. Physicians engaged in the medical care of elderly patients promote research to advance scientific knowledge of the aging process and the treatment of its diseases. A number of nurses are associate members. The society publishes the *American Journal of Geriatrics.*

The Gerontological Society, Incorporated. The Gerontological Society was organized in 1944. This society has a broader base of interest in all aspects of aging, and a wider membership of interested health professionals. The Committee on Aging of this group has stimulated increased interest among other related organizations and community and government agencies in the problems of the aging person in our society. The organization publishes the *Journal of Gerontology.*

The local community groups representing other health professions such as the Medical Society, the nursing organizations, and the Dietetic Association, sponsor a variety of programs to help meet the needs of the aged people in their respective communities. For example, the Dial-a-Dietition program of the Dietetic Association provides sound information concerning nutritional needs.

Government agencies

Federal legislation. The impact in the United States of recent federal legislation covering aid to elderly persons for medical care under the Social Security Act can hardly be minimized. The so-called Medicare bill (Title XIX) has increased the demand for high quality medical care and its availability to elderly persons. The pressure upon community nursing homes, hospitals, and related medical care resources is already being felt. Additional medical assistance programs in a number of states augment the community resources on the state and local level.

The Department of Health, Education and Welfare. In August of 1950 the first national conference on aging was held in Washington, D. C. As a result of this beginning activity and stimulus of interest, in 1956 the President appointed a federal council on aging to coordinate and broaden federal activities under the Department of Health, Education and Welfare. This council publishes the news letter *Aging* and provides many other resource materials for community workers.

Department of Agriculture. The Department of Agriculture through its Agriculture Extension Services in state universities and county home advisors on the local level provides much practical aid for elderly persons and community workers.

Public health departments. Skilled health professionals work in the community through local and state public health departments. Much health guidance for elderly persons is available through their resources. Many chronic disease programs or related programs are in operation.

Volunteer organizations

Many activities of volunteer health organizations such as the Heart Association and the Diabetes Association relate to the needs of older persons. Also, two particular national organizations sponsor local community groups: (1) Senior Citizens of America, organized in 1954; and (2) American Society for the Aged, Incorporated, organized in 1955. Additional resources are provided in some larger urban centers, such as the Meals-on-Wheels program which prepares and delivers hot meals to persons in need of such services, who are referred to the group by their physicians.

Industry

A number of industry-related groups such as the Dairy Council and pharmaceutical firms provide educational materials and sponsor research and workshops.

References
Specific
1. Yerushalmy, J.: Factors in human longevity, Amer. J. Public Health **53**:148, 1963.
2. Austin, C. L.: The basic six needs of the aging, Nurs. Outlook **7**:138, 1959.
3. Shock, N. W.: Some biological aspects of aging, Nutr. News **26**:1, 1963.
4. Morgan, A. F.: The San Mateo study of the nutritional status of the aging, Calif. Health **13**:65, 1955.
5. Horwitt, M. K.: Dietary requirements of the aged, J. Amer. Diet. Ass. **29**:443, 1953.
6. Mayer, J.: Nutrition in the aged, Postgrad. Med. **32**:394, 1962.

General
Albanese, A. A., and others: Protein requirements of old age, Geriatrics **7**:109, 1952.
Amer. J. of Public Health, Vol. 57, No. 7, 1957 (entire issue).
Ashbrook, J. B.: Not by bread alone, Amer. J. Nurs. **55**:164, 1955.
Baker, D. A., and LeBovit, C.: The nutritional adequacy of diets of older people, Family Economics Review, Agricultural Research Service **62**:10, 1963.

Barry, M. C.: Planning for older persons in an urban community, Geriatrics **13**:535, 1958.

Batchelder, E. L.: Foods for the upper age group and nutritional implications, Amer. J. Public Health **46**:1329, 1956.

Batchelder, E. L.: Nutritional status and dietary habits of older people, J. Amer. Diet. Ass. **33**:471, 1957.

Beeuwkes, A. M.: Studying food habits of the ꞏ elderly, J. Amer. Diet. Ass. **37**:215, 1960.

Blumenthal, G. W.: Emotional aspects of feeding the aged, J. Amer. Diet. Ass. **32**:829, 1956.

Campbell, V. A., and Dodds, M. L.: Collecting dietary information from groups of older people, J. Amer. Diet. Ass. **51**:29, 1967.

Chinn, A. B.: Some problems of nutrition in the aged, J.A.M.A. **162**:1511, 1956.

Chope, H. G.: Relation of nutrition to health in aging persons—a four-year follow-up of a study in San Mateo County, Calif. Med. **81**:335, 1954.

Cowdry, E. V., editor: The care of the geriatric patient, St. Louis, 1958, The C. V. Mosby Co.

Davidson, C. S., and others: The nutrition of a group of apparently healthy aging persons, Amer. J. Clin. Nutr. **10**:181, 1962.

Dietary habits of elderly people, Nutr. Rev. **13**:81, 1955.

Food and Agriculture Organization of the United Nations, Calorie Requirements, FAO Nutritional Studies No. 5.

Gillum, H. L., Morgan, A. F., and others: Nutritional status of the aging, J. Nutr. **55**:265, 1955.

Hayes, O. B., and others: Relation of dietary intake to bone fragility in the aged, J. Geront. **11**:154, 1956.

Jans, P.: Meals on wheels, Nurs. Outlook **3**:130, 1955.

Jordan, M., and others: Dietary habits of persons living alone, Geriatrics **9**:230, 1954.

Kelley, L., and others: Food selection and well-being of aging women, J. Amer. Diet. Ass. **33**:466, 1957.

Keys, A.: Nutrition for later years of life, Public Health Reports **67**:484, 1952.

Kinnaman, J. H., and others: Attending the nutritional needs of patients in nursing homes—theory and practice, Amer. J. Public Health **45**:627, 1955.

LeBovit, C.: The food of older persons living at home, J. Amer. Diet. Ass. **46**:285, 1965.

Lissitz, S.: Food symbolization within a geriatric hospital, J. Rehab. **29**:23, 1963.

Lyons, J. S., and Trulson, M. F.: Food practices of older people living at home, J. Geront. **11**:66, 1956.

Mayer, J.: Nutrition in the aged, Postgrad. Med. **32**:394, 1962.

Mead, M., editor: Cultural patterns and technical change, Paris, 1955, United Nations Educational, Scientific, and Cultural Oganization.

Mitchell, D. L., and Goldfarb, A. I.: Psychological needs of aged patients at home, Amer. J. Public Health **56**:1716, 1966.

Moss, B. B.: Caring for the aged, Garden City, N. Y., 1966, Doubleday and Co., Inc.

Newton, K.: Geriatric nursing, ed. 3, St. Louis, 1960, The C. V. Mosby Co.

Nyhus, D.: How Medicare is affecting a public health nutrition program, J. Amer. Diet. Ass. **51**:143, 1967.

Ohlson, M. A., Jackson, L., and others: Nutrition and dietary habits of aging women, Amer. J. Public Health **40**:1101, 1950.

Phillips, E.: Meal à la car, Nurs. Outlook **8**:76, 1960.

Pollack, H.: Nutritional problems in the aging and the aged, J.A.M.A. **165**:257, 1957.

Pyke, M., and others: Nutritional value of diets eaten by old people in London, Lancet **253**:461, 1947.

Report, Committee on Guidelines for Home Delivered Meals, National Council on the Aging, Inc., Amer. J. Pub. Health (supplement), 1965.

Schwartz, D.: Nursing needs of chronically ill ambulatory patients, Nurs. Res. **9**:185, 1960.

Schwartz, D., Henley, B., and Zeitz, L.: The elderly ambulatory patient: nursing and psychosocial needs, New York, 1964, The Macmillan Company.

Shock, N. W.: Symposium on biology of aging, Fed. Proc. **15**:938, 1956.

Steinkamp, R. C.: Resurvey of an aging population—fourteen year follow-up, J. Amer. Diet. Ass. **46**:103, 1965.

Swanson, P.: Nutritional needs after 25. In Stefferud, A.: Food, the yearbook of agriculture, 1959, Washington, D. C., 1959, U. S. Department of Agriculture.

Swanson, P., Smith, T. A., Ohlson, M. A., and others: Food intakes of 2,189 women in five North Central states, Iowa Home Economics Experimental Station Bulletin 1959.

Swartz, F. C.: Medical aspects of aging, J. Amer. Diet. Ass. **33**:461, 1957.

Tibbitts, C.: Economic and social adequacy of older people, J. Home Econ. **54**:695, 1962.

Tibbitts, C.: Social change, aging, and public health nursing, Nurs. Outlook **6**:144, 1958.

Tibbitts, C.: Committee on Aging, The states and their programs in aging, Washington, D. C., 1956, U. S. Department of Health, Education, and Welfare.

Vaughn, M. E.: An agency nutritionist looks at home health care under Medicare, J. Amer. Diet. Ass. **51**:146, 1967.

Vedder, C. B., editor: Problems of the middle-aged, Springfield, Illinois, 1965, Charles C Thomas, Publisher.

Vinther-Paulsen, N.: Investigation of actual food

intake of elderly chronically hospitalized patients, J. Geront. **5**:331, 1950.

Weife, S. O.: Nutrition needs of maturing men, J. Amer. Geriat. Soc. **6**:190, 1958.

Walker, D. M.: New findings in nutrition of older people, Amer. J. Public Health, **55**:548, 1965.

Watkin, D. M.: Nutrition for the aging and the aged. In Wohl, M. G., and Goodhart, R. S., editors: Modern nutrition in health and disease, ed. 3, Philadelphia, 1964, Lea & Febiger.

CHAPTER 21

Nutrition in rehabilitation nursing

At any one of the stages of the normal growth and development span of man's life, in addition to his common human developmental struggles, an individual may face the added stress of a disabling physical condition or mental illness and need special care. It is usually a situation of more or less profound trauma and calls for tremendous resources on the patient's part to cope with the condition. These patients are essentially the same persons with the same basic age group needs as the nurse has encountered in previous study and will care for on other clinical services. Here, however, they face added physical and psychologic problems. Such a situation requires of the nurse special knowledge and skills, sympathetic insights, and personal strengths.

Nursing care of patients undergoing such severe difficulties involves certain nutritional components. In this chapter nutritional principles in rehabilitation nursing will be identified, and practical means offered to apply them in the very necessary daily activity of eating.

These are questions to which realistic answers will be sought:

1. What positive concept underlies all of rehabilitation nursing? How does this concept affect nutrition and feeding?
2. What social, economic, and psychologic problems does the patient face?
3. How does the physical problem affect his nutritional needs? What solutions are there for his practical eating problems?
4. What special clinical problems may require particular dietary management?

GOALS AND METHODS

Rehabilitation is a concept and a process. It involves a positive philosophy based on optimum potential and a cooperative approach built on a learning objective.

A positive concept. Basic to an understanding of rehabilitation needs is the concept of the patient's optimum potential. The nurse sees her patient not primarily from the usual view of the public of what his disability prevents him from doing; rather, she considers what maximum function his disability will allow him to achieve. There is an important difference in perspective and philosophy. One breeds increasing dependence and is negative. The other is a reaching for independence and is positive.

Specialists in rehabilitative medicine and nursing speak of this positive role as being both *preventive* and *restorative*.[1] Many of the techniques of care that have been developed are designed to prevent further disability and also to restore maximum potential use. Both of these key principles of prevention and restoration apply also to nutritional care.

A team approach. How is the twin goal embodied in this concept to be realized? In some cases, obstacles seem almost insurmountable. Often the patient's initial reaction is one of defeat. Certainly he cannot accomplish the goal alone. Such a complex and complicated endeavor requires *team* approach. Several skilled health specialists lend their particular training, insights, and resources to identify specific needs and seek solutions. This *multidisciplinary* team of specialists, under the direction of the internist—a specialist in physical medicine—

447

includes psychiatrists, clinical and social psychologists, nurses, social workers, physical therapists, occupational therapists, speech therapists, nutritionists, special school teachers for handicapped children, and others according to special needs such as orthopedists, plastic surgeons, dentists, and orthodontists. Additional health workers such as licensed vocational nurses, hospital aids, volunteers, and vocational counselors provide essential services.

The most important member of the health team, however, is the patient himself, and with him, his family. The patient is the focus of the team effort. Goal setting is always done *with*, not for, the patient and his family. These three, therefore—the health specialists, the patient, and the patient's family—together form a greater health team. It is a shared undertaking.

SOCIOECONOMIC AND PSYCHOLOGIC FACTORS

Social attitudes. The all-too-common attitude of society toward a disabled person is one of overprotection or avoidance. Some people are repelled by gross deformities. Others completely ignore them. The first attitude builds dependence and sometimes smothers the all-important *will* of the patient to fight against the odds that surround him and develop self-acceptance. The second attitude creates problems in everyday living. Like the left-handed child who finds himself in a world built for right-handed people, the disabled person faces doorways not built for wheelchairs, stairs, curbings, and a multitude of articles encountered in everyday living all designed for simple neuromotor controls which he lacks. One of these simple, everyday activities that sometimes becomes a monumental task for the disabled person is *eating*—and food he must have.

Increasingly, however, through the work of many realistic, accepting, and knowledgeable people, the public is being educated to the fact that disabled persons are human beings, and that they do have potential with which they can find useful and productive roles in society. Perhaps in the process some doorways will be widened and some ramps built, as well as some minds opened and some attitudes lifted.

Economic problems. Rehabilitation care is a long and costly process. A major area of exploration for the health team is one of financial resources and assistance needed. Also, continuing long-term economic problems will revolve around employment capabilities or earning capacities, or of the means for providing care.

Living situations. The disabled person faces many practical problems of everyday living. Whether the individual needs institutional care or can maintain independent living, perhaps with an attendant, depends upon a number of physical and situational factors. If with help he is able to maintain his own home, the necessary special equipment for maximum self care and his additional care by the attendant must be provided.

Psychologic barriers. Tremendous psychologic adjustment is required of the disabled person to resolve the problems he faces. The trauma to self-image as well as to the physical body, and the regressive tendency that he must struggle against constantly, may leave him withdrawn, defeated, and exhausted. Often personality changes occur during the rehabilitation process. The patient's inner strength and resources, as well as his physical stamina, are tested and tried, and, depending upon the nature of his coping resources and defenses, he will be able to function or not. Much of the health team's keen insight and concern is directed toward supporting the patient in *his* efforts to meet his own needs. That many disabled persons do achieve this goal is evident by the repeated monumental achievements these persons do attain despite—or perhaps because of—their difficulties.

BASIC PRINCIPLES OF NUTRITIONAL CARE

Two basic principles of nutritional care evolve from the goals of rehabilitation, prevention and restoration.

Prevention of malnutrition

Calories. The rehabilitation process of physical therapy often involves hard work. The patient may tire easily and his energy must be sufficient to meet the demands. Excess calories, however, must be avoided to prevent obesity. Also, sufficient energy for metabolic tissue demands is important.

Protein. Tissue and organ integrity is a bulwark against skin breakdown, decubitus ulcers, infections, and negative nitrogen balance. Protein in optimum quantity and quality must be assured in the diet. Essential amino acids are required for tissue synthesis. Negative nitrogen balance is often seen in disabled persons, especially in the early stages following the initial injury. The negative balance occurs because the rate of breakdown of tissue proteins (catabolism) exceeds that of building them up (anabolism). It almost always occurs after spinal cord injury. The metabolic process usually follows three stages:

1. *Early catabolic period*—peaks about two weeks after the injury and may remain for several more weeks; nitrogen replacement needs are high, and usually plasma transfusions are required

2. *Late catabolic period*—nitrogen excretions lessen; this period may remain for some weeks or months, especially if it is complicated by infections or decubiti

3. *Positive nitrogen balance period*—finally reached after protein therapy by dietary means and clearing of any infection or ulcers; sometimes as much as 150 to 300 gm. of protein are required daily, and protein supplements will need to be used

Carbohydrates. The proper metabolism of carbohydrate may also be impaired in the early stages following a severe injury. The oxidation of glucose by the cell is dependent upon the presence of the specific enzyme glucokinase. This enzyme controls the initial phosphorylation reaction which attaches phosphate to glucose (p. 21). Without being phosphorylated, glucose cannot be oxidized for energy. The activity of glucokinase and other similar enzymes is in turn controlled by hormone regulators from the pituitary and the adrenal cortex and from the pancreatic islet cells (insulin). The increased activity of the pituitary and in turn the adrenal gland, following the stress of injury (p. 170) inhibits the proper functioning of the cellular enzyme systems and prevents adequate phosphorylation and oxidation of glucose. More breakdown of tissue protein and fat occurs to provide needed energy, thus effectively adding further to the negative nitrogen balance. Sufficient carbohydrate foods are therefore important in the diet to help provide needed energy.

Fats. Essential fatty acids (linoleic acid) are needed by the body for its metabolism and have also been associated with skin integrity, especially in children. The National Research Council recommends for adults that about 20% of the total day's calories will be supplied by fats and that 1% of the total calories be essential fatty acids. Enough fat for food palatibility aids appetite, which tends to be poor in the course of long, confining illness.

Vitamins and minerals. Optimum intake for metabolic activity and nutritional maintenance is essential. The normal age group allowances are adequate unless therapeutic needs such as anemia indicate individual increases. In some rehabilitation centers, however, multivitamin preparations are given routinely as insurance against deficiences. How necessary this is may be questionable; however, all steps warranted to maintain optimum nutrition should be taken as the physician deems wise.

Restoration of eating ability. The maximum use is made of individual available motor resources. These resources are aided by self-feeding devices as needed.

ACTIVITIES OF DAILY LIVING—EATING

The achievement of nutritional goals rests upon adequate food intake. The achievement of rehabilitation goals rests upon development of maximum individual potential. Eating, therefore, is an important part of learning. Persons with disabilities affecting use of the upper body and extremities will have need for retraining as much as is possible to manage the daily task of eating. Four considerations are involved in planning such a teaching program. These are the basic principles of specific individual need and related equipment, the use of self-help devices, the learning process, and a satisfactory place to eat.

Principles

Determining the specific individual needs. How much can the patient do? What use does he have of his hands and what reaching capacity does he have? Also, what ability does he have in getting to the place he wants to eat? What muscles are involved? What muscle development or aid does he need?

Providing equipment to meet needs. What specific self-help devices does his particular disability require? How may these be procured or constructed? What tables or trays or other furniture is needed? For home use, what storage facilities might the necessary equipment require?

Self-help devices

Food textures. You may have heard at one time or another this little rhyme:

> Don't puree the food if ground will do;
> Don't grind the food if chopped will do;
> Don't chop the food if whole will do;
> Do all you can to make them chew.°

It is important to keep the patient as independent as possible for as long as possible, particularly in the very personal activity of eating.

The food should be kept as nearly "regular" food as the individual patient can handle. Besides the physical benefit of needed bulk and some degree of chewing (even "gumming") the patient gets an added

°I am indebted to my friend and colleague, Delores Nyhus, Nutrition Consultant, California Department of Public Health, for this pointed reminder that pureed foods have little valid use in adult diets, and in this case are self-defeating in result.

psychologic boost from not having to have baby food. Many toothless patients can manage most stews, soft fish and poultry, or moist meatloaf without difficulty. If foods do have to be pureed, patients would prefer having the regular food put through a sieve or blender, rather than eating the commercial baby food.

Grasping and holding devices. With the proper approach and attitudes, and with the help of a few simple, well-planned devices, many patients can bridge the gap between discouraging dependency and independent self-help. These devices may well make the difference between utter frustration and a renewed interest in eating. Some of these self-help devices for eating include the following:

Hand cuff with palm pocket to hold eating utensil. The cuff is made of wide elastic to fit over the back of the hand. The palm piece has a pocket or slot formed by sewing together two pieces of leather, leaving an opening into which the fork or spoon handle fits.

Thickened handle. When painful fingers or weakened muscles make it difficult to grasp objects, often simply thickening the handle of the utensils will enable the patient to manage holding his fork, spoon or knife. The following are suggested ways of thickening the handle:

1. Foam rubber strips wrapped around handles
2. Handle inserted into center space of large-size foam rubber or plastic hair curlers after removal of the clip part
3. Use of bicycle handlebar grip after wrapping to make a still larger handle
4. Use of file handle attached for length as well as thickness.

All these gadgets can be removed for washing of the utensil.

Lengthened handle. If range of motion is limited, handles may be lengthened, or the direction of the tines of the fork or the bowl of the spoon can be altered. Some of these long-handled utensils are also collapsible for carrying.

Curved knife. A knife with a curved

blade to cut meat and other food is useful for a patient with weak hands or where the patient has only one hand. These knives are sometimes called rocker knives.

Plate modifications. Plate guards that attach to the side of the plate, or scoop-type dishes and spoons are available to enable the patient to corner his food rather than have it go round and round as he tries to get it up. Often simple rounded bowls or ones with straight edges, such as Pyrex baking dishes, can help him just as well. Also, the dish should be stationed firmly. It can be anchored with ordinary suction cups, adhesive tape, or a tray insert can be made by cutting out holes or building up rims to fit dishes.

Devices to aid drinking. Liquids often present difficulty, not only in swallowing, but also in grasping and lifting the container. Thus, the container should be as lightweight as possible.

Drinking straws and straw-holders. When a patient cannot use his hands or has difficulty in using a glass, the problem of grasping and lifting can be eliminated by the wise use and placement of drinking straws. Usually plastic tubing can be purchased in about five-foot lengths and cut to any desired size, then bent to the most satisfactory angle for approach to the mouth. Two simple devices will help to stabilize the straw in the glass: (1) a "bulldog clip" can be clamped to the glass and the straw fitted through; or (2) a common pencil clip can be used the same way on the edge of the glass with the straw fitted through the space ordinarily provided for the pencil.

Coasters or jackets for glasses. If a patient can achieve some degree of grasp and lift of the glass, simple coasters or jackets fitted over the glass will often help him to hold on to it better. These can be crocheted or straw matted, or stocking type. The rougher surface, free of moisture, will give him a more secure grip. And where color is used, it adds a bright note to the tray or to the table.

Tilt and swallow. The swallowing reflex is frequently diminished or absent in dis-

abled persons. The reflex may be enhanced, however, by the use of an ice collar or by brushing the neck with a small brush (such as a ten-cent paint brush) just before eating. The liquid should be placed behind the front teeth, and the patient should slowly tilt his head back and swallow. He can learn this routine as the nurse goes over it several times with him, saying "Tilt and swallow . . . . tilt and swallow . . . . tilt and swallow . . . ."

Cups. Cups should have large enough handles for the entire hand to be placed in it so the cup can be grasped more securely.

Paper cups are difficult to manage and should not be attempted. Some patients, however, want to practice despite extensive hand involvement from high cervical traumatic lesions. All materials used should be unbreakable to reduce the patient's fear and anxiety.

The learning process

Learning to eat is often a frustrating and tedious process for the disabled person. However, it is worth the effort. A more independent patient, doing as much as possible to help himself, is a happier patient.

Evaluation of patient's abilities. The patient's ability to move effectively, to use his hands, and to reach for things must be evaluated. He should be helped into the most comfortable position or helped to get to the place where he wants to eat. The nurse should acquaint the patient with the various utensils and tableware, their nature, the materials from which they are made, their shapes, possible adjustments, and uses they serve. Additional special equipment and devices may be necessary to facilitate the use of the hands.

Usually it is easier to start with the spoon and work up to the use of forks and knives.

Arm support. The nurse should see that the patient has good forearm support, perhaps with his elbows on the table. Some patients may need more elaborate support such as a rocker splint.

Use of real food. Applesauce is a good

food to start with, because it is easily managed and the temperature does not matter. It is good either warm or cold. As the learning process proceeds, there should be a happy medium in the consistency of food as patients try to feed themselves. Foods should not be too soft (liquid or gruel consistency) or too dry. For example, mashed potatoes, fairly firm puddings, and other such foods adhere more easily to the utensils. But such foods as rice or green peas may prove difficult to manage. If it sticks together and sticks to the utensil, it is easier to eat.

Continued use of devices. Later on, the devices may be discarded, or their use may be necessary on a permanent basis. In this case the patient may use a small plastic bag to carry them, and he may want to include a large napkin as protection against spills.

A place to eat

The table. From the beginning the table is the best place to use for eating, if it is at all possible. It helps to develop skills and has psychologic value. The nurse should help the patient assume the best posture possible for reaching, as he may have need.

The bed. If the patient is eating in bed, he must have adequate support. An overbed table should be provided for the tray. Trays should be used that are stable and do not tip.

A wheel chair. When the patient is eating in a wheel chair an over-bed table or the regular wheel chair tray may be used. Frequently wheel chair patients enjoy eating out-of-doors when weather permits, to have the social value in eating together. A regular table with legs spaced apart to give room for the wheel chair may be used also. The height of the table should be sufficient to allow the arms of the wheel chair underneath it, so that the patient may get close enough to the table for comfort.

CLINICAL PROBLEMS

Injuries producing prolonged immobility or enervation of muscles controlling normal elimination create additional problems for some disabled persons. With adequate medical and nursing care, much difficulty can be avoided.

Elimination

Constipation. Constipation and fecal impaction occur frequently following disabling illnesses and injuries. Careful attention to simple measures is imperative.

Fluid intake. Adequate fluid intake is an important nutritional principle at all times, both in health and in disease. It becomes of prime significance in disabling injuries. Assuming a normal renal function, two to three liters of total fluid intake daily should be assured. Water should be placed in convenient reach of the patient. If he cannot use his upper extremities in cases of severe disability, a plastic water bottle may be arranged with a drinking tube fixed in place, and positioned at the bedside so that the patient may take frequent sips. In some rehabilitation centers a one-inch layer of water in the bottom of the bottle is first frozen, then the bottle is filled with water and attached at the bedside. This practice helps to keep the water cool and makes it more tasteful to the patient.

Careful records of fluid intake should be kept and continuing supportive encouragement given to the patient to assure an adequate amount of fluid intake.

Elimination aids. According to the physician's direction additional aids to elimination may be used, such as mineral oil, wetting agents to maintain a soft stool, or occasional bulk-producing agents when natural bulk in foods is limited or impossible. Intravenous or tube feeding may be necessary in early stages after injury, but a return to a regular diet should follow as soon as possible to aid normal peristalsis. Glycerine suppositories or a suppository of bisacodyl (Dulcolax) may be ordered by the physician in constipation problems involving impaction. These should only be used under medical supervision.

Bowel and bladder training. Fluid intake is an important aspect of a bowel and bladder training program. Such training should be encouraged when possible to give the patient a greater degree of independence, particularly if he has employment potential. A bowel training program to establish regular evacuation, similar to that used in many rehabilitation centers, follows:

Bowel rehabilitation routine

1. Daily intake of adequate fluids should be maintained (2 to 3 liters); a record should be kept to ensure knowledge of optimum amount.

2. A diet high in natural residue foods should be given.

3. A regular time should be scheduled for defecation. In rehabilitation centers this may be in the evening. For a home patient the more practical time may be in the morning.

4. According to the individual schedule, 4 oz. prune juice (a little lemon juice improves the flavor and is also an elimination aid) should be given about twelve hours before the scheduled defecation time. For the evening evacuation plan, the prune juice would be taken before or with breakfast. For the morning evacuation plan, it would be taken the night before.

5. Twenty to thirty minutes before the scheduled evacuation time, glycerine suppositories (one or two according to individual need) should be inserted. These should be placed well above the internal sphincter, at least 2½ inches into the rectum, against the rectal mucosa.

6. The patient should be placed in a relaxed sitting position on the toilet or bedside commode. Care should be taken to see that he has adequate support as needed.

7. The schedule and recording of results should be maintained with no interruption by enemas.

Renal calculi

Prolonged enforced immobilization and certain paralytic disorders usually cause calcium withdrawal from the bones. Apparently bone integrity and homeostasis, a balance between calcium accretions and calcium withdrawal, is maintained by a combination of weight bearing and muscle tension. The needed muscle tension comes from the natural pull on origin and insertions of muscles produced by normal motion and activity. When the operation of these factors is prevented by paralyzing or immobilizing injuries, or by treatment such as extensive body casting, bone calcium withdrawal increases. This imbalance produces excessive urinary excretions of calcium and consequent danger of stone formation.

Early use of tube feeding or subsequent regular dietary management should give attention to the calcium content of the diet. In prolonged inactivity it may need to be reduced and a low-calcium regimen (about 400 to 500 mg. of calcium) followed. In less severe cases, the average normal adult intake of calcium (about 800 mg.) is sufficient. In any case, *excess* calcium should be avoided, and individual therapeutic needs should be treated accordingly. A review of the metabolism of calcium in Chapter 8, and of diet therapy for renal calculi in Chapter 29 will help clarify these nutritional principles.

Obesity

Perhaps the one most common nutritional problem in rehabilitation is obesity. Even a small amount of excess weight in patients with severe disabilities may hinder their progress. If caloric intake is not adapted to energy expenditure level, a gradual gain in weight will follow. Individual need is important. The amount of possible exercise and activity varies. Thus, weight control by a balanced diet, adjusting its caloric value to the need of the patient, is essential.

Overweight patients should have sufficient calorie reduction to effect a gradual weight loss. Stringent weight reduction programs are usually unwise and should be used with caution. A 1,000 calorie diet may be effective to bring about the desired results. In some cases, however (such as elderly paralyzed patients), a diet as low as 400 calories may be required to reduce weight. In these cases, strict attention must be given to dietary nutrient intake, with supplementary vitamins and minerals given as needed.

Indiscriminate fasting programs are unwise. Important protein tissue (muscle mass) needed in the rehabilitation program may be lost, especially by the more inactive patients. Also, a large part of the loss in such a program is only temporary water loss.[2] However, some clinicians feel that there may be some possible advantage in a fasting program in cases of extreme obesity, built on noncaloric fluids, vitamins, and physical activity.[3]

The nutritional principles of weight control and various dietary reduction programs are given in greater detail in Chapter 24.

References
Specific

1. Hirschberg, G. G., Lewis, L., and Thomas, D.: Rehabilitation: a manual for the care of the disabled and elderly, Philadelphia, 1964, J. B. Lippincott Co., p. 6.
2. Wishnofsky, M.: Caloric equivalents of gained or lost weight, Amer. J. Clin. Nutr. **6**:542, 1958.
3. Hirschberg, G. G., Lewis, L., and Thomas, D.: Rehabilitation: a manual for the care of the disabled and elderly, Philadelphia, 1964, J. B. Lippincott Co., p. 48.

General

Balsam, F. J.: The team approach to the rehabilitation program, J. Ass. Phys. Ment. Rehab. **7**:18, 1953.
Chatton, M. J., Margen, S., and Brainerd, H.: Current diagnosis and treatment, Los Altos, Calif., 1963, Lange Medical Publications.
Deaver, G. C.: Rehabilitation, a philosophy; Jerome, M. M.: The bed patient; Taylor, W.: The ambulatory patient, Amer. J. Nurs. **59**: 1278-1281, 1959.
Elliot, J. S., and others: Mineralogical studies of urine, J. Urol. **80**:269, 1958.
Elliot, J. S., and others: Urinary pH, J. Urol. **81**:339, 1959.
Heather, A. J.: Manual of care for the disabled patient, New York, 1960, The Macmillan Company.
Hirschberg, G. G., Lewis, L., and Thomas, D.: Rehabilitation, a manual for the care of the disabled and elderly, Philadelphia, 1964, J. B. Lippincott Co.
Larson, C. B., and Gould, M.: Calderwood's orthopedic nursing, ed. 4, St. Louis, 1957, The C. V. Mosby Co.
Lawton, E. B.: Activities of daily living for physical rehabilitation, New York, 1963, McGraw-Hill Book Company.
Morrissey, A. B.: The procedures of urinary and bowel rehabilitation, Amer. J. Nurs. **51**:194, 1951.
Priest, P. I.: Teaching patients to take care of themselves, Amer. J. Nurs. **52**:1492, 1952.
Prinzing, D. M.: Cleft palate habilitation, Nurs. Outlook **7**:577, 1959.
Rusk, H. A., and others: Rehabilitation medicine, St. Louis, 1958, The C. V. Mosby Co.
Sain, U.: The rehabilitation nurse, Rehab. Rec. **8**:39, 1967.
Self-help devices for rehabilitation (booklet), Institute of Physical Medicine and Rehabilitation, New York University, Bellevue Medical Center, New York.
Terry, F. J., and others: Principles and technics of rehabilitation nursing, ed. 2, St. Louis, 1961, The C. V. Mosby Co.
Turner, G. E.: The cerebral vascular accident patient, Nurs. Outlook **8**:326, 1960.
Wohl, M. G., editor: Long-term illness, Philadelphia, 1959, W. B. Saunders Company.

CHAPTER 22

Nutrition in psychiatric nursing

Psychiatric principles in nursing are not confined merely to the care of patients with manifest mental illness. They are an integral part of all nursing care. They were introduced in the beginning of the nurse's general clinical experience, although she may not have identified them as such at that time. They have continued to be woven throughout nursing education and they form a large base for all nursing practice. Perhaps the only difference in the application of these principles in the care of patients with mental illness is that the basic human psychologic need is much more acute at this point, and has led to pathologic symptoms, thus making the principles of care that much more evident.

The individual gains certain masteries and controls and coping mechanisms at each stage of his individual development. These strengths vary with individuals according to their unique life experiences and relationships. However, everyone deals with the same essential human problems of self— the problems of meaning, relationship, and communication. Numerous psychiatrists and psychologists have added insights concerning these basic human needs. For example, Jurgen Ruesch[1,2] has developed his theory and approach to mental illness basically around success or failure in communication. Carl Rogers[3] has focused attention upon the patient and his own essential capacities for psychologic growth.

Increasingly, nursing has based its approaches to general patient care upon psychiatric principles. Nutrition, as an essential part of total patient care, is applied, there-

fore, in the light of these basic human needs. Many of these relationships between food and feeding and individual psychosocial needs have been developed in the previous chapters. They will focus here upon the patient with mental illness, the goals and methods of psychiatric care, the problems the psychiatric patient faces in the community, and the many opportunities the nurse finds to apply principles of nutrition to her day-to-day care.

The same principles stated at the beginning of Chapter 21 on "Nutrition in Rehabilitation Nursing" apply to psychiatric nursing. Realistic answers should be sought to the following questions:

1. How do rehabilitation principles apply to psychiatric nursing?
2. What social attitudes, economic problems, and psychologic barriers does the patient with mental illness face?
3. What are the basic principles of nutritional care of psychiatric patients? What practical approaches may help overcome feeding problems?
4. What special clinical problems may involve particular dietary management?

GOALS AND METHODS
A positive concept

As in rehabilitation, psychiatric care is based on a positive concept of the healing potential within the patient himself. To this end, the psychiatric hospital community seeks to establish a therapeutic environment to support the patient in his effort to regain health.

455

A team approach

The skills of many health professionals are used in a group effort to work *with* the patient and guide his way back to health. He is the focus of the team. They work with him in individual and group relationships and many of their techniques are based on the therapeutic value of this human relationship of finding meaning in human experience through relating to another person. The psychiatric health team is guided by the psychiatrist who coordinates the overall plan for individual patient care. Other specialists who work with him in this effort include clinical psychologists, nurses, social workers, technicians, vocational nurses, aides, occupational and recreational therapists, and others. The dietitian in the psychiatric hospital is a special resource person to the psychiatric team, and is in a key position to help make experiences with food have meaningful therapeutic value for the individual patients.

SOCIOECONOMIC AND PSYCHOLOGIC FACTORS

Many interrelated socioeconomic and psychologic factors surround the psychiatric patient and account for his responses. Human behavior has causes, both rational and irrational, and can be understood if its background is known.

Social attitudes. Although social attitudes toward mental illness are increasingly more enlightened, they still convey a negative stigma of guilt, shame, or fear. Many feel that mental illness is something to be hidden as if one were less a person because of his illness. Moreover, many attitudes prevail in American society today such as prejudice, discrimination, segregation, injustice, and lack of communcation, all of which devalue and alienate the individual. These unaccepting and somewhat moralistic views create problems for the patient and for those who would help him in his effort to function in society again.

Economic problems. Because of these attitudes, the patient faces economic problems in future employment and in finding

a productive role in his group. Also, anxieties concerning the cost of psychiatric care may prevent the patient having need for such care from seeking it. In addition, such burdens may create anxieties which further complicate his treatment and cause him to respond to his environment in a negative way.

Care facilities. Some of the related social problems involve facilities for care of the person with mental illness. Public education concerning mental health is helping to bridge the gap and many community counseling activities are being provided for those in need. There are clinics for treatment of alcoholism, family case work, pastoral counseling, marital counseling, work through the courts with juvenile offenders, and public health programs. For the most part, however, the initial clinical care of patients with mental illness will concern those hospitalized in psychiatric institutions. Through many activities of daily living in this group situation, the nurse will relate to patients and aid in their recoveries. One of these basic activities is nutritional— eating.

BASIC PRINCIPLES OF NUTRITIONAL CARE

The same two basic principles of nutritional care that governed activities in rehabilitation, also operate in the care of psychiatric patients.

Prevention of malnutrition

Many surveys and general observations have indicated that patients in hospitals for the mentally ill, especially in large, overcrowded state hospitals, frequently suffer from varying degrees of malnutrition. Because the number of personnel is often inadequate and the patient's needs are so great, a far from ideal environment sometimes prevails. Persons with severe illness and consequent eating problems may not receive the close attention and care they require to help them eat. The resulting chronic malnutrition adds to their generally poor state of health and in turn to their mental illness. Sometimes these groups of patients are called "the forgotten back ward," a label that indicates their great need for care. That even these seemingly hopeless situations are amenable to improvement, however, is evident through the experience of one large state hospital. A few concerned staff members with help from interested volunteers from the community found that a custodial ward could be changed to a treatment ward and self-respect restored for patients and aides.[4]

General mental illness per se does not require an increase in nutrients. Normal age group needs are sufficient. The value of sound nutrition lies in the contribution it makes to general physical health, and the increasing sense of strength and well-being such a state gives an individual to aid his efforts to recovery.

Restoration of eating abilities and satisfactions

The positive goal of nutritional care is achieved through restoration of the disturbed patient's ability to eat and to receive both physical and emotional satisfaction from his food. Often with increased interest in eating comes increased interest in other aspects of his environment, and positive steps are taken toward health.

APPLICATION OF NUTRITIONAL PRINCIPLES IN PATIENT CARE
Food as a therapeutic tool

In the discussion of influences on eating habits in Chapter 13, it was found that a great many cultural, social, and psychologic factors influence response to food. Certain foods and food patterns have meaning largely as a result of past experiences in human relationships. From earliest infancy, food is a vehicle of relationship, first between the infant and his mother, then between the growing child and his family, and finally between the adult and his wider social relationships in the enlarging community. Food is one of the earliest means of building trust. Early feeding experiences can either build warmth, satisfaction, com-

fort, and a sense of being cared for, or they can build anxiety, frustration, and a sense of rejection and neglect. These are the sorts of underlying psychic patterns which become perpetuated with age and adult relationships. In the mentally ill person, they become even more exaggerated by the kind of interpersonal relations the person is now maintaining. If early feeding experiences were negative, they may express themselves in negative attitudes toward his food and toward the person offering it.

Thus, because food does carry meaning—often great symbolic meaning—for the patient, the nature of it and the way it is offered can have great therapeutic significance. Often it is simply the persistent sympathetic manner in which a nurse helps a person to eat that says to him "I care," and helps him to overcome his projected feelings.

Feeding problems

A number of feeding problems may exist among psychiatric patients. Solutions for these problems must be found individually by understanding of the factors behind such food behavior.

Refusal to eat. Severely disturbed patients may reject food completely, not because they are unwilling to eat, but because their illness makes eating on their own initiative impossible. The extreme form of inability to eat, *anorexia nervosa*, is a somewhat uncommon psychophysiologic reaction, and is seen mostly in adolescent girls or young adult single women. As described by Sir William Gull in his original classic paper (1858), these patients are usually of high intelligence, introverted, perfectionistic, compulsive, and overly sensitive. Their response to food is one of revulsion and disgust with vomiting usually following any forced feeding. Sometimes there is a preceding history of the opposite reaction to food, overeating and obesity, with shame at being fat following. Usually there is hostility in parental relations at home, especially with the mother, or in sibling rivalry and jealousy. Occasionally a pregnancy fantasy may have triggered the desire to "diet," with complete refusal of food developing as a result. During treatment with psychotherapy, the nurse may give support to the patient by offering intimate personal attention at meals. Often this is done in many small ways. She may first be able to feed the patient herself in an unhurried and accepting manner, gradually encouraging self-feeding. Small doses of insulin before meals may sometimes be a part of the treatment to stimulate need and desire for food. Some patients, however, will require tube feeding.

Refusal to eat in other patients may have a number of conscious and unconscious psychologic roots. It may stem from a suicidal death wish. It may result from feelings of guilt or personal unworthiness with the denial of food as the means of self-punishment. The patient's delusional beliefs that the food is poisoned, that he has no stomach to hold or digest it, or that he is eating various body parts, may cause him to reject the food. Hallucinations such as hearing voices commanding no food intake or preoccupation, depression, withdrawal, and catatonic states may influence the patient's reaction to food and make it impossible for him to eat.

Approach. The patient's physical survival, however, depends upon food. On his own he would starve. He must have nourishment. Treatment is aimed at seeking to determine the reasons for his rejection of food and to support all individual efforts in retraining to eat. If tube feeding must be used as a last life-saving resort, the procedure should be done in a therapeutic manner—*never* in a punitive manner. Since the nursing aim is to help the patient assume responsibility for his own eating, there should be a consistent approach involving patience and understanding. The patient should be involved in the care plan, given the reasons for it, and helped to see that he is accepted and cared for as a person. His refusal to eat must be recognized as his inability to do otherwise, not as a perverse unwillingness to do so. As a relationship of confidence and trust builds, the patient may be led to become more actively involved in self-feeding and eventually in group eating.

Reluctant or anxious eating behavior. The anxious patient finds decision-making difficult. As a result, food intake may be inadequate because in his confusion he hesitates and questions whether he should eat or not, what items he should eat, and how much he should eat. He takes a long time over his food, eats very slowly, if at all, and resists being hurried or pushed. Sometimes he may hide food, give it away or try to bargain with the nurse to avoid pressures concerning eating.

In caring for such patients, the wise nurse will recognize that through such seemingly reluctant food behavior, the patient is trying to communicate other unmet personal needs. By accepting the behavior as such a reflection, therefore, the nurse may help him to express his real needs and explore with him actions or activities that will help to meet these needs. The nurse may need to help feed him at first. She should give support and assurance as he assumes more and more of the responsibility for food choices, and help him toward the social value of group eating as soon as he is able.

Bizarre food behavior. Other bizarre food behavior may take the form of general destructiveness or personal untidiness. The patient may throw food or dishes; he may grab at other patient's food. He may mix all his food up on his plate, play with it, drop it on the floor. He may eat his food in an unconventional manner—spitting it up, stuffing it in his mouth, gulping it down.

Again, the nurse will approach such a patient with an effort to understand the personal needs expressed by such behavior. Punitive reactions or disgust only reinforce his behavior and worsen his condition. In periods of destructiveness, brief use of paper food containers may be helpful. The essential aim of nursing care, however, is to help the patient get personal and social satisfactions from the experience of eating, and to assume an increasing responsibility for achieving this goal.

Food and food service. Administrative and medical personnel in psychiatric hospitals are increasingly recognizing the therapeutic value of good food served in pleasant, comfortable, and attractive surroundings. Cafeterias that offer a variety of food choices are being used to help develop the patient's confidence in his ability to make decisions. In many hospitals the food is appetizing, attractive, and tasteful. Old drab dining rooms with long bare tables and benches are being replaced by colorful rooms with draperies, wall pictures, and modern small tables and comfortable chairs. In these situations, eating becomes a major support of therapy and a way of sharing with the patient a meaningful activity, one which is vital to his welfare. Around the dining table in small group situations, the patient finds in sharing food a way of relating to others. Such experiences strengthen his efforts to reach out for personal relationships and give him a foundation for future satisfying relations with others.

NUTRITIONAL THERAPY IN CLINICAL PROBLEMS
Alcoholism

Alcoholism is a symptom of underlying emotional difficulties. Experienced psychiatric personnel point out that it often represents problems of hostility, a masochistic need for rejection, and excessive dependency.[5] According to one study,[6] the incidence of alcoholism in large urban cities such as San Francisco, is about one in every six adults. It is rated as the number 4 public health problem in the United States.

Often malnutrition compounds the basic psychosocial problem of the alcoholic, and his physical health deteriorates. His medical program of treatment will include optimum nutritional therapy and help in building better food habits. Usually his diet is poor. He frequently skips meals, using alcohol instead, or goes without food for longer periods of time during drinking bouts. As a result, his body is depleted of needed nutrients, especially proteins and vitamins. Increased amounts of protein, carbohy-

drates, and vitamins should be given, unless advanced liver disease calls for a reduced protein intake (see Chapter 27).

General care. In her nursing care and discussions with the patient concerning his nutritional needs, the nurse will remember the principles of learning (Chapter 14). An individual must learn for himself and accept the responsibility of his own personal choices in the light of facts presented him. The patient's basic need is to develop self-respect and responsibility. The nurse will, therefore, avoid moralistic judgments. She will provide sound, straightforward information. She will give emotional support with acceptance and understanding. To the question once asked a psychiatric social worker, "Do you hold your patient's hand?" her wisdom borne of much experience in helping alcoholics gave the reply, "Yes, and we let go finger by finger."[7]

Korsakoff's psychosis. Acutely ill hospitalized patients, suffering from the effect of prolonged alcoholism, may display symptoms of Korsakoff's psychosis. This syndrome is named for the Russian physician, Sergei Korsakoff, who first described its clinical nature in 1887. Due to the nutritional deficiency imposed by excess alcohol intake, especially of the vitamins thiamine and niacin, degenerative changes occur in the long peripheral nerves and the nerve cells of the cerebral cortex. A neuritis develops with pain and tingling in the feet and legs. The calves of the legs are tender to pressure, and foot drop occurs. The leg muscles may even atrophy and produce painful contractures. The patient is treated initially with intravenous glucose solutions containing large amounts of thiamine chloride and nicotinic acid. Electrolytes and fluids are also given to combat dehydration and to increase the alkaline reserves. Insulin may be used to accelerate the metabolism of the alcohol of the body. As the patient is able to take oral feeding, he is given large amounts of fluid (3,000 to 4,000 ml. daily), much of it as orange juice and milk. If symptoms of impending hepatic coma occur, he is changed to a low-protein or protein-free diet with large amounts of carbohydrate. These symptoms are not confined, however, to alcoholism and may occur in other vitamin B deficiency states from other causes.

Insulin coma therapy in schizophrenia

Insulin shock therapy is frequently used as a treatment for schizophrenia in supportive preparation for psychotherapy. It was initially developed and used in the early 1930's by Sakel and has since come to be considered by many as the most effective therapy in this type of mental disorder. Patients are carefully selected according to their physical condition and age, and most of them are over forty years old. The patient is given injections of insulin beginning with about 40 units daily, and continuing until the desired coma stage is reached. He is held in this stage for thirty to sixty minutes. If the coma deepens during this period, it is terminated immediately. Over a period of weeks, the course of treatment may involve thirty to forty comas, depending upon individual need and response. The amount of regular crystalline insulin necessary to produce the coma generally varies from 80 to 600 units. The coma is terminated by an injection (0.25 to 0.50 mg.) of glucagon (p. 21). During the period of treatment, the staff team maintains close contact with the patient, and opportunity for closer therapeutic communication is experienced.

Nursing care is essential to help prepare the patient for the treatment, explaining its general nature and effectiveness. The nurse should be well versed in the symptoms of insulin shock, the levels of coma, and alert to the progress of the desired coma stage. She should maintain a quiet therapeutic environment during the awakening periods. The first meal following a treatment may be high in carbohydrate to replenish glycogen stores and blood glucose levels.

Mental retardation

Nutritional care of mentally retarded children is based upon meeting the physical growth and development needs of the individual child according to his age-group needs. These growth needs have been outlined in Chapter 18. Sometimes in the presence of profound disabilities, concern for the child's disability may overshadow his basic physical needs and care for these primary needs may be neglected. Approaches to feeding will be adapted to each child's need, with emotional support or physical aid as he may require.

Particular disabilities may require additional nutritional care. In *cerebral palsy,* for example, the uncontrollable body motions of *athetoids* necessitates a diet high in calories for simple physical maintenance. (Athetoid motions are repeated involuntary muscular distortions of the limbs—legs, arms, hands, fingers—and sometimes involve the entire body. They are caused by the brain lesion.) Also, the child with cerebral palsy may have great difficulty chewing and swallowing. Anorexia or obesity may be additional complications requiring individual nutritional planning.

General clinical situation involving the central nervous system

Chorea. Chorea is an infectious disease of the central nervous system, and affects both the brain cortex and the basal ganglia. Chorea is believed to be caused by the same organism that causes rheumatic fever. Danger lies in involvement of valvular heart disease. The child displays muscular incoordination in jerky, involuntary movements. A quiet environment of physical and mental rest is essential. The diet should be of high nutritional quality and may require extra calories because of the hyperactivity.

Delirium from general systemic infection. Delirium from systemic infection is seen more often in general hospitals, but it may be observed on psychiatric wards. The patient requires a high fluid intake (3,000 to 5,000 ml. daily). Cool beverages and fruit juices are desirable. The calories should be high, and the food texture should be liquid to soft. Caution must be exercised in feeding to prevent choking.

Traumatic coma. Following injury to the brain, a patient may remain in coma for a number of days. Usually tube feedings (Chapter 30) are required to sustain his nutritional requirements.

Cerebral arteriosclerosis. In older patients damage to brain function may occur from arteriosclerosis. The diet may be modified in fat or sodium according to individual situations. In any case, it should be of optimum general nutrition. The brain damage may involve paralysis—a cerebrovascular accident ("stroke")—and the patient will need to be fed. A patient, unhurried, kind approach to the feeding of these patients is a highly significant part of their nursing care.

Epilepsy. The general term epilepsy (Gr. *epilepsia,* a seizing) refers to several types of recurrent seizures of varying intensities produced by excessive neuronal discharges in different parts of the brain. It may be caused by a number of cerebral and general physical disorders. Usually drug therapy controls the convulsive seizures, and there is no dietary modification required. However, treatment of children may sometimes involve a *ketogenic* diet, one high in fat content and relatively low in carbohydrate sufficient to produce a pronounced state of ketosis. Because of the large amount of fat, the diet is unpleasant, even to the point of nausea. It is therefore difficult to maintain, and hence, is seldom used.

References
Specific

1. Ruesch, J., and Bateson, G.: Communication, the social matrix of psychiatry, New York, 1951, W. W. Norton & Company, Inc.
2. Ruesch, J., and Kees, W.: Nonverbal communication, Los Angeles, 1959, University of California Press.
3. Rogers, C.: Client-centered therapy, Boston, 1957, Houghton Mifflin Company.
4. Ruhlman, R. G., and Ishiyama, T.: Remedy for the forgotten back ward, Amer. J. of Nurs. 64:109, 1964.
5. Quiros, A.: Adjusting nursing techniques to the treatment of alcoholic patients, Nurs. Outlook 5:276, 1957.
6. Keller, M., and Efron, V.: Alcoholism in the big cities of the United States, Quarterly Journal of Studies on Alcoholism 17:63, 1956.
7. Peltenburg, C. M.: Casework with the alcoholic patient, Social Casework 37:81, 1956.

General

Bermosk, L. S., and Mordan, M. J.: Interviewing in nursing, New York, 1964, The Macmillan Company.

Bojar, S.: The psychotherapeutic function of the general hospital nurse, Nurs. Outlook 6:151, 1958.

Cherescavich, G., and Tieger, M.: Coffee break therapy, Nurs. Outlook 5:227, 1957.

Chinque, K.: The management of children with phenylketonuria, Nurs. Outlook 10:328, 1962.

Farnsworth, D. L.: Mental health—a point of view, Amer. J. Nurs. 60:688, 1960.

Galdston, I.: Nutrition from the psychiatric viewpoint, J. Amer. Diet. Ass. 28:405, 1952.

Garrett, A.: Interviewing: its principles and methods, New York, 1942, Family Service Association of America.

Gilmore, E., and Braun, M.: Advances in insulin coma therapy, Amer. J. Nurs. 60:1626, 1960.

Golder, G.: The nurse and the alcoholic patient, Amer. J. Nurs. 56:436, 1956.

Guide for nutrition services for mentally retarded children, Children's Bureau, U. S. Department of Health, Education, and Welfare, Washington, D. C., 1964.

Haun, P.: Are you a hostess to your patient-guests? J. Amer. Diet. Ass. 30:1140, 1954.

Haun, P.: Food and the mentally ill, Ment. Hosp. 5:18, 1954.

Hofling, C. K., Leininger, M., and Bregg, E.: Basic psychiatric concepts in nursing, ed. 2, Philadelphia, 1967, J. B. Lippincott Company.

Horwitt, M. K.: Nutrition and mental health, Nutr. Rev. 23:289, 1965.

Johnson, D.: The significance of nursing care, Amer. J. Nurs. 61:65, 1961.

Jubenville, C. P.: Day care centers for severely retarded children, Nurs. Outlook 8:371, 1960.

Kunkel, F.: In search of maturity, New York, 1943, Charles Scribner's Sons.

Lewis, J. A.: Alcoholism, Amer. J. Nurs. 56:433, 1956.

Manfreda, M. L.: Psychiatric nursing, ed. 7, Philadelphia, 1964, F. A. Davis Co.

Matheney, R. V., and Topalis, M.: Psychiatric nursing, ed. 4, St. Louis, 1965, The C. V. Mosby Co.

Mereness, D., and Karnosh, L. J.: Essentials of psychiatric nursing, ed. 6, St. Louis, 1962, The C. V. Mosby Co.

Noyes, A. P., Camp, W. P., and Sickel, M. V.: Psychiatric nursing, ed. 6, New York, 1964, The Macmillan Company.

Orlando, I. J.: The dynamic nurse-patient relationship, New York, 1961, G. P. Putnam's Sons.

Owens, L., and White, G. S.: Observations on food acceptance during mental illness, J. Amer. Diet Ass. **30:**1110, 1954.

Rinkel, M., and Himwich, H. E.: Insulin treatment in psychiatry, New York, 1959, Philosophical Library, Inc.

Sapir, J. V.: Relationship factors in the treatment of the alcoholic, Social Casework **34:**297, 1953.

Schwartz, D.: Nursing needs of chronically ill ambulatory patients, Nurs. Res. **9:**185, 1960.

Schwartz, D., Henley, B., and Zeitz, L.: The elderly ambulatory patient: nursing and psycho-social needs, New York, 1964, The Macmillan Company.

Schwartz, M. S., and Shackley, E. L.: The nurse and the mental patient, New York, 1956, Russell Sage Foundation.

Sorensen, K., and Fagan, R.: The hospitalized skid row alcoholic, Nurs. Forum **2:**48, 1963.

Walker, G. H.: Nutrition in mentally deficient children, J. Amer. Diet. Ass. **31:**494, 1955.

Woodfall, R.: A retarded child at home, Amer. J. Nurs. **63:**80, 1963.

Wright, M.: Care for the mentally retarded, Amer. J. Nurs. **63:**70, 1963.

UNIT **IV**

NUTRITION IN
MEDICAL-SURGICAL NURSING

Up to this point in the study of nutrition and its role in nursing practice, the important basic principles of nutritional science and their role in human life have been discussed. In Unit I each of the vital nutritional elements and the dynamic metabolic interrelationships that give life to the human body were explored. Unit II was concerned with people in their communities, and applying these principles in practical everyday living and learning better ways of using them to meet life's needs. Unit III concerned the continuum of man's whole life span and his needs throughout that cycle for normal growth and development, with the possible added stress from some traumatic disability or mental illness.

The final unit, "Nutrition in Medical-Surgical Nursing," completes the whole of man's nutritional needs—his modified needs in illness. Like the iceberg whose cap is seen above water, therapeutic nutrition is but a small portion of the whole basic structure of nutrition which sustains it. A therapeutic diet is but a modification of an individual's normal nutritional needs only insofar as is necessary to meet a specific disease requirement.

This significant concept of diet therapy may be pictured as a pyramid. Forming the broad base of the triangle on which the whole superstructure rests is the foundational metabolic chemistry of all human life, the essential nutrients and their dynamic interdependent reaction. Rising above this, and built upon it, is man's life cycle needs for these essential nutrients through-

out his total growth and development. Finally, at the apex of the structure, formed and positioned by the foundation beneath, and having its major strength in its roots therein, is therapeutic nutrition, those nutritional modifications which an individual person may require as treatment during an illness. Therefore, the principles of diet therapy have meaning only in terms of normal nutrition. Indeed, they exist only to the degree that there is a specific disease-related necessity for them. An understanding of diet therapy lies, therefore, in an understanding of normal human nutrition and metabolism. This has been the emphasis and order of study in this book.

Therefore, this final unit applying basic nutritional principles in medical-surgical nursing will form a brief manual of diet therapy—the modifications of normal nutrition which may be required in a particular disease condition. Many of the clinical applications in reference to specific nutrients were discussed in earlier chapters of the book. Moreover, the study of the disease entity, its anatomy and physiology, its clinical manifestations and related nursing care, are the core of the medical-surgical nursing course. These details need not be repeated here but should be reviewed carefully as diet therapy is correlated with other treatment in the study of particular patient needs. The discussion of the disease here will focus on its metabolic aspects, and the related clinical symptoms and rationale for nutritional modifications.

Thus, the general format followed in each

discussion will outline three areas of knowledge needed to answer basic questions raised.

1. *Disease*—how does this disease affect the body and its normal metabolic functioning?
2. *Diet therapy*—how and why does the diet need to be modified (in terms of its nutritional components) to meet the needs created by this particular disease?
3. *Diet guidelines*—how do these necessary nutritional modifications affect daily food choices.

It is evident that three tools will be valuable in this study: (1) bibliographies listed at the end of each chapter will give additional reference sources for background reading; (2) the appendix given at the back of the book will provide numerous tables as tools for study of specific diet therapy modifications; and (3) the book's index and the cross-references throughout will provide valuable assistance in locating correlated discussions concerning individual nutrient modifications in clinical situations.

CHAPTER 23

Principles of diet therapy in patient care

THE HOSPITALIZED PATIENT—FACTORS IN HIS CARE

The basis of care given hospital patients is the need each individual presents in the course of his illness and its medical treatment. In her excellent book, *Newer Dimensions of Patient Care*,[1] Esther Lucile Brown has stressed the positive concepts that the environment of the general hospital *can* be therapeutic, that staff motivation and competence *can* be improved, and—most important of all—that *patients are people,* by which she does not mean the idea of "collective people," but rather the very human dimension of *individual persons.* Sometimes in the idealistic and diffuse "service to humanity" notions, the nurse forgets that she cares for *individual persons,* one at a time, and that each one is unique. Thus, to give good patient care she needs to understand factors at work in the patient and in the hospital setting which influence his reactions. On this basis she may be able to identify personal health needs and plan relevant individual care to meet these needs.

The patient

From his perspective, the uninitiated patient in the hospital milieu often faces a formidable environment. His illness and his anxieties create psychologic tensions, and various coping mechanisms result within him. Also, he brings with him his socioeconomic and cultural molding, and in whatever nature and degree they may have been developed, his spiritual resources. He is a whole person. Physical, psychologic, social and economic, and cultural factors are parts of the whole and need to be considered in the total care of the patient.

Physical factors

One of the physician's first acts is to examine his patient physically. He knows that this is an imperative initial step in planning his medical care. The nurse also must have knowledge of physical details such as age, sex, general physical condition, and presence and degree of signs and symptoms of illness. She may learn much through alert observation during such general nursing care as bathing and moving in bed: for example, skin conditions, injuries or irritations, disabilities, and general nutritional status (p. 372).

Psychologic factors

The stress an individual faces causes him to use various mental mechanisms developed over his growing years in his attempt to relieve tension. These mechanisms may be observed in patients. They are often the only means of making a painful situation psychologically tolerable.

Depression. Responses may vary from a quiet downheartedness, feelings of general pessimism, and inadequacy and discouragement, to a hopeless despair. The patient is quiet, restrained, and inhibited.

Repression. The patient may completely repress painful aspects of the environment, pushing them out of his conscious awareness. They remain within him, however, and may manifest their influence in various personality traits.

Suppression. Undesired strivings not possible in his present situation may be suppressed by the patient on a more conscious level, only to have them come out later, perhaps in a different form of behavior.

Identification. The patient may find support through identifying with persons or associations in his environment. He may *transfer* a past role image to the nurse, for example, his mother; or he may be able to project his feelings as warmth and empathy for another patient; or may *introject* (direct to himself) aspects of another person's personality.

Reaction-formation. Sometimes inappropriate perfectionistic or rigid responses may be observed. These may be reactions formed as opposites of the natural desire in the circumstance.

Compensation. Inadequacies or inabilities in one area may lead to compensating developments in another. This is often observed in patients with physical disabilities, for example, who have developed other capacities in remarkable ways. In some cases, the loss of prestige and self-esteem which often accompanies the indignities of the patient role, will lead a patient to compensate with boastings or constant commands for attention.

Rationalization. Perhaps more operative in everyone is the mental mechanism of rationalizing to prevent guilt feelings or loss of self-respect. It is the well-known "sour grapes" response. After first responding to something simultaneously without clear motives, a person then offers "reasons" for his act, presentable and reasonable motives to excuse his behavior. These usually have a portion of truth in them and are hence admissible to his consciences. Such rationalization often serves a useful protective function to the psyche and gives comfort.

Substitution. To combat frustration, if one desired goal is not obtainable in his situation, the patient may substitute an alternative gratification. Sometimes it does not necessitate a changed goal but a different means of achieving it.

Displacement. Sometimes a deeper anxiety is handled by transferring the emotional feeling from its real object to a substitute object. This may take the form of phobias such as that associated with extreme cleanliness in constant hand washing, or of symbolization. Food sometimes serves as such a symbol and the patient may use it as his language of communication.

Projection. A common defense mechanism is a person attributing to others traits in himself which he dislikes. A person's severe criticism of another's weak points may indicate the presence of these very weaknesses in himself.

Withdrawal. If the situation remains unresolved and too stressful, the patient may withdraw. Mild withdrawal protects one's resources, but can develop to undesirable extremes and prevent the healthy involvement of the patient in his own recovery.

Social and economic factors

Family. Persons live in families, be they near, or far, or no longer present. These family relationships, derived or present, directly influence the patient's development and his present living situation.

Group memberships. Memberships in various community group situations outside the family also influence a patient's responses or provide supportive group resources for him. These groups may be business or professional, volunteer service groups, social, civic, or religious groups.

Occupation. Occupational roles in society develop related behavior patterns. One's occupation also determines a person's social class status and income level (pp. 250 and 251).

Financial resources. Direct pressures may result from anxieties concerning the high cost of medical care and limited personal financial resources to pay the bills. Often help may be worked out for some source of financial assistance through consultation with the social workers on the hospital staff.

Housing. The patient's living situation may have been a factor in his illness. It may still offer problems in planning his continuing care.

Cultural factors

A person is a direct product of his culture, ethnic and religious, and bears the imprint of its values, attitudes, and behaviors. Within the broad culture there are also significant influential subculture groups (p. 250).

The hospital setting

The hospital setting itself imposes other limiting factors upon the patient. Often he is no longer a person; he is a case. No matter what his illness, he is immediately bed-bound, stripped of clothing and other personal identification, and all rights of decision or independent action are removed. Even such a homely and necessary task as going to the toilet is listed on his chart as a "privilege." He is punctured, plumbed and palpated with innumerable, fearsome-looking gadgets and machines, with little or no explanation of what is happening to him. Or he is repeatedly given lectures as if he had no knowledge at all.

The often complicated structure of the modern community hospital, especially in larger cities, bewilders and confuses many patients. It is both a medical compex devoting its energies and resources to healing and at the same time a large social community with many overt and subtle networks of relationships.

Complex medical center. Many departments contribute specialized medical and allied services. Numerous medical specialty groups work with laboratory, x-ray, nursing service, dietary, social service, pharmacy, publications, medical records, library, and other groups. Also, necessary departments to carry on the day-to-day business of the hospital include accounting, reception, maintenance, central supply, purchasing, housekeeping, and many others. A representative procession of these persons file in and out of the patient's room with a confusing and often conflicting array of requests and a denial of privacy. Through a labyrinth of corridors, doorways, and elevators, he may be wheeled or escorted by or to these various hospital staff members for vague and undefined purposes.

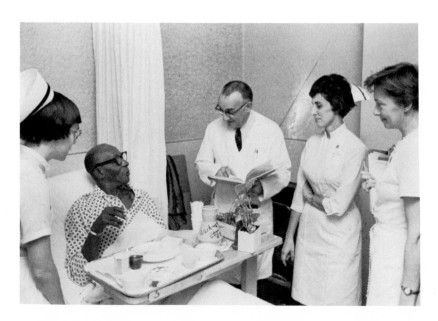

Fig. 23-1. The health team on ward rounds. Here the physician, nurse, dietitian, and student nurse confer with a patient recovering from a coronary occlusion.

The hospital hierarchy. Among the many groups of persons comprising the hospital's staff and personnel, there are numerous intra- and interrelationships. Sometimes the patient may find himself caught in the middle of conflicts between these groups, and his interests suffer. A distinct hospital hierarchy assigns status rights and privileges, eating areas, use of facilities, with an infinite number of admission symbols ranging from the dangling stethescope to the enveloping apron. In his book *Games People Play,* psychiatrist Eric Berne describes many of the common human patterns in social relationships, maneuvers, and manipulations. L. I. Stein[2] sees the easily recognizable flow of communication between doctors and nurses as the "doctor-nurse game." This is perhaps a necessary relationship played by both to preserve the physician's psychic strength for the responsibility he carries for the patient's life.

That such forces do operate in many complex hospital communities is evident by what Dr. Brown calls "competing chain of command" between medical and hospital administrations.[1] Increasingly, however, positive changes which she describes as being possible are being made. Cooperative group efforts are helping to meet personal needs of the staff for recognition and a sense of accomplishment, and at the same time provide for the patient the high quality care he must have.

The health team. One such positive change is the increasing use of the health team in the various aspects of the patient's care. This approach, described in previous chapter (p. 281), recognizes the unique contribution of special skills and knowledge, and the value to the patient and to the health workers of a team effort. In the care of the hospitalized patient, key persons related to his day-to-day welfare include the physician, the nurse, the dietitian, the social worker, and in many places, the hospital chaplain, who is an especially trained person in pastoral counseling. Provision in many hospitals for such a significant new health team member indicates the close relationship of human spiritual needs to mental health and to physical health. Public health workshops for representatives from both groups—mental health and religion—are being held in many centers to discuss common areas of patients' needs to which both may contribute insights and resources.

Many other administrative level conferences and other small group sessions are being organized in many hospitals to facilitate communication between these groups and improve patient care.

The patient's health needs— nursing diagnosis

In the setting provided by the individual hospital, with its strengths and despite its shortcomings, the nurse must care for her patient. The diagnosis of the patient's nursing care needs will be her initial responsibility. Useful and necessary background knowledge may come from several sources such as the patient, the patient's chart, the patient's family or other relatives, oral or written communication with other hospital personnel, and related research. In determining her present patient care it may be helpful for the nurse to think of the patient's needs in three areas—past, present, and future. The following outline may be used as a guide:

I. Influence of past experience on present needs. (Interviewing is an important communicative skill in nursing [Fig. 23-2]. Here the skill is history taking to obtain needed information relevant to the patient's care.)

A. Social history—general socioeconomic and cultural background (family, living situation, occupations, and any other important individual information)

B. Medical history—previous illnesses, surgery, reactions (including drug sensitivities), hospitalization, treatments

C. Nutrition history and analysis—general diet habits, marketing and cooking methods, food behavior,

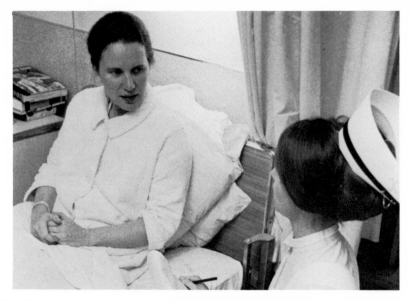

Fig. 23-2. Student nurse interviewing her patient to plan nursing care.

likes, dislikes, food meanings; typical day's food intake, and analysis of nutritional status (Review the discussion in Chapter 18 to provide background materials for nutrition history and analysis.)

II. Present needs
  A. General nursing needs of hospitalized patients
    1. Physical safety and comfort needs
    2. Basic physiologic needs
      a. Nutrition (including water and electrolytes)
      b. Hygiene—cleanliness, elimination
      c. Rest, sleep
      d. Exercise, body mechanics
    3. Basic psychosocial needs
      a. Minimal stress—nonthreatening environment
      b. Effective communication, meaning
      c. Integrity, fulfillment
  B. Nursing needs of present illness (classic picture and individual patient response)
    1. Nature of the illness and its

effect on the body, clinical signs and symptoms
    2. Treatments and medications; patient responses
    3. Diet therapy—specific order, rationale for each principle, and foods affected; meals planned (selected menu), mode of food service and any needs for eating aids; patient response

III. Future needs for continuing care
  A. The physician's plan of continuing medical care
  B. Care facilities—home, relative, nursing home
  C. If indicated, the person responsible for care, to discuss the patient's care plans—family member, visiting nurse, home aide

**The patient's health care—
nursing care plan**

Communications skills. On the basis of background information (knowledge of specific nursing care relative to present illness and general needs) the nurse will make her nursing care plan for the patient. It will need to be flexible. Results must be checked

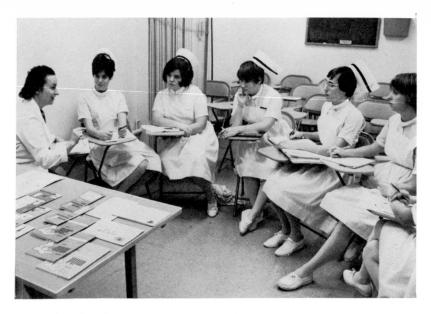

Fig. 23-3. A clinical conference with the teaching dietitian.

from day to day, even hour to hour, and the plan reevaluated according to need. Involvement of the patient in the plan is essential. Communication skills in interviewing and alert observation are vital parts of good nursing care.

Points to consider. Generally, the plan will consider these points:

1. Identified needs
2. Goals related to specific needs
3. Relevant background knowledge
4. Related nursing activity
5. Results

Nutritional needs will be a part of the total nursing care. They will be found as identified needs. Goals in relation to them will be established (in relation to present meals served or instruction concerning special diet needs). Related background knowledge of nutritional science and dietetics will apply. The related nursing activity will involve getting a diet history, analyzing the patient's food intake, planning instructional needs, and following through with him to determine future care needs. In clinical conferences with the teaching dietitian these activities will be clarified and enlarged (Fig. 23-3).

DIET THERAPY
Basic concepts

Normal nutrition base. The primary concept of diet therapy should be reviewed again as stated in the introduction to Unit IV (p. 463). This is an important initial fact to grasp, and to impart to the patients. For example, it is a great source of encouragement to the mother of a newly diagnosed diabetic child that his diet plan will be based on his normal growth and development needs and will use regular foods. Again, a therapeutic diet is but a modification of normal nutritional needs, modified only insofar as the specific disease in the specific individual necessitates.

The disease application. The principles of a specific therapeutic diet will be based upon modifications of the nutritional components of the normal diet. These changes may include:

1. Nutrients—modifications in one or more of the basic nutrients (protein, carbohydrate, fat, minerals, vitamins)
2. Energy—modification in energy value (calories)
3. Texture—modification in texture or

Table 23-1. Routine hospital diets

Food groups	Clear liquid	Full liquid	Soft	Light	General
Soup	Broth, bouillon	Same, plus strained soups	Same	All	All
Cereal			Refined cooked cereals, cornflakes, rice, noodles, macaroni, spaghetti	Same	All
Bread			White bread, crackers, Melba, Zwieback	Same, plus graham and rye bread	All
Protein foods		Milk, cream, milk drinks	Same, plus eggs (not fried), mild cheese, fowl, fish, sweetbreads, tender beef, veal, lamb, liver, bacon, gravy	Same	All
Vegetables			Potatoes—baked, mashed, creamed, steamed, escalloped; tender cooked whole bland vegetables (may be strained or pureed)	Same, cooked whole bland	All
Fruit and fruit juices	Apple juice	All fruit juices	Same, plus bland cooked fruit; peaches, pears, applesauce, peeled apricots, white cherries, bananas, orange and grapefruit sections without membrane	All	All
Desserts, gelatin	Plain gelatin, water ice	Same, plus sherbet, ice cream, puddings, custard	Same, plus plain sponge cakes, plain cookies, plain cake, simple puddings	Same	All
Miscellaneous	Ginger ale, carbonated water, coffee, tea	Same	Same, plus butter, salt, pepper	Same	All

seasoning (liquid, bland, low residue, and so on)

The individual patient adaptation. A diet may be theoretically correct and contain well-balanced food plans, but if these plans are unacceptable to the patient, they will not be followed. Careful planning *with* the patient, based on an initial interview to obtain a diet history and knowledge of general food habits, living conditions, and related factors, is necessary. Thus, the diet principles may be understood and motivation secured to follow through. It will be a workable plan adapted to his particular needs and desires. Individual tailoring of the diet to individual needs is imperative to successful therapy.

Routine "house" diets. A schedule of routine "house" diets is followed in hospitals for those patients not requiring a so-called special diet modification. According to general patient need and tolerance, the diet ordered for him may be liquid (clear liquid or full liquid, milk being used on the full liquid diet), soft (no raw foods, generally bland in seasoning), and regular (a full, normal for age, diet). Occasionally an interval step between soft and regular will be used—the light diet. Table 23-1 indi-

cates the usual progression and food choices in each stage.

Role of the nurse. The role of the nurse in the nutritional care of her patient is three-fold. She is the coordinator, interpreter, and teacher.

Coordinator. The nurse is best able, because of her close relationship to the patient and her more constant attendance, to coordinate the special services and treatments he may require. She may be the one to help schedule his activities to prevent conflicts, or secure needed consultation for him with the social worker, the dietitian, or other member of the health team. Thus, she may help to remove unnecessary confusion surrounding him.

Interpreter. Because of her relationship with the patient and his confidence in her, the nurse can help reduce his tension by careful, brief, easily understood explanations to him concerning his various treatments and plan of care. This will include basic interpretation of his therapeutic diet order and resulting food selections on his tray, and seeing that he gets his proper diet.

Teacher. The nurse's most significant role in nutritional care is that of teacher. She

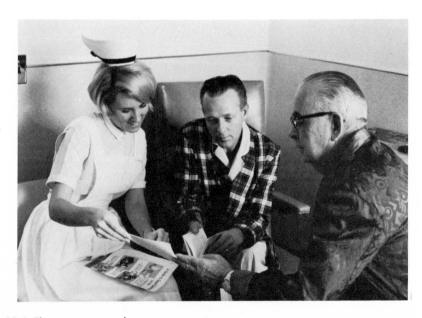

Fig. 23-4. The nurse as a teacher.

will have innumerable informal opportunities during daily nursing care for planned conversation about sound nutritional principles. In addition, according to patient situations, she may plan periods of instruction concerning the principles of his therapeutic diet integrated with general health teaching about his disease (Fig. 23-4). She will work in close cooperation with the patient's physician, to coordinate her efforts with the physician's medical management of the patient's illness. She will also work closely with the hospital's therapeutic dietitians to support and supplement additional instruction from them. The dietitian will also be an excellent resource for teaching materials and needed information.

It is evident that learning about the patient's needs should be a continuing activity beginning with his hospital admission. It should follow through and include plans for continuing application in the home environment. Follow-up care may be provided by the outpatient dietitian, by public health nutritionists or nurses, or by referrals to various community resource groups.

That this optimum learning situation does not prevail in all hospitals is a concern of many nurses, physicians, and dietitians. There are many reasons and they vary in different situations. One reason, however, is very pertinent here—the negative attitude of many nurses about their own nutrition and the negative patient responses to their nutrition education efforts. A recent two-year study in California hospitals,[3] sociologic and anthropologic in orientation, not only indicated this fact of negative attitudes and responses but also that physician information was preferred, that printed diet lists were the main means of conveying information to patients, and that the nurses closest to the patient placed the least priority value on nutrition in patient care.

Perhaps through the different concepts and perspectives presented here, the nurse will be able to venture into new approaches. The patient is her concern, and his care is her responsibility.

References
Specific

1. Brown, E. L.: Newer dimensions of patient care, New York, 1964, Russell Sage Foundation.
2. Stein, L. I.: The doctor-nurse game, Arch. Gen. Psychiat. (Chicago) **16**:699-703, 1967.
3. Newton, M. E., Beal, M. E., and Strauss, A. L.: Nutritional aspects of nursing care, Nurs. Res. **16**:46, 1967.

General

Abdellah, F. G., and others: Patient-centered approaches to nursing, New York, 1960, The Macmillan Company.

Ahart, H. E.: Assessing food intake of hospital patients, J. Amer. Diet. Ass. **40**:114, 1962.

Aldrich, C. K.: Prescribing a diet is not enough, J. Amer. Diet. Ass. **33**:785, 1957.

Babcock, C. G.: Comments on human interrelations, J. Amer. Diet. Ass. **33**:871, 1957.

Babcock, C. G.: Food and its emotional significance, J. Amer. Diet. Ass. **24**:390, 1948.

Babcock, C. G.: Problems in sustaining the nutritional care of patients, J. Amer. Diet. Ass. **28**:222, 1952.

Babcock, C. G.: Psychologically significant factors in the nutrition interview, J. Amer. Diet. Ass. **23**:8, 1947.

Balsley, M.: A look at selected diet manuals, J. Amer. Diet. Ass. **47**:123, 1965.

Bean, W. B.: The clinician interrogates nutrition, Amer. J. Clin. Nutr. **13**:263, 1963.

Bergevin, P.: Telling vs. teaching-learning by participation, J. Amer. Diet. Ass. **33**:781, 1957.

Blecha, E. E.: Dietary study methods. IV. The dietary history for use in diet therapy, J. Amer. Diet. Ass. **27**:968, 1951.

Brandt, M. B.: Perspective on diet manuals, J. Amer. Diet. Ass. **47**:121, 1965.

Brener, R.: Dietitian and patient: evaluation of an interpersonal relationship, J. Amer. Diet. Ass. **28**:515, 1952.

Coston, H. M.: Dining room service for hospital patients, Nurs. Outlook **7**:425, 1959.

Dawson, M. J.: New patients dine with the nurse, Amer. J. Nurs. **66**:287, 1966.

Derrington, P., and others: What opportunities do general duty nurses have to teach patients about diet and nutritional needs? Amer. J. Nurs. **56**:1139, 1956.

Downing, C. B.: What is programmed instruction?, J. Amer. Diet. Ass. **46**:39, 1965.

Duncan, G. C.: Some nutritional hazards of the hospitalized patient, J. Amer. Diet. Ass. **25**:330, 1949.

Editorial: The unpalatability of therapeutic diets, J.A.M.A. **164**:53, 1957.

English, O. S.: Psychosomatic medicine and dietetics, J. Amer. Diet. Ass. **27**:721, 1951.

Food and Nutrition Board, National Academy of

Science, National Research Council, Recommended dietary allowances, Rev. 1968.

Gebbard, B.: Exhibit planning and analysis, J. Amer. Diet. Ass. **24**:394, 1948.

Germain, L. D.: Dietetic aspects of nursing care, J. Amer. Diet. Ass. **29**:906, 1953.

Goodhart, R. S., and Wohl, M. G.: Manual of clinical nutrition, Philadelphia, 1964, Lea & Febiger.

Hall, M. N.: Home health aide services are here to stay, Nurs. Outlook **14**:44, 1966.

Hashim, A.: The difficult patient: how do you feed him?, Nutr. Rev. **20**:1, 1962.

Hathaway, M. L.: Heights and weights of children and youth in the United States, Home Economics Research Reports No. 2, U. S. Department of Agriculture, Washington, D. C., 1957.

Hildreth, H. M.: Hunger and eating, J. Amer. Diet. Ass. **31**:561, 1955.

Hospital dietitians: do you chart?, J. Amer. Diet. Ass. **44**:361, 1964.

Ingles, T.: Do patients feel lost in a general hospital?, Amer. J. Nurs. **60**:648, 1960.

Johnson, D.: Present concepts in diet therapy. In Bourne, G. H.: World review of nutrition and dietetics, Vol. 5, New York, 1965, Hafner Publishing Co., Inc., pp. 79-131.

Johnson, J. A.: The nurse-dietitian team, J. Amer. Diet. Ass. **32**:940, 1956.

Kelly, C. W.: Nurses, nutrition and the general public, Amer. J. Nurs. **58**:217, 1958.

Knutson, A. L., and Newton, M. E.: Behavioral factors in nutrition education, J. Amer. Diet. Ass. **37**:222, 1960.

Kreitlow, B. W.: Teaching adults democratically, J. Amer. Diet. Ass. **33**:788, 1957.

Larsen, V. L.: What hospitalization means to patients, Amer. J. Nurs. **61**:44, 1961.

Leach, J. M.: Motivating people to use educational material, J. Amer. Diet. Ass. **29**:245, 1953.

Lewis, M. N., and Pevsner, E.: How to make nutrition education effective, Hospitals **30**:70, 1956.

Mohammed, M. F. B.: Patients' understanding of written health information, Nurs. Res. **13**:100, 1964.

Moore, H. B.: Psychological fact and dietary fancies, J. Amer. Diet. Ass. **28**:789, 1952.

Morris, E.: How does a nurse teach nutrition to patients? Amer. J. Nurs. **60**:67, 1960.

Newton, M. E., and Knutson, A. L.: Nutrition education of hospitalized patients, J. Amer. Diet. Ass. **37**:226, 1960.

Piper, G. M.: Survey of home-delivered meals programs, Public Health Reports **80**:432, 1965.

Pragoff, H.: Areas of cooperation between medical social workers and dietitians, J. Amer. Diet. Ass. **24**:485, 1948.

Robinson, C.: Dietary nomenclature, J. Amer. Diet. Ass. **28**:640, 1952.

Robinson, C.: Food therapy begins with the normal diet, Amer. J. Clin. Nutr. **1**:150, 1953.

Rogers, C. R.: A counseling approach to human problems, Amer. J. Nurs. **56**:997, 1956.

Sebrell, W. H.: Adequate therapeutic diets, J. Amer. Diet. Ass. **30**:1256, 1954.

Sense, E.: Clinical studies in nutrition, Philadelphia, 1960, J. B. Lippincott Co.

Seymour, M.: Current practices, research and education in diet therapy, Amer. J. Clin. Nutr. **14**:233, 1964.

Skiff, A. W.: Programmed instruction and patient teaching, Amer. J. Public Health **55**:409, 1965.

Tarnower, W.: Psychological needs of the hospitalized patient, Nurs. Outlook **13**:28, 1965.

Turner, D.: Handbook of diet therapy, ed. 4, Chicago, 1965, The University of Chicago Press.

Walsh, E.: Nutritionists and social workers cooperate on mutual problems, J. Amer. Diet. Ass. **25**:681, 1949.

Walsh, H. E.: The changing nature of public health, J. Amer. Diet. Ass. **46**:93, 1965.

Wayler, T. J., and Klein, R. S.: Applied nutrition, New York, 1965, The Macmillan Company.

Weber, K. B.: Diet instruction for patients at home, Nurs. Outlook, **4**:39, 1956.

Wellin, E.: In-patient dietary instruction and the hospital setting, J. Amer. Diet. Ass. **34**:1179, 1958.

What 200 agencies are saying about Medicare, Nurs. Outlook **14**:30, 1966.

White, G.: The patient as the focus of attention, J. Amer. Diet. Ass. **30**:25, 1954.

Wohl, M. G., and Goodhart, R. S.: Modern nutrition in health and disease, Philadelphia, 1964, Lea & Febiger.

Wood, C. L.: How the chaplain and the dietitian can cooperate, J. Amer. Diet. Ass. **35**:821, 1959.

Young, C. M.: Diet therapy—interviewing the patient, Amer. J. Clin. Nutr. **8**:523, 1960.

Young, C. M.: The interview itself, J. Amer. Diet. Ass. **35**:677, 1959.

Young, C. M.: Teaching the patient means reaching the patient, J. Amer. Diet. Ass. **33**:52, 1957.

CHAPTER 24

The problem of obesity and weight control

BASIS OF THE PROBLEM OF OBESITY

Obesity is a problem of affluent societies. Abundant statistical evidence indicts it as a health hazard. It increases the risk of a number of diseases such as diabetes mellitus, gout, gallbladder disease, coronary atherosclerosis, and hypertension. It complicates respiratory difficulties such as emphysema, chronic bronchitis, and asthma. It increases surgical risk, complicates pregnancy, and disturbs growing adolescence. It reduces life expectancy.

Rare forms of obesity due to endocrine disorders exist, but it is the so-called simple obesity constantly seen in everyday clinical practice, that concerns both patient and practitioner. In the face of overwhelming and obvious evidence of its effect upon health, the obesity problem continues to plague victims and health authorities alike, and efforts to combat it are largely frustrating to both. It soon becomes evident, therefore, that so-called simple obesity is not so simple after all. The enigma of the problem stems generally from two factors—its unsure definition and its multiple etiology.

Definitions

Ideal weight. The clinical term obesity is given to the presence of excess body weight (15% or more above the ideal weight). The problem, however, lies in defining the word "ideal." It is generally defined in reference to average weight according to height and frame, but in reality there is no such thing as an average person. Each

person is individual, and normal values in healthy persons vary over a wide range. And how does one precisely measure *frame?* Current research studies at the University of California's School of Public Health employing anthropometric methods to determine body build and composition use from thirty-three to thirty-eight separate measures.[1] Also, tables of "ideal" weight usually use figures based on "average" activity. This factor, too, may be an unrealistic one. Individuals vary widely in the amount of their physical exercise, and the majority of them are becoming increasingly sedentary, as is indicated by many studies and by general observation. An old general rule of thumb, however, for measuring ideal weight is: for women, beginning with a height of five feet use 100 pounds, and add five pounds for every inch over five feet; for men, beginning at five feet use 110 pounds, and add five pounds for every inch over five feet.

Types of obesity. Recognition of different types of obesity adds to the problem of definition. It is not merely a matter of total weight. The ratio of lean body mass (muscle) to body fat is involved. For example, a *developmental* type of obesity, beginning early in life and steadily continuing into adult years produces a higher ratio of lean body mass, whereas the *reactive* type associated with emotional stress of growth years produces an excess ratio of fat (p. 431). Therefore, body composition must be considered in making more precise definitions. Tests being used today by researchers to

Table 24-1. General approximations for daily adult basal and activity energy needs

Basal energy needs (av. 1 cal. per kg. per hr.)		Man (70 kg.) calories 70 × 24 = 1,680	Woman (58 kg.) calories 58 × 24 = 1,392
Activity energy needs			
Very sedentary	+20% basal	1,680 + 336 = 2,016	1,392 + 278 = 1,670
Sedentary	+30% basal	1,680 + 504 = 2,184	1,392 + 418 = 1,810
Moderately active	+40% basal	1,680 + 672 = 2,352	1,392 + 557 = 1,949
Very active	+50% basal	1,680 + 840 = 2,520	1,392 + 696 = 2,088

measure this variation in body composition include:

1. Skin-fold thicknesses—measures subcutaneous or surface fat, adipose tissue
2. Anthropometric measures—measures size of body frame and body contours
3. Water displacement—measures total fat content of the body
4. Radio-active potassium count—measures amount of lean body tissue
5. X-ray defraction (shadows)—measures fat surrounding organs, minimal fat deposits

Etiology

The complexity of "simple" obesity is further increased by its multiple etiology. Among these factors are the following.

Physical factors. The basic physical laws of energy exchange (Chapter 8) account for obesity—an intake of more energy potential (calories) in food than output (calories) in total energy metabolism, including basal needs and physical activity. Table 24-1 indicates a general scheme for measuring basal energy needs and additions for activities. The statement concerning the balance of energy exchange, however, simple as it seems, is more complex. The maintenance level of calories varies widely with individuals in like circumstances. It is also influenced by their activity level. Numerous investigators report that obese subjects generally consume fewer calories than non-obese ones, but their activity level is usually lower also.[2] Obese sedentary persons, there-

fore, simply cannot afford to eat as much as their leaner counterparts.

Physiologic factors. The normal physiology of the growth years contributes to accumulation of fat tissue deposits. Numerous studies and surveys[2-4] indicate that there are critical periods for the development of obesity. For children the critical periods are very early infancy and early stages of puberty. For the female, a critical period is after age 21 because of less activity with no adjustment of caloric intake. Other times are during the first pregnancy and after menopause, due to the hormonal factors that are operating. For the male, a critical period is between the ages of twenty-five and forty, generally caused by decreasing activity with no consequent change in the large food habits formed during adolescence. Both men and women tend to gain weight after the age of fifty because of the lowered basal metabolic rate and decreased exercise, with failure to adjust calories accordingly.

Practical factors that influence physical obesity are the overfeeding of infants and children, and lack of dietary adjustment by adults during periods of increased susceptibility to weight gain.

Inheritance factors. Some experimental studies with mice[5] seem to indicate a genetic factor in obesity, but the significance of these results for human obesity is unknown. It is true that obese children are more likely than nonobese children to have obese parents. Surveys indicate that where one parent is obese, approximately 40% of the offspring are obese; where both parents are obese, 80% of the offspring are obese. It is probable, however, that the familial influence is a situational one that molds food habits. Excessive food preparation and consumption is the normal family habit pattern, one which tends to be perpetuated in adulthood and passed on to successive generations.

Social factors. The class values placed upon the obese state by different social groups will also influence the incidence of obesity. A recent study by Goldblatt's group at the University of Pennsylvania[6] surveyed 1,660 representative adults in an urban residential area. These subjects were grouped according to socioeconomic status and their rates of obesity were compared. A greater number of obese persons were found in the lower socioeconomic status group than in the higher one. Also, it was found that with increasing upward mobility, the incidence of obesity declined; there was a more noticeable difference being seen in women than in men. With increasing social status, the women moved from the "obese" to the "thin" category; the men moved from the "obese" to the "normal" category. These investigators concluded that movement *among* social classes as well as membership *in* a social class influences obesity. In the lower socioeconomic status groups, obesity was common and therefore, considered normal, whereas greater social value was placed on the nonobese state in higher groups. The length of exposure to these values and their pressure upon the individual determine his reaction to them.

Psychologic factors. The relation of emotional factors to obesity is well established. The obese state may well be the individual's protective resolution of deeper emotional problems. In such cases, to remove it without providing an alternative and satisfying resolution may well create still further problems. Hilda Bruch[7] (p. 430) indicates from her many studies of children that such obesity problems may develop through the growth years when normal psychosocial struggles of children are not positively supported by the child's environment. Studies with college students at Cornell University revealed that success or failure in a weight reduction program could be predetermined by measures of the individual's degree of emotional stability. [8,9]

DIET THERAPY

By and large, two general approaches to the control of obesity are found in clinic practice, depending upon the orientation of

Table 24-2. Principles and rationale for the Gordon diet for treatment of obesity*

Diet principles			Rationale theory
1. Initial 48 hour total fast			Breaks the metabolic pattern of augmented lipogenesis (based on rat experiments)
2. Diet:	gm.	calories	
High protein	100	400	High satiety value and specific dynamic action
Moderate fat	80	720	Satiety value; 15 to 20% as UFA supplement
Low carbohydrate	50	200	Close relation of glucose to fat formation
Total calories		1,320	
3. Six-meal pattern (equal)			Reduce lipogenesis from smaller glucose loads
4. Low salt (2 to 3 gm.)			Water produced by fat oxidation
			Slow disposal of sodium loads
5. Supplement of polyunsaturated fatty acids (vegetable oil); 15 to 20% of fat calories			Accelerates oxidation of body fat

*Adapted from Gordon, E. S., and others: A new concept in the treatment of obesity, J.A.M.A. 186:50, 1963.

the clinician and the type of patient and obesity with which he is dealing. For the type of obesity that has been labeled 'intractable" or "biochemically resistant," the approach of some researchers is based upon the apparent metabolic etiology.

Metabolic approach

Principles and rationale. The metabolic approach is illustrated by the research of Gordon's group at the University of Wisconsin Medical School.[10] Based on their studies and resulting theories, this group has developed a dietary program around several metabolic principles:

1. Lipogenesis
   a. The close relation of glucose and fat metabolism, the conversion of glucose to fatty acid, and the subsequent formation of triglycerides
   b. The influence of meal distribution (glucose load) on the conversion of glucose to fat
   c. The influence of brief fasting upon

The Gordon diet for treatment of obesity[*]

Foods to include daily

1. One egg
2. Eleven ounces (cooked weight) lean meat
3. Seven teaspoons of margarine or oil or equivalent
4. Two cups skimmed milk
5. Two servings of fruit
6. Two to four cups vegetables from list A[†]
7. One-half slice bread

Menu plan (minimum of six meals a day)

Breakfast	Lunch	Dinner
½ cup vitamin C fruit or juice	3 oz. meat	3 oz. meat
1 egg	vegetable A	vegetable A
1 oz. meat	1 tsp. margarine	1 tsp. margarine
1 tsp. margarine	2 tsp. corn oil	2 tsp. corn oil
½ slice bread	coffee or tea	1 serving fruit
coffee or tea		coffee or tea

Mid morning	Mid afternoon	Evening
1 cup skimmed milk	½ cup skimmed milk	½ cup skimmed milk
1 oz. meat	2 oz. meat	1 oz. meat

"Free" foods

1. Clear fat-free broth (homemade)
2. Unsweetened plain gelatin
3. Artificially sweetened gelatin products
4. Lemon
5. Vinegar
6. Spices and herbs
7. Carbonated beverages prepared with noncaloric sweeteners

Foods to avoid

1. Sugar, syrups, molasses, honey, candy, cake, cookies, ice cream, potato chips, crackers, gelatin products sweetened with sugar, puddings, pies, gravy, alcoholic beverages
2. Highly salted foods (use salt *lightly* in cooking; no added salt)
3. Any foods which are not included in the diet list above

[*]Adapted from Gordon, E. S., and others: A new concept in the treatment of obesity, J.A.M.A. 186:50, 1963.
[†]See Food Exchange Groups, p. 483.

the breaking of this lipogenesis chain

2. Lipolysis—the influence of unsaturated fatty acids upon the oxidation of saturated fat or body fat
3. Water metabolism—sodium and water retention (100 gm. of fat when oxidized yields 112 gm. of water)

Diet plan. The resulting diet therapy principles and rationale of the Gordon program are summarized in Table 24-2. The suggested dietary regimen such as may be used with medically selected and supervised patients in a clinical setting is given on p. 478.

General clinical approach

Principles and rationale. In common practice, the general approach to the control of simple obesity (excluding that form in subjects with more pronounced psychological or metabolic problems) is based upon the underlying energy exchange etiology and the patient's situational needs. It has three main principles:

1. Individual decision and support
2. Individual diet with calorie and situational adaptations
3. A planned follow-up program

Motivation and support. The degree of patient motivation is a prime factor. The initial interviews seek to determine individual needs, attitudes toward food, and the meaning food has for the patient. Recognition is given the emotional factors involved in a reduction program and support is provided by the team of physician, nutritionist and nurse, to meet the patient's particular needs. Shame or scare tactics generally have no place in such a program.

DIET THERAPY

Initial interview. Upon the basis of careful interviewing, the patient's food habits

---

TO PROBE FURTHER
The exchange system of dietary control

The exchange system, set up by professional organizations including the American Dietetic Association, is based upon a simple grouping of common foods according to generally equivalent nutritional values. This system may be used for any situation requiring calorie and food value control.

The foods are divided into six basic groups, called the exchange groups (pp. 483 and 484). Each food within a group contains approximately the same food value as any other food item in that same group, allowing for free exchange *within any given group.* Hence the term *food exchange* is used throughout. The total number of exchanges per day depends upon individual nutritional needs, based always upon normal nutritional recommendations of the Food and Nutrition Board, National Research Council.

Although there is some variation in the composition of foods within the exchange groups, for simplicity the following values for carbohydrate, protein, and fat are used:

Food	Approx. measure	Carbohydrate gm.	Protein gm.	Fat gm.	Calories
Fruit exchange	Varies	10	—	—	40
Bread exchange	1 slice	15	2	—	70
Meat exchange	1 oz.	—	7	5	75
Vegetable B exchange	½ cup	7	2	—	40
Milk exchange	1 cup	12	8	10	170 (skimmed = 80)
Fat exchange	1 tsp.	—	—	5	45

Table 24-3. Calorie adjustment required for weight loss

To lose 1 pound a week—500 fewer calories daily
Basis of estimation

1 lb. body fat	= 454 grams
1 gm. pure fat	= 9 calories
1 gm. body fat	= 7.7 calories (some water in fat cells)
454 gm. × 9 cal. per gm.	= 4,086 calories per lb. fat (pure fat)
454 gm. × 7.7 cal. per gm.	= 3,496 calories per lb. body fat (or 3,500 calories)
500 cal. × 7 days	= 3,500 calories = 1 lb. body fat.

Table 24-4. Weight reduction diets using the exchange system of dietary control

Food exchange group*	Approx. measure	800 calories	1,000 calories	1,200 calories	1,500 calories
Total number of exchanges per day					
Milk (nonfat)	1 cup	2	2	2	2
Vegetable A	As desired	Free	Free	Free	Free
Vegetable B	½ cup	1	1	1	1
Fruit	Varies	3	3	3	4
Bread	1 slice	1	3	4	4
Meat	1 ounce	6	6	7	9
Fat	1 teaspoon	1	1	2	4
Distribution of food exchanges					
Breakfast					
Fruit		1	1	1	1
Meat		1	1	1	1
Bread		1	1	1	1
Fat		1	1	1	1
Lunch and dinner					
Meat		2 to 3	2 to 3	3	4
Vegetable A		Any	Any	Any	Any
Vegetable A (either meal)		1	1	1	1
Bread		0	1	1 to 2	1 to 2
Fat		0	0	0 to 1	1 to 2
Fruit		1	1	1	1 to 2
Milk		1	1	1	1

*See Food Exchange Groups, pp. 483 and 484.

and situational factors are determined. A balanced diet is made out for him, based on normal nutritional needs, and the calorie level is adjusted to meet his individual weight reduction requirement. One thousand fewer calories daily is the necessary adjustment to lose about two pounds a week; 500 fewer calories to lose one pound a week. The basis of this calculation is given in Table 24-3. Usually the energy value of the adjusted diet will range between 800 and 1,500 calories.

Individual diet plan using exchange system. Using the basic exchange system of dietary control given in Table 24-4, a meal pattern is made out with the patient which will meet his individual living situation, individual desires, and cultural patterns.

TO PROBE FURTHER
Practical suggestions to dieters

Goals

Be realistic. Don't set your goals too high. Adapt your rate of loss to one to two pounds per week. If visible tools are helpful motivation techniques, use them.

Calories

Don't be an obsessive calorie counter. Simply become familiar with the food exchanges in your diet list and learn the general calorie values of some of your favorite home dishes in order that you might occasionally make substitutions.

Plateaus

Anticipate plateaus. They happen to everyone. They are related to water accumulation as fat is lost. During these periods, increase your exercise to help you get started again.

Binges

Don't be discouraged when you break over and have a dietary binge. This, too, happens to most people. Simply keep them infrequent and when possible, plan ahead for special occasions. Adjust the following day's diet or remaining part of the same day accordingly.

Special diet foods

There is no need to purchase special low-calorie foods. Learn to read labels carefully. Most special diet foods are expensive and many are not much lower in calories than regular foods.

Home meals

Try to avoid a separate menu for yourself. Adapt your needs to the family meal, adjusting seasoning or method of preparing family dishes to lower caloric values of added fats and starches.

Eating away from home

Watch portions. When a guest, limit extras such as sauces and dressings, trim meat well. In restaurants select singly prepared items rather than combination dishes. Avoid items with heavy sauces or fat seasoning. Select fruit or sherbet as desserts rather than pastries.

Appetite control

Avoid dependence on appetite depressant medications. Usually they are only crutches. Beginning efforts to control appetite may be aided by nibbling on food from the free list or by saving over meal items for use between meals such as the fruit.

Meal pattern

Eat three or more meals a day. If you are used to three meals, then leave it at that. If you are helped by snacks between meals then plan part of your day's allowance to account for them. The main thing is that you do not take all of your calories at one sitting. Avoid the all-too-common pattern of no breakfast, little or no lunch, and a huge dinner!

Continued.

Practical suggestions to dieters—cont'd

Artificial sweeteners	On the basis of much research, there is no reason to question the safety of such products. If you like, use any of the foods sweetened with these products as you desire, accounting for the calories and food value in the base food to which they may be added, such as fruit. Artificially sweetened soft drinks may help as occasional between meal carry-overs.
Alcohol	Remember that alcohol has an energy value of 8 calories per gram, nearly that of fat. The details of the metabolic pathways by which alcohol is oxidized are not clear, but it is known that the calories are available.

Food choices for meals are taken from the Food Exchange Groups listed on pp. 483 and 484.

Follow-up appointments. A follow-up schedule of appointments is outlined and its values are discussed with the patient. On subsequent clinical visits progress records are kept, problems discussed, and solutions to them mutually decided. Continuing support is given. A number of practical suggestions to dieters have evolved from much experience (p. 481). These may help the patient to anticipate needs, avoid pitfalls, and sustain his motivation.

Essential characteristics of sound diet for weight control

Experience in many clinics has shown that there are no real short-cuts. In the face of many periods of discouragement, the patient may be harried and vexed, tempted to grab for a plethora of pills, formulas, and fads. However, a sound dietary approach to weight control which holds hope of achieving a degree of *lasting* success, must be based upon five characteristics.

1. *Realistic goals.* Goals must be realistic in terms of overall loss and rate of loss.
2. *Calories lowered according to need.* The diet must be low enough in calories in relation to individual expenditure levels of energy to effect a gradual weight loss. Usually a rate of one to two pounds a week is recommended.
3. *Nutritional adequacy.* The diet must be nutritionally adequate. Lower caloric levels may need supplementation. The nutrient ratio should supply no less than 12 to 15% of the calories as protein; no more than 35% of the calories as fat, with reduced intake of saturated fats; and the rest of the calories as carbohydrate, using little sucrose and including a variety of food sources.
4. *Culturally desirable.* The food plan must be enough like the cultural eating pattern of the individual to form the basis for *permanent* re-education of his eating habits. In other words, he must be able to live with it.
5. *Calorie readjustment to maintain weight.* When the desired weight level is reached, the calories are adjusted accordingly, but the re-education achieved in basic habits is the continuing means of weight control.

Best approach—prevention. In the last analysis, in the approach to the problem of obesity and its control, it would seem that the best work would be aimed at *prevention* —early nutrition education and support to young mothers and children before the obese condition becomes a reality.

Food exchange groups

List 1. *Milk exchanges.*

Whole	1 cup	(Cream portion of whole milk equals
Skim milk	1 cup	two fat exchanges. One cup of
Buttermilk	1 cup	whole milk equals 1 cup of skim
Evaporated milk	½ cup	milk plus two fat exchanges.)
Powdered skim milk	¼ cup	
Yogurt, plain	1 cup	

List 2. *Vegetable exchanges (as served plain, without fat seasoning or dressing). (Any fat used is taken from fat exchange allowance).*

Group A. (Use as desired. Negligible carbohydrate, protein, and fat in amounts commonly eaten.)

Asparagus	Greens	Mushrooms
Bak choi, Gai choi	Beet greens	Okra
Bamboo shoots	Chard	Peppers (Bell, Chili, etc.)
Broccoli	Collards	Radishes
Brussel sprouts	Kale	Sauerkraut
Cabbage	Mustard	String Beans, young
Cauliflower	Spinach	Summer squash
Celery	Turnip greens	Tomatoes
Chicory		Watercress
Chinese cabbage	Salad greens	Parsley
Cucumbers	Lettuces	Pimientoes
Escarole, endive		
Eggplant		

Group B. (½ cup equals one serving)

Artichoke (1 medium)	Peas, green	Squash, winter
Beets	Pumpkin	Turnip
Carrots	Rutabaga	
Onions		

List 3. *Fruit exchanges (unsweetened—fresh, frozen, canned, cooked). (One exchange is portion indicated by each fruit.)*

Berries		Dried fruits		Others	
Blackberries	1 cup	Apricots	4 halves	Apple	1 small
Blueberries	⅔ cup	Dates	2	Apple Juice	⅓ cup
Raspberries	¾ cup	Figs	1 small	Applesauce	½ cup
Strawberries	1 cup	Prunes	2 medium	Apricots (fresh)	2 med.
		Raisins	2 tablespoons	Banana	½ small
Citrus fruits				Cherries	10 large
Grapefruit	½ small			Fig (fresh)	1
Grapefruit				Grapes	12 med.
juice	½ cup			Grape Juice	¼ cup
Orange	1 small			Peach	1 medium
Orange				Pear	1 small
juice	½ cup			Pineapple	½ cup, 1 slice
Tangerine	1 large			Pineapple	
				juice	⅓ cup
Melons				Plums	2 medium
Cantaloupe	¼ med.			Prunes (fresh)	2
Honeydew	⅛ med.			Prune juice	¼ cup
Watermelon	½ center slice				

Continued.

Food exchange groups—cont'd

List 4. Bread exchanges (equivalent portions indicated by each item).

Bread		Cereal	
Bagel	½	Cereal, cooked	½ cup
Biscuit, roll (2 in. diam.)	1	Cereal, dry (flakes, puffed)	¾ cup
Bread (white or dark)	1 slice	Flour	2½ tablespoons
Cornbread (1½ in. cube)	1	Rice, grits (cooked)	½ cup
Frankfurter roll	1 small	Corn	⅓ cup
Hamburger roll	½ large	Spaghetti, macaroni,	
		noodles (cooked)	½ cup

Crackers		Vegetables, and other	
Animal	8	Baked beans, no pork	¼ cup
Graham (2½ in. square)	2	Beans, peas, dried, cooked	½ cup
Oyster	½ cup	Corn on the cob	½ large ear,
Round, thin (½ in. diam.)	6-8		1 small ear
Saltines (2 in. square)	5	Popcorn (popped)	1 cup
Soda (2½ in. square)	3	Parsnips	⅔ cup
Matzos (6 in. diam.)	1 piece	Potatoes, white	1 small
Muffin (2 in. diam.)	1	Potatoes, mashed white	½ cup
Melba thins	4	Potatoes, sweet or yams	¼ cup
Pretzels (22 per lb.)	1 med.	Sponge cake, plain (1½ in.	
Pretzel sticks (av. thin)	14	cube)	
		Ice cream, vanilla (omit	
		2 fat exch.)	½ cup
		Ice milk, vanilla	½ cup

List 5. Meat exchanges (all items refer to cooked weight).

Lean meat, poultry	1 ounce	Fish	
Cold cuts (4½ in. x ⅛ in.)	1 slice	Cod, halibut	1 oz.
Frankfurter (8-9/lb.)	1	Salmon, tuna, crab, lobster	¼ cup
Egg	1	Shrimp, clams, oysters, etc.	5 small
Cheese, cheddar type	1 ounce	Sardines	3 medium
Cheese, cottage	¼ cup	Scallops (12 pcs. per lb.)	1 large
Sausage (3 in. x ½ in.)	2	Peanut butter (limit 1 exch.	
		per day)	2 tablespoons

List 6. Fat exchanges

Avocado (4 in. diam.)	⅛	French dressing	1 tablespoon
Bacon, crisp	1 slice	Half and half (10% cream	
Butter or margerine	1 teaspoon	and milk)	4 tablespoons
Cream, light (20%)	2 tablespoons	Mayonnaise	1 teaspoon
Cream, heavy (40%)	1 tablespoon	Nuts	6 small
Cream cheese	1 tablespoon	Oil or cooking fat	1 teaspoon
Cheese spreads	1 tablespoon	Olives	5 small
		Sour cream	2 tablespoons

Miscellaneous foods allowed as desired (negligible carbohydrate, protein, fat).

Artificial sweeteners	Gelatin, plain	Rennet tablets, plain
Bouillion, fat-free	Lemon	Rhubarb
Broth, clear	Mustard	Spices
Coffee	Pepper	Tea
Cranberries, unsweetened	Pickle, dill and sour	Vinegar
Catsup		

References
Specific

1. Hampton, M. C., Huenemann, R. L., Shapiro, L. R., Mitchell, B. W., and Behnke, A. R.: A longitudinal study of gross body composition and body conformation and their association with food and activity in a teen-age population. II. Anthropometric evaluation of body build, Amer. J. Clin. Nutr. **19**:422, 1966.
2. Huenemann, R. L., Shapiro, L. R., Hampton, M. C., and Mitchell, B. W.: Teen-agers' activities and attitudes toward activity, J. Amer. Diet. Ass. **51**:433, 1967.
3. Forbes, G. B.: Overnutrition for the child: blessing or curse?, Nutr. Rev. **15**:193, 1957.
4. Heald, F. P., and Hollander, R. J.: The relationship between obesity in adolescence and early growth, J. Pediat. **67**:35, 1965.
5. Mayer, J.: An experimentalist's approach to the problem of obesity, J. Amer. Diet. Ass. **31**:230, 1955.
6. Goldblatt, P. B., Moore, M. E., and Stunkard, A. J.: Social factors in obesity, J.A.M.A. **192**:1039, 1965.
7. Bruch, H.: The importance of overweight, New York, 1957, W. W. Norton & Company, Inc.
8. Darling, C. D., and Summerskill, J.: Emotional factors in obesity and weight reduction, J. Amer. Diet. Ass. **29**:1204, 1953.
9. Young, C. M., and others: Psychologic factors in weight control, Amer. J. Clin. Nutr. **5**:186, 1957.
10. Gordon, E. S., Goldberg, M., and Chosey, G. J.: A new concept in the treatment of obesity, J.A.M.A. **186**:50, 1963.

General

Astwood, E. B.: Heritage of corpulence, Endocrinology **71**:337, 1962.
Ayers, W. M.: Changing attitudes toward overweight and reducing, J. Amer. Diet. Ass. **34**:23, 1958.
Bayles, S., and Ebough, F. G.: Emotional factors in eating and obesity, J. Amer. Diet. Ass. **26**:430, 1950.
Blondheim, S. H., and others: Comparison of fasting and 800-1000 calorie diet in treatment of obesity, Lancet **1**:250, 1965.
Bruch, H.: The importance of overweight, New York, 1957, W. W. Norton & Company, Inc.
Cohn, C., and Joseph, D.: Effects on metabolism produced by rate of ingestion of diet, Amer. J. Clin. Nutr. **8**:682, 1960.
Conrad, S. W.: Resistance of the obese to reducing, J. Amer. Diet. Ass. **30**:581, 1954.
Drenick, E. J., and others: Prolonged starvation as treatment for severe obesity, J.A.M.A. **187**:100, 1964.
Duncan, G. G., et al.: Correction and control of intractable obesity, J.A.M.A. **181**:309, 1962.

Elsbach, P., and Schwartz, I. L.: Salt and water metabolism during weight reduction, Metabolism **10**:595, 1961.
Eppright, E. S., Swanson, P., and Iverson, C. A.: Weight control, Ames, Iowa, 1955, The Iowa State College Press.
Fryer, J. H.: The effects of a late-night calorie supplement upon body weight and food intake in man, Amer. J. Clin. Nutr. **6**:354, 1958.
Gray, F. I., and Little, D. E.: It's not just a matter of will power, Amer. J. Nurs. **61**:101, 1961.
Hamburger, W. W.: The psychology of weight reduction: the initial nutritional interview; the nutritionist-patient relationship; and the complications of weight reduction, J. Amer. Diet. Ass. **34**:17, 1958.
Hampton, M. C., Huenemann, R. L., Shipiro, L. R., and Mitchell, B. W.: Caloric and nutrient intakes of teen-agers, J. Amer. Diet. Ass. **50**:385, 1967.
Leverton, R. M.: Food needs and energy use in weight reduction, J. Amer. Diet. Ass. **49**:23, 1966.
Mayer, J.: Obesity, cardiovascular diseases, and the dietitian, J. Amer. Diet. Ass. **52**:13, 1958.
Mayer, J.: Obesity: causes and treatment, Amer. J. Nurs. **59**:1732, 1959.
Mayer, J.: Obesity control, Amer. J. Nurs. **65**:112, 1965.
Mayer, J.: Some aspects of the problem of regulation of food intake and obesity, N. Eng. J. Med. **274**:610, 1966.
Mayer, J.: Treatment of obesity, N. Eng. J. Med. **274**:722, 1966.
Mayer, J., and Stare, F. J.: Exercise and weight control: frequent misconceptions, J. Amer. Diet. Ass. **29**:340, 1953.
Montagu, A.: Obesity and the evolution of man, J.A.M.A. **195**:105, 1966.
Nordsick, F. W.: An epidemiologic approach to obesity, Amer. J. Public Health **54**:1689, 1964.
Parson, W., and Crispell, K. R.: Obesity, Med. Clin. N. Amer. **36**:385, 1952.
Peckos, P. S., and Spargo, J. A.: For overweight teen-age girls, Amer. J. Nurs. **64**:85, 1964.
Randle, P. J., and others: Glucose fatty acid cycle, Lancet **1**:785, 1963.
Sebrell, M. H., Jr.: Weight control through prevention of obesity, J. Amer. Diet. Ass. **34**:920, 1958.
Shipmen, W. C., and Plesset, M. R.: Predicting the outcome for obese dieters, J. Amer. Diet. Ass. **42**:383, 1963.
Stare, F. J.: Overnutrition, Amer. J. Public Health **53**:1795, 1963.
Steinberg, A. G.: Comments on genetics of human obesity, Amer. J. Clin. Nutr. **8**:752, 1960.
Stunkard, A. J., and others: The night-eating syndrome, Amer. J. Med. **19**:78, 1955.
Swenseid, M. E., and others: Nitrogen and weight

losses during starvation and realimentation in obesity, J. Amer. Diet. Ass. **46:**276, 1965.

Symposium on over-nutrition, Amer. J. Clin. Nutr. **9:**525, 1961.

Young, C. M.: Weight reduction using a moderate fat diet. I. Clinical responses and energy metabolism, J. Amer. Diet. Ass. **28:**410, 1952.

Young, C. M., Ringler, I., and Greer, B. J.: Reducing and past-reducing maintenance on the moderate fat diet, metabolic studies, J. Amer. Diet. Ass. **29:**890, 1953.

CHAPTER 25

Diabetes mellitus

HISTORY

Diabetes is an ancient disease. Its symptoms have been found described on an Egyptian papyrus—the Ebers Papyrus—dating about 1500 B.C. In the first century the Greek physician Aretaeus wrote of a malady in which the body "ate its own flesh" and gave off large quantities of urine. He gave it the name *diabetes*, from the Greek word meaning "siphon" or "to pass through." Much later, in the 17th century, the word *mellitus*, from the Latin word for honey, was added because of the sweet nature of the urine. This addition distinguished it from *diabetes insipidus*, another disorder in which the passage of copious amounts of urine was observed.

Over the years many scientists and physicians continued to puzzle over the mystery of diabetes, but the cause remained obscure. For physicians and their patients these years could be called the "Diabetic Dark Ages." Patients had short lives and were maintained on a variety of semi-starvation regimens.

A beginning clue pointing to the involvement of the pancreas in the disease was provided by a young German medical student, Paul Langerhans. He found special clusters of cells scattered about the pancreas, so-called cellular islands or islets. These cells were different from the rest of the tissue. Though their function was still then unknown, these islet cells were named for their young discoverer—the islets of Langerhans. Soon after, in 1922, following this lead, two Canadian scientists, F. G. Banting and his assistant, C. H. Best, isolated and identified the special substance secreted by these islet cells. It proved to be a hormone which regulates the oxidation of blood sugar and helps convert it to heat and energy. They called the new hormone *insulin*, from the Latin word *insula* meaning "island." For his discovery, Banting received a Nobel prize and was knighted by his government.

Insulin now continues to be the tool of control for diabetes, but the underlying metabolic problem, even yet, is unsolved. Recent insulin assay tests developed to measure the level of insulin activity in the blood (I.L.A.) have found insulin-like activity levels in early diabetes to be two or three times the normal insulin levels. Investigators have postulated that the insulin is present but bound with a protein, hence making it unavailable.[1] Diabetes, therefore, results from the lack of insulin; whether the lack is in production by the pancreatic islet cells, or at the level of availability in the blood is not entirely clear.

DESCRIPTION
Clinical manifestations

Diabetes has been found to be a hereditary disease. It is defined in terms of the clinical symptoms produced as a result of the lack of insulin. These symptoms appear as the diabetes develops.

A. Initial complaints
1. Increased thirst (polydipsia)
2. Increased urination (polyuria)
3. Increased hunger (polyphagia)

487

4. Weight loss (maturity onset frequently is opposite—the patient may be obese)
B. Clinical laboratory test data
  1. Glycosuria (sugar in the urine)
  2. Hyperglycemia (elevated blood sugar level)
  3. Abnormal glucose tolerance tests (With a glucose load, the blood sugar rises to a higher level and takes a longer period to return to normal.)
C. Other possible overt symptoms
  1. Blurred vision
  2. Skin irritation or infections
D. If the diabetes continues uncontrolled
  1. Fluid and electrolyte imbalance
  2. Acidosis (ketosis)
  3. Loss of strength (weakness)
  4. Coma

Because the apparent symptoms, glycosuria and hyperglycemia, are related to excess glucose, diabetes has been called a disease of carbohydrate metabolism. However, as more has been learned about the intimate interrelationships of carbohydrate metabolism with fat and protein metabolism, it is increasingly viewed as a general

metabolic disorder resulting from an insulin lack (absolute, partial, or due to its unavailability) affecting more or less each of the basic nutrients.

Classification

Juvenile onset. In its juvenile form diabetes develops fairly rapidly and is more severe and unstable; the child is usually underweight. Acidosis is fairly common, and insulin therapy is required.

Maturity onset. In its maturity onset form, diabetes develops more slowly, is usually milder and more stable, and the patient may be overweight. Acidosis is infrequent, and the majority are maintained on oral hypoglycemics and diet therapy, or by diet therapy alone.

Metabolic pattern

Normal blood sugar controls. A knowledge of the controls for maintaining a normal blood sugar level (70 to 120 mg. per 100 ml.) is essential to an understanding of the impairment of these controls in diabetes. The basic metabolism of carbohydrates in Chapter 2 should be reviewed carefully. In Fig. 25-1, these normal control

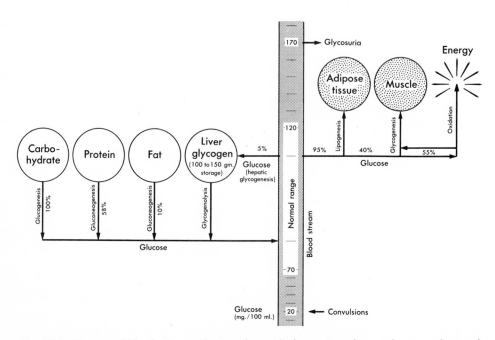

Fig. 25-1. Sources of blood glucose (food and stored glycogen) and normal routes of control.

routes may be visualized. Entry of blood glucose from dietary carbohydrates, protein, and fat, and from liver glycogen (glycogenolysis) maintains a steady supply of blood glucose. To prevent a continued rise above 120 mg. percent, several routes of glucose use are active:

1. Conversion to glycogen for storage in the liver (glycogenesis)
2. Conversion to fat (lipogenesis) and storage in adipose tissue
3. Conversion to muscle glycogen
4. Cell oxidation for energy

Insulin. Although its precise role is not entirely clear, insulin has an effect on these control mechanisms. It is believed to function in several ways (p. 21).

1. It facilitates the transport of glucose through the cell membrane.
2. It enhances the conversion of glucose to glycogen and its storage in the liver (glycogenesis).
3. It stimulates the conversion of glucose to fat (lipogenesis).
4. It influences glucose oxidation through the main glycolytic pathway by aiding the necessary initial phosphoryla-

tion reaction catalyzed by the enzyme glucokinase.

Glucagon. Recently another pancreatic hormone has been discovered, secreted by the alpha cells in the islets of Langerhans. Insulin is produced by adjacent beta cells. The new hormone was given the name *glucagon,* because of its stimulating effect on *glycogenolysis,* the conversion of glycogen to glucose. It has an opposite action to insulin and is sometimes used to control more brittle or unstable diabetes. It acts as a counterbalance to excess insulin, that is, as treatment for insulin shock or hypoglycemic reactions.

Metabolic changes in diabetes. In uncontrolled diabetes insulin is lacking to facilitate the operation of normal controls of the blood sugar level. Glucose cannot be oxidized properly through the main glycolytic pathway in the cell to furnish energy, and it therefore builds up in the blood (hyperglycemia). Fat formation (lipogenesis) is curtailed and fat breakdown (lipolysis) increases, leading to excess ketone formation and accumulation (ketosis). The appearance of one of these ketones—*acetone*—in

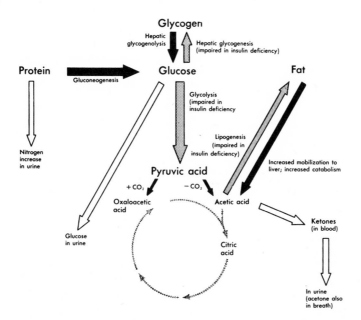

Fig. 25-2. Abnormal metabolism in uncontrolled diabetes. (From Harper, H. A.: Review of physiological chemistry, ed. 10, Los Altos, California, Lange Medical Publications, 1963.)

the urine indicates the development of ketosis. Tissue protein is also broken down in an effort to secure energy, causing weight loss and nitrogen excretion in the urine. These changes from normal metabolic pathways which operate in uncontrolled diabetes are illustrated in Fig. 25-2.

MEDICAL TREATMENT

Objectives of medical care. The physician has three basic objectives in his medical care of the diabetic patient.

The first objective is to maintain optimum nutrition. The patient's basic requirement is adequate nutrition for growth and development, and the maintenance of an *ideal* weight. The leaner side of the average weight for height is wise, and any degree of overweight is to be avoided.

The second objective is to keep the patient relatively free of symptoms such as glycosuria, hyperglycemia.

The third is to prevent complications in tissues such as the eye (retinopathy), in nerve tissue (neuropathy), and in renal tissue (nephropathy). Coronary artery disease occurs in diabetics about four times as often as in the general population, and peripheral vascular disease about forty times as often. These chronic manifestations may be reduced by good care and control.

Philosophies of control. Physicians vary as to their approaches to control measures. Some follow a philosophy of strict *chemical control,* seeking to maintain a sugar-free urine constantly. Others follow a more moderate *clinical control* approach, seeking to maintain the patient *relatively* free of clinical symptoms. Still others follow a *free control* approach, placing little or no control on the patient's diet and administering insulin if necessary accordingly. Whatever philosophy of diabetic management a particular physician may use, the basic *consistency* of habit prevails. Someone has expressed this important characterization as the three R's: *regulation, regularity,* and *routine.*

Whatever the individual physician's approach, the basic control of diabetes rests upon a balance of three important interrelated factors: (1) diet, (2) insulin, and (3) exercise.

DIET THERAPY
Nutritional needs

The fundamental principle of the diet for an individual diabetic patient may be stated simply. *It is always based upon the normal nutritional needs of that individual.* His diet is expressed in terms of his total requirement of calories, and a ratio of these calories in grams of carbohydrates, protein, and fat.

Calories. Calorie specifications are based on *ideal weight,* with allowances for physical activity or added stress, such as growth. If the patient is obese, as many adult diabetics are, then the diet prescription would indicate a sufficient reduction in calories to effect a gradual weight loss (no more than 1,200 to 1,500 calories per day). If the patient is a fast-growing, lean, adolescent boy, the calories may need to be as high as 4,000. As a general rule of thumb, the protein (grams) is about 5% of the number of total calories (in a 1,500 calorie diet there would be 75 gm. of protein).

Protein. Normal age-group requirements for protein govern the amount indicated for the individual patient, with perhaps the optimum or upper range being the guideline. For the adult man, an average of 65 gm. is the National Research Council's recommended daily allowance. For the diabetic, 65 to 80 gm. may be used daily.

Carbohydrate. Carbohydrates should be adequate for need but not excessive. The range is from 100 to 250 gm. As a general rule, the carbohydrate (grams) is about 10% of the number of calories (in a 1,500 calorie diet, there would be 150 gm. of carbohydrate). Refined or "free" sugars should be avoided in habitual use. Sugar substitute sweeteners may be used as desired.

Fat. Fats also should be adequate, but *moderation* is the guideline. Some clinicians advise substitution of vegetable fats for some of the animal fats in the diet to increase the ratio of unsaturated fatty acids. This is based on the general indication of a relationship between saturated fats and coronary artery disease, and the greater risk factor of such disease in diabetes.

A general rule of thumb for outlining the final prescription is the setting of calories and protein according to known standard individual requirements. Then, after the protein calories have been deducted from the total calories, the remaining calories are divided approximately half and half between carbohydrate and fat. Roughly, the carbohydrate to protein to fat dietary ratio will be about 2:1:1. For example, an average 1,500 calorie diet may be divided approximately into 150 gm. of carbohydrate, 75 gm. of protein, and 75 gm. of fat. Another general rule is that the fat (grams) is about 5% of the number of total calories. (In a 1,500 calorie diet, there would be 75 gm. of fat.)

Meal distribution

An important consideration is the distribution of the total diet through the day. This will be influenced by the type of control used—insulin, oral hypoglycemic agent, or diet alone.

Insulin. The schedule of the day's food intake pattern should be balanced with the type of insulin used and its pattern of absorption and activity peaks.

Short-acting insulin—regular crystalline, semilente. Short-acting insulins cover about a four-hour period of time, and thus only the one meal following their use. These insulins are usually used in situations where short term periods of control are indicated, such as in surgery, during labor and delivery, or in periods of illness.

Medium-acting insulin—NPH (neutral protamine Hagerdorn), lente, globin. NPH is the most widely used insulin preparation. Medium-acting insulins usually are given in the morning a half hour before breakfast, reach their peak of activity in eight to ten hours (about mid-afternoon), and last from twenty to twenty-four hours. The meal distribution may be considered a $\frac{1}{5}$, $\frac{2}{5}$, $\frac{2}{5}$ pattern, with allocations for a mid-afternoon and evening snack, or with the snacks coming from lunch and dinner as three fairly equal meals. For some patients, particularly adult patients, the afternoon snack may not be as important, depending on the interval of time between lunch and dinner.

Long-acting insulin—PZI (protamine zinc insulin). PZI is rarely used now. Long-acting insulins require a more substantial evening meal and bedtime snack to cover the more prolonged period of activity through the sleep hours. The meal distribution is a $\frac{1}{7}$, $\frac{2}{7}$, $\frac{2}{7}$, $\frac{2}{7}$ pattern for each of the three meals and the bedtime snack.

Mixtures of insulin. Occasionally two types of insulin may be mixed in one syringe and given in one injection. For example, regular insulin may be mixed with NPH if more immediate morning coverage is required. In such cases, a more substantial breakfast may be given and a mid-morning snack as well as mid-afternoon and bedtime snacks. The morning snack is usually more necessary only for the younger child.

Oral hypoglycemic drugs. Sulfonylureas may be used with some adult diabetics. General indications for the use of these medications include: (1) maturity onset type of diabetes, (2) no history of ketosis or coma, and (3) the diabetes has been present for less than ten years. Examples of these drugs are tolbutamide (Orinase), chlorpropamide (Diabinese), and acetohexamide (Dymelor). An additional oral hypoglycemic agent is phenformin (DBI). Sometimes the gastrointestinal disturbances which have been encountered as a side effect with phenformin may be avoided by the use of its modified form, a slow-release preparation, DBI-TD. With all of these oral medications, a fairly even distribution of the diet is also important. These medications are thought to operate on the basis of stimulation they provide for the limited function of insulin-producing cells in the pancreas. There is insulin activity going on as a result of their use and distribution of food to balance with this activity would naturally follow.

Diet alone. Even if the diabetes requires only diet control, there is still need to consider distribution through the day in a fairly consistent balance of meals. Since there is a limited tolerance for handling glucose, a load of glucose at any one point is to be avoided. There is better overall con-

trol with a balance of meals through the course of the day.

Diet management with exchange system

Recognizing the need for a more flexible and realistic approach to the dietary management of diabetes, a joint national committee with representatives from the American Diabetes Association and the American

Table 25-1. Food exchange groups

Food group	Unit of exchange	Composition				Characteristic items
		Carbohy-drate (gm.)	Protein (gm.)	Fat (gm.)	Calories	
Milk						
Whole	1 cup	12	8	10	170	Equivalents to 1 cup whole milk listed; 1 cup skimmed and 2 fat exchanges = whole milk
Skimmed	1 cup	12	8	—	80	
Vegetables						
A	as desired	—	—	—	—	Free use: 3% carbohydrates and below (tomatoes, green beans, leafy vegetables)
B	½ cup	7	2	—	35	Medium carbohydrate: pod and root varieties (green peas, carrots)
Fruit	Varies	10	—	—	40	Fresh or canned without sugar Portion size varies with carbohydrate value of item. All portions equated at 10% carbohydrate
Bread	Varies; 1 slice bread	15	2	—	70	Variety of starch items, breads, cereals, vegetables; portions equal in carbohydrate value to 1 slice bread
Meat	1 oz.	—	7	5	75	Protein foods, exchange units equal to protein value of 1 oz. lean meat (cheese, egg, seafood)
Fat	1 tsp.	—	—	5	45	Fat food items equal to 1 tsp. butter or margarine (bacon, oil, mayonnaise, olives, avocado)

Dietetic Association formulated a system of dietary control based upon the concept of food equivalents. This system of control was introduced in 1950. In this system, foods commonly used were grouped according to like nutrient composition and designated "Food Exchange Groups." Six food groups were listed: milk, vegetables A and B, fruit, bread, meat, and fat. Within any one group, food items can be freely exchanged, since all foods in that group, in the portion indicated, are of approximately the same food value.

Since the introduction of the Food Exchange System it has been widely accepted and used in health centers of all kinds for care and teaching of the diabetic patient. It has provided a simple and sound means of dietary regulation which is easily understood and flexible enough to meet a wide variety of living situations.

The food exchange groups. The six food groups of the exchange system (see also Table 24-4 and the Food Exchange Groups listed on pp. 483 and 484) form the basic tools with which health workers may calculate diet needs and make wise food selections and substitutions. The composition and characteristics of these food groups are given in Table 25-1.

Calculation. Using the food exchange groupings, the individual diabetic patient's diet may easily be calculated by a short method illustrated in Table 25-2.

Steps in calculation

1. The food groups listed in Table 25-2 and nutrient columns arranged in the order given should be used.
2. The diet prescription (calories; grams of carbohydrate, protein, fat) is placed in spaces indicated. If only calories are given in the diet order, the ratio distribution guides given on p. 490 should be used.
3. Estimates of general use of first three food items—milk, vegetable B (group A is free and not calculated), and fruit should be made. The allowance estimate is based on the general caloric level.

4. Nutrient values of the milk, vegetable B, fruit are filled in from values for single items given in Table 25-1.
5. To calculate number of bread exchanges:
   a. Add carbohydrate in first three items (milk, vegetable, fruit), and subtract this amount from the total day's allowance of carbohydrate. The remaining carbohydrate will be used in bread exchanges.
   b. Divide the carbohydrate value of one bread exchange (15 gm.) into the remaining carbohydrate to be used. This will give the total number of bread exchanges. Fill in this number of exchanges and its nutrient values, found by multiplying the single bread exchange values in Table 25-1.
   c. Total carbohydrate column. (Totals in each nutrient within 3 to 4 grams of indicated prescription are satisfactory.)
6. To calculate number of meat exchanges:
   a. Add protein in items used thus far (milk, vegetable, bread) and subtract this amount from the day's total allowance of protein. The remaining protein will be used in meat exchanges.
   b. Divide the protein value of one meat exchange (7 gm.) into the remaining protein to be used. This will give the total number of bread exchanges. Fill in this number of exchanges and its nutrient values, found by multiplying the single meat exchange values in Table 25-1.
   c. Total protein column.
7. To calculate number of fat exchanges:
   a. Add fat in items used thus far (milk, meat) and subtract from day's total fat allowance.
   b. Divide value of one fat exchange (5 gm.) into the remaining fat to be used. This will give the total

Table 25-2. Calculation of diabetic diet—short method using exchange system (2,200 calories)

Food group	Total day's exchanges	Carbo-hydrate 230 gm.	Protein 90 gm.	Fat 100 gm.	Bkfst.	Lunch	Dinner	Snacks PM	Snacks HS
Milk	2	24	16	20	1				1
Vegetable A	as desired	—	—	—		as desired	as desired	as desired	
Vegetable B	1	7	2				1		
Fruit	6	60 ____ 91			1	1	2	1	1
Bread	9	135 ____ 226	18 ____ 36		2	2	2	1	1
Meat	8		56 ____ 92	40 ____ 60	1	3	4		
Fat	8			40 ____ 100	2	3	3		

fat exchanges. Fill in this amount and its nutrient value.

c. Total fat column.

Meal pattern. The total number of exchanges calculated for each food group are distributed into the day's meal pattern according to the insulin used. (The example given above is the general pattern for use with medium-acting insulin.) If insulin is not used, as with many adult diabetics, meals should be divided fairly evenly and a consistent pattern should be maintained.

Individual menus should be made each day by the pattern for each meal, choosing a variety of foods from the food exchange groups (pp. 483 and 484) in the amounts indicated in the basic meal pattern.

Individual adaptation. Each patient's diet must be tailored to fit his individual needs, his living situation, and his general eating habits. Therefore, a careful diet history is an important first step in adapting the needed dietary pattern to the individual patient's life situation. If the diet is to be a useful therapeutic tool in the care of his diabetes, it must be realistic and workable for him.

Using the patient's diet history as a guide, his diabetic diet needs are outlined and discussed with him, determining what limited modifications of his present habits are wise. After the diet plan is in use, follow-up counseling will determine any further adjustments or changes that are needed.

American Diabetes Association diets. For the convenience of physicians, a series of nine diet plans have been outlined by the National Planning Committee of the American Diabetes Association. These diets, ranging in caloric value from 1,200 to 3,000, including several adapted for children, are given in Table 25-3. Copies of these A.D.A. Diet Plans may be obtained inexpensively from the American Diabetes Association or the American Dietetic Association. An illustrated booklet, "Meal Planning with Ex-

Table 25-3. A.D.A. meal plans, for diabetics

Diet plan number	1	2	3	4	5*	6*	7*	8	9
Calories	1,200	1,500	1,800	2,200	1,800	2,600	3,500	2,600	3,000
Carbohydrate (gm.)	125	150	180	220	180	250	370	250	300
Protein (gm.)	60	70	80	90	80	100	140	115	120
Fat (gm.)	50	70	80	100	80	130	165	130	145
Total Food Exchanges									
Milk	2	2	2	2	4	4	4	2	2
Vegetable A	†	†	†	†	†	†	†	†	†
Vegetable B	1	1	1	1	1	1	1	1	1
Fruits	3	3	3	4	3	4	6	4	4
Bread	4	6	8	10	6	10	17	12	15
Meat	5	6	7	8	5	7	10	10	10
Fat	1	4	5	8	3	11	15	12	15

*These diets contain more milk and are planned for children.
†As desired.

change Lists" is also available, as well as modified lists for use in low sodium or bland diabetic diets.

PATIENT EDUCATION

The key to satisfactory management of diabetes lies in sound, realistic patient education, initiated early and followed up as needed for reevaluation and reinforcement and support. A general admonition to stay away from starches and sweets is wholly inadequate and may well lead to bizarre food choices. Wise teaching based on a well-planned diet program is sound nutrition education. Frequently the nutrition of the whole family improves when the home meals are planned around the well-balanced outline given the diabetic member. Also, because the patient has a flexible plan that allows a variety of food choices, he is far more likely to follow it and build the consistent food habits that will give better long-range diabetic control.

What the diabetic patient must know

Education of the diabetic patient should include a thorough knowledge of all those factors he must understand in order to care for his diabetes himself. These factors are:
1. The disease—general facts of diabetes, its nature, symptoms and care

2. The diet—basic knowledge of food values, individual diet plan, and ways of using substitutes; practical guides in marketing and food preparation may be needed
3. Insulin or oral hypoglycemics—details of insulin administration and care of equipment, or use of oral drugs; relation to food intake and exercise
4. Urine testing—methods of testing urine for sugar and acetone, and recording of results
5. Exercise—its value in diabetic control and general health; its relation to balance with insulin and food
6. Skin care and hygiene—for control of infection and maintenance of good circulation
7. Insulin shock—recognition of symptoms and knowledge of action to counteract those symptoms
8. Diabetic acidosis—recognition of symptoms and the need for immediate medical care
9. Personal identification—the necessity for a card or tag identifying diabetic needs, especially if on insulin
10. Educational resources—reading materials, and community organizations providing services

Diet instructions

Methods

Individual counseling. The skilled personal diet counseling given a patient with newly-diagnosed diabetes is the most valuable means of initiating a stable course. Regulation of the diabetes depends upon securing the necessary cooperation of the patient himself. Sound knowledge is the basis of wise action and consistent habits. Therefore, the initial dietary interview and the planning of the diet *with* the patient to meet his individual needs are of primary importance.

Follow-up program. Follow-up interviews continue the learning process. Adjustments may be made, new material introduced, and former knowledge corrected or reinforced. Emotional support is provided for acceptance of the disease and the working-out of personal adjustments to its care. Involving other family members in the discussions strengthens the instructions and clarifies home needs.

Group instruction. Group instruction and discussion is a helpful adjunct to personal counseling. Classes are regularly held in many clinics. Physicians, nurses, and dietitians share in the teaching responsibilities. The group discussions often reinforce personal decisions, and the exchange of ideas and experiences provides resources for learning.

Teaching materials

Visual aids and equipment. A number of visual-aid materials are available or can easily be constructed, which enhance and clarify instruction. Wax, plastic, or cardboard food models help to picture portion sizes. Food models may also be prepared by dipping a measured portion of the real food (held in a strainer) into hot paraffin, then placing the mound of food on a cardboard circle to set and harden.[2] Later the hardened food portion may be encased in a very thin film of plastic for cleanliness and protection. Different sizes of cups, glasses and spoons will also help the patient to determine standard portion sizes.

Charts, diagrams, and pamphlets help to clarify factual material. Exhibits prepared around a basic facet of care provide additional background information. Films, filmstrips, and slides are useful for group discussion. Also, demonstration equipment for practice in insulin administration and urine testing is needed.

Programmed instruction. Teaching machines are used in some clinics to augment the patient education program. Usually this teaching method is well-accepted by patients and is effective. Although it cannot replace the necessary personal instruction—nor is it so intended—it is a helpful reinforcement, freeing the dietitian and the nurse from repetitive routine teaching so that they may do more creative work with patients. Some clinics are also expanding their education program to include the use of closed-circuit television in teaching.

Reading and reference material. A number of standard reference books have been provided for diabetic patients. Some of these are listed in the patient-education references at the end of the chapter. Two are particularly useful—*A Pilgrim's Progress, with Further Revelations, for Diabetics* by Duncan,[3] and Danowski's[4] clear and practical guide for self-care, covering all facets of diabetes.

Community resources. Other helpful pamphlets and booklets are provided by pharmaceutical firms, professional groups, and health organizations. Materials available from the American Diabetes Association are listed in the chapter references. Local chapters of the American Diabetes Association are active in many communities with annual detection drives, conferences, group meetings, and classes cooperatively sponsored by adult evening schools.

Medic Alert. An identification program for alerting medical personnel to the needs of persons with hidden health problems has been provided through the creative efforts of a California physician, Dr. Marion Collins. When his own daughter, a student nurse, suffered a near-fatal reaction to horse serum given in a routine post-injury tetanus injection, he designed for her an identifying metal disc to protect her from similar danger again in the course of routine care. Afterward he began to prepare identifying discs for his patients who had drug allergies or other hidden medical problems. In 1956 his plan was officially endorsed by the American College of Surgeons and is now a nonprofit service foundation with more than 150,000 American members and affiliated groups in a number of foreign countries.

The small stainless steel medallion, worn on a bracelet or necklace, carries the individual's assigned identification serial number, a brief warning of the medical problem, and a telephone number. The telephone number may be called collect, day or night, to reach the Central Answering Service in the foundation's Turlock, California, headquarters, where all members' records are on file and are available to medical personnel.

The membership fee of $5.00 is paid only once. It includes the stainless steel medallion with emblem and a supplemental wallet card. Additional information may be obtained by writing Medic Alert Foundation International, Turlock, California 95380.

References
Specific

1. Antoniades, H. N., and others: Studies on the state of insulin in blood, New Eng. J. Med. **267**:953, 1962.
2. Moore, M. C., and others: Using graduated food models in taking dietary histories, J. Amer. Diet. Ass. **51**:447, 1967.
3. Duncan, G. G.: A modern pilgrim's progress—with further revelations—for diabetics, ed. 2, Philadelphia, 1967, W. B. Saunders Company.
4. Danowski, T., editor: Diabetes mellitus: diagnosis and treatment, New York, 1964, The American Diabetes Association.

General
   Diabetes

Allen, F. A.: Education of the diabetic patient, New Eng. J. Med. **268**:93, 1963.
Beeuwkes, A. M., editor: Education of the diabetic and his family, Institute Proceedings (1965), Continuing Education Service, School of Public Health, University of Michigan, 1967, Ann Arbor, J. Amer. Diet. Ass., p. 342.

Beaser, S. B.: Oral Treatment of diabetes mellitus, J.A.M.A. **187**:887, 1964.
Bergen, S. S., Jr., and Van Itallie, T. B.: The glucagon problem, New York J. Med. **61**:779, 1961.
Calculation of diabetic diets, J. Amer. Diet. Ass. **24**:218, 1948.
Carrington, E.: Pregnancy and diabetes, Ann. Int. Med. **59**:120, 1963.
Caso, E. K.: Diabetic meal planning: a good guide is not enough, Amer. J. Nurs. **62**:76, 1962.
Caso, E. K.: Supplements to diabetic diet material, J. Amer. Diet. Ass. **32**:929, 1956.
Caso, E. K., and Stare, F. J.: Simplified method for calculating diabetic diets, J.A.M.A. **133**:169, 1947.
Chidester, F. H.: Programmed instruction: past, present, and future, J. Amer. Diet. Ass. **51**:413, 1967.
Coultas, R.: Patients use props to plan diabetic menus, Amer. J. Nurs. **63**:104, 1963.
Daughaday, W. H.: Dietary treatment of adults with diabetes mellitus, J.A.M.A. **167**:859, 1958.
Ellenberg, M.: Diabetes in the older age group, Geriatrics **19**:47, 1964.
Farkas, C. S., and Forbes, C. E.: Do non-caloric sweeteners aid patients with diabetes to adhere to diets?, J. Amer. Diet. Ass. **46**:482, 1965.
Hamwi, G. J.: Treatment of diabetes, J.A.M.A. **181**:124, 1962.
Hinkle, L. E.: Customs, emotions, and behavior in the dietary treatment of diabetes, J. Amer. Diet. Ass. **41**:341, 1962.
Hodges, R. E.: Present knowledge of nutrition in relation to diabetes mellitus, Nutr. Rev. **24**:257, 1966.
Il'in, V. S.: The mechanism of action of insulin: primary and secondary metabolic disturbances in experimental diabetes, Fed. Proc. **25**:1034 (Part II, Translation supplement), 1966.
Johnson, D.: Effective diet counseling begins early in hospitalization, Hospitals **41**:94, 1967.
Johnson, D.: Planning a restricted sodium diet and bland, low fiber diet for the diabetic patient, Amer. J. Clin. Nutr. **5**:569, 1957.
Kaufman, M.: The many dimensions of diet counseling for diabetes, Amer. J. Clin. Nutr. **15**:45, 1964.
Kaufman, M.: Newer programs for patients with diabetes, J. Amer. Diet. Ass. **44**:277, 1964.
Kaufman, M.: Programmed instruction material on diabetes, J. Amer. Diet. Ass. **46**:36, 1965.
King, L. S.: Empiricism, rationalism, and diabetes, J.A.M.A. **187**:521, 1964.
Kinsell, L. W.: The case for routine use of diets high in polyunsaturated fat for diabetics, Diabetes **11**:338, 1962.
Krysan, G. A.: How do we teach four million diabetics?, Amer. J. Nurs. **65**:105, 1965.
Levine, R., and Sobel, G. W.: Mechanism of action

of the sulfonylureas in diabetes mellitus, Diabetes **6**:263, 1957.

Lozano-Castanedo, O., and others: Two year's experience with acetobexamide, Metabolism **8**: 99, 1964.

Martin, M. M.: Diabetes mellitus: current concepts, Amer. J. Nurs. **66**:510, 1966.

Martin, M. M.: The unconscious diabetic patient, Amer. J. Nurs. **61**:92, 1961.

Moore, A. N.: Problems in producing programs for auto-instruction, J. Amer. Diet. Ass. **51**:420, 1967.

O'Sullivan, J. B., and Mahan, C. M.: Factors related to development of diabetes mellitus, J.A.M.A. **194**:587, 1965.

Parente, B. P., and others: Adaptation of exchange lists—use in planning ward diets, J. Amer. Diet. Ass. **46**:267, 1965.

Review: Coronary disease and preclinical diabetes, Nutr. Rev. **23**:323, 1965.

Seltzer, H. S.: Treatment of unstable (brittle) diabetes in children and adults, Modern Treatm. **2**:623, 1965.

Sharkey, T. P.: Recent research developments in diabetes mellitus. J. Amer. Diet. Ass. **48**:281, 1966.

Stenzel, K. H., and others: Diabetic ketoacidosis, J.A.M.A. **187**:372, 1964.

Stone, D.: A rational approach to diet and diabetes in 1964, J. Amer. Diet. Ass. **46**:30, 1965.

Teaching diabetic self-care, New Eng. J. Med. **276**:182, 1967.

Thrush, R. S., and Lanese, R. R.: The use of printed material in diabetic education, Diabetes **11**:133, 1962.

Tolstoy, E.: The free diet for diabetic patients, Amer. J. Nurs. **50**:652, 1950.

Wagner, D. H.: The preparation and care of diabetic patients requiring surgery, Surg. Clin. N. Amer. **39**:161, 1959.

Waife, S. O., editor: Diabetes mellitus, Indianapolis, 1967, Lilly Research Laboratories, Eli Lilly and Company.

Weller, C.: Oral hypoglycemic agents, Amer. J. Nurs. **64**:90, 1964.

Wilder, R. M.: Adventures among the islands of Langerhans, J. Amer. Diet. Ass. **36**:309, 1960.

Patient education

ADA Forecast, magazine published bimonthly by the American Diabetes Assoc., Inc., 18 E. 48th St., New York, New York 10017.

ADA Meal Planning Booklet, The American Diabetes Association, 18 E. 48th Street, New York, New York 10017. Also: Diabetic Diet Card for Physicians.

ADA Meal Plans Nos. 1-9, The American Diabetes Association, 18 E. 48th St., New York, New York 10017; The American Dietetic. Association, Chicago, Illinois, 1956.

Behrman, Sister M.: A cookbook for diabetics, American Diabetes Association, Inc., New York, 1959.

Danowski, T. S.: Diabetes as a way of life, ed. 2, New York, 1964, Howard-McCann, Inc.

Dolger, H., and Seeman, B.: How to live with diabetes, New York, 1958, W. W. Norton & Company, Inc. (Paperback edition, New York, 1964, Pyramid Books).

Duncan, G. G.: A modern pilgrim's progress—with further revelations—for diabetics, ed. 2, Philadelphia, 1967, W. B. Saunders Company.

Public Health Service, U. S. Dept. of Health, Education, and Welfare, Washington, D. C.: (Booklets) Are you related to a diabetic? Pub. No. 726, rev. 1964. Diabetes, Pub. No. 137, 1964. Diabetes mellitus, a guide for nurses, Pub. 861, 1963. Taking care of diabetes, Pub. No. 567, 1963.

Rosenthal, H., and Rosenthal, J.: Diabetic care in pictures, Philadelphia, 1960, J. B. Lippincott Company.

Strachan, C. B.: The diabetic's cookbook, Houston, Texas, 1955, Medical Arts Publishing Foundation.

CHAPTER 26

Gastrointestinal diseases

GENERAL DIETARY CONSIDERATIONS

Personal needs. The gastrointestinal tract is a sensitive mirror of the individual human condition. Its physiologic functioning reflects both physical and psychologic conditioning. In adapting diet therapy for patients with gastrointestinal disorders, the nurse is dealing not so much with a specific food item per se, as with the state of the body that receives it. There is far more truth than mere humor to the statement, "Surrounding every stomach there is a person."

Physiologic functions. The digestion and absorption of the food a person eats is accomplished in the gastrointestinal tract through a series of intimately related secretory and neuromuscular mechanisms. In Chapter 10 this normal network of functions was summarized and forms the basis for understanding general dietary modifications used in disease states which hinder the normal operation of these mechanisms.

Factors involved in diet therapy. Diet therapy for various gastrointestinal disorders, therefore, will be determined by a consideration of four basic factors involved. Three of these factors are physiologic:

1. The secretory functions which provide the necessary environment and agents for chemical digestion
2. The neuromuscular functions which provide the necessary motility for mechanical digestion and move the food mass along
3. The absorptive functions which enable the end products of digestion (the nutrients) to enter the body's circulation and nourish the cells

The fourth factor affects each of the others. It is *the psychologic influence.* The individual's particular emotional make-up and his manner of dealing with life's day-to-day problems and challenges, will often be reflected in the functions of his digestive tract. Here again, it is not what he eats, it's what is eating him that is important.

The principles of nutritional care in each of the gastrointestinal disorders discussed here will concern in some way: (1) chemical secretions, (2) degree of motility, (3) absorbing mucosa, and (4) the person himself.

PEPTIC ULCER
Etiology

Peptic ulcer is the general term given to an eroded mucosal lesion in the stomach or the duodenum. Gastric ulcers are less common; the majority occur in the duodenal bulb where the gastric contents emptying into the duodenum through the pyloric valve are most concentrated.

The fundamental cause of peptic ulcer is not clear. However, two factors seem to be involved: (1) the amount of gastric acid and pepsin secreted, and (2) the degree of tissue resistance to withstand the digestive action of these secretions. In the development of gastric ulcers, although the presence of acid is essential, the degree of tissue sensitivity seems to be the paramount factor. In the patient with duodenal ulcer, excess production of acid and pepsin is the primary factor. In either case, hydrochloric acid in the gastric juice is generally acknowledged to be the essential factor in

499

the development, perpetuation, and recurrence of peptic ulcer.

The psychogenic factor in peptic ulcer is variable. The so-called ulcer personality has been described in many texts. Though overdrawn, perhaps, in some sources, the ulcer-prone individual does tend to be anxious or tense, aggressive, and competitive. Peptic ulcer usually occurs in men between the ages of 20 and 50 years, a time in life when career and personal strivings may be at a peak.

Clinical manifestations

Increased gastric tone and painful hunger contractions when the stomach is empty are cardinal symptoms of peptic ulcer. The amount and concentration of hydrochloric acid is increased in duodenal ulcer, but may be normal in gastric ulcer. Nutritional deficiencies may be manifest in low plasma protein levels, anemia, and loss of weight. Hemorrhage may be the first sign of the ulcer in some patients. Confirmation of the diagnosis comes from clinical findings, x-ray tests, or visualization by gastroscopy.

General medical management

Three factors form the basis of medical care: (1) *drug therapy* and antacids, to counteract hypermotility and hypersecretions, (2) *rest*, both physical and mental, aided as needed by sedative therapy, and (3) *diet therapy*, to provide maximum restorative powers and prevent further tissue damage.

Diet therapy

The general term "bland" has been used to describe the various ulcer regimens found in common practice. The word comes from the Latin word *blandus* meaning "a smooth tongue," or "soothing" and has taken on the connotation of something insipid, dull, uninteresting, and unattractive. Such meanings are all too often conveyed by the ulcer routines in many hospitals, diets which are nutritionally inadequate, esthetically repelling, scientifically unsound, and emotionally disturbing. That such a state need not be is

increasingly made evident by research that indicates that the usual rigid and restrictive approach is based more on tradition and assumption than on scientific fact. Perhaps a better perspective may be gained by seeing the background development of diet therapy for peptic ulcer, the rationale given for the traditional conservative management, and the current challenge of the liberal individual approach.

History of dietary treatment for peptic ulcer. The roots of diet manipulation in the treatment of patients with peptic ulcer extend far back in medical history. As early as the first century, Celsus ordered smooth diets free of "acrid" food, and practitioners of the seventh century wrote of their belief in "special healing properties" of milk for patients with digestive disturbances. In the first half of the nineteenth century, peptic ulcer became established as a pathologic and clinical entity, and physicians generally advocated a liberal dietary regimen with frequent feedings.

However, in the latter part of the nineteenth century, a radical change developed in medical opinion concerning peptic ulcer treatment. The belief spread that food was harmful to the ulcer, and only complete rest—meaning an empty stomach—would allow the stomach to heal itself. Semistarvation regimens became the accepted practice among European physicians and were soon introduced in the United States.

In 1915 an American physician, Bertram Sippy[1], broke the common practice of initial starvation treatment and established the beginning principle of continuous control of gastric acidity through diet and alkaline medication. However, his rather rigidly outlined program of milk and cream feedings with slow additions of single soft food items over a prolonged period of time allowed little variation for individual need or nutritional adequacy. Some increase in diet was made in 1935 by a Danish physician, Meulengracht,[2] who introduced a more liberal approach in feeding peptic ulcer patients, especially as treatment for hemorrhage. In the main, however, Sippy's regi-

Graduated bland diet for peptic ulcer

General description:

1. Avoid overeating at any one meal. It is better to eat smaller amounts more often.
2. Eat slowly and chew thoroughly. Sip liquids slowly, especially hot or cold ones.
3. Avoid worry, tension, argument, hurry, and fatigue, particularly at mealtime.
4. Avoid monotony in diet by varying the foods used as much as the diet allows.
5. Use no spices or seasonings except salt. Avoid concentrated sweets. Small amounts of sugar may be used.
6. Do not drink over a glass of liquid with each meal, but drink as much as desired between meals.
7. Take medications regularly as directed.
8. Follow all directions carefully and include only that part of the following diet list which is prescribed. Make the additions to the diet only as the physician advises it.
9. Maintain regular hours for eating, and take meals regularly.

Stage I

Food	*Allowed*	*Not allowed*
Milk	Regular or homogenized, buttermilk	
Cream	Plain or mixed with milk	
Fats	Fresh butter or fortified margarine	Any others
Eggs	Boiled, poached, coddled; plain omelet or scrambled in double boiler; eggnog with vanilla only	Fried eggs
Cereals	Cooked refined or strained; oatmeal, cream of wheat, Farina, Wheatena, precooked infant cereals; also plain buttered noodles, macaroni, spaghetti, or white rice Dry cereals such as cornflakes, puffed rice, Rice Krispies, without bran	Whole grain cereals; cereals containing bran or shredded wheat
Desserts	Plain custard, Jell-o, rennet, plain cornstarch, tapioca or rice puddings; plain vanilla ice cream (if allowed to melt in mouth)	Any other
Bread	Enriched white; fine rye or fine whole wheat bread at least one day old (may be plain or toasted); soda crackers, zwieback, melba toast, hard rolls	Whole wheat and other whole grain bread; graham or coarse crackers; hot or fresh bread
Cheese	Cream, cottage cheese, mild processed American and Swiss	All other
Sweets	Jelly (clear, plain) honey, sugar (in moderation), strained cranberry sauce	Any other
Potato	White, baked, boiled, creamed; boiled or baked sweet potatoes or yams in moderate amounts	Any other
Cream soups	Homemade cream soups from the following pureed vegetables: asparagus spinach pea potato green bean tomato	Canned cream soups; soups from any other vegetables; dehydrated soups, chicken soups, broths, meat stock, bouillon

Continued.

Graduated bland diet for peptic ulcer—cont'd

Stage II

Food	Allowed	Not allowed
Fruit juices	Strained orange juice, beginning with ¼ cup, diluted with water and taken at the end of the meal Later can be undiluted; prune juice if necessary for bowel regulation; grapefruit juice may be added later if tolerated	Any other
Plain cake	Angel food, sponge, pound, butter cake (without frosting)	Any cakes made with nuts, dates, spices, frostings
Vegetables (Group 1)	Winter squash, banana squash, or acorn squash; tomato juice if tolerated The following cooked and strained, or prepared infant strained vegetables: asparagus, peas, carrots, green beans, beets, spinach	Any other, also raw or coarse vegetables
Fruits (Group 1)	The following stewed, cooked fruits which have been strained (or prepared strained infant fruits): pear, peach, prune, apricot, applesauce	All other

Stage III

Food	Allowed	Not allowed
Fowl	Tender white or dark meat boiled, broiled, roasted, or baked; of turkey, chicken, squab, or pheasant	Fried, braised, or in any other form; skin, gristle or fat.
Fish	Fresh or frozen; boiled, broiled or baked; scalded canned tuna or salmon; oysters, fresh or canned.	Other canned fish or prepared in any other manner; smoked, pickled, preserved fish, crab, lobster, sardines
Meats	At first, only finely ground, plain beef; later, tender cuts of beef, veal, lamb; also liver, sweetbreads, brains (boiled, broiled, creamed, roasted)	Fried, smoked, pickled, cured; skin, gristle, fat, meats with tough fiber; delicatessen pork, ham, bacon, salami, weiners

Stage IV

Food	Allowed	Not allowed
Desserts	Prune or apricot whip, plain vanilla, chocolate or sugar cookies or wafers; plain sherbet, water ices, ice cream, if eaten slowly; fine graham crackers	Rich pastries or pies, nuts, raisins, coconut; gingerbread, spice cake, candy
Vegetables (Group 2)	Tender whole cooked vegetables: asparagus squash carrots spinach peas string beans beets mushrooms tomatoes, peeled	Onions, celery, sauerkraut, cucumbers, peppers, turnips, radishes, cabbage, cauliflower, broccoli, brussel sprouts; any coarse vegetables; hull or fiber of green vegetables; salads or coleslaw

Graduated bland diet for peptic ulcer—cont'd

Food	Allowed	Not allowed
Fruits (Group 2)	Canned or cooked without skins or seeds: pear, apricot, peach, persimmon; Nectar from pear, peach or apricot; juices of apple, grapefruit or orange	
Beverages	Weak tea, weak cocoa, Sanka, Postum; plain milkshakes	Coffee, strong tea or coffee, iced drinks, soft drinks, alcoholic beverages of any kind.
Miscellaneous	Homemade mayonnaise without spices; duck; crisp bacon; vegetable oils or shortening; less tender cuts of meat (properly prepared) such as beef round, cutlet; sour cream, yogurt; brown sugar, powdered sugar; mint jelly	Spices or condiments, pepper, horseradish, meat sauces, catsup, mustard, vinegar, pickles, relishes, olives; spicy foods of any kind; fried foods of any kind; gravies; hot cakes and other hot breads; chewing gum

men, though clearly establishing the important acid neutralizing principle of frequent feedings, continued to place rigid restrictions on the traditional dietary programs followed in common practice.

Traditional conservative dietary management. Although many changes in details of management have occurred since Sippy's day, his general restrictive pattern has been the mold for much of the traditional conservative management used today. This traditional diet therapy is based on several principles. The food must be both acid neutralizing and nonirritating.

Acid neutralizing. This therapy begins with milk and cream feedings every hour or so, to neutralize free acid with the milk protein, suppress gastric secretion with the cream, and generally soothe the ulcer by coating the stomach. These assumptions have not been supported by research.

There are gradual additions of soft bland foods over a period of time, keeping some food in the stomach at all times to mix with the acid to prevent its corrosive action on the ulcer. These bland foods are usually limited to choices of white toast or crackers, refined cereals, egg, mild cheeses, a few cooked pureed fruits and vegetables, and later, ground meat.

Nonirritating. This therapy is concerned with eliminating chemical, mechanical, and thermal irritation.

CHEMICAL IRRITATION. Any food believed to stimulate gastric secretions is prohibited. These include highly seasoned foods, meat extractives, coffee, tea, alcohol, citrus fruit juices, fried foods, spices, and flavorings.

MECHANICAL IRRITATION. Any food believed to be abrasive in its effect upon the ulcer is prohibited. These include all raw foods, plant fibers (strained fruits and vegetables are used), coarse or rough foods, whole grains, and "gas-forming" or strongly flavored foods.

THERMAL IRRITATION. Any very hot or cold food believed to irritate the lesion by its effect on surface blood vessels is prohibited. These include hot beverages and soups, frozen desserts or iced beverages.

After initial hourly milk and cream only, the diet is gradually increased as the ulcer heals. The routine usually follows a progressive four stage pattern similar to that shown on pp. 501-503.

Liberal individual approach. Accumulating experience and research, however, has begun to challenge the validity of some of these beliefs. In the 1940's, the classic experiments of Wolf and Wolff[3] with their fistulous subject demonstrated the influence of various environmental stimuli. The irritating effect of emotional tension was verified by their observations of engorged blood vessels of the stomach fistula mucosa, increased acid production, and active motility when the man was provoked and anxious. Wolf[4] later fed a variety of highly seasoned foods to his fistulous subject whose stomach and duodenum were normal, and to a second patient with a gastric fistula who also had an active duodenal ulcer. No evidence of irritation to the gastric mucosa appeared in either subject. Wolf even applied several chemicals, including strong condiments, directly through the fistulas to the gastric mucosa of the two subjects. At the same time he also applied the same materials to the skin of their forearms. There was no remarkable effect on the gastric mucosa; the greater reaction was on the skin.

Several other English physicians followed up Wolf's studies with experiments of their own. Gill[5] reported a series of studies with chronic ulcer patients, whose ulcers healed in four to eight weeks with placebo treatment of a daily injection of 1 ml. of distilled water and no diet or exercise restrictions or medications. He concluded that ulcers healed not by manipulation of the various common therapies used but because, ". . . the man with the ulcer comes under the care of a physician who is able to transmit some of his own confidence to the patient." Larger groups of patients with gastric and duodenal ulcers were studied by Lawrence,[6] Todd,[7] and Doll's group.[8] In each instance the results were the same. They each concluded that the current concept of rigid dietary treatment was not verified as superior or sound therapy. Bland foods did not increase the rate of healing, nor was there any particular benefit from avoidance of all foods thought to be commonly irritating.

Studies by American physicians supported these results of English workers. Kramer[9] treated a group of clinic patients with duodenal ulcers with a routine sched-

ule consisting of milk, antacid, and the regular ingestion of foods as desired. There was no dietary restriction. Each patient ate as he chose. Relief and healing in these patients was the same as with those on a strict bland diet. Miller and Berkowitz[10] demonstrated the same results in large series of patients. Satisfactory healing in peptic ulcer disease was obtained on a much more liberal dietary regimen than is conventionally prescribed.

The question of food influence on gastric acidity and irritation has been investigated by several workers. Schneider's group[11] tested a number of spices and herbs on patients with active and healing ulcers and checked the responses by gastroscopy and personal patient reactions. There was no irritating effect from a number of common spices and herbs (allspice, caraway seeds, cinnamon, mace, paprika, thyme, sage) when they were used with foods. Only slight effects were noted by some patients from chili powder, nutmeg, mustard seeds, cloves, and black pepper. The effect of foods on the gastric acidity was studied by Saint-Hilaire's group.[12] The sight, smell, and taste of most food normally initiated gastric secretion. But no significant change in gastric pH was noted with any items, except in the case of alcohol, caffeine, meat extractives, and black pepper. Also, no food is sufficiently acid of itself to effect a significant pH change or cause direct irritation of an ulcer.

Protein foods are effective buffering agents because of their amphoteric nature (p. 45). Milk has some buffering effect, but other protein foods seem to be as effective or more so. All proteins influence acid secretion, however, more than do carbohydrates and fats. Any form of fat tends to suppress gastric secretion and motility through the enterogastrone mechanism (p. 188). Volume of any food sufficient to exert antrum pressure stimulates gastric secretion through the gastrin mechanism (p. 188).

The routine omission of any fiber in the diet also seems to have no basis in fact. Individual modes of eating, improper mastication, and rapid consumption of meals are more involved as sources of irritation. Many clinicians, such as Shull,[13] contend from their experiences with individual patients that so-called course or rough foods, such as lettuce, raw fruits, celery, cabbage, and nuts, do not necessarily traumatize a peptic ulcer when they are properly chewed and mixed with saliva. Grinding or straining of food is needed only when teeth are poor or absent.

Foods labeled "gas-formers" also are questionable routine omissions for all patients with peptic ulcers. Koch and Donaldson[14] found little consistency in the replies of 655 hospitalized patients concerning individual tolerances for standard foods such as onions, fried foods, cabbage, coffee, baked beans, orange juice, milk, nuts, and spiced foods. Symptoms and responses varied widely among the patients, with no greater frequency of intolerance in those with gastrointestinal disease than in those with no disorder of the gastrointestinal tract. It was entirely a matter of individual response.

Basic principles of liberal dietary management. In the light of studies such as the preceding and the accumulative experiences of many physicians in daily practice, what reasonable principles of diet therapy for peptic ulcer disease may be concluded? Certainly, more extensive and controlled research will continue to give needed knowledge on which to base treatment, and will aid in distinguishing between assumption and fact, and between traditional belief and scientific finding. That sound dietary management does play an important part in total therapy is clear. But it seems equally clear that the individual must be the focus of treatment. It is not *an* ulcer; it is *his* ulcer. It is conditioned by his unique make-up and life situation, and the presence of the ulcer in turn affects the patient's life.

Therefore, two basic principles guide the more liberal approach:

1. *The individual must be treated as such.* A careful initial history will give information about daily living situations, attitudes, food reactions, and tolerances. On the basis of such a history a reasonable and adequate dietary program *which he can follow* may be worked out.

2. *The activity of the patient's ulcer will influence dietary management.* During acute periods of active ulceration more vigorous treatment is necessary to control acidity and initiate healing. However, when pain disappears, feedings should be liberalized according to individual tolerance and desire, using a variety of foods. Optimum nutrition and emotional outlook—hence, recovery—are more likely to be supported by such a program. During quiescent periods and for long term prophylaxis when the patient is asymptomatic, he fares best from judicious choice of a wide range of foods and the establishment of regular, unhurried eating habits.

Summary of general diet therapy

The following is a summary of the diet therapy principles for peptic ulcer:

1. There must be *optimum total nutrition* to support recovery and maintenance of health, based on individual needs and food tolerances.

2. *Protein* must be adequate for tissue healing needs and for buffering capacity.

3. *Fat* should be used in moderate amounts for suppression of gastric secretion and motility. Where cardiovascular disease is a concern, reduction of saturated fat may be desired and substitutions made of polyunsaturated fat.[15,16]

4. *Meal intervals and size* should be adequate to maintain individual control of gastric secretions. There should be frequent, small feedings during more active stress periods. Regular meals, moderate in size and sufficient in number for individual need, should be an established habit.

5. *Positive individual needs on a flexible program* rather than negative blanket restrictions on a rigid regimen should be the guide. In any event, picayune

dictums and uncompromising pro-
hibitions have no place. Objective research that eliminates prejudiced ideas
and individual counseling that meets
personal needs together form the keystone of wise peptic ulcer therapy.

INTESTINAL DISEASES
General functional disorders

General functional disorders of the intestine, such as "irritable colon," constipation, or diarrhea, are treated by attention to
underlying cause and symptomatic care.
Adjunct therapy with diet may involve fluid
intake, modification of the diet's fiber content, and adjustment of specific foods according to individual tolerances.

Organic diseases

Organic diseases of the intestine may be
classified in three general groups: (1) anatomical changes, as in diverticulosis, (2)
malabsorption difficulties, as in sprue, and
(3) inflammatory and infectious mucosal
changes, as in ulcerative colitis.

Diverticulosis and diverticulitis

Etiology. Diverticula (L. *diverticulare,*
to turn aside) are small tubular sacs
branching off from a main canal or cavity
in the body. The formation of these small
protrusions from the intestinal lumen,
usually the colon, produces the condition
diverticulosis. More often diverticulosis occurs in older people, and develops at
points of weakened musculature in the
bowel wall.

Clinical manifestations. The condition is
asymptomatic unless the diverticula become
inflamed, a state called *diverticulitis.* Fecal
residue causes increased irritation. There
is pain and tenderness usually localized in
the lower left side of the abdomen, nausea,
vomiting, distention, and intestinal spasm,
accompanied by fever. If the process continues, intestinal obstruction or perforation
may necessitate surgery.

Treatent. During acute periods oral feedings may be limited to clear liquids with
gradual progression to full liquids (p. 471).

Follow-up diet therapy is based on texture
modification, using at first a residue-free
diet, if necessary, then maintenance according to individual need on a low residue
dietary regimen. An outline of a suitable
low residue diet plan is given on p. 507.

Malabsorption syndrome (sprue)

Etiology. The general classification of
malabsorption conditions manifesting the
common characteristic of steatorrhea is
given on p. 403. Adult nontropical sprue is
similar in nature to childhood celiac disease.
In fact, most adults with sprue give a history of having had episodes of celiac disease as a child. A review of the discussion
of celiac disease in Chapter 19 will be
helpful here.

Clinical manifestations. The characteristic diarrhea in sprue consists of multiple
foamy, malodorous, bulky, and greasy
stools. Poor absorption of fat is evident in
the large amounts appearing in the stools
as soaps (saponification of fatty acids with
calcium salts) and fatty acids. Poor absorption of iron produces a microcytic hypochromic anemia. In other persons, a lack of
folic acid will produce a macrocytic anemia.
Poor absorption of vitamin K may lead to
hemorrhagic tendencies. Poor calcium absorption may produce a disturbed serum
calcium to phosphorus ration with resulting
tetany (p. 338). The condition varies widely
among individuals with subsequent differences in severity of symptoms and nature
of treatment.

Treatment—diet therapy. Since the discovery that gluten is an important factor in
the etiology of nontropical sprue (p. 404),
the gluten-free or low gluten diet has been
widely used with marked remission of
symptoms. Gluten is a protein found mainly
in wheat, with additional amounts in rye
and oat. The gliadin fraction of the gluten
protein seems to be the offending agent in
sensitive individuals (p. 404). A regimen
similar to that used by many clinics is the
wheat-, rye-, and oat-free diet given on p.
508. Compare this with the low gluten diet
therapy outlined for children in Chapter 19.

Low residue diet

	Allowed	*Not allowed*
Beverages	Only 2 glasses of milk, if allowed, boiled or evaporated; fruit juices, coffee, tea, carbonated beverages	Alcohol
Eggs	Prepared in any manner, except fried	Fried eggs
Cheese	Cottage, cream, mild American, Tillamook (use in small amounts)	Highly flavored cheeses
Meat or poultry	Roasted, baked, or broiled tender beef, bacon, ham, lamb, liver, veal, fish, chicken, or turkey	Tough meats, pork; no fried meats or highly spiced.
Soup	Bouillon, broth, strained cream soups from the foods allowed	Any others
Fats	Butter, margarine, oils, 1 oz. cream daily	None
Vegetables	Canned or cooked strained vegetable such as asparagus, beets, carrots, peas, pumpkin, squash, spinach, young string beans, tomato juice	Raw or whole cooked vegetables
Fruits	Strained fruit juice, cooked or canned apples, apricots, Royal Anne cherries, peach, pear; dried fruit puree; ripe banana and avocado; all without skins or seeds	All other raw fruits, other cooked fruits
Breads and crackers	Refined bread, toast, rolls, crackers	Pancakes, waffles, whole grain bread or rolls
Cereals	Cooked cereal as Cream of Wheat, Maltomeal, strained oatmeal, cornmeal, cornflakes, puffed rice, Rice Krispies, puffed wheat	Whole grain cereals; other prepared cereals
Potatoes and substitute	Potatoes, white rice, macaroni, noodles, spaghetti	Fried potato, potato chips, brown rice
Desserts	Gelatin desserts, tapioca, angel food or sponge cake, plain custards, water ice or ice cream without fruit or nuts, rennet or simple puddings	Rich pastries, pies, anything with nuts, or dried fruits
Sweets	Sugar, jelly, honey, syrups, gumdrops, hard candy, plain creams, milk chocolate	Other candy; jam, marmalade
Miscellaneous	Cream sauce, plain gravy, salt	Nuts, olives, popcorn, rich gravies, pepper, spices, vinegar

Gluten-free diet for nontropical sprue

Characteristics

1. All forms of *wheat, rye, oat, buckwheat, and barley* are omitted except gluten-free wheat starch (Cellu Products Co.).
2. All other foods are permitted freely, unless specified otherwise by the doctor.
3. The diet should be high in protein, calories, vitamins and minerals.

Foods	Allowed	Not allowed
Milk (2 glasses or more)	As desired	
Cheese	Any, as desired	
Eggs (1 or 2 daily)	As desired	
Meat, fish, fowl (1 or 2 servings)	Any plain meat	Breaded, creamed, or with thickened gravy; no bread dressings.
Soups	All clear and vegetable soups; cream soups thickened with cream, cornstarch, or potato flour only	No wheat flour thickened soup; no canned soup except clear broth
Vegetables (2 servings of green or yellow daily, at least)	As desired, except creamed	No cream sauce or breading
Fruits (At least 2 or 3 daily, including 1 citrus)	As desired	
Bread	Only that made from rice, corn, or soybean flour, or gluten-free wheat starch	All bread, rolls, crackers, cake and cookies made from wheat and rye, Ry-Krisp, muffins, biscuits, waffles, pancake flour and other prepared mixes, rusks, Zwiebach, pretzels; any product containing oatmeal, barley or buckwheat; no breaded food, or food crumbs
Cereals	Cornflakes, cornmeal, hominy, rice, Rice Krispies, Puffed Rice, precooked rice cereals.	No wheat or rye cereals, wheat germ, barley, buckwheat, kasha.
Pastes		No macaroni, spaghetti, noodles, dumplings
Desserts	Jell-o, fruit jell-o, ice or sherbet, homemade ice cream, custard, junket, rice pudding, cornstarch pudding (homemade)	Cakes, cookies, pastry; commercial ice cream and ice cream cones; prepared mixes, puddings; homemade puddings thickened with wheat flour

Gluten-free diet for nontropical sprue—cont'd

Foods	Allowed	Not allowed
Beverages	Milk, fruit juices, gingerale, cocoa (read label to see that no wheat flour has been added to cocoa or cocoa syrup); Coffee (made from ground coffee), tea, carbonated beverages	Postum, malted milk, Ovaltine. (Read labels on instant coffees to see that no wheat flour has been added)
Condiments and sweets	Salt; sugar, white or brown; molasses; jellies and jams; honey, corn syrup	Commercial candies containing cereal products (read labels)
Fats	Butter, margarine, oils	Commercial salad dressings, except pure mayonnaise (read labels)

Caution: Read labels on all packaged and prepared foods.

Ulcerative colitis

Etiology. The cause of ulcerative colitis is unknown and no specific cure has been devised. However, treatment today is far more helpful than in years past, as it is based upon a better understanding of the clinical types of ulcerative colitis and how the pathology involved develops. New drug therapy with more patent antibiotics and endocrine agents has improved the condition in many patients.

Ulcerative colitis usually occurs in young adulthood. In a group of 220 patients studied by Hightower's group[17] the average age at onset for the men was thirty-one and for the women was twenty-nine. Some observers describe a psychogenic overlay in the development of the disease, with patients manifesting various degrees of anxiety and insecurity. However, this is by no means true in all cases.

Clinical manifestations. The common clinical manifestation is a chronic bloody diarrhea which occurs at night as well as during the day. Ulceration of the mucous membrane of the intestine leads to various associated nutritional problems such as anorexia, nutritional edema, anemia, avita-

minosis, protein losses, negative nitrogen balance, dehydration, and electrolyte disturbances. There is weight loss, often general malnutrition, fever, skin lesions, and arthritic joint involvement.

Principles of treatment. The management of patients with active but uncomplicated chronic ulcerative colitis involves the three important factors of rest, nutritional therapy, and sulfanamides. There must be physical, gastrointestinal, and emotional rest. There must be vigorous nutritional therapy. Indeed, many physicians have identified nutrition as the key to successful medical treatment.

Diet therapy. Nutritional therapy for ulcerative colitis is based upon restoration of nutrient deficits and prevention of local trauma to the inflamed area.

High protein. The raw surface of the inflamed colon may be regarded as equivalent to an extensive wound or burn of the skin. There are massive losses of protein from the colon tissue by exudation and bleeding. Also, there are losses associated with impaired intestinal absorption. Only if adequate protein is provided for tissue synthesis can healing take place. The diet

Graduated low residue diet for ulcerative colitis

General directions

1. Monotony in diet should be avoided by varying the foods as much as the diet prescription allows.
2. There is an individual variation in the tolerance to certain foods. If any of the foods in this diet disagrees with the patient, it may require some change in the diet schedule.

Food	Allowed	Not Allowed
Beverages	Carbonated drinks (not iced) in small amounts; coffee or substitutes, tea, special mixtures as prescribed	Milk in any form; fruit juices
Bread	Enriched white or fine rye bread, plain or toasted; plain or salted crackers, Zweibach, melba toast, plain muffins	Whole wheat, dark rye, pumpernickel, or any hot breads
Cereal	Cooked refined or strained—Oatmeal, cream of wheat, cream of rice, Farina, Wheatena; precooked cereals; Pablum, Pabena, Cerevim Dry cereals without bran or shredded wheat; noodles, spaghetti, macaroni, plain rice	Cereals containing bran or shredded wheat; unrefined rice, hominy
Meat	Ground or tender beef, lamb, pork, veal; sweetbreads, brains, liver; may be baked, boiled, broiled or roasted; crisp bacon	Fried, smoked, pickled or cured meats, meat with long fibers, gristle, skin, delicatessen rare meats
Fish	Fresh fish, boiled, broiled or baked; canned, scalded tuna or salmon; crab meat, oysters	Fried fish, lobster, other canned, smoked, pickled, preserved, or gefilte fish
Fowl	Any boiled, broiled, baked or roasted	Gristle, skin, or fat; fried fowl
Egg	Soft or hard, boiled, poached, coddled, plain omelet, scrambled, creamed	Fried
Cheese	Cream, cottage, mild cheddar or American	All other cheeses
Milk	None	
Fat	Butter, or margarine in limited amounts, cream for beverage or cereal; crisp bacon; plain gravies in small amounts	Any other
Soup	Bouillon, broth, meat or poultry; may add strained vegetable juices	Cream soup, vegetable soup
Vegetables	Potatoes without skins	All others
Fruit	None	All
Dessert	Plain angel food, butter, sponge or pound cakes, plain cookies, plain sherbet or water ice, plain ice cream, plain smooth puddings, (rice, tapioca, bread, starch, custard), plain jello in small quantities; gelatin flavored with coffee, strained fruit juices	Nuts, coconut, raisins

Graduated low residue diet for ulcerative colitis—cont'd

Foods	Allowed	Not allowed
Sweets	Plain jelly, sugar, honey, syrup, plain hard candies, in *limited* amounts	Large amounts of any sweets, jam, or marmalade, candy with nuts or fruit, concentrated sweets, rich pastry or candy
Miscellaneous	Spices and seasonings in moderation	Nuts, olives, pickles, popcorn, horseradish, relishes

Additions:

The following foods may be added, in order, only when prescribed. Add each food in small amounts at first until tolerance is assured.

1. Banana, ripe
2. Orange juice—strained and diluted at first—begin with ¼ glass at end of a main meal and gradually increase to full glass
3. Vegetable juice, including tomato—canned, or vegetable juices prepared in a Waring blender and strained
4. Other fruit juices—as with orange juice
5. Vegetables—cooked and strained, or prepared strained baby vegetables
6. Fruits—cooked or stewed, and strained; or prepared strained baby fruits; canned pears; strained applesauce; baked apple without skin or seeds; no dates, figs, or other raw fruits
7. Milk—boiled for three minutes. May be served hot or cold. Begin with ½ glass once daily. May be used in creamed soups, creamed sauce, milk toast, or plain pancakes. Increase slowly to ½ glass three times daily, and finally to one glass at a time as prescribed. May be used with flavoring nutrient powders or cream.
8. Vegetables—tender, whole cooked or canned, not strained. Gradually introduce asparagus tips, carrots, beets, spinach, squash, string beans, peas, and pumpkin. Avoid skin and seeds. No cabbage, cauliflower, onions, radishes, and turnips.
9. Raw, crisp lettuce (finely shredded); raw tomato; no other raw vegetables
10. Unboiled milk

should supply from 120 to 150 gm. of protein per day. Protein supplements, such as between meal feedings using skimmed milk powder, Sustagen, Geveral, Protenum, or Meritene are helpful to achieve the necessary intake. Tasteful ways of including protein foods of high biologic value (egg, meat, cheese) must be devised. Milk causes some difficulty with many patients, so it is usually omitted at first, then gradually added in cooked form, such as cream soups or puddings.

High calorie. At least 3,000 calories a day are needed to restore nutritional deficits from daily losses in the stools and the consequent weight loss. Also, only if sufficient calories are present to support and protect

protein's main catabolic function will the negative nitrogen balance be overcome.

Increased minerals and vitamins. When anemia is present, iron supplements may be ordered. However, in many patients oral iron preparations are poorly tolerated and blood transfusions are used instead. Extra vitamins associated with the healing process and with the metabolism of the increased calories and protein are especially needed. These are ascorbic acid and the B vitamins thiamine, riboflavin, and niacin. Usually additional supplements of these vitamins are ordered. Potassium therapy may also be indicated due to losses from diarrhea and tissue destruction.

Low residue. To avoid irritation to the

colon, the diet is fairly low in residue. In acute stages, it may be almost residue-free (based mainly on lean meat, rice, white bread, Italian pasta, strained cereal, cooked eggs, sugar, butter, and cream). The graduated low residue diet (p. 510) may be used initially, with additional protein and calorie additions in interval feedings. As soon as tolerated, a full bland diet with high protein feedings should be attained. Only heavy roughage need be avoided, as the primary concern is the positive supply of necessary nutrition in as appetizing a manner as possible.

Perhaps no other condition better illustrates the need for a close working relationship between physician, nurse, dietitian, and patient than does chronic ulcerative colitis. The appetite is poor but the nutritional intake is imperative. In many creative ways, individually explored and implemented, the fundamental therapeutic needs may be met—through attractive, nourishing food, given with supportive warmth and encouragement.

References
Specific

1. Sippy, B. W.: Gastric and duodenal ulcers: medical cure by an efficient removal of gastric juice erosion, J.A.M.A. **64**:1625, 1915.
2. Meulengracht, E.: Treatment of haematemesis and malaena with food: mortality, Lancet **2**:1220, 1935.
3. Wolf, S., and Wolff, H. G.: Human gastric function: experimental study of man and his stomach, ed. 2, London, 1947, Oxford University Press, pp. 187-191.
4. Wolf, S.: A clinical appraisal of the dietary management of peptic ulcer and ulcerative colitis, Amer. J. Clin. Nutr. **2**:1, 1954.
5. Gill, A. M.: Pain and healing of peptic ulcer, Lancet **1**:291, 1947.
6. Lawrence, J. S.: Dietetic and other methods in treatment of peptic ulcer, Lancet **1**:482, 1952.
7. Todd, J. W.: Treatment of peptic ulcer, Lancet **1**:291, 1952.
8. Doll, R., Friedlander, P., and Pygott, F.: Dietetic treatment of peptic ulcer, Lancet **1**:5, 1956.
9. Kramer, P.: Symposium on specific methods of treatment: medical treatment of peptic ulcer, Med. Clin. N. Amer. **39**:1381, 1955.
10. Miller, T. G., and Berkowitz, D.: Analysis of results of conservative peptic ulcer therapy, Gastroenterology **20**:353, 1955.
11. Schneider, M. A., DeLuca, V., Jr., and Gray, S. J.: The effect of spice ingestion upon the stomach, Am. J. Gastroent. **26**:722, 1956.
12. Saint-Hilaire, S., Lavers, M. K., Kennedy, J., and Code, C. F.: Gastric acid secretory value of different foods, Gastroenterology **39**:1, 1960.
13. Shull, H. J.: Diet in the management of peptic ulcer, J.A.M.A. **170**:1068, 1959.
14. Koch, J. F., and Donaldson, R. M.: A survey of food intolerances of hospitalized patients, New Eng. J. Med. **271**:657, 1964.
15. Kinsell, L. W., and others: Dietary considerations with regard to type of fat, Amer. J. Clin. Nutr. **15**:198, 1964.
16. Hartroft, W. S.: The incidence of coronary artery disease in patients with Sippy diet, Amer. J. Clin. Nutr. **15**:205, 1964.
17. Hightower, N. C., Jr., and others: Chronic ulcerative colitis. I. Diagnostic considerations, Amer. J. Dig. Dis. 3(n.s.):722, 1958.

General

Abowd, M.: Low gluten diets with recipes, Ann Arbor, University Hospital, University of Michigan, 1958.

Andresen, A. F. R.: Results of treatment of massive gastrict hemorrhage, Amer. J. Dig. Dis. **6**:641, 1939.

Baker, H., et al.: Mechanisms of folic acid deficiency in nontropical sprue, J.A.M.A. **187**:119, 1964.

Clifton, J. A.: Intestinal absorption and malabsorption, J. Amer. Diet. Ass. **39**:449, 1961.

Duncan, G. C.: Some nutritional hazards of the hospitalized patient, J. Amer. Diet. Ass. **25**:330, 1949.

Editorial: Is there a rationale for the bland diet?, J. Amer. Diet. Ass. **33**:608, 1957.

Emàs, S., and Fyrö, B.: Antral gastrin activity in duodenal and gastric ulcers, Gastroenterology **46**:1, 1964.

Frohman, I. P.: Constipation, Amer. J. Nurs. **55**:65, 1955.

Fullerton, D. T., and others: A clinical study of ulcerative colitis, J.A.M.A. **181**:463, 1962.

Gardner, F. H.: Nutritional management of chronic diarrhea in adults, J.A.M.A. **180**:147, 1962.

Green, P. A., and others: Nontropical sprue, J.A.M.A. **171**:157, 1959.

Hardinge, M. G., Swarner, J. B., and Crooks, H.: Carbohydrate in foods, J. Amer. Diet. Ass. **46**:197, 1965.

Hartroft, W. S.: The incidence of coronary artery disease in patients treated with the Sippy diet, Amer. J. Clin. Nutr. **15**:205, 1964.

Hightower, N. C., Jr., and others: Chronic ulcerative colitis. II. Complications, Amer. J. Dig. Dis. 3:861, 1958.

Hightower, N. C., Jr., and others: Chronic ulcerative colitis. III. Treatment, Amer. J. Dig. Dis. 3:931, 1958.

Hock, C. W.: Peptic ulcer—a curse of modern civilization, Amer. J. Clin. Nutr. 15:223, 1964.

Jay, A. N.: Colitis, Amer. J. Nurs. 59:1133, 1959.

Jay, A. N.: Is it indigestion?, Amer. J. Nurs. 58: 1552, 1958.

Kiefer, E. D.: The management of chronic ulcerative colitis, Surg. Clin. N. Amer. 35:809, 1955.

Kirsner, J. B.: Facts and fallacies of current medical therapy for uncomplicated duodenal ulcer, J.A.M.A. 187:423, 1964.

Kramer, P., and Caso, E. K.: Is the rationale for gastrointestinal diet therapy sound?, J. Amer. Diet. Ass. 42:505, 1963.

Marshall, E. A., and Sass, M.: Treatment of peptic ulcer in the aged with unrestricted diet, Geriatrics 4:498, 1956.

McKittrick, J. B., and Shotkin, J. M.: Ulcerative colitis, Amer. J. Nurs. 62:60, 1962.

Mike, E. M.: Practical management of patients with the celiac syndrome, Amer. J. Clin. Nutr. 35:1184, 1959.

Moeller, H. C.: Conventional dietary teatment of peptic ulcer, Amer. J. Clin. Nutr. 15:194, 1964.

Pinter, K. G., and others: Fat absorption studies in various forms of steatorrhea, Amer. J. Clin. Nutr. 15:293, 1965.

Report, Joint Committee on Diet as Related to Gastrointestinal Function of The American Dietetic Association and The American Medical Association, Diet as related to gastrointestinal function, J. Amer. Diet. Ass. 38:425, 1961.

Rider, J. A., and Moeller, H. C.: Food hypersensitivity in ulcerative colitis, Amer. J. Gastroent. 37:497, 1962.

Robinson, C. H.: Fiber in the diet, Amer. J. Clin. Nutr. 4:288, 1956.

Robinson, C. H.: The bland diet, Amer. J. Clin. Nutr. 2:206, 1954.

Rubin, C. E.: Malabsorption: celiac sprue, Ann. Rev. Med. 12:39, 1961.

Rubin, C. E., and others: Studies of caeliac disease, Gastroenterology 38:28, 1960.

Ruffin, J. M., and others: Gluten-free diet for nontropical sprue, J.A.M.A. 188:42, 1964.

Rynbergen, H. J.: In gastrointestinal disease—few dietary restrictions, Amer. J. Nurs. 63:86, 1963.

Schiff, L.: The Meulengracht diet in the treatment of bleeding peptic ulcer, J. Amer. Diet. Ass. 18:298, 1942.

Selesnick, S.: Psychotherapy in chronic peptic ulcer, Gastroenterology 14:364, 1950.

Seymour, C. T., and Weinberg, J. A.: Emotion and gastric activity, J.A.M.A. 171:1193, 1959.

Shiner, M.: Duodenal biopsy, Lancet 1:17, 1956.

Shiner, M.: Effect of a gluten-free diet in 17 patients with idiopathic steatorrhea: a follow-up study, Amer. J. Dig. Dis. 8:969, 1963.

Shiner, M., and Daniach, I.: Histopathological studies in steatorrhea, Gastroenterology 38:419, 1960.

Sleisenger, M. H., and others: A wheat-, rye-, and oat-free diet, J. Amer. Diet. Ass. 33:1137, 1957.

Woldman, E. E.: Peptic ulcer: current medical treatment, Amer. J. Nurs. 59:222, 1959.

Zetzel, L.: Current concepts—treatment of ulcerative colitis, New Eng. J. Med. 271:891, 1964.

CHAPTER 27

Diseases of the liver and gallbladder

METABOLIC FUNCTIONS OF THE LIVER

The liver is a highly active, vital metabolic organ. Through its vast network of biochemical reactions it controls a major portion of the body's internal environment and its functions are intimately related to those of other organ systems. Therefore, when the liver is diseased and its usual cellular activities do not proceed normally, repercussions of this diminished capacity are reflected in numerous metabolic difficulties and clinical manifestations.

Essentially the functions of the liver may be divided into three groups: (1) metabolic functions relating to the majority of the metabolic systems of the entire body, (2) secretory function of producing bile for the gastrointestinal tract, and (3) vascular functions for storing and filtering blood. The first two of these functional categories are of concern here. They bear a direct relationship to the nutritional therapy required by a patient with liver disease.

Therefore, a careful review and clear understanding of the normal metabolic functions of the liver are essential first steps in establishing valid rationale for nutrient modifications in liver disease. These metabolic functions have been discussed at length in previous portions of this text. To guide a review, the outline below is given as a summary of the normal metabolic functions of the liver:

I. Carbohydrate metabolism (Chapter 2)
   A. Formation and storage of glycogen—glycogenesis
   B. Conversion of galactose and fructose to glucose
   C. Conversion of amino acid residues to glucose—gluconeogenesis
   D. Formation of many important chemical compounds from carbohydrate intermediates.

II. Fat metabolism (Chapter 3)
   A. Fat conversion to transport form—formation of lipoproteins
   B. Oxidation of fatty acids to acetoacetic acid, hence to acetyl CoA (active acetate), and into the Krebs' cycle to yield energy
   C. Formation of cholesterol and phospholipids
   D. Formation of bile salts
   E. Conversion of carbohydrate and protein intermediates to fat—lipogenesis

III. Protein metabolism (Chapter 4)
   A. Deamination of amino acids
   B. Provision of lipotropic factor for fat conversion to lipoproteins
   C. Formation of plasma proteins
   D. Urea formation for removal of ammonia from body fluids
   E. Many amino acid interconversions; transamination, amination; synthesis of non-essential amino acids, purines, pyrimidines, creative phosphate, and so on

IV. Other related functions
   A. Vitamin storage—A, D, B_{12} and other B-complex vitamins, K
   B. Conversion of carotene to vitamin A

C. Blood coagulation factors—forms prothrombin in presence of vitamin K; also forms other blood factors such as fibrinogen, accelerator globulin, factor VII
D. Storage of iron as ferritin
E. Conjugation and excretion of steroid hormones.
F. Detoxification of certain drugs—morphine, barbituates

DISEASES OF THE LIVER
Hepatitis

Several types of hepatitis exist, mainly epidemic or infectious hepatitis (IH) and homologous serum or serum hepatitis (SH). However, the resulting clinical syndrome is very much the same, and the two diseases may be considered essentially identical in terms of medical management.

Etiology. The exact organism responsible for hepatitis is not clearly defined. It is probably one of a group of related viruses. In infectious hepatitis the viral agent is transmitted by the oral-fecal route, a common one in many epidemic diseases. Thus, the usual entry is through contaminated food or water. In serum hepatitis the organism is usually transmitted in infected blood (transfusions) or by contaminated instruments[1] (syringes, needles).

Clinical manifestations. The viral agents of hepatitis produce diffuse injury to liver cells, especially the parenchymal cells. In milder cases, the tissue injury is largely reversible, but with increasing severity more extensive necrosis occurs. Massive necrosis in some cases leads to liver failure and death. Thus, varying clinical manifestations appear depending on the degree of liver injury. *Jaundice*, the most obvious manifestation, serves as a rough index of the severity of the disease. However, jaundice is frequently not seen; 80% of the infected individuals in an outbreak of hepatitis may be nonicteric, and thus go undiagnosed and untreated.[2]

After an incubation period of two to six weeks in infectious hepatitis and ten to seventeen weeks in serum hepatitis, manifestations develop. These include general malaise, lassitude, anorexia, diarrhea, headache, fever, enlarged and tender liver, and enlarged spleen. When jaundice develops, it usually follows a preicteric period of five to ten days, deepens for one to two weeks, then levels off and decreases. At this crisis point, sufficient recovery of injured cells has taken place to begin the convalescent period. Convalescence varies from three weeks to three months and is a significant period. Optimum care is essential to avoid relapse.

Treatment. The importance of *bed rest* in the treatment of acute hepatitis has been clearly demonstrated by observations during World War II among groups of infected soldiers.[3] Physical exercise increased both severity and duration of the disease.

A daily intake of 3,000 to 3,500 ml. *fluid* guards against dehydration and gives a general sense of well being and improved appetite.

Optimum nutrition provides the foundation for recovery of the injured liver cells and overall return of strength. It is the major therapy. The principles of diet therapy relate to the liver's function in the metabolism of each nutrient.

Principles of diet therapy

High protein. Protein is essential for liver cell regeneration. It also provides lipotropic agents such as methionine and choline (p. 38) for the conversion of fats to lipoproteins and removal from the liver, thus preventing fatty infiltration. The diet should supply from 75 to 100 gm. of protein daily.

High carbohydrate. Sufficient available glucose must be provided to restore protective glycogen reserves and meet the energy demands of the disease process. Also, an adequate amount of glucose ensures the use of protein for vital tissue regeneration, the so-called protein-sparing action of carbohydrate. The diet should supply from 300 to 400 gms. of carbohydrate daily.

Moderate fat. An adequate amount of fat in the diet makes the food more palatable

Table 27-1. High protein, high caloric formula for milkshakes

Ingredients	Amount	Approximate food value	
Milk	1 cup	Protein	40 gm.
Eggs	2	Fat	30 gm.
Skimmed milk powder or	6 to 8 tbsp.	Carbohydrate	70 gm.
Casec	2 tbsp.	Calories	710
Sugar	2 tbsp.		
Ice cream	1 in. slice or 1 scoop		
Cocoa or other flavoring	2 tbsp.		
Vanilla	few drops, as desired		

and hence the anorexic patient will be more encouraged to eat. Former regimens limited the fat on the basis of preventing fat accumulation in the diseased liver. However, values of better overall nutrition from improved food intake outweigh these concerns, and a moderate amount of easily utilizable fat (whole milk, cream, butter, margarine, vegetable oil, cooking fats) is beneficial. The diet should incorporate from 100 to 150 gm. of such fat daily.

High calorie. From 2,500 to 3,000 calories are needed daily to furnish energy demands of the tissue regeneration process, to compensate for losses due to fever and general debilitation, and to renew strength and recuperative powers.

Meals and feedings. The problem of supplying a diet adequate to meet the increased nutritive demands to a patient whose illness makes food almost repelling to him is a delicate one calling for creativeness and supportive encouragement. The food may need to be in liquid form at first, using concentrated formulas such as the one in Table 27-1 for frequent feedings. As the patient can better tolerate solid food, every effort should be made to prepare and serve appetizing and attractive food. Nutritional therapy is the key to recovery. Therefore, a major nursing responsibility is the devising of ways to encourage an optimal food intake approximating the amount given on p. 517. The nurse and the dietitian

will work closely together to achieve this goal.

Cirrhosis

Liver disease may advance to the chronic state of cirrhosis. The French physician Läennec first named the disease, from the Greek word *kirrhos,* meaning "orange," because the cirrhotic liver was a firm, fibrous mass with orange-colored nodules projecting from its surface. The nutritional or alcoholic form of cirrhosis bears his name, Läennec's cirrhosis.

Etiology. Some forms of cirrhosis result from biliary obstruction or liver necrosis from undetermined causes (idiopathic postnecrotic cirrhosis), or in some cases from previous viral hepatitis. The most common problem, however, is fatty cirrhosis associated with malnutrition. The associated malnutrition may develop from other causes, but usually is the result of a long history of alcoholism. The fatty liver and early cirrhosis may appear within five years from the onset of the alcoholism, but more often 10 to 15 years is required. Increasingly poor food intake as the excessive drinking continues leads to multiple nutritional deficiencies. Damage to the liver cells occurs as fatty infiltration causes cellular destruction and fibrotic tissue changes.

Clinical manifestations. Early signs include gastrointestinal disturbances including nausea, vomiting, anorexia, distention,

High protein, moderate fat, high carbohydrate diet

Daily food plan:
   1 quart milk
   1 to 2 eggs
   8 oz. lean meat, fish, poultry
   4 servings vegetables:
      2 servings potato or substitute
      1 serving green leafy or yellow vegetable
      1 to 2 servings of other vegetables, including 1 raw
   3 to 4 servings fruit (include juices often)
      1 to 2 citrus fruit (or other good source of ascorbic acid)
      2 servings other fruit
   6 to 8 servings bread and cereal (whole grain or enriched)
      1 serving cereal
      5 to 6 slices bread, crackers
   2 to 4 tablespoons butter or fortified margarine
   Additional jam, jelly, honey, and other carbohydrate foods as patient desires and is able to
      eat them. Sweetened fruit juices increase both carbohydrate and fluid.

and epigastric pain. In time, jaundice may appear, increasing weakness, edema, ascites, gastrointestinal bleeding tendencies, and iron-deficiency or hemorrhagic anemia. A macrocytic anemia from folic acid deficiency is also frequently observed.[4]

The protein deficiency produces multiple problems. (1) Low plasma protein levels lead to failure of the capillary fluid shift mechanism (p. 162) when decreased colloidal osmotic pressure causes *ascites* to develop. (2) Lipotropic agents are not supplied to effect fat conversion to lipoproteins and damaging fat accumulates in the liver tissue. (3) Blood clotting mechanisms are impaired as factors such as prothrombin and fibrinogen are not adequately produced. (4) General tissue catabolism and negative nitrogen balance continue the overall degenerative process.

As the disease progresses, fibrous scar tissue increasingly impairs blood circulation through the liver, and portal hypertension develops. Contributing further to the problem is *ascites,* localization of edema fluid within the peritoneal cavity. The impaired portal circulation may lead to *esophageal varices,* with danger of rupture and fatal massive hemorrhage.

Treatment. Treatment is difficult when alcoholism is the underlying problem. Each patient requires individual supportive care and approach (p. 459). Usually therapy is aimed at correction of fluid and electrolyte problems, and nutritional support to encourage hepatic repair as much as is possible.

Principles of diet therapy

Protein according to tolerance. In the absence of impending hepatic coma, the daily protein intake should be 80 to 100 gm. to correct the severe undernutrition, regenerate functional liver tissue, and replenish plasma proteins. However, if signs of hepatic coma appear, the protein is adjusted to individual tolerance.

Low sodium. Sodium is usually restricted to 500 to 1,000 mg. daily to reduce the fluid retention. Outlines of these low sodium diet plans are given in Chapter 28, p. 533.

Texture. If esophageal varices develop, it may be necessary to give soft foods that are smooth in texture to prevent the danger of rupture.

Optimum general nutrition. The remaining overall diet principles outlined for hepatitis are continued for cirrhosis for the same reasons. Calories, carbohydrate, and vitamins are supplied according to individual need and deficiency. Moderate fat is used. Alcohol is strictly forbidden.

Hepatic coma

Etiology. As cirrhotic changes continue in the liver, and portal blood circulation diminishes, collateral circulation develops bypassing the liver. The normal liver, by means of its urea cycle, is by far the most important organ in the body for the removal of ammonia from the blood, converting it to urea for excretion. In the diseased liver, these normal reactions cannot take place. Ammonia-laden blood approaches the liver, cannot follow the usual portal pathways, and is detoured through the collateral circulation. It reenters the systemic blood flow still carrying its ammonia load and produces ammonia intoxication.

Ammonia is formed predominantly in the gastrointestinal tract as the result of enzymatic action on dietary protein. Gastrointestinal bleeding adds still another source, and intestinal bacteria produce more ammonia.

Thus, three variables combine to produce hepatic coma: (1) hepatic functioning of the urea cycle, (2) extent of collateral circulation, and (3) the amount of nitrogenous material in the intestine from dietary protein, blood, and ammonia produced by bacteria.

Low protein diets—15 gm., 30 gm., 40 gm., and 50 gm. protein

General description:
1. The following diets are used when dietary protein is to be restricted.
2. The patterns limit foods containing a large percent of protein, such as milk, eggs, cheese, meat, fish, fowl, and legumes.
3. Avoid meat extractives, soups, broth, bouillon, gravies, and gelatin desserts.

Basic meal patterns: (Contains approximately 15 gm. of protein)

Breakfast	Luncheon	Dinner
½ cup fruit or fruit juice	1 small potato	1 small potato
½ cup cereal	½ cup vegetable	½ cup vegetable
1 slice toast	salad (vegetable or fruit)	salad (vegetable or fruit)
butter	1 slice bread	1 slice bread
jelly	butter	butter
sugar	1 serving fruit	1 serving fruit
2 tbsp. cream	sugar	sugar
coffee	coffee or tea	coffee or tea

For 30 gm. protein
Add: ½ pint milk
    1 ounce meat, 1 egg,
      or equivalent

Examples of meat portions
    1 oz. meat = 1 thin slice roast—2″ x 1½″
      1 rounded tbsp. cottage
        cheese
      1 slice American cheese

For 40 grams protein
Add: ½ pint milk
    2½ oz. meat or 1 egg and
    1½ oz. meat

    2½ oz. meat = Ground beef patty (5
      from 1 lb.)
    1 slice roast

For 50 grams protein
Add: ½ pint milk
    4 oz. meat or 2 eggs and
    2 oz. meat

    4 oz. meat = ¼ lb. meat
    2 lamb chops
    1 average steak

Clinical manifestations. Typical response of the patient involves disorders of consciousness and alterations in motor function. There is apathy, mild confusion, inappropriate behavior, and drowsiness, progressing to coma. Facial expressions are described as an absent stare. The speech may be slurred and monotonous. A typical motor-system change is the coarse, flapping tremor (*asterixis*) observed in the outstretched hands. The breath may have a fecal odor(*fetor hepaticus*).

Treatment. The fundamental principle of therapy is the removal of the sources of excess ammonia. A Sengstaken-Blakemore tube may be used to depress varices and stop bleeding. Antibiotics such as neomycin as well as purgation by enema and a suitable laxative may be administered to reduce ammonia-producing bacteria. Diet adjustments will focus upon reduced intake of protein and control of fluid and electrolytes.

Principles of diet therapy

Low protein. Protein intake is reduced as individually necessary to restrict the exogenous source of nitrogen in amino acids. The amount of restriction will vary with the circumstances. The unconscious patient will receive no protein, but the usual amounts given range from 15 to 50 gm. depending upon whether symptoms are severe or mild. A simple method for controlling the protein intake is given on p. 518. A base meal pattern containing approximately 15 gm. of protein is used, adding small items of protein foods according to the level of total protein desired.

Calories and vitamins. The amount of calories and vitamins are ordered according to need. About 1,500 to 2,000 calories are sufficient to prevent tissue catabolism (a source of more amino acids and available nitrogen). Carbohydrates and fats sufficient for energy needs are essential. Vitamin K is usually given parenterally, along with other vitamins that may be deficient.

Fluid intake. Fluid is carefully controlled in relation to output.

DISEASES OF THE GALLBLADDER
Functions of the gallbladder

Bile produced by the hepatic cells is concentrated and stored in the gallbladder. Liver bile consists largely of bile salts, with additional amounts of bilirubin (a major end-product of hemoglobin decomposition), cholesterol, fatty acids and the usual plasma electrolytes (Na^+, K^+, Ca^{++}, Cl^-, HCO_3^-). When bile is concentrated in the gallbladder, water and most of the electrolytes are reabsorbed by the gallbladder mucosa, leaving the remaining ingredients, especially the bile salts, in a highly concentrated form in the gallbladder bile. The liver secretes about 600 to 800 ml. of bile daily, which the gallbladder normally concentrates five- to ten-fold. Thus, this constant concentrating power enables the gallbladder to accommodate the daily bile in its small 40 to 70 ml. capacity. Through the cholecystokinin mechanism (p. 192), the presence of fat in the duodenum stimulates contraction of the gallbladder and the consequent release of bile into the common duct and then into the small intestine.

Cholecystitis and cholelithiasis

Cholecystitis is an inflammation of the gallbladder, usually resulting from a low grade chronic infection. The infectious process produces changes in the gallbladder mucosa which affect its absorptive powers. Normally, the cholesterol in bile, which is insoluble in water, is kept in solution by the hydrotropic action of the other bile ingredients, especially the bile acids. However, when mucosal changes occur in cholecystitis, the absorptive powers of the gallbladder may be altered, affecting the solubility ratios of the bile ingredients. Excess water may be absorbed, or excess bile acids may be absorbed.

Under these abnormal absorptive conditions, cholesterol may precipitate, causing gallstones (almost pure cholesterol) to form, a condition called *cholelithiasis*. Also, a high dietary fat intake over a long period of time predisposes to gallstone formation because of the constant stimulus to produce

Low fat and fat free diets

General description:
1. This diet contains foods that are low in fat.
2. Foods are prepared without the addition of fat.
3. Fatty meats, gravies, oils, cream, lard, and desserts containing eggs, butter, cream, nuts, and avacados are avoided.
4. Foods should be used in amounts specified and only as tolerated.
5. The sample pattern contains approximately 85 grams protein, 50 grams fat, 220 grams carbohydrate, and 1,670 calories.

	Allowed	*Not allowed*
Beverages	Skimmed milk, coffee, tea, carbonated beverages, fruit juices	Whole milk, cream, evaporated and condensed milk
Bread and cereal	All kinds	Rich rolls, breads, waffles, pancakes
Desserts	Jell-o, sherbet, water ices, fruit whips made without cream, angel food cake, rice and tapioca puddings made with skimmed milk	Pastries, pies, rich cakes, and cookies, ice cream
Fruits	All fruits, as tolerated	Avocado
Eggs	3 allowed per week, cooked any way except fried	Fried eggs
Fats	3 tsp. butter or margarine daily	Salad and cooking oils, mayonnaise
Meats	Lean meat such as beef, veal, lamb, liver, lean fish and fowl, baked, broiled, or roasted without added fat	Fried meats, bacon, ham, pork, goose, duck, fatty fish, fish canned in oil, cold cuts
Cheese	Dry or fat-free cottage cheese	All other cheese
Potato or substitute	Potatoes, rice, macaroni, noodles, spaghetti, all prepared without added fat	Fried potatoes, potato chips
Soups	Bouillon or broth, without fat; soups made with skimmed milk	Cream soups
Sweets	Jam, jelly, sugar, sugar candies without nuts or chocolate	Chocolate, nuts, peanut butter
Vegetables	All kinds as tolerated	The following should be omitted if they cause distress: broccoli, cauliflower, corn, cucumber, green pepper, radishes, turnips, onions, dried peas, and beans
Miscellaneous	Salt in moderation	Pepper, spices; highly spiced food, olives, pickles, cream sauces, gravies

Low fat and fat free diets—cont'd

	Suggested menu pattern	
	Breakfast	*Lunch and dinner*
	Fruit	Meat, broiled or baked
	cereal	potato
	toast, jelly	vegetable
	1 teaspoon butter or margarine	salad with fat-free dressing
	egg 3 times per week	bread, jelly
	skimmed milk, 1 cup	1 teaspoon butter or margarine
	coffee, sugar	fruit or dessert, as allowed
		skimmed milk, 1 cup
		coffee, sugar

Fat free diet

General description:
The following additional restrictions are made to the low fat diet to make it relatively fat free:
1. Meat, eggs, and butter or margarine are omitted
2. Three ounces of fat-free cottage cheese are substituted for meat at the noon and evening meal

more cholesterol as a necessary bile ingredient to metabolize the fat.

Clinical manifestations. When either inflammation, stones, or both are present in the gallbladder, contraction from the cholecytokinin mechanism causes pain. Sometimes the pain is severe. There is fullness and distention after eating, and difficulty particularly with fatty foods.

Treatment. Surgical removal of the gallbladder is usually indicated. However, the surgeon may wish to postpone surgery until the inflammation has subsided. If the patient is obese, as many persons with gallbladder disease are, some weight loss before surgery is advisable. Thus, the supportive therapy is largely dietary.

Principles of diet therapy

Fat. Because fat is the principal cause of contraction of the diseased organ and the subsequent pain, it should be greatly reduced. Calories should come principally from carbohydrate foods, especially during acute phases. The day's diet should be limited in fat to 20 to 30 gm. Later, the patient may tolerate 50 to 60 gm., so that the

diet may be made more palatable. A diet plan for a low fat regimen is given on p. 520.

Calories. If weight loss is indicated, the calories will be reduced according to need. Principles of weight reduction regimens are given in Chapter 24. Usually, such a low calorie reduction diet will have a low fat ratio and meet the needs of the patient with gallbladder disease for fat restriction.

Cholesterol and "gas formers." Two additional modifications usually found on traditional low fat diets for gallbladder disease concern restriction of foods containing cholesterol and foods labeled "gas-formers." Neither modification has valid rationale; the body synthesizes daily several times more cholesterol than is present in an average diet. Thus, restriction of exogenous cholesterol in food has no appreciable effect in reducing gallstone formation.[5] Total dietary fat reduction is more to the point.

Blanket restriction on so-called gas-formers seem unwarranted also. Food tolerances are highly individual (p. 505). A recent survey of hospitalized patients failed to show any differences in food tolerances attributable to the presence of gastrointestinal disorders. Patients with gallbladder disease had no more incidence of specific food intolerances than patients without gastrointestinal disease.[6]

References
Specific

1. Capps, R. B., Sborov, V. M., and Scheiffley, C. H.: A syringe transmitted epidemic of infectious hepatitis, J.A.M.A. **136**:819, 1948.
2. Capps, R. B.: Acute hepatitis, Mod. Treatm. **1**: 393, 1964.
3. Barker, M. H., and others: Acute infectious hepatitis in the Mediterranean theater, J.A.M.A. **128**:997, 1945.
4. Herbert, V., and others: Correlation of folate deficiency with alcoholism and associated macrocytosis anemia and liver disease, Ann. Int. Med. **58**:977, 1963.
5. Committee on Dietary Fat Levels: The regulation of dietary fat, J.A.M.A. **181**:411, 1962.
6. Koch, J. F., and Donaldson, R. M.: A survey of food intolerances of hospitalized patients, New Eng. J. Med. **271**:657, 1964.

General

Bielski, M. T., and Molander, D. W.: Laennec's cirrhosis, Amer. J. Nurs. **65**:82, 1965.
Capps, R. B., and Stokes, J. Jr.: Epidemiology of infectious hepatitis and problems of prevention and control, J.A.M.A. **149**:557, 1952.
Crews, R. H., and Faloon, W. W.: The fallacy of a low-fat diet, J.A.M.A. **181**:754, 1962.
Davidson, C. S.: Cirrhosis in alcoholics. Protein nutrition and hepatic coma, J.A.M.A. **160**:390, 1956.
Davidson, C. S.: Cirrhosis of the liver treated with prolonged sodium restriction. Improvement in nutrition, hepatic function, and portal hypertension, J.A.M.A. **159**:1257, 1955.
Davidson, C. S.: Diet in the treatment of liver disease, Amer. J. Med. **25**:690, 1958.
Flynn, B. M.: Esophageal varices, components of nursing care, Amer. J. Nurs. **64**:107, 1964.
Girolami, M.: Medical management of cirrhosis of the liver, Postgrad. Med. **35**:87, 1964.
Glenn, F.: Surgical treatment of biliary tract disease, Amer. J. Nurs. **64**:88, 1964.
Grollman, A.: Diuretics, Amer. J. Nurs. **65**:84, 1965.

Harper, H. A.: Protein intake in liver disease, J. Amer. Diet. Ass. **38**:350, 1961.
Henderson, L. M.: Nursing care in acute cholecystitis, Amer. J. Nurs. **64**:93, 1964.
Hoffbauer, F. W.: Cirrhosis: general considerations, Mod. Treatm. **1**:434, 1964.
Jones, D. P., and Davidson, C. S.: The treatment of hepatic coma, New Eng. J. Med. **267**:196, 1962.
Kaplan, M. H., and Bernheim, E. J.: Esophageal varices, Amer. J. Nurs. **64**:104, 1964.
Klatskin, G.: Effect of alcohol on the liver, J.A.M.A. **170**:1671, 1959.
LaLonde, J. B., and others: Hepatic regulation of sodium and water in ascites, J.A.M.A. **187**:117, 1964.
Lambert, M.: Fundamental concepts of liver disease, J. Amer. Diet. Ass. **33**:1005, 1957.
Laragh, J. H., and Ames, R. P.: Physiology of body water and electrolytes in hepatic disease, M. Clin. N. Amer. **47**:587, 1963.
Leevy, C. M., and others: B-complex vitamins in liver disease in the alcoholic, Am. J. Clin. Nutr. **16**:339, 1965.
Leevy, C. M.: Portal hypertension and bleeding, Mod. Treatm. **1**:462, 1964.
Nefzger, M. D., and Chalmers, T. C.: The treatment of acute infectious hepatitis. Ten-year follow-up study of the effects of diet and rest, Amer. J. Med. **35**:299, 1963.
Review: Nutritional cirrhosis of the liver, Nutr. Rev. **21**:175, 1963.
Sborov, V. M.: Treatment of chronic viral hepatitis, Mod. Treatm. **1**:410, 1964.
Schiff, L., editor: Diseases of the liver, ed. 2, Philadelphia, 1963, J. B. Lippincott Co.
Summerskill, W. H. J.: Management of the hepatic coma syndromes, Mod. Treatm. **1**:420, 1964.
Victor, M.: Alcohol and nutritional diseases of the nervous system, J.A.M.A. **167**:65, 1958.
Volwiler, W.: Cirrhosis: fluid retention, Mod. Treatm. **1**:451, 1964.
Watson, C.: Current status of treatment of cirrhosis of the liver, J.A.M.A. **166**:764, 1958.
Westerfeld, W. W., and Schulman, M. P.: Metabolism and caloric value of alcohol, J.A.M.A. **170**:197, 1959.

CHAPTER 28

Cardiovascular diseases

Cardiovascular disease is a health problem of major proportion. Its incidence in the United States continues to increase, causing more deaths than all other diseases together,[1] and accounting for cardiac symptoms in about 75% of all adult patients under care in general hospitals. The pattern is the same in other developed countries. It is a problem of wide scope in all of Western society.

Although much has been learned by tremendous research efforts in many areas of the world, the precise etiology of cardiovascular disease is still obscure. Multiple factors have emerged as contributory such as hypercholesteremia, obesity, hypertension, lack of exercise, cigarette smoking, stress. Recent work[2,3] suggests additional links with two other factors—heavy coffee drinking and insufficient sleep—although the association is unclear. Mayer[4] suggests the commonly observed relationship of heavy coffee use to heavy cigarette smoking and insufficient sleep to sedentary late-night television habits.

Three of the established contributory factors have definite dietary relationships. Studies have linked hypercholesteremia to high fat intake, as well as to lack of exercise. The incidence of hypertension is related to high salt use with food. Obesity is the result of calorie intake, especially in carbohydrate foods, in excess of energy expenditure needs, and lack of exercise. Therefore, current diet therapy for patients with heart disease centers on modification of these three factors—fat, sodium, and calories.

The metabolism of these nutrients is associated with problems in atherosclerosis, congestive heart failure, hypertensive cardiovascular disease, and acute myocardial infarction.

THE PROBLEM OF ATHEROSCLEROSIS

Atherosclerosis, a basic pathologic process in coronary heart disease, remains an enigma in modern medicine. Fatty degeneration and thickening occurs in arterial walls with plaque formations, narrowing of the vessel lumen, development of blood clots, and eventual occlusion of the involved artery. The tissue area serviced by the involved artery is deprived of its vital oxygen and nutrient supply (ischemia) and the cells die. The localized area of dying or dead tissue is called an *infarct*. When the artery is one supplying the cardiac muscle (myocardium), the result is an acute myocardial infarction.

Etiology—relation to lipid metabolism. A search for the cause of atherosclerosis, the underlying disease process, has focused attention on *lipid metabolism* for two reasons: (1) the artery deposits and plaque formations are largely cholesterol and other fatty materials, and (2) an elevated blood cholesterol level (hypercholesteremia) and elevation of other serum lipids (hyperlipidemia, hypertriglyceridemia) is usually present. A number of large-scale studies have demonstrated a definite association between types of dietary fat and effect on elevated blood lipid levels. Dietary substitution of foods high in polyunsaturated fatty acids for foods high in saturated fatty acids produced a lowering of blood cholesterol. However, what the significance of lowered cholesterol levels is in terms of the disease process is unknown. If the serum cholesterol value returns to normal, is further atherosclerosis prevented? Is the disease process reversed? These are the important questions to which answers have not been found. But the mass of clinical and experimental data does suggest some disorder related to lipid metabolism.

Chapter 3 on fat metabolism should be reviewed carefully. The concepts of fatty acid saturation and unsaturation, essential fatty acid, and related fat substances such as cholesterol and lipoproteins should be

Table 28-1. Fat controlled diets on three calorie levels*

Diet plans	Total calories from fat	Total day's exchanges		
		1,200 calories P/S ratio 1.1:1	1,800 calories P/S ratio 1.3:1	2,400 calories P/S ratio 1.5:1
I. Modified fatty acid content	40%			
Milk		2	2	2
Vegetables A		As desired	As desired	As desired
Vegetables B		1	1	1
Fruit		3	5	5
Bread and cereals		4	6	8
Meat, fish, poultry		5	6	7
Eggs (if desired, as part of the meat exchange)		4 per week	4 per week	4 per week
Fat		5	9	15
Special margarine		1		3
Sugar, sweets			9	12
II. Moderate fat reduction	25%			
Milk		2	2	2
Vegetables A		As desired	As desired	As desired
Vegetables B		1	1	1
Fruit		6	8	10
Bread and cereals		3	5	6
Meat, fish, poultry		6	7	9
Eggs (if desired, as part of the meat exchange)		4 per week	4 per week	4 per week
Fat		3	6	8
Sugar, sweets		—	8	22
III. Severe fat reduction	10%			
Milk		2	2	2
Vegetables A		As desired	As desired	As desired
Vegetables B		1	1	1
Fruit		5	8	9
Bread and cereals		4	7	7
Meat, fish, poultry		6	7	9
Eggs (if desired, as part of the meat exchange)		4 per week	4 per week	4 per week
Fat		—	—	—
Sugar, sweets		8	15	36

*Adapted from The regulation of dietary fat, Food and Nutrition Council, American Medical Association, J.A.M.A. 181:411-429, 1962.

Food exchange lists for fat controlled diets.*

List 1—Milk exchanges

Nonfat dried milk	¼ cup
Skimmed milk	1 cup
Buttermilk (made from skimmed milk)	1 cup

List 2—Vegetable exchanges

Vegetable A	As desired
Asparagus	
Beans, string, young	
Broccoli	
Brussels sprouts	
Cabbage	
Lettuce	
Mushrooms	
Okra	
Pepper	
Radishes	
Califlower	
Celery	
Chicory	
Cucumber	
Escarole	
Eggplant	
Sauerkraut	
Squash, summer	
Tomatoes	
Watercress	
Greens (beet greens, chard, collard,)	
Vegetable B	½ cup per serving
Beets	
Carrots	
Onions	
Peas, green	
Pumpkin	
Rutabaga	
Squash, winter	
Turnip	

List 3—Fruit exchanges

Apple (2 in. diameter)	1
Applesauce	½ cup
Apricots	
fresh	2 medium
dried	4 halves
Banana	½ small
Blackberries	1 cup
Blueberries	⅔ cup
Cantaloupe (6 in. diameter)	¼
Cherries	10 large
Dates	2

*Adapted from The regulation of dietary fat, Food and Nutrition Council, American Medical Association, J.A.M.A. **181**(5):411, 1962.

Continued.

Food exchange lists for fat controlled diets—cont'd

List 3—Fruit exchanges—cont'd.

Figs	
fresh	2 large
dried	2
Grape juice	½ cup
Grapefruit	½ small
Grapefruit juice	½ cup
Grapes	12
Honeydew melon (7 in. diameter)	⅛
Mango	½ small
Orange	1 small
Orange juice	½ cup
Papaya	⅓ medium
Peach	1 medium
Pear	1 small
Pineapple	½ cup
Pineapple juice	⅓ cup
Plums	2 medium
Prunes, dried	2 medium
Raisins	2 tbsp.
Raspberries	1 cup
Strawberries	1 cup
Tangerine	1 large
Watermelon	1 cup

List 4—Bread exchanges

Bread	1 slice
†Biscuit, muffin, roll (2 in. diameter)	1
†Cornbread (1½ in. cube)	1
Cereal, cooked	⅓ cup
dry, flake or puffed	¾ cup
Rice, grits, cooked	½ cup
Spaghetti, noodles, cooked	½ cup
Macaroni, cooked	½ cup
Crackers, graham	2
saltines	5
soda	3
Beans, peas, dried, cooked	½ cup
Corn, sweet	⅓ cup
Corn on the cob, medium ear	½
Potatoes, white (2 in. diameter)	1
Potatoes, sweet	½ cup
Parsnips	⅔ cup

List 5—‡Meat, fish, and poultry exchanges

(Select meat from this group for 3 meals a week)	
Beef, eye of round, top and bottom round, lean, ground round, lean rump, tenderloin	1 oz.
Lamb, leg only	1 oz.
Pork, lean loin	1 oz.
Ham, lean and well trimmed	1 oz.

†Made with corn or cottonseed oil. Diets planned according to American Diabetes Association exchange system.
‡Meat exchanges were calculated as containing 3 gm. fat instead of ADA value of 5 gm.

Food exchange lists for fat controlled diets—cont'd

List 5—‡Meat, fish, and poultry exchanges—cont'd

(Make selections from this group for 11 meals a week)

Chicken, no skin	1 oz.
Turkey, no skin	1 oz.
Veal	1 oz.
Fish	1 oz.
Shellfish	1 oz.
Meat substitute, cottage cheese, preferably uncreamed	¼ cup

List 6—Eggs

Four eggs per week allowed (as part of meat exchanges) in each diet plan at discretion of physician

List 7—Fat exchanges

50% polyunsaturated

Corn oil	1 tsp.
Cottonseed oil	1 tsp.
Safflower oil	1 tsp.
Mayonnaise made with corn or cottonseed oil	1 tsp.
French dressing made with corn or cottonseed oil	2 tsp.

30% to 40% polyunsaturated

Special margarines	1 tsp.
Special shortenings	1 tsp.

List 8—§Sugar exchanges

White, brown, or maple sugar	1 tsp.
Corn syrup, honey, molasses	1 tsp.
Candy (no chocolate)	
gum drops	1 medium or six small
hard-type	6 to 8 small fruit drops
mints, cream	3—4
marshmallow, plain	1 average
jelly, jams, all varieties	1 tsp.
sherbet	1 tbsp.
carbonated beverages	2 oz.

‡Meat exchanges were calculated as containing 3 gm. fat instead of ADA value of 5 gm.
§1 oz. alcohol = 1 sugar exchange and may be substituted at discretion of physician.

clearly understood in theory and in terms of foods. Patients will need brief, concise explanations of their diet and its rationale. Misunderstandings gained from lay articles or public advertising of food products may need to be corrected and clarified. The food fat spectrum, Fig. 3-2, p. 31, will be a useful tool in teaching.

Principles of diet therapy— fat-controlled diets

Amount of fat. About half the calories of the average American's diet is contributed by fat. It is suggested that this be moderated to about 35%, or lower if weight reduction is needed.

Kind of fat. About two-thirds of the total

fat in the American diet is of animal origin, and therefore is mainly saturated fat. The remaining one-third comes from vegetable sources, and is mainly unsaturated fat. The fat-controlled diet reduces the animal fat and uses instead more plant fat, bringing the ratio of polyunsaturated fat calories to about half of the total fat calories.

American Medical Association fat-controlled diets. The Council on Foods and Nutrition of the American Medical Association has outlined a series of three fat-controlled diets, each one on three calorie levels, with the ratio of polyunsaturated fatty acids to saturated fatty acids ranging from 1:1 to 1.5:1.[5] These diets may serve as guides for physicians who wish to use them with indicated patients:

1. Modified fatty acid content—35% fat, 40% of total calories.
2. Moderate fat reduction—fat, 25% of total calories
3. Severe fat reduction—fat, 10% of total calories.

The basic food exchange groups of the American Diabetes Association exchange system of dietary control (p. 483) are modified for fat content and an additional list of sugar exchanges outlined. These groups provide a basis for food choices on each of the three calorie levels—1,200 calories for weight reduction, 1,800 calories for reduction or maintenance, and 2,400 calories for maintenance. The day's food plan for each diet is given in Table 28-1. The modified food exchange groups are listed in the box on p. 525. A simplified fat-controlled diet list for general use without specific calorie modification is given on p. 529.

EDEMA CONTROL IN CONGESTIVE HEART FAILURE

In congestive heart failure the weakened myocardium is unable to maintain an adequate cardiac output to sustain a normal blood circulation. The resulting fluid imbalances cause edema to develop (p. 169) bringing problems in breathing and placing added stress on the laboring heart.

Etiology—relation to sodium and water metabolism

Imbalance in capillary fluid shift mechanism. As the heart fails to pump out the returning blood fast enough, the venous return is retarded and a disproportionate amount of blood accumulates in the vascular system concerned with the right side of the heart. The venous pressure rises, overcoming the balance of filtration pressures necessary to maintain the normal capillary fluid shift mechanism. (See Fig. 9-5, p. 162 for a diagram of this mechanism.) Fluid which normally would flow between the interstitial spaces and the blood vessels is held in the tissue spaces, rather than being returned to circulation.

Hormonal mechanisms. The aldosterone mechanism (Fig. 9-8, p. 169) compounds the edema problem. As the heart fails to propel the blood circulation forward, the deficient cardiac output effectively reduces the renal blood flow. The decreased renal blood pressure triggers the release of renin, an enzyme from the renal cortex that combines in the blood with its substrate, angiotensinogen, to produce angiotensin I and II. Angiotensin II acts as a stimulant to the adrenal gland. It causes the adrenals to produce aldosterone, the hormone which in turn effects a reabsorption of sodium in an ion exchange with potassium in the distal tubules of the nephrons, and water absorption follows. Ordinarily, this is a life-saving mechanism to protect the body's water supply. In congestive heart failure, however, it only adds to the edema problem.

The ADH mechanism, (Fig. 9-9, p. 170) adds to the edema also. The cardiac stress and the reduced renal flow cause the release of *vasopressin,* the antidiuretic hormone from the pituitary gland. This hormone stimulates still more water reabsorption in the distal tubules of the nephrons.

Increased cellular free potassium. As the reduced blood circulation depresses cellular metabolism, protein catabolism releases protein-bound potassium in the cell, increasing intracellular osmotic pressure from free potassium. Sodium ions in the sur-

Controlled fat diet—high polyunsaturated fatty acids diet

	Foods allowed	*Foods not allowed*
Soups	Bouillon cubes, vegetables and broths from which fat has been removed. Cream soups made with nonfat milk	Meat soups, commercial cream soups and cream soups made with whole milk or cream
Meat, fish, poultry	One or two servings daily (not to exceed a total of 4 oz.) lean muscle meat, broiled or roasted; beef, veal, lamb, pork, chicken, turkey, lean ham, organ meats (all visible fat should be trimmed from meat); all fish and shell fish	Bacon, pork sausage, luncheon meat, dried meat, and all fatty cuts of meat; weiners, fish roe, duck, goose, skin of poultry, and T. V. dinners
Milk and milk products	At least one pint nonfat milk or nonfat buttermilk daily; nonfat cottage cheese, Sap Sago cheese	Whole milk and cream; all cheeses (except nonfat cottage cheese), ice cream, imitation ice cream (except that containing safflower oil), ice milk, sour cream, commercial yogurt
Eggs	Egg whites only	Egg yolks
Vegetables	All raw or cooked as tolerated (leafy green and yellow vegetables are good sources of vitamin A)	No restrictions
Fruits	All raw, cooked, dried, frozen or canned; use citrus or tomato daily; fruit juices	Avocado and olives
Salads	Any fruit, vegetable, and gelatin salad	
Cereals	All cooked and dry cereals; serve with nonfat milk or fruit; macaroni, noodles, spaghetti, and rice	
Breads	Whole wheat, rye, enriched white, French bread, English muffins, graham crackers, saltine crackers	Commercial pancakes, waffles, coffee cakes, muffins, doughnuts and all other quick breads made with whole milk and fat; biscuit mixes and other commercial mixes, cheese crackers, pretzels
Desserts	Fruits, tapioca, cornstarch, rice, Junket puddings all made with nonfat milk and without egg yolks; fruit whips made with egg whites, gelatin desserts, angel food cake, sherbet, water ices, and special imitation ice cream containing vegetable safflower oil; cake and cookies made with nonfat milk, oil, and egg white; fruit pie (pastry made with oil)	Omit desserts and candies made with whole milk, cream, egg yolk, chocolate, cocoa butter, coconut, hydrogenated shortenings, butter and other animal fats

Continued.

Controlled fat diet—high polyunsaturated fatty acids diet—cont'd

	Foods allowed	*Foods not allowed*
Concentrated fats	Corn oil, soybean oil, cotton seed oil, sesame oil, safflower oil, sunflower oil, walnuts and other nuts except cashew and those commercially fried or roasted	Butter, chocolate, coconut oil, hydrogenated fats and shortenings, cashew nuts; mineral oil, olive oil, margarine, except as specified; commercial salad dressings, except as listed; hydrogenated peanut butter; gravy, except as specified
	Margarine made from above oils, such as Award, Mazola, Emdee, Fleishmann's, and Kraft Corn Oil	
	Commercial French and Italian salad dressing if not made with olive oil	
	Gravy may be made from bouillon cubes, or fat-free meat stock thickened with flour and add oil if desired	
	Freshly ground or old fashioned peanut butter	
Sweets	Jelly, jam, honey, hard candy, and sugar	
Beverages	Tea, coffee, or coffee substitutes; tomato juice, fruit juice, cocoa prepared with non-fat milk	Beverages containing chocolate, ice cream, ice milk, eggs, whole milk or cream

If the diet is also to be high in unsaturated fat it should include liberal amounts of:
1. Oils allowed which can be incorporated in salad dressings, or added to soups, to nonfat milk, to cereal, to vegetables
2. Walnuts, almonds, Brazil nuts, Filberts, pecans
3. Extra margarine in or on foods

rounding extracellular fluid increase to prevent hypotonic dehydration (pp. 161 and 180). The increased extracellular sodium in time adds to more water retention.

The metabolism of sodium, potassium, and water in Chapter 9 should be reviewed. These mechanisms are discussed there in greater detail with diagrams, and will help clarify the abnormal shifts and balances involved in cardiac edema which produce a serious dislocation in the body water compartments.

Principles of diet therapy—sodium restricted diets

Because of the role of sodium in water balance, the diet used to treat cardiac edema restricts the sodium intake. Four levels of dietary sodium restriction have been outlined by the American Heart Association and are in common use throughout the United States. They may best be understood in reference to the usual range of dietary sodium and the common food items each level of restriction would affect.

Sodium in general diet. The taste for salt is an acquired one. Some persons salt food heavily and habituate their taste to high salt levels. Others acquire lighter tastes and use smaller amounts. Common daily adult intakes of sodium range rather widely from about 3 or 4 gm. with lighter tastes to as high as 10 to 12 gm. with heavy use.

Sodium-restricted diets. The main source of dietary sodium is in sodium chloride, common table salt. Many other lesser-used sodium compounds (baking powder, baking soda) contribute small amounts. Other-

Restrictions for a mild low sodium diet (2 to 3 gm. sodium)

Do not use:

1. Salt at the table (use salt lightly in cooking)
2. Salt preserved foods such as salted or smoked meat (bacon and bacon fat, bologna, dried or chipped beef, corned beef, frankfurters, ham kosher meats, luncheon meats, salt pork, sausage, smoked tongue); salted or smoked fish (anchovies, caviar, salted and dried cod, herring, sardines; sauerkraut, olives)
3. Highly salted foods such as crackers, pretzels, potato chips, corn chips, salted nuts, salted popcorn
4. Spices and condiments such as bouillon cubes,* catsup,* chili sauce,* celery salt, garlic sauce, onion salt, monosodium glutamate, meat sauces, meat tenderizers,* pickles, prepared mustard, relishes, worcestershire sauce, soy sauce
5. Cheese,* peanut butter*

*Dietetic low sodium kind may be used.

Restrictions for a moderate low sodium diet (1,000 mg. sodium)

Do not use:

1. Salt in cooking or at the table
2. Salt preserved foods such as salted or smoked meat (bacon and bacon fat, bologna, dried or chipped beef, brains, corned beef, frankfurters, ham, kosher meats, luncheon meats, salt pork, sausage, smoked tongue, kidneys); salted or smoked fish (anchovies, caviar, salted and dried cod, herring, sardines, frozen fish fillets, canned salmon,* tuna*); sauerkraut, olives
3. Highly salted foods such as crackers, pretzels, potato chips, corn chips, salted nuts, salted popcorn
4. Spices and condiments such as bouillon cubes,* catsup,* chili sauce,* celery salt, garlic salt, onion salt, monosodium glutamate, meat sauces, meat tenderizers,* pickles, prepared mustard, relishes, worcestershire sauce, soy sauce
5. Cheese,* peanut butter*
6. Buttermilk (unsalted buttermilk may be used) instead of skimmed milk
7. Canned vegetables* or canned vegetable juices*
8. Frozen peas, frozen limas, frozen mixed vegetables or any frozen vegetables to which salt has been added
9. More than one serving of any of these vegetables in one day—artichokes, beet greens, beets, carrots, celery, dandelion greens, kale, mustard greens, spinach, swiss chard, turnips (white)
10. Regular bread, rolls,* crackers*
11. Dry cereals,* except puffed rice, puffed wheat, and shredded wheat
12. Quick cooking cream of wheat
13. Shell fish—clams, crab, lobster, shrimp (oysters may be used)
14. Salted butter, salted margarine, commercial French dressings,* mayonnaise,* or other salad dressings*
15. Regular baking powder,* baking soda or anything containing them; self-rising flour
16. Prepared mixes—Pudding,* gelatin,* cake, biscuit
17. Commercial candies

*Dietetic low sodium kinds may be used

wise, the remaining dietary source is sodium occurring in foods as a natural mineral. The four levels of sodium-restricted diets delete in turn an increasing number of food items or ways of food preparation.

Mild sodium restriction (2 to 3 gm. sodium). Salt may be used *lightly* in cooking, but no *added* salt is allowed. Obviously, salty foods (salt used as a preservative or flavoring agent) are deleted such as pickles, olives, bacon, ham, and potato chips. A list for mild sodium restriction is shown on p. 531.

Moderate sodium restriction (1,000 mg.). There may be no salt in cooking, no added salt, and no salty foods. Beginning with this level, some control of natural sodium foods is evident. Higher sodium vegetables

are limited in use, salt-free canned vegetables are substituted for regular canned ones, salt-free baked products are used, and meat and milk are used in moderate portions. The moderate sodium restriction list is shown on p. 531.

Strict sodium restriction (500 mg.). In addition to the deletions thus far, meat, milk and egg are allowed in smaller portions. Milk is limited to two cups total in any form, meat to 5 to 6 oz. total, and no more than one egg. Higher sodium vegetables are deleted. A list of restrictions for a strict low sodium diet is shown below.

Severe sodium restriction (250 mg.). No regular milk may be used; low sodium milk is substituted. Meat is limited to 2 to 4 oz. total, and egg to about three a week. It

---

Restrictions for a strict low sodium diet (500 mg. sodium)

Do not use:

1. Salt in cooking or at the table
2. Salt preserved foods such as salted or smoked meat—bacon and bacon fat, bologna, dried or chipped beef, brains, corned beef, frankfurters, ham, kosher meats, luncheon meats, salt pork, sausage, smoked tongue, kidneys; salted or smoked fish—anchovies, caviar, salted and dried cod, herring, sardines, frozen fish fillets, canned salmon,* tuna*; sauerkraut; olives
3. Highly salted foods such as crackers, pretzels, potato chips, corn chips, salted nuts, salted popcorn
4. Spices and condiments such as bouillon cubes,* catsup,* chili sauce,* celery salt, garlic salt, onion salt, monosodium glutamate (M.S.G., Accent, etc.), meat sauces, meat tenderizers,* pickles, prepared mustard, relishes, worcestershire sauce, soy sauce
5. Cheese,* peanut butter*
6. Buttermilk (unsalted buttermilk may be used) instead of skimmed milk
7. More than one pint skimmed milk a day, including that used on cereal
8. Any commercial foods made of milk (ice cream, ice milk, milk shakes)
9. Canned vegetables* or canned vegetable juices*
10. Frozen peas, frozen limas, frozen mixed vegetables, or any frozen vegetables to which salt has been added
11. These vegetables—artichokes, beet greens, beets, carrots, celery, dandelion greens, kale, mustard greens, spinach, swiss chard, turnips (white)
12. Regular bread,* rolls,* crackers*
13. Dry cereals,* except puffed rice, puffed wheat, and shredded wheat
14. Quick cooking cream of wheat
15. Shell fish—clams, crab, lobster, shrimp (oysters may be used)
16. Salted butter, salted margarine, commercial French dressings,* mayonnaise,* or other salad dressings*
17. Regular baking powder,* baking soda, or anything containing them; self-rising flour
18. Prepared mixes—pudding,* gelatin, cake, biscuit
19. Commercial candies

---

*Dietetic low sodium kinds may be used

Low sodium diet (500 mg. sodium)

General description:

1. All foods are to be prepared and served without the addition of salt, baking powder or baking soda.
2. Take only those foods which are tolerated and in the amounts specified.
3. Read all food labels for the *addition of salt or sodium in form.*
4. Avoid medications and laxatives unless approved by your doctor.
5. The suggested menu pattern for 500 mg. sodium contains approximately 275 grams carbohydrate, 85 grams protein, 130 grams fat, and 2,300 calories. All menu patterns meet the recommended allowances of vitamins and minerals.

	Daily allowance	*Foods to avoid*
Milk	Limit to 2 cups milk daily—frozen, powdered, or canned or as 1 cup evaporated milk, used as beverage or in cooking; 2 tbsp. cream (1 ounce)	Malted milk, sour cream, butter-milk, condensed milk, milk-shakes, chocolate milk, fruit flavored beverage powders, whipped toppings
Eggs	One daily	
Meat, poultry fish	Six ounces cooked daily; fresh beef, lamb, liver, pork, veal, rabbit, chicken, duck, goose, quail, turkey, cod, halibut, filet sole, tuna, salmon or meats canned without salt, frozen meat containing no salt or sodium (beef or calf liver allowed not more than once in two weeks)	All meat, poultry, fish not listed; avoid meat, fish or poultry that is smoked, cured, canned, frozen, containing salt or sodium, pickled, salted or dried (bacon, ham, luncheon meats, sausages, salt pork, canned salmon and tuna, sardines), clams, crabs, lobsters, (oysters Eastern), scal-lops, shrimp, anchovies, salted dried cod, frozen fish fillets, com-mercial meat pies, T. V. dinners
Cheese	Special dietetic low sodium cheese may be used as a meat substitute as part of the daily allowance	Any other.
Fruit	Three servings daily including one citrus fruit—½ cup per serving, fresh, canned or frozen.	Dried figs, raisins containing sodium sulfite.
Vegetables	Four servings daily (fresh, frozen, or dietetic canned vegetables only)—½ cup per serving; asparagus, green beans, wax beans, lima beans, navy beans, broccoli, cauliflower, corn, cucumber, endive, egg plant, lentils, onions, parsnips, peppers, radishes, rutabagas, cabbage, brussel sprouts, lettuce, mushrooms, okra, soybeans, squash, tomatoes, unsalted tomato juice, turnip greens	Canned vegetables or juices con-taining salt (V-8 juice), sauer-kraut, white turnip, beets, celery, carrot, artichoke; greens —beets, spinach, chard, dande-lions, kalo, mustard greens; frozen peas, frozen lima beans, frozen mixed vegetables
Potato or substitute	Two servings daily of potato, rice, macaroni, spaghetti, noodles, fresh sweet potatoes	Potato chips, corn chips

Continued.

Low sodium diet (500 mg. sodium)—cont'd

	Daily allowance	Foods to avoid
Cereal	One serving daily shredded wheat, puffed rice, puffed wheat, or cooked cereals which contain no added salt or sodium as regular Cream of Wheat, cornmeal, Maltomeal, rice, Wheatena, Pettijohns, Ralston, oatmeal.	Quick-cooking Cream of Wheat and all other ready to eat cereals not listed; selfrising flour
Breads	Low sodium bread or unsalted matzoth; low sodium crackers.	Potato chips, salted crackers, salted pop corn, pretzels, regular bread, roll, biscuits, or muffins, waffles, commercial mixes
Fats	Sweet butter, lard, salad oils, shortening, low sodium salad dressing as desired; unsalted margarine (check label and brand)	Salted nuts, salted butter, bacon fat, margarine, salted peanut butter, gravies and commercial salad dressings
Soup	Homemade soup made with allowed meat, vegetables, and milk	Broth, bouillon, consomme, and canned soups.
Sweets	Jelly, jam, sugar, honey, gumdrops, marshmallows as desired; small amounts of brown sugar	Any commercial jam and jelly containing a sodium preservative, molasses, candy, candy bars
Desserts	Fruit, gelatin dessert made with plain gelatin and fruit juice, fruit pie made without salt; rice, tapioca or cornstarch pudding made with low sodium milk and/or fruit and fruit juices, desserts made with sodium free baking powder	All others, ice cream, sherbet, desserts made with regular baking powder, baking soda, rennet tablets, pudding mixes; commercial gelatin desserts, pudding and cake mixes
Beverages	Tea, coffee, postum, sanka, cocoa, (except Dutch process) made with low sodium milk allowance, fruit juice	Instant cocoa mix, prepared beverage mixes
Condiments	Allspice, bay leaves, caraway seeds, cinnamon, curry powder, garlic, mace, marjoram, mustard powder, nutmeg, paprika, parsley, pimiento, rosemary, sage, sesame seeds, thyme, tumeric, ginger, pepper, vinegar; extracts of almond, lemon, vanilla, peppermint, walnut, maple	Celery salt, garlic salt, catsup, prepared mustard, salt, meat sauces, meat tenderizers, monosodium glutamate, soy sauce, pickles, relishes, olives, prepared horseradish, worcestershire sauce, chili sauce, seasoning salts
Miscellaneous		Baking powder, baking soda, chewing tobacco

500 mg. sodium diet suggested menu pattern

Breakfast	Lunch	Dinner
1 fruit	3 ounces unsalted meat	3 ounces unsalted meat
1 egg	unsalted potato	unsalted potato
Low sodium cereal	low sodium vegetable	low sodium vegetable
1 low sodium bread	low sodium vegetable salad	low sodium salad
1 unsalted butter	1 low sodium bread	1 low sodium bread

Low sodium diet (500 mg. sodium)—cont'd

500 mg. sodium diet suggested menu pattern—cont'd

	Daily allowance	*Foods to avoid*
jelly	1 unsalted butter	1 unsalted butter
½ cup milk	jelly	jelly
coffee	1 fruit	1 cup milk
2 tbsp. cream (1 oz.)	½ cup milk	coffee
	coffee	fruit

Modifications for a 250 mg. sodium diet

The 250 mg. sodium diet is essentially the same as the 500 mg. sodium diet except:
1. Use low sodium milk (2 or more glasses) instead of regular milk.
2. Use only 5 ounces of meat instead of 6 ounces.
3. Omit the cream.

Modifications for a 1,000 mg. sodium diet

One of the three following modifications may be used to raise the sodium content in the 500 mg. sodium diet to 1,000 mg.

Modification I
1. 2 slices regular bread are allowed daily
2. 2 teaspoons only regular butter (above this amount, unsalted butter must be used)
3. One serving (½ cup) is allowed daily of spinach, celery, carrots, beets, artichoke, white turnip

Modification II (high protein)
1. 10 oz. of meat are allowed instead of 6 oz.
2. 1 serving of prepared or milk dessert, such as ice cream, custard, gelatin, or 1 cup milk
3. 2 eggs instead of 1
4. One serving of spinach, celery, carrots, beets or artichoke is allowed

Modification III
1. 3 slices regular bread may be used in place of the low sodium bread (above this amount, unsalted bread must be used)

becomes more important, therefore, to devise ways of incorporating adequate low sodium milk to ensure adequate protein intake. The liquid beverage forms (whole and skimmed), available from processing plants in most larger urban centers, are quite acceptable if well chilled and served immediately upon thawing. Because these fresh milk products deteriorate rapidly after the sodium is removed, the milk is usually frozen and delivered to consumers in this form. If it is thawed just before using, and consumed immediately while still icy, it is very palatable.

The lists of foods that should not be used for each sodium-restricted diet level have proved to be useful tools in patient education to identify for them key foods affected in maintaining a particular sodium intake. The lists also are helpful for general comparison of the diets when changes are made from one level to another.

HYPERTENSIVE CARDIOVASCULAR DISEASE

Hypertension alone is not a disease. It is a symptom complex that may be present in a number of disorders. It is a common clinical problem in cardiovascular disease. Little is known of its etiology. However,

Dahl's[6] studies have linked hypertension to a sensitivity to high salt use.

Other investigators have observed clinical improvement of hypertensive patients through use of a low sodium dietary regimen. In 1944, Kempner[7] proposed a strict rice-fruit diet and administered it to his patients with beneficial effects to the hypertension. However, it was in reality a barren, semistarvation regimen without realistic application in common use. Other clinicians[8] used a more liberal diet than Kempner's, but still the diet was a severe one, limiting sodium to 200 mg. daily.

With the advent of potent antihypertensive drugs in the past two decades, such severe diets are no longer necessary. However, the effectiveness of these drugs is enhanced and the hypertensive condition improved by moderate restriction of sodium from 500 to 1,000 mg., depending upon individual need and response. The 500 mg. and 1,000 mg. sodium diets given on pp. 533 to 535 may be used.

ACUTE CARDIOVASCULAR DISEASE

In the acute phase of cardiovascular disease, myocardial infarction, or congestive failure, additional dietary modifications are usually indicated. The basic therapeutic objective is cardiac rest. Hence, all care is given to assure this requirement for restoring the damaged heart to adequate functioning. The diet will be modified, therefore, in energy value and texture.

Calories. A brief period of undernutrition during the first few days after the attack is advisable. The metabolic demands for digestion, absorption, and utilization of food require a generous cardiac output. Small intakes of food decrease the level of metabolic activity to one which the weakened heart can accommodate. A century ago in 1866 a French physician recognized this principle and, during this acute period, fed his patients only four glasses of milk a day. Even today such a regimen is ordered by his name—The Karrell Diet; or some physicians may simply request milk only for the first day or so, and then progress to more food as the patient improves. During the recovery stages the calories may be limited to 800 to 1,200, to continue cardiac rest from metabolic loads. If the patient is obese, as is frequent, this caloric level may be continued for a longer period to effect desired weight loss.

Texture. Early feedings will be soft in nature, or easily digested, to avoid effort in eating. Smaller meals served more frequently may give needed nutrition without undue strain or pressure.

PATIENT EDUCATION

Since cardiovascular disease assumes more or less a chronic nature, an important responsibility of the health team is education of the patient and his family concerning continuing needs for health care. Such teaching should not wait for discharge instructions, but should begin early in convalescence and give the patient a clear knowledge of positive needs. Such an approach will provide resources for sound and vigorous self-care within the limits of individual capacity, and help avoid the negative apprehension of a cardiac cripple.

Many excellent resources for patient education are provided by the American Heart Association through their national and regional offices. Practical discussions need to center on food buying and preparation to make the diets palatable and acceptable to the patients. Many helpful suggestions are included in the Heart Association booklets and in the listed cookbooks. A survey of local markets will give guidance concerning commercial products and label reading.

Modified low-sodium food exchange groups are listed on p. 537. These may be used to guide patients on calorie controlled low sodium diets. The 800 to 1,500 calorie diet plans are on p. 480, and can be used to make food choices from these low-sodium food groups.

Low sodium food exchange groups

Foods permitted	*Foods to avoid*

Group A vegetables

Raw, cooked or canned without salt or fat; may be eaten as desired; one serving contains little or no calories and 9 mg. sodium

Asparagus	Canned vegetables (unless canned without
Beans, green	salt)
Broccoli	
Brussel sprouts	The following vegetables are high in natural
Cauliflower	salt and must be omitted from the diet:
Celery*	
Cabbage, fresh	Beet greens
Chicory	Chard
Cucumbers	Swiss kale
Eggplant	Sauerkraut
Endive	
Escarole	
Lettuce	
Mushrooms	
Okra	
Parsley	
Peppers	
Radishes	
Squash, summer	
Spinach*	
Tomatoes	
Salt-free tomato juice	
Watercress	

Group B vegetables

Only ½ cup of one of the following vegetables may be used per day; contains approximately 9 mg. sodium per serving; 7 gm. carbohydrate, 2 gm. protein and 35 calories

Beets*	White turnips
Carrots*	Frozen peas
Onions	
Peas	
Pumpkin	
Artichokes	
Rutabagas	
Winter squash	

Fruits

Fresh, dried, cooked or canned without added sugar; this list shows the amount of fruit to use for one serving; contains 2 mg. sodium; one serving contains 10 gm. carbohydrate and 40 calories.

Apple	1 small	Canned tomato juice or vegetable juices.
Applesauce	½ cup	Fruit or fruit products which contain
Apricots, fresh	2 medium	sodium bensoate, maraschino cherries;
Apricots, dried	4 halves	dried fruit sometimes has sodium sulfate
Banana	½ small	added, these should be avoided, read
Blackberries	1 cup	label (use only sundried fruits)
Raspberries	1 cup	
Blueberries	⅔ cup	
Strawberries	1 cup	

*Vegetables allowed once a day if sodium allowance is 1,000 mg.   *Continued.*

Low sodium food exchange groups—cont'd

Foods permitted		*Foods to avoid*
Fruits—cont'd		
Cantaloupe	¼ medium	
Cherries	10 large	
Dates	2	
Figs, fresh	2 large	
Watermelon	1 cup	
Grapefruit juice	½ cup	
Grapes	12	
Grape juice	¼ cup	
Honeydew melon	⅛ medium	
Orange	1 small	
Orange juice	½ cup	
Peach	1 medium	
Pear	1 small	
Pineapple	½ cup	
Pineapple juice	⅓ cup	
Plums	2 medium	
Prunes, dried	2 medium	
Tangerine	1 large	

Bread

One serving contains 15 gm. carbohydrate; 2 gm. protein; 70 calories; 5 mgs. sodium (substitute the following for one slice salt-free bread)

Foods permitted		Foods to avoid
Salt-free passover Matzoth,	½	Regular bread and rolls
		Biscuit and popovers
Salt-free melba toast,	3	Salted or soda crackers
Low sodium toast (Nabisco),	2	Pastries and cakes
		Prepared muffins, waffles, cakes
Cooked cereals (without salt),	½ cup	Pancake and pastry mixes
		Self-rising flour
Pearl barley, rice, noodles,	½ cup	Cornmeal
		Quick' cooking (5 minute) hot cereals
Macaroni, spaghetti,	½ cup	Dry cereals except those listed
Lima beans, fresh,	½ cup	Pretzels, potato chips
Navy beans, dried,	½ cup	Salted popcorn
Soybeans, cowpeas,	½ cup	Frozen lima beans
Potato (white),	1 small	
Potato (sweet),	¼ cup	
Parsnips,	⅔ cup	
Corn (fresh, frozen, or canned unsalted or 1 small ear),	⅔ cup	
Puffed Wheat, Puffed Rice,	¾ cup	
Shredded Wheat	1 biscuit	
Popcorn, unsalted	1 cup	

Low sodium food exchange groups—cont'd

Foods permitted		*Foods to avoid*

Meats

One ounce contains 7 gm. protein; 5 gm. fat; 25 mgs. sodium; 75 calories; substitute the following for one ounce salt-free meat, (baked, broiled, stewed or pan broiled)

Fresh or frozen beef, lamb, liver, pork, rabbit, veal, or tongue	1 ounce	All smoked, processed or canned meats, fish, or fowl, such as anchovies, caviar, herring, salted dry cod, bacon, oysters
		Cold cuts
Fresh fish (except shellfish)	1 ounce	Cornbeef or chipped beef
		Frankfurters or sausages
Fresh or frozen chicken, duck, turkey or quail	1 ounce	Brain, kidney
		Ham, smoked tongue, sausage
		All cheese except salt-free cheese
Canned salt-free tuna or salmon	¼ cup	Frozen fish fillets, clams, crab, lobster, shrimp, sardines, oysters, kosher meats.
Salt-free peanut butter	1 tbsp.	Peanut butter, except salt-free
Salt-free American cheese	1 ounce	
Salt-free cottage cheese (dry curd)	¼ cup	
Egg (no more than one a day)		

Fats

One serving contains 5 gms. fat; little or no sodium and 45 calories. Substitute the following for 1 teaspoon salt-free butter:

Butter, salt-free	1 tsp.	Salted butter, oleomargarine
Cream, light (sweet or sour)	2 tbsp.	Commercial mayonnaise or french dressing
Cream, heavy	1 tbsp.	Bacon fat and salty meat drippings and olives
Avocado	⅛	Salted nuts
French dressing, salt-free	1 tbsp.	Salt pork
Mayonnaise, salt-free	1 tsp.	
Oil or cooking fat	1 tsp.	
Nuts, unsalted	6 small	

Seasonings

Allspice	Rennet tablets
Baking yeast	Salt in any form
Caraway	Baking soda and baking powder
Cinnamon	Prepared mustard, ketchup, meat sauces, chili sauce, horseradish
Curry powder	
Garlic	Bouillon or canned soups
Ginger	Olives and pickles and relishes
Herbs	Celery salt, celery seed, onion salt, garlic salt
Horseradish (fresh grated)	

Continued.

Low sodium food exchange groups—cont'd

Foods permitted	Foods to avoid
Seasonings—cont'd	
Lemon juice or extract	
Mace	Accent, Zest, Tok
Mustard, dry	Salted meat tenderizers
Nutmeg	Prepared horseradish
Paprika	Worchestershire sauce
Parsley	Meat extracts
Peppermint extract	Meat sauces
Sage	
Saccharine	
Thyme	
Tumeric	
Vanilla extract	
Walnut extract	
Pepper, black	
Pepper, red	
Pepper, white	
Vinegar	

References
Specific

1. The heart and circulation: report of the Second National Conference on Cardiovascular Diseases, Washington, D. C., 1965, U. S. Government Printing Office.
2. Bellet, S., and others: Comparative human study: coffee linked to free fatty acid increase, J.A.M.A. **197**:37, 1966.
3. Jankelson, O. M., and others: The effect of coffee on glucose tolerance and circulating insulin in men with maturity-onset diabetes, Lancet **1**:527, 1967.
4. Mayer, J.: Obesity and cardiovascular disease, J. Amer. Diet. Ass. **52**:13, 1968.
5. Council on Foods and Nutrition, American Medical Association, The regulation of dietary fat, J.A.M.A. **181**:411, 1962.
6. Dahl, L. K.: Role of dietary sodium in essential hypertension, J. Amer. Diet. Ass. **34**:585, 1958.
7. Kempner, W.: Rice diet in the treatment of hypertension and vascular diseases, N. Carolina Med. J. **5**:125, 1944; **6**:61, 1945.
8. Grollman, A., and others: Sodium restriction in the diet for hypertension, J.A.M.A. **129**:533, 1945.

General

Ahrens, E. H., Jr., and others: Symposium on significance of lowered cholesterol levels, J.A.M.A. **170**:2198, 1959.
Albrink, M. J.: Diet and cardiovascular disease, J. Amer. Diet. Ass. **46**:26, 1965.

Baker, B. M., and others: The national diet-heart study, J.A.M.A. **185**:105, 1963.
Bills, C. E., and others: Sodium and potassium in foods and water, J. Amer. Diet. Ass. **25**:304, 1949.
Brown, H. B., and others: Design of practical fat-controlled diets. Foods, fat composition and serum cholesterol content, J.A.M.A. **196**:205, 1966.
Bruce, T. A., and Bing, R. J.: Clinical management of myocardial infarction, J.A.M.A. **191**:136, 1965.
Cantoni, J.: Adding flavor to sodium-restricted meals in the hospital, J. Amer. Diet. Ass. **30**:1146, 1954.
Christakis, G., and others: The anti-coronary club: a dietary approach to the prevention of coronary heart disease—a seven-year report, Amer. J. Public Health **56**:299, 1966.
Council on Foods and Nutrition: Diet and the possible prevention of coronary atheroma, J.A.M.A. **194**:1149, 1965.
Council on Foods and Nutrition, Fats in human nutrition, with particular attention to fats, cholesterol, and atherosclerosis, Chicago, 1957, American Medical Association.
Council on Foods and Nutrition: Low sodium milk, J.A.M.A. **163**:739, 1957.
Council on Foods and Nutrition: Special shortenings, J.A.M.A. **187**:766, 1964.
Council on Foods and Nutrition: The regulation of dietary fat, J.A.M.A. **181**:411, 1962.
Danowski, T. S.: Low sodium diets—physiological

adaptation and clinical usefulness, J.A.M.A. **168:**1886, 1958.

Davidson, C. S., and others: Sodium-restricted diets: the rationale, complications and practical aspects of their use, Pub. 325, Washington, D. C., 1954, Food and Nutrition Board, National Research Council.

Dustan, H. P.: Diet and diuretics in the treatment of hypertensive cardiovascular disease, J.A.M.A. **172:**2052, 1960.

Food and Nutrition Board: Dietary fat and human health, Pub. No. 1146, Washington, D. C., 1966, National Academy of Sciences, National Research Council.

Friedman, G. J.: Nutrition in relation to atherosclerosis. In Wohl, M. and Goodhart, R., editors: Modern nutrition in health and disease, ed. 3, Philadelphia, 1964, Lea & Febiger.

Goldsmith, G. A.: Highlights on the cholesterol-fats, diets and atherosclerosis problem, J.A.M.A. **176:**783, 1961.

Griffith, W. H.: Fats in the diet, J.A.M.A. **164:**411, 1957.

Hashim, S. A.: Medium-chain triglycerides-clinical and metabolic aspects, J. Amer. Diet. Ass. **51:**221, 1967.

Hashim, S. A.: The relation of diet to atherosclerosis and infarction, Amer. J. Nurs. **60:**348, 1960.

Hayter, J.: Acute myocardial infarction, Amer. J. Nurs. **59:**1602, 1959.

Heap, B.: Sodium restricted diets, Amer. J. Nurs. **60:**206, 1960.

Heap, B., and Robinson, C.: New diet booklets for cardiac patients and sodium restriction, J. Amer. Diet. Ass. **34:**277, 1958.

Hodges, R. E., and Krehl, W. A.: The role of carbohydrates in lipid metabolism, Amer. J. Clin. Nutr. **17:**334, 1965.

Holinger, B. W., and others: Analyzed sodium values in foods ready to serve, J. Amer. Diet. Ass. **48:**501, 1966.

Keys, A.: Blood lipids in man—a brief review, J. Amer. Diet. Ass. **51:**508, 1967.

Kinsell, L. W., and others: Essential fatty acids, lipid metabolism, and atherosclerosis, Lancet **1:**334, 1958.

Modell, W., and others: Handbook of cardiology for nurses, ed. 5, New York, 1966, Springer Publishing Co., Inc.

Newburgh, L. H., and Reimer, A.: The rationale and administration of low sodium diets, J. Am. Diet. Ass. **23:**1047, 1947.

Nite, G., and Willis, F. N.: The coronary patient: hospital care and rehabilitation, New York, 1964, The Macmillan Company.

Ostwald, R.: Fatty acids in eleven brands of margarine, J. Amer. Diet. Ass. **39:**313, 1961.

Reimer, A., and others: Sodium-restricted diets: a bookshelf, J. Amer. Diet. Ass. **33:**104, 1957.

Review: Cardiovascular disease—the picture in the United States, J. Amer. Diet. Ass. **46:**394, 1965.

Review: Fat and cholesterol in the diet, Nutr. Rev. **23:**3, 1965.

Schizas, A., and others: Medium-chain triglycerides—use in food preparation, J. Amer. Diet. Ass. **51:**228, 1967.

Sodium Restricted Diets: The rationale, complications, and practical aspects of their use, Pub. #325, 1954, Food and Nutrition Board, National Research Council.

Stamler, J., and others: Coronary risk factors, Med. Clin. N. Amer. **50:**229, 1966.

Stare, F. J., and others: Nutritional studies relating to serum lipids and atherosclerosis: therapeutic implications, J.A.M.A. **164:**1920, 1957.

Talbot, G. D.: Influence of environmental factors on lipid-response curves. Cigarette smoking, salt, alcohol, and high fat diet affecting healthy males, Geriatrics **19:**575, 1964.

Trulson, M. F., and others: Comparison of siblings in Boston and Ireland, J. Amer. Diet. Ass. **45:**225, 1964.

Van Itallie, T. B., and Hashim, S. A.: Diet in heart disease, J. Amer. Diet. Ass. **38:**531, 1961.

Weller, J. M., and Hoobler, S. W.: Salt metabolism in hypertension, Ann. Int. Med. **50:**106, 1958.

Wood, P. D.: Dietary regulation of cholesterol metabolism, Lancet **2:**604, 1966.

Zukel, M. C.: Fat-controlled diets, Amer. J. Clin. Nutr. **16:**270, 1965.

Patient education materials

American Heart Association, New York, N. Y., (or local Heart Association),
Booklets:
Planning Fat-Controlled Meals for Unrestricted Calories, 1962.
Planning Fat-Controlled Meals for 1,200 and 1,800 calories, rev. 1966.
Your Sodium-Restricted Diet: 500 mg., 1000 mg., and Mild Restriction, 1958.
Fold-out Charts:
Sodium-Restricted Diet, 500 mg., 1965.
Sodium-Restricted Diet, 1,000 mg., 1966.
Sodium-Restricted Diet, mild, 1967.

Heap, B., and others: Simplifying the sodium-restricted diets, J. Amer. Diet. Ass. **49:**327, 1966.

Keys, A., and Keys, M.: Eat well and stay well, Garden City, New York, 1963, Doubleday & Company, Inc.

Payne, A. S., and Callahan, D.: The low-sodium, fat-controlled cookbook, Boston, 1965, Little, Brown and Company.

Public Health Service, The food you eat and heart disease, Pub. 537, 1963, U. S. Department of Health, Education, and Welfare.

Stead, E. S., and Warren, G. K.: Low-fat cookery, New York, 1959, McGraw-Hill Book Company, Inc.

Waldo, M.: Cooking for your heart and health, New York, 1961, G. P. Putnam's Sons.

CHAPTER 29

Renal disease

PHYSIOLOGY OF THE KIDNEY

Knowledge of the normal functions of the kidney forms an essential background for relating therapy in renal disorders to the organ's impaired functioning in disease. In Chapter 9 these functions are discussed in detail in relation to fluid and electrolyte balance. This basic section should be reviewed and the diagram of the nephron in Fig. 9-6, p. 166 should be carefully studied.

Basic renal functions

The nephron is an exquisite example of a highly complex, minute tissue unit, adapted in fine structural detail to its vital function—maintaining an internal fluid environment compatible with life. Through the successive sections of some one million nephrons in each kidney, important body fluid flows. The nephrons *filter* from the entering blood most of its constituents except red cells and protein, *reabsorb* needed substances as the filtrate continues along the winding tubules, *secrete* additional ions to maintain acid-base balance, and finally *excrete* unneeded materials in a concentrated urine.

Nephron structures. Several nephron structures perform unique homeostatic and metabolic tasks.

Glomerulus. At the head of the nephron, an entering arteriole breaks up into a group of collateral capillaries which rejoin to form the efferent or leaving arteriole. The tuft of collateral capillaries is held closely applied in a cupped membrane. This capsule is named for the young English physician, Sir William Bowman, who in 1843 first clearly established the basis of plasma filtration and consequent urine secretion upon this intimate relationship of blood-filled glomeruli and enveloping membrane. The filtrate formed here is cell-free and virtually protein-free. Otherwise it carries the same constituents as does the entering blood.

Tubules. Continuous with the base of Bowman's capsule, the nephron's tubule winds in a series of convolutions toward its terminal in the kidney pelvis. Specific reabsorption functions are performed by the sections of the tubule.

PROXIMAL TUBULE. In the first section, major nutrient reabsorption occurs. Essentially 100% of the glucose and amino acids, 80 to 85% of the water, sodium, potassium, chloride, and most other substances are absorbed. Only 15% to 29% of the filtrate remains to enter the loop of Henle.

LOOP OF HENLE. Midway, the tubule narrows and its thin loop dips into the central renal medulla. Through a balanced system of water and sodium exchange in the limbs of the loop (the counter-current system, p. 167), important interstitial fluid densities are created in the medulla to concentrate the urine by osmotic pressure as it later passes through the environment in the collecting tubule.

DISTAL TUBULE. The latter portion of the tubule functions primarily in acid-base balance through secretion of ionized hydrogen and in conservation of sodium through the influence of aldosterone.

COLLECTING TUBULE. In the final section of the tubule water is absorbed under the influence of vasopressin (ADH) and the osmotic pressure of the surrounding interstitial fluid. The resulting volume of urine, now concentrated and excreted, is only 0.5 to 1.0% of the original filtered water.

• • •

Inflammatory and degenerative diseases of the kidney diffusely involve entire nephrons or nephron segments. In such conditions, the normal functions of the nephron are disrupted and nutritional disturbances in the metabolism of protein, electrolytes, and water follow. Several of these diseases are discussed here as representative of the correlation of diet therapy to impaired renal function and resulting clinical symptoms. These include acute glomerulonephritis, the nephrotic syndrome, acute renal failure, and chronic uremia.

ACUTE GLOMERULONEPHRITIS
Etiology

Usually some antecedent streptococcal infection is related to the onset of glomerulonephritis. It has a more or less sudden onset, and, after a brief course, the majority of the cases (especially those among children) recover completely. In others the disease may progress or become latent only to develop later into chronic glomerulonephritis. There is some dispute, however, as to whether acute and chronic glomerulonephritis are one continuous disease. The inflammatory process involves primarily the glomeruli; as a result of loss of glomerular function, degeneration of the conjoined tubules follows.

Clinical symptoms

Classic symptoms include hematuria, proteinuria, and varying degrees of edema, hypertension, and renal insufficiency. There may be oliguria or anuria (acute renal failure) and chronic renal failure.

Diet therapy

Protein. Much controversy exists concerning the use of a low protein diet. Studies seem to indicate, however, that no advantage is found in restricting protein.[1] In short-term acute cases in children, pedia-tricians in general favor overall optimum nutrition with adequate protein, unless oliguria or anuria develop. This complication usually lasts no more than two or three days and is managed by conservative treatment.

Sodium. Salt, also, is usually not restricted unless complications of edema, hypertension, or oliguria become dangers. In such cases, 500 to 1,000 mg. sodium diet may be used (p. 533). In most patients, especially in children with acute post-streptococcal glomerulonephritis, diet modifications are not crucial. Treatment centers upon bed rest and drugs.

Water. Intake should be adjusted to output, as a rule, including losses in vomiting or diarrhea. During periods of oliguria the intake of water may be 500 to 700 ml. a day.

THE NEPHROTIC SYNDROME
Etiology

The nephrotic syndrome may result from many causes. Kark[2,3] identifies some of these causes as infective (syphilis, malaria, bacterial endocarditis), allergic (bee sting, serum sickness), mechanical (renal vein thrombosis, congestive heart failure), generalized disease processes (amyloidosis, systemic lupus erythematosus, diabetic glomerulosclerosis, arteriolar nephrosclerosis), and intrinsic renal disease (membranous or proliferative glomerulonephritis, tubular degeneration—lipoid nephrosis). However, in a number of cases no underlying cause is recognized. Whether or not the nephrotic syndrome represents a stage of chronic glomerulonephritis is unclear. Some patients do show progressive renal failure as in chronic glomerulonephritis. Others, however, respond to treatment with complete recoveries.

Formerly it was believed that the disease process in nephrosis affected primarily the tubular epithelium. Now it is recognized that the primary degenerative defect is in the capillary basement membrane of the glomerulus, which permits the escape of large amounts of protein into the filtrate. The tubular changes are probably secondary to the high protein concentration in the filtrate, with some protein uptake from the tubule lumen.

Clinical symptoms

The primary symptom in the nephrotic syndrome is massive albuminuria. Other findings include additional protein losses in the urine, including globulins, and specialized binding proteins for thyroid and iron, which sometimes produce signs of hypothyroidism and anemia. Blood levels of plasma proteins drop and serum cholesterol levels rise.

As serum protein losses continue, tissue proteins are broken down and general malnutrition ensues. There are fatty tissue changes in the liver, sodium retention, and edema. Severe ascites and pedal edema mask gross tissue wasting.

Diet therapy

Treatment is directed toward control of the major symptoms—edema and malnutrition—from the massive protein losses.

Protein. Replacement of the prolonged nitrogen deficit is a fundamental and immediate need. The plasma albumin level may have been reduced to 20% or less of its normal value. This is a major factor in the development of nephrotic ascites and edema. Daily protein allowances of 100 to 150 gm. or more will be needed.

Calories. To ensure protein use for tissue synthesis, sufficient calories must always be given. High calorie intakes daily of 50 to 60 calories per kilogram body weight are essential. Every effort must be made to ensure that the patient actually consumes the diet. Since appetite is usually poor, much encouragement and support are needed. The food must be appetizing and in a form most easily tolerated.

Sodium. To combat the massive edema, sodium levels in the diet must be sufficiently low. Usually the 500 mg. sodium diet (p. 533) is satisfactory to help initiate diuresis.

The dietary management is similar to that given for hepatitis (p. 517) with added need for sodium restriction. The use of low-sodium milk is indicated to help maintain the desired high protein intake and yet restrict sodium to the more severe levels.

CHRONIC RENAL FAILURE—UREMIA
Etiology

Progressive degenerative changes in renal tissue bring marked depression of all renal functions. Few functioning nephrons remain, and these gradually deteriorate. Uremia is the term given the symptom complex of advanced renal insufficiency. Although the name derives from the common finding of elevated blood urea levels, the symptoms result not so much from urea concentrations per se as from disturbances in acid-base balance and in fluid and electrolyte metabolism, and from accumulation of other obscure toxic substances not clearly identified.

Clinical symptoms

Individual patients vary in degree of symptoms and must be managed individually according to laboratory test indications of renal function. Usually there is anemia, lassitude, weakness, loss of weight, and hypertension. Sometimes aching and pain in bone and joints are present. Later signs in progressive illness include skin, oral, and gastrointestinal bleeding from increased capillary fragility, muscular twitching, uremic convulsions, pericarditis, Cheyne-Stokes respiration (an irregular, cyclic type of breathing), ulceration of the mouth, and fetid breath. Resistance to infection is low.

Treatment objectives

The variables of treatment center primarily upon protein, sodium, potassium, and water. Levels of each nutrient will need to be individually adjusted according to progression of the illness, type of treatment being used, and the patient's response to treatment. In general, however, overall treatment has several basic objectives:

1. To reduce and minimize protein catabolism
2. To avoid dehydration or overhydration
3. To carefully correct acidosis

4. To correct electrolyte depletions and avoid excesses
5. To control fluid and electrolyte losses from vomiting and diarrhea
6. To maintain nutrition and weight
7. To maintain appetite and morale
8. To control complications such as hypertension, bone pain, and central nervous system abnormalities

Principles of diet therapy

In many of these general therapy objectives, nutritional care plays a large role. Principles of therapeutic nutrition involve variable nutrient adjustments according to individual need.

Protein. The knotty problem is to provide sufficient protein to prevent tissue protein catabolism, yet avoid an excess which would elevate urea levels. A number of years ago Borst,[4] an English physician, proposed a zero-protein, nonpotassium regimen composed of butter, sugar, and cornstarch served as soup, pudding, or butterballs. However, the diet is drastic and intolerable and is rarely administered except in extreme cases (see box below).

With recent advances in the use of hemodialysis, some kidney treatment centers have outlined a more liberal but moderate protein intake for their patients undergoing intermittent dialysis for chronic uremia. Cimino[5] recommends a carefully controlled 70 to 75 gm. protein diet. Bakke[6] reports the use of a 40 to 60 gm. protein diet at The Seattle Artificial Kidney Center. Mitchell and Smith[7] describe a protein intake adjusted according to weight: 0.2 to 0.5 gm. per kilogram body weight. Merrill[8] advises a diet of 35 to 50 gm. protein, chiefly of animal origin, for the average patient with advanced renal failure.

Thus, according to individual need and response to treatment, protein will in any event be closely controlled, and will range in quantity from 30 to 70 gm. and have a high biological value to supply essential amino acids.

Sodium. The recommendations for sodium intake vary also. Both severe restriction and excess are to be avoided. Since sodium is the chief determinant of extracellular fluid osmolarity, the dietary need is closely related to the patient's handling of water.

Borst nonprotein, nonpotassium diet for renal shutdown (uremia)

I. *Borst butter soup*
  150 gm. sugar
  150 gm. salt-free butter
  20 gm. flour
  300 gm. water
  Coffee extract, vanilla or lemon flavoring
  Serve hot
  Divide into 6 feedings

II. *Borst pudding or soup*
  720 ml. cold water
  85 gm. salt free butter
  18 gm. cornstarch
  60 gm. sugar
  2 drops vanilla
  May be served hot as a soup or cold as a pudding.
  Add peppermint extract when served as a pudding.

III. *Butter balls*
  168 gms. salt free butter—1,250 calories
  100 gms. powdered sugar—400 calories
  Makes 60 butter balls

Table 29-1. Basic pattern for a controlled protein, sodium, and potassium diet*

Food	Protein gm.	Sodium mg.	Potassium mg.	Calories	Water ml.
Breakfast					
Scrambled egg (1 med.)	6.0	61.0	64.5	80	36.9
Puffed wheat (1 oz. or substitute from cereal list)	4.0	1.1	95.2	102	1.0
Whole milk (⅓ C.)	3.0	40.5	117.1	53	71.1
Unsalted bread (1 slice)	2.0	5.2	7.2	60	8.2
Unsalted butter (2 tsp.)	—	7.6	3.2	70	2.2
Jam or preserves (1 tbsp. or substitute from sweets list)	—	2.4	17.6	54	5.8
Noon meal					
Roast beef (3 oz. or substitute from meat list)	22.0	51.0	314.5	245	46.5
Green beans, low-sodium canned (½ c. or substitute from vegetable list)	1.5	2.0	95.0	25	58.3
Rice, cooked (½ c. or substitute from rice list)	1.7	0.5	23.5	92	60.9
Unsalted bread (1 slice)	2.0	5.2	7.2	60	8.2
Unsalted butter (2 tsp.)	—	7.6	3.2	70	2.2
Jelly (1 Tbsp. or substitute from sweets list)	—	3.4	15.0	55	5.8
Apricots, canned (4 halves or substitute from fruit list)	0.4	0.6	142.7	52	46.9
Evening meal					
Broiled chicken (3 oz. or substitute from meat list)	20.0	56.0	233.0	185	60.4
Mixed vegetables, frozen (½ c. or substitute from vegetable list)	2.4	40.5	146.0	48	63.2
Unsalted bread, (1 slice)	2.0	5.2	7.2	60	8.2
Unsalted butter (2 tsp.)	—	7.6	3.2	70	2.2
Apple, fresh (1 2-in. diameter or substitute from fruit list)	0.2	1.0	110.0	70	126.6
Sugar (6 tsp.)	—	0.2	0.4	92	trace
Fat, cooking (4 tbsp.)	—	—	—	442	—
Total	67.2	298.6	1,405.7	1,985	614.6

*Jordan, W. L., Cimino, J. E., Grist, A. C., McMahon, G. E. and Doyle, M. M.: Basic pattern for a controlled protein sodium and potassium diet, J. Amer. Diet. Ass. **50**:138, 1967.

Some patients may tolerate little sodium, whereas others waste salt excessively in their urine and require a high salt intake of 4 or 5 gm. daily to achieve balance. Usually, however, the sodium intake is controlled between 400 and 2,000 mg.

Potassium. In renal failure, the patient's potassium levels may be depressed or elevated. Guided by blood potassium determinations, the physician adjusts potassium intake to maintain normal levels. The damaged kidney cannot clear potassium adequately, so the daily dietary intake is kept at about 1,500 mg.

Water. Much care must be exercised to avoid water intoxication from overloading, or dehydration from too little water. The capacity of the damaged kidney to handle water is limited, and in many cases solids can actually be excreted better with a controlled amount of water. As little as 600 ml. daily may be indicated for some patients to prevent dilution of sodium ions and further fall in the filtration rate. The usual recommendation is from 800 to 1,000 ml. daily. Careful records of total fluid intake and output are necessary.

Carbohydrate and fat. The diet must supply sufficient nonprotein calories to ensure protein use for tissue protein synthesis and to supply energy. Carbohydrate should always be given with protein food to increase utilization of the amino acids. About 300 to 400 gm. of carbohydrate is the average daily need. Sufficient fat is added (75 to 90 gm.) to give the patient 2,000 to 2,500 total calories daily.

Summary of average dietary needs in chronic renal failure

Protein	30 to 50 gm.
Carbohydrate	300 to 400 gm.
Fat	70 to 90 gm.
Calories	2,000 to 2,500
Sodium	400 to 2,000 mg. (4 gm. salt)
Potassium	1,300 to 1,900 mg.

Dietary management

General protein and electrolyte control. New treatments, such as hemodialysis, have prolonged life in patients with chronic renal disease. Such treatment has also made necessary a more rigidly controlled diet to prevent serum electrolytes and the products of protein catabolism from reaching fatal heights during the intervals between treatments. Therefore, to achieve a two-fold objective, rigid control and patient acceptance, diets for uremia patients are being organized on the exchange system of control. A basic daily food pattern is outlined, and food exchange groups are listed from which to make equivalent food choices. An example of such a plan is given in Table 29-1. Individual patient adjustments may be made from such a plan. For example, salt may be added if increased sodium chloride is needed; protein food allowances may be decreased and low-protein bread[9] used if less protein is desired; carbohydrate foods may be increased if added calories and protein-sparing effect is required. Basic food exchange lists for use with this diet plan are given in Table 29-2.

The low protein-essential amino acid diet (modified Giordano-Giovannetti regimen). The recent separate work of two Italian physicians, Carmelo Giordano[10] at the University of Naples and Sergio Giovannetti[11] at the University of Pisa, has given an encouraging dietary base to sustain patients with uremia and alleviate many of their difficult symptoms. In 1963 Dr. Giordano reported an experiment with eight uremia patients using a synthetic diet of carbohydrate (starch and sugar) and fat (margarine or vegetable oil) made into a flavored pudding, served with an additional vegetable and fruit, and supplemented with a formula of essential amino acids. All the patients improved clinically, azotemia was lowered, and positive nitrogen balance was achieved. He formulated his approach on the principle of feeding only essential amino acids, which caused the body to use its own excess urea nitrogen to synthesize the nonessential amino acids needed for tissue protein production.

Using a similar principle, Dr. Giovannetti treated chronic uremia patients, some of whom were on dialysis, with a low protein basal diet composed of bread and Italian

Table 29-2. Food exchange lists for use with controlled protein, sodium, and potassium diet*

Food	Protein gm.	Sodium mg.	Potassium mg.	Water ml.
Meat list—select 2 items daily				
Beef				
Ground, commercial (2 oz.)	14.0	26.7	255.1	30.4
Loin roast (3 oz.)	20.0	51.0	314.5	37.3
Pot roast (3 oz.)	22.0	51.0	314.5	46.5
Rib roast (3 oz.)	17.0	51.0	314.5	34.0
Cheese, low-sodium dietetic (2 oz.)	17.0	7.0	17.5	22.5
Chicken				
†Broiled (3 oz.)	20.0	56.0	233.0	60.4
Dark meat, boned, no skin (2½ oz.)	22.0	62.3	233.8	45.1
White meat, no skin (2 oz.)	18.1	38.4	244.9	38.2
Lamb				
Leg, roast (3 oz.)	20.0	59.5	246.5	42.8
Loin chops, without bone (3 oz.)	16.5	58.5	243.6	35.0
Shoulder, roast (3 oz.)	18.0	59.5	246.5	39.3
†Perch, breaded (3 oz.)	17.0	57.8	195.5	50.0
Pork				
Chops, without bone (2½ oz.)	16.0	45.5	272.9	29.4
Roast (2 oz.)	13.0	36.6	221.3	25.3
Turkey, roast (2 oz.)	17.4	42.0	147.0	31.0
Veal roast or cutlet (2 oz.)	15.0	45.3	283.3	32.9
Vegetable list—select 2 items daily				
Asparagus				
Canned, low sodium (1½ oz.)	1.3	1.5	79.5	39.3
Fresh (1½ oz.)	0.9	0.4	80.0	39.3
Frozen (1½ oz.)	1.4	0.4	96.3	38.9
Beans				
Green, canned, low-sodium (½ C.)	1.5	2.0	95.0	58.3
Lima, canned, low-sodium (¼ C.)	2.3	1.6	88.8	30.2
Beets				
Canned, low-sodium (½ C.)	0.7	37.9	138.0	74.1
Fresh, cooked (¼ C.)	0.5	17.8	85.8	37.5
Broccoli, fresh, cooked (¼ C.)	1.2	3.8	100.0	34.2
Brussels sprouts				
Fresh, cooked (¼ C.)	1.4	3.3	88.5	28.7
Frozen (¼ C.)	1.1	4.5	96.5	29.0
Cabbage				
†Cooked (½ C.)	0.9	11.0	128.0	80.2
raw (½ C.)	0.7	10.0	117.0	46.0
Carrots				
Canned, low-sodium (½ C.)	0.6	28.3	87.0	67.4
fresh, cooked (¼ C.)	0.4	11.9	81.0	33.1
raw, (half, 1 oz.)	0.3	11.7	85.5	24.7
Cauliflower				
fresh, cooked (½ C.)	1.4	5.4	124.0	55.7
frozen (½ C.)	1.1	6.0	124.0	56.4
Celery (1 stalk, 8 x 1½ in.)	0.4	50.4	136.0	37.6

*Jordan, W. L., Cimino, J. E., M. D., Grist, A. C., McMahon, G. E., and Doyle, M. M.: Basic pattern for a controlled protein, sodium and potassium diet, J. Amer. Diet. Ass. **50**:138-140, 1967.
†If these items (highest in fluid in each list) are selected, fluid intake for the day would be approximately 1,000 ml.

Table 29-2. Food exchange lists for use with controlled protein, sodium, and potassium diet.*—cont'd.

Food	Protein gm.	Sodium mg.	Potassium mg.	Water ml.
Vegetable list—select 2 items daily—cont'd				
Corn, fresh, cooked (¼ C.)	2.1	trace	105.5	48.9
Cucumber, raw (1½ oz.)	0.3	3.1	82.4	40.9
Endive or escarole (1 oz.)	0.5	3.9	83.7	26.5
Kale, fresh, cooked (½ C.)	2.5	23.6	121.5	50.1
Lettuce (⅛ head, 1 oz.)	0.2	2.5	48.1	26.3
Mixed vegetables, frozen (½ C.)	2.4	40.5	146.0	63.2
Okra				
fresh, (8 pods, 3 oz.)	1.7	1.7	147.9	77.4
frozen (8 pods, 3 oz.)	1.9	1.7	139.4	75.1
†Onions, mature, cooked (½ C.)	1.3	7.4	115.5	96.4
Peas				
Early June, canned, low-sodium (¼ C.)	3.0	1.9	60.0	50.1
fresh (¼ C.)	2.2	0.4	78.4	32.6
frozen (¼ C.)	2.0	46.0	54.0	32.8
Spinach, fresh, cooked (¼ C.)	1.3	22.5	146.0	41.4
Squash				
summer, fresh, cooked (¼ C.)	0.5	0.5	74.0	50.1
winter, fresh, cooked (¼ C.)	0.6	0.5	132.3	46.2
Tomatoes				
Canned, low-sodium (¼ C.)	0.6	1.8	131.5	56.9
raw (¼ of 2 x 2½ in.)	0.4	1.2	91.5	35.1
Turnips, fresh, cooked (½ C.)	0.6	26.0	145.7	73.0
Fruit list—select 2 items daily				
Apple				
Juice, canned (⅓ C.)	0.1	0.7	77.1	73.0
†Raw, (1 small, 2-in. diameter)	0.2	1.0	110.0	126.6
Apricots, canned, heavy syrup (4 halves)	0.4	0.6	142.7	46.9
Blackberries				
Canned, heavy syrup (½ C.)	1.0	1.3	136.0	92.6
Raw (½ C.)	0.9	0.7	122.4	60.8
Blueberries				
Canned, heavy syrup (½ C.)	0.5	1.3	68.8	72.3
Raw (½ C.)	0.5	0.7	56.7	58.2
Cherries				
Raw, sweet or sour (½ C.)	0.7	1.1	108.8	45.8
Royal Ann, canned, heavy syrup (¼ C.)	0.6	0.6	78.1	48.4
Grapes				
Juice, canned (⅓ C.)	0.4	0.8	134.5	70.5
Raw (½ C.)	1.0	2.3	120.9	62.4
Grapefruit sections, syrup pack (¼ C.)	0.4	0.6	84.0	50.5
Peach, raw (1 small, 2-in. diameter)	0.3	0.6	115.0	101.6
Pears				
Canned (2 halves)	0.2	1.2	98.3	93.4
†Raw (1 small, 3 x 2½ in.)	0.6	1.8	118.0	151.4
Pineapple				
Canned, heavy syrup (2 slices)	0.4	1.2	117.0	97.5
Juice, canned (⅓ C.)	0.3	0.7	110.8	71.4
Raw (½ C.)	0.3	0.7	102.0	59.7

*Jordan, W. L., Cimino, J. E., M. D., Grist, A. C., McMahon, G. E., and Doyle, M. M.: Basic pattern for a controlled protein, sodium and potassium diet, J. Amer. Diet. Ass. **50**:138-140, 1967.
†If these items (highest in fluid in each list) are selected, fluid intake for the day would be approximately 1,000 ml.

Continued.

Table 29-2. Food exchange lists for use with controlled protein, sodium, and potassium diet.*—cont'd.

Food	Protein gm.	Sodium mg.	Potassium mg.	Water ml.
Fruit list—select 2 items daily—cont'd				
Plums				
Greengage, raw (½ C.)	0.5	1.3	105.0	99.1
Not Damson (1 raw, 2-in. diameter)	0.3	0.6	102.0	51.9
Raisins, dried, seedless (2 tbsp.)	0.4	4.0	144.0	1.8
Raspberries				
Black, raw (½ C.)	0.9	0.6	123.0	50.1
Red, raw (½ C.)	0.7	0.6	104.0	50.1
Strawberries				
Frozen (2½ oz.)	0.3	0.7	74.0	49.9
Raw (½ C.)	0.5	0.7	122.2	66.9
Tangerine (1 small, 2½-in. diameter, 5 oz.)	0.9	2.3	144.0	99.2
Cereal list—select 1 item daily				
Cornflakes (½ oz.)	1.0	140.5	16.8	0.5
†Corn grits, cooked (1 C.)	3.0	—	26.6	210.8
Farina, enriched, uncooked, unsalted (1 oz.)	3.4	0.6	24.9	23.4
Oatmeal, cooked, unsalted (¾ C.)	3.4	0.5	84.5	152.2
Puffed Wheat, low-sodium (1 oz.)	4.0	1.1	95.2	0.9
Shredded Wheat, low-sodium (1 oz.)	3.0	0.8	97.4	1.8
Rice list—select 1 item daily				
Macaroni, cooked, unsalted (½ C.)	2.5	0.7	42.7	50.4
Noodles, cooked, unsalted (½ C.)	3.5	1.6	35.2	56.3
Rice, cooked, unsalted (½ C.)	1.7	0.5	23.5	60.9
†Spaghetti, cooked, unsalted (½ C.)	2.5	0.7	42.7	82.8
Sweets list—select 2 items daily				
Cookie, plain assorted (one)	1.0	91.0	16.8	1.6
†Jams or preserves (1 tbsp.)	trace	2.4	17.6	5.8
†Jelly (1 tbsp.)	0	3.4	15.0	5.8
†Honey (1 tbsp.)	trace	1.0	10.7	3.6
Sugar, powdered (¼ C.)	0	0.3	0.9	trace

*Jordan, W. L., Cimino, J. E., M. D., Grist, A. C., McMahon, G. E., and Doyle, M. M.: Basic pattern for a controlled protein, sodium and potassium diet, J. Amer. Diet. Ass. **50**:138-140, 1967.
†If these items (highest in fluid in each list) are selected, fluid intake for the day would be approximately 1,000 ml.

pastes made with a special low protein wheat starch, fats and sugars, selected low protein vegetables, and fruit, supplemented with essential amino acids and small amounts of egg protein (selected because it has the highest biological value of the protein foods, p. 58). His report in 1964 indicated the same positive effects. Blood urea concentrations decreased, nitrogen balance became positive and reached equi-

librium, and clinical symptoms such as anorexia, vomiting, fatigue, and twitching disappeared or improved. The diet effectively reduced the production of protein catabolites and prevented wastage of body protein.

In 1965 confirmation of these original results of Giordano and Giovannetti was reported in England by Berlyne's group at the Manchester Royal Infirmary.[12-14] Adapting

Basic food plan for modified Giovannetti diet (20 gm. protein, 1,500 mg. potassium)

Daily food plan

1 egg
6 ounces milk or 1 additional egg*
Low protein bread—1 loaf (½ lb.; approximately 650 calories and 1.5 gm. protein)
Fruit: 2 to 4 servings from fruit list
Vegetables: 2 to 4 servings from vegetable list (fruit and vegetable choices to total 3 to 12 gm. of protein and 1,300 to 1,900 mg. of potassium)
Free food list: Use as desired for extra calories

Nutrient supplements as prescribed

*Amino acid supplement: Formula of minimum adult requirements of essential amino acids, or only methionine 0.5 gm. if additional food source given in milk or egg
Multivitamin supplement
Iron supplement

Sample meal plan

Breakfast

Fruit or juice
1 egg
2 slices low protein bread,†
  butter, jelly
Amino acid supplement

Lunch

Vegetable
Rice (or substitute starch)
Pudding‡ (wheat starch, fruit)
2 slices low protein bread,†
  butter, jelly

Dinner

Clear broth (rice or pastes, if desired)
Vegetable salad
Cooked vegetable
2 slices low protein bread,†
  butter, jelly
Fruit

Snacks

Tea with milk
Low protein bread,†
  butter, jelly, fruit

Basic pudding and bread recipes for use with modified Giovannetti diet

Low protein pudding*
(makes six servings)

Ingredients	Amount
Butter or margarine	5 oz.
Sugar	¾ cup
Cornstarch (or tapioca)	2 tbsp.
Water	1¼ cups
Lemon extract (see other variations of flavors below)	⅛ tsp.

Method

Combine sugar and cornstarch.
Melt butter or margarine and add above mixture.
Stir well.
Add hot water, blend.
Cook until mixture is thick and clear.
Remove from heat and add flavoring.
Pour into individual cups and chill.

---

*Paygel, P. General Mills, Inc., or Cellu.
†Steele, B. F., and others: A yeast-leavened, low-protein bread for research diets, J. Amer. Diet. Ass. 47:405-6, 1965.

Continued.

Basic food plan for modified Giovannetti diet (20 gm. protein, 1,500 mg. potassium)—cont'd

Variations

Instead of lemon extract use: lemon juice, peppermint extract, rum extract, orange peel, vanilla extract, or a combination of two or three extracts.

Instead of the water, or instead of part of the water, substitute part of the fruit juice allowance for the day (examples: pineapple juice, drained fruit cocktail juice, apricot juice). Red sour pitted cherries are good with tapioca pudding.

Add to the pudding: crushed peppermint stick candy, crushed pineapple, sliced peaches, fruit cocktail.

Garnish with: Gum drops, a tablespoon of whipped cream (0.3 gm. of protein), maraschino cherry, fruit cocktail. Serve in half of a pear. Serve with a slice of candied ginger on top.

Low protein bread†

Ingredient	*Amount*
	gms.
Granulated sugar	12
Salt	3
Water (100° F.)	105
Yeast, compressed‡	9
Butter	5
Hydrogenated vegetable fat§	5
Glyceryl monostearate	0.5
Glycerol, pure	2 drops
Wheat starch*	150

Method

The amount of each ingredient needed for one batch of rolls or one loaf of bread is given in above table. Procedures are as follows:

1. Place sucrose and sodium chloride in mixing bowl; add water.
2. Dissolve yeast in above solution.
3. Melt butter and vegetable fat together; add glyceryl monostearate (GMS) to hot fat mixture and stir until dissolved. Add glycerol.
4. Add mixture (3) to (2).
5. Add wheat starch to (4), one-half at a time, stirring gently at low speed with an automatic mixer until the starch is well moistened.
6. Mix for 5 to 7 min. (use either a rotary beater or paddle) with automatic mixer. Scrape sides and bottom of bowl with spatula once during mixing. Do not scrape any material adhering to beaters into the batter at end of the mixing period.
7. Scrape mixture adhering to sides of bowl into the mass of material at bottom of bowl. Cover bowl with a damp cloth and allow mixture to ferment for 30 min. at 82° F.
8. At end of 30-min. period, stir the mixture thoroughly, by hand, until the batter returns to the fluid but plastic state it had before fermentation.
9. If making rolls, divide mixture equally between six heavy aluminum muffin cups (3 in. diameter by 1½ in. deep) greased with vegetable fat. Brush top of each roll with melted butter. If making loaf, pour mixture into a heavy aluminum pan (7½ by 3½ by 2½ in.) greased with vegetable fat. Brush top with melted butter.
10. Cover with a damp cloth and let rise for 45 min. at 82° F.
11. Bake rolls at 400° F. for 20 min.; place under broiler for 2 min. to brown tops of rolls. Bake loaf at 550° F. for 5 min., then at 400°F. for 30 to 35 min.; place under broiler for 2 min. to brown top of loaf.
12. Remove rolls or loaf from oven; remove from pan and cool on a wire rack.

*Paygel, P. General Mills, Inc., or Cellu.
†Steele, B. F., *et al.*: A Yeast-Leavened, Low-Protein Bread for Research Diets, J. Amer. Diet. Ass. **47:**405-6, 1965.
‡Fleischmann's cake yeast.
§Crisco.

Food exchange lists* for use with modified Giovannetti diet (1 gm. protein)

List 1—fruits and fruit juices

Food	Description	Amount containing 1 gm. protein	Potassium mg.
Applesauce	canned or fresh	1⅔ cups	325
Apricots	fresh, medium	2 to 3	281
	canned in heavy syrup, medium halves	5	390
Banana	small, 6 inches long	1	370
Blackberries	fresh	½ cup	136
	canned	½ cup	215
	frozen	½ cup	115
Blueberries	fresh, canned, frozen	1 cup	128
Cantaloupe	fresh, diced	⅔ cup	401
Sweet cherries	fresh, large	13	165
	fresh, small	21	161
	canned in heavy syrup	½ cup	124
Maraschino cherries	large	60	
Figs, fresh	large	2	194
	small	3	194
Fruit cocktail	canned	1¼ cups	363
Grapefruit	white or pink, medium 4 inches in diameter	1	270
Grapes	American type	½ cup	158
	Thompson seedless, canned or fresh	1 cup	220
Orange	small	1	200
	segments	½ cup	194
Papaya	fresh	½ cup	(290)
Peaches	fresh, sliced	1 cup	340
	canned, heavy syrup, medium halves	5	325
Pears	small halves	10	420
Pineapple	fresh, diced	2 cups	390
	canned, in heavy syrup, large slices	3	300
Strawberries	fresh, stems removed, or sliced, and frozen	1 cup	246-286
	whole, frozen, sugar added, 10 oz. carton	1	295
Tangerine	large	1	126
	small	2	126
Tomato	small	1	244
Watermelon	balls or cubes	1 cup	200
Fruit juice or nectar			
Apple juice		1 cup	250
Apricot juice		1 cup	
Apricot nectar		1¼ cups	469
Cranberry juice		5 cups	125
Grapefruit juice	canned	1 cup	360
	fresh	1 cup	405
Grapefruit-orange juice		¾ cup	345
Grape juice		2 cups	580
Orange juice		¾ cup	375

*Figures from Bowes, A. D. and Church, C. F.: Food values of portions commonly used, ed. 10. Revised by Church, C. F., and Church, H. N., Philadelphia, 1968, J. B. Lippincott Co.   *Continued.*

Food exchange lists* for use with modified Giovannetti diet (1 gm. protein)—cont'd

List 1—fruits and fruit juices—cont'd

Food	Description	Amount containing 1 gm. protein	Potassium mg.
Peach nectar		2 cups	390
Pear nectar		1¼ cups	125
Pineapple juice		1 cup	375
Prune juice		1 cup	600
Tangerine juice		1 cup	450
Tomato juice		½ cup	273

List 2—vegetables

Food	Description	Amount containing 1 gm. protein	Potassium mg.
Beans	green snap or yellow wax, cooked and drained	½ cup	114
Beets	red, diced, canned, drained	½ cup	138
Cabbage	head green, cooked	⅗ cup	163
Chinese cabbage	raw, shredded	2¼ cups	253
	cooked	½ cup	(253)
Carrots	cooked, drained	⅔ cup	222
	fresh, 1 large, 2 small		341
Celery	diced	1 cup	341
Cucumber	fresh, pared, medium	1½	240
pickles	dill or sweet, large	1½	300
Eggplant	cooked, drained	½ cup	150
Lettuce	large, outer leaves	2	264
	coarsely broken	1¼ cups	264
	finely cut	½ cup	264
Mushrooms	canned and drained	⅓ cup	164
Pepper	green: fresh or cooked large, empty shell	1	213
Onion	fresh, 1½ inch in diameter	1	104
	cooked	½ cup	110
	scallions, 5 inches long, ½ inch in diameter	5	231
Potatoes	crisp chips, 2 inches in diameter	10	226
Rutabagas	cooked cubes	½ cup	167
Sauerkraut	drained	⅔ cup	140
Summer squash	fresh, cooked	½ cup	202
Sweet potato	canned, syrup pack	1 small with syrup	120
Tomato	ripe, fresh, small	1	244
Turnip	cooked, diced	⅔ cup	188

List 3—vegetables and other foods containing two grams of protein in amounts listed

Food	Description	Amount containing 2 gm. protein	Potassium mg.
Vegetables			
Asparagus	Cooked, cut pieces	½ cup	140
	Canned, medium spears	5	160

*Figures from Bowes, A. D. and Church, C. F.: Food values of portions commonly used, ed. 10. Revised by Church, C. F., and Church, H. N., Philadelphia, 1968, J. B. Lippincott Co.

Food exchange lists* for use with modified Giovannetti diet (1 gm. protein)—
cont'd

*List 3—vegetables and other foods
containing two grams of protein in amounts listed—cont'd*

Food	Description	Amount containing 1 gm. protein	Potassium mg.
Beans	green snap or yellow wax, fresh, canned, frozen, cooked and drained	1 cup	243
Red cabbage	raw, shredded	1 cup	268
Corn	canned, drained	½ cup (scant)	81
Okra	cooked pods	8 to 9	174
Potato	boiled or baked, 2¼ inches in diameter	1	285
	french fries: pieces ½ inch by ½ inch by 2 inches	10	427
Other foods			
Bacon	Slice (1 oz. before cooking)	1	16
Bread	average slice	1	20-30
Danish	small sweet roll	1	39
Zweiback	piece	2	
Melba toast	slice	2	
Raspberries	frozen, sugar added, 10 oz. carton	1	284
Rice	cooked, white or brown	⅔ cup	105
Spaghetti	cooked, tender (not firm)	½ cup (scant)	50
Macaroni	cooked, tender	⅓ cup	45
Noodles	cooked	⅓ cup	25
Myost	cheese product	1 oz.	—

List 4—free list (foods containing little or no protein)

Foods	Exceptions
Butter	
Oil	
Vinegar	
Jelly	No jams
Honey	
Alcoholic beverages	No beer or ale
Soy sauce	
Tea, coffee, sanka, carbonated beverages	
Herbs and spices (pepper, oregano, cinnamon, etc.)	
Candy: hard candy, sour balls, butterscotch, cream mints (no chocolate coating), lollipops, jelly beans, gum drops, fondant	No chocolate candy
Sugar: white, powdered, brown, sugar syrup, corn syrup.	
Limeade	
Cornstarch	
Tapioca	

*Figures from Bowes, A. D. and Church, C. F.: Food values of portions commonly used, ed. 10. Revised by Church, C. F., and Church, H. N., Philadelphia, 1968, J. B. Lippincott Co.

the Giovannetti diet to British tastes (milk for tea; a low protein bread product and wafers instead of Italian pastes), they observed the same clinical improvement in chronic uremia patients treated with the modified diet of 18 to 20 gm. protein. The protein was of animal source—6½ oz. of milk and one egg—and vegetable protein, and included minimal requirements of all the essential amino acids except methionine. This one essential amino acid was added as a dietary supplement. In 1966, Schloerb[15] also reported confirmation of these results in studies at the University of Kansas with uremic patients using the low protein (20 gm.) high caloric (2,000) diet with amino acid supplementation.

A number of U. S. clinics have since used the modified Giovannetti diet for uremic patients and observed similar relief of clinical symptoms. Practical diet plans and food exchange lists, recipes and food preparation suggestions have helped to make the diet useful in the home situation. Careful instruction is given the patient and his family, with much follow-up help and support to carry out the plan. The basic diet pattern is given on p. 551, and food lists on pp. 553-555.

RENAL CALCULI
Etiology

Although the basic cause of renal calculi is unknown, many factors contribute directly or indirectly to their formation. These factors relate to the nature of the urine itself or to the conditions of the urinary tract environment.

Concentration of urinary constituents

Calcium. By far the majority of renal stones—about 96%—are composed of calcium compounds. The normal excretion of calcium on a relatively moderate calcium diet of about 400 mg. daily is 100 to 175 mg. every twenty-four hours. On an average adult intake of 800 mg. or more of calcium, homeostatic mechanisms regulate the amount of calcium excretion. In some persons, however, hyperexcretion of calcium

may occur, which produces supersaturation of the urine with crystalloid elements. Apparently in persons who form stones there is a greater precipitating tendency caused by the lack of substances in normal urine which prevents agglomeration of these crystals. Excess urinary calcium may result from the following.

1. *Excess calcium intake.* Prolonged use of large amounts of milk and alkali therapy for peptic ulcer, or of a hard water supply, contribute to excess calcium loads.
2. *Hypervitaminosis D.* Excess Vitamin D may cause increased calcium absorption from the intestine as well as increased calcium withdrawal from bone.
3. *Prolonged immobilization.* Body casting or immobilization in illness or disability may lead to withdrawal of bone calcium and increased urine concentration (p. 453).
4. *Hyperparathyroidism.* Primary hyperparathyroidism causes excess calcium excretion (p. 123). About two-thirds of the persons with this endocrine disorder have renal stones, but this disorder accounts for only a small number (about 5%) of the total calcium stones.
5. *Renal tubular acidosis.* Excess excretion of calcium is caused by defective ammonia formation.
6. *Idiopathic hypercalciuria.* Some persons, even on a low calcium diet, and for unknown reasons, may excrete as much as 500 mg. of calcium daily.
7. *Oxalate.* Due to some error in handling oxalates, about half the calcium stones are compounds with these materials. Oxalates occur naturally in only a few food sources, such as rhubarb, spinach, tomatoes, and others. These foods are listed on p. 557.
8. *Uric acid.* Excess uric acid excretion may be caused by a derangement in the intermediary metabolism of purines, as in gout. It may also result

Food sources of oxalates

Fruits	*Vegetables*
Currants	Beans, green and wax
Concord grapes	Beets
Figs	Beet greens
Gooseberries	Chard
Plums	Endive
Raspberries	Okra
Rhubarb	Spinach
	Sweet potato
	Tomato
Nuts	*Beverages*
Almonds	Chocolate
Cashew nuts	Cocoa
	Tea

from rapid tissue breakdown as in wasting diseases.

Cystine. A hereditary metabolic defect in renal tubular reabsorption of the amino acid cystine causes it to accumulate in the urine (cystinuria).

Urinary tract conditions

Physical changes in the urine. Physical changes in the urine may predispose susceptible persons to stone formation.

Concentration of urine may result from a lower water intake or from excess water loss, as in prolonged sweating, fever, vomiting, or diarrhea.

Changes in urinary pH from its mean of 5.85 to 6.00 may be influenced by diet or altered by the ingestion of acid or alkaline medications.

Organic stone matrix. Formation of an organic stone matrix provides the core or nucleus (nidus) which acts as a seed crystal for precipitation. This organic matrix is a mucoprotein-carbohydrate complex in which galactose and hexosamine are the principal carbohydrates. The source of these organic materials is obscure. Some possible factors include: (1) bacteria masses from recurrent urinary tract infections, (2) renal epithelial tissue of urinary tract which has sloughed off, possibly due

to vitamin A deficiency, and (3) calcified plaques (Randall's plaques) formed beneath the renal epithelium in hypercalcinuria. Irritation and ulceration of overlying tissue causes the plaques to slough off into the collecting tubules.

Clinical symptoms

Severe pain and numerous urinary symptoms may result. There is general weakness, and sometimes fever. Laboratory examination of urine and chemical analysis of any stone that is passed help to determine treatment.

Principles of treatment

Fluid intake. A large fluid intake produces a more dilute urine and helps to prevent concentration of stone constituents.

Urinary pH. An attempt to control the solubility factor is made by changing the urinary pH to an increased acidity or alkalinity, depending upon the chemical composition of the stones formed.

Stone composition. Dietary constituents of the stone are controlled to reduce the amount of the substance available for precipitation.

Binding agents. Materials which bind the stone elements and prevent their absorption in the intestine cause fecal excretion. For

Low calcium diet (approximately 400 mg. of calcium)

	Foods allowed	*Foods not allowed*
Beverage*	Carbonated beverage, coffee, tea	Chocolate flavored drinks, milk, milk drinks
Bread	White and light rye bread or crackers	
Cereals	Refined cereals	Oatmeal, whole-grain cereals
Desserts	Cake, cookies, gelatin desserts, pastries, pudding, sherbets, all made without chocolate, milk or nuts. If egg yolk is used, it must be from 1 egg allowance.	
Fat	Butter, cream, 2 tbsp. daily; French dressing, margarine, salad oil, shortening	Cream, except in amount allowed, mayonnaise
Fruit	Canned, cooked or fresh fruit or juice except rhubarb	Dried fruit, rhubarb
Meat, eggs	8 ounces daily of any meat, fowl or fish except clams, oysters, or shrimp; not more than 1 egg daily including those used in cooking	Clams, oysters, shrimp cheese
Potato or substitute	Potato, hominy, macaroni, noodles, refined rice, spaghetti	Whole grain rice
Soup	Broth, vegetable soup made from vegetables allowed	Bean or pea soup, cream or milk soups
Sweets	Honey, jam, jelly, sugar	
Vegetables	Any canned, cooked or fresh vegetables or juice except those listed	Dried beans, broccoli, green cabbage, celery, chard, collards, endive, greens, lettuce, lentils, okra, parsley, parsnips, dried peas, rutabagas
Miscellaneous	Herbs, pickles, popcorn, relishes, salt, spices, vinegar	Chocolate, cocoa, milk gravy, nuts, olives, white sauce

*Depending upon calcium content of local water supply; in instances of high calcium content, distilled water may be indicated.

example, sodium phytate is used to bind calcium, and aluminum gels are used to bind phosphate. Glycine may have a similar effect on oxalates.

Diet therapy

Diet therapy is directly related to the stone chemistry.

Calcium stones. A low calcium diet of about 400 mg. daily is usually given. This is an amount about half that of an average adult intake of 800 mg. The lower level is achieved mainly by removal of milk and dairy products. Other calcium food sources affected are leafy vegetables and whole grains. An outline for a low calcium diet is given above. If the stone is calcium-phosphate, phosphorus foods will be low (p. 559). Diets with other calcium levels may occasionally be used. Shorr[16] has recommended a moderately lowered calcium and phosphorus intake (700 mg.

Low phosphorus diet (approximately 1 gm. phosphorus and 40 gm. protein)

	Foods allowed	*Foods not allowed*
Milk	Not more than 1 cup daily; whole, skimmed or butter milk, or 3 tbsp. powdered including the amount used in cooking	
Beverages	Fruit juices, tea, coffee, carbonated drinks, postum	Milk and milk drinks except as allowed
Breads	White only. Enriched commercial, French, hard rolls, soda crackers, rusk	Rye and whole grain breads, cornbread, buscuits, muffins, waffles
Cereals	Refined cereals, such as Cream of Wheat, Cream of Rice, rice, cornmeal, dry cereals, cornflakes, spaghetti, and noodles	All whole grain cereals
Desserts	Berry or fruit pie, cookies, cakes in average amounts; Jell-o, gelatin, angel food cake, sherbet, meringues made with egg whites; puddings if made with 1 egg or milk allowance	Desserts with milk and eggs, unless made with the daily allowance
Eggs	Not more than 1 egg daily including those used in cooking; extra egg whites may be used	
Fats	Butter, margarine, oils, shortening	
Fruits	Fresh, frozen, canned, as desired	Dried fruits, such as raisins, prunes dates, figs, apricots
Meats	One large serving or two small servings daily of beef, lamb, veal, pork, rabbit, chicken, or turkey	Fish, shellfish (crab, oyster, shrimp, lobster, etc.) Dried and cured meats (bacon, ham, chipped beef, etc.) liver, kidney, sweetbreads, brains
Cheese	None	Avoid all cheese and cheese spreads
Vegetables	Potatoes as desired; at least 2 servings per day of any of the following: asparagus, carrots, beets, green beans, squash, lettuce, rutabagas, tomatoes, celery, peas, onions, cucumber, corn. No more than 1 serving daily of either cabbage, spinach, broccoli, cauliflower, brussels sprouts, artichokes	Dried vegetables such as peas, mushrooms, lima beans
Miscellaneous	Sugar, jams, jellies, syrups, salt, spices, seasonings, condiments in moderation	Chocolate, nuts, and nut products, such as peanut butter; cream sauces

Sample menu pattern

Breakfast	*Lunch*	*Dinner*
Fruit Juice	Meat, 2 oz.	Meat, 2 oz.
Refined cereal	Potato	Potato
Egg	Vegetable	Vegetable
White toast	Salad	Salad
Butter	Bread, white	Bread, white
½ cup milk	Butter	Butter
Coffee or tea	½ cup milk	Dessert
	Dessert	Coffee or tea
	Coffee or tea	

Low calcium test diet (200 mg. calcium)

	Gm.	Mg. calcium	
Breakfast			
Orange juice, fresh	100	19.00	
Bread (toast) white	25	19.57	
Butter	15	3.00	
Rice Krispies	15	3.70	
Cream, 20% butter fat	35	33.95	
Sugar	7	0.00	
Jam	20	2.00	
Distilled water, coffee, or tea*		0.00	
			81.22
Lunch			
Beef steak, cooked	100	10.00	
Potato	100	11.00	
Tomatoes	100	11.00	
Bread	25	19.57	
Butter	15	3.00	
Honey	20	1.00	
Applesauce	20	1.00	
Distilled water, coffee, or tea		0.00	
			56.57
Dinner			
Lamb chop, cooked	90	10.00	
Potato	100	11.00	
Frozen green peas	80	10.32	
Bread	25	19.57	
Butter	15	3.00	
Jam	20	2.00	
Peach sauce	100	5.00	
Distilled water, coffee, or tea		0.00	
			60.89
Total		198.68 mg. calcium	

*Use distilled water only, for cooking and for beverages.

Acid and alkaline ash food groups

Acid ash	Alkaline ash	Neutral
Meat	Milk	Sugars
Whole grains	Vegetables	Fats
Egg	Fruit (except cran-	Beverages (coffee and tea)
Cheese	berries, prunes,	
Cranberries	and plums)	
Prunes		
Plums		

Acid ash diet

The purpose of this diet is to furnish a well-balanced diet in which the total acid ash is greater than the total alkaline ash each day. It lists:

    I.   Unrestricted foods
    II.   Restricted foods
    III.   Foods not allowed
    IV.   Sample of a day's diet

I. *Unrestricted foods:* You may eat all you want of the following foods:

1. Breads: any, preferably whole grain; crackers, rolls
2. Cereals: any, preferably whole grain
3. Desserts: angel food or sunshine cake; cookies made without baking powder or soda; cornstarch pudding, cranberry desserts, custards, gelatin desserts, ice cream, sherbet, plum or prune desserts; rice or tapioca pudding
4. Fats: any, as butter, margarine, salad dressings, Crisco; Spry, lard, salad oils, olive oil, etc.
5. Fruits: cranberries, plums, prunes
6. Meat, egg, cheese; any meat, fish or fowl, 2 servings daily; at least one egg daily
7. Potato substitutes: corn, hominy, lentils, macaroni, noodles, rice, spaghetti, vermicelli
8. Soup: broth as desired; other soups from foods allowed
9. Sweets; cranberry or plum jelly; sugar, plain sugar candy
10. Miscellaneous: cream sauce, gravy, peanut butter, peanuts, popcorn, salt, spices, vinegar, walnuts

II. *Restricted foods:* Do not eat any more than the amount allowed each day

1. Milk: 1 pint daily (may be used in other ways than as beverage)
2. Cream: $\frac{1}{3}$ cup or less daily
3. Fruits: 1 serving of fruit daily (in addition to the prunes, plums, and cranberries); certain fruits listed below in paragraph IV are not allowed at any time
4. Vegetables including potato: two servings daily; certain vegetables listed below in paragraph IV are not allowed at any time

III. *Foods not allowed:*

1. Carbonated beverages, as ginger ale, coca cola, root beer
2. Cakes or cookies made with baking powder or soda
3. Fruits: dried apricots, bananas, dates, figs, raisins, rhubarb
4. Vegetables: dried beans, beet greens, dandelion greens, carrots, chard, lima beans
5. Sweets; chocolate or other candies than those in Group I; syrups
6. Miscellaneous: other nuts, olives, pickles

IV. *Sample menu:*

Breakfast	Lunch	Dinner
Grapefruit	Creamed chicken	Broth
Wheatena	Steamed rice	Roast beef, gravy
Scrambled Eggs	Green beans	Buttered noodles
Toast, butter, plum jam	Stewed prunes	Sliced tomato
Coffee, cream, sugar	Bread, butter	Mayonnaise
	Milk	Vanilla ice cream
		Bread, butter

Low purine diet (approximately 125 mg. purine)

General directions
1. During acute stages use only List 1.
2. After acute stage subsides and for chronic conditions use the following schedule:
    (a) Two days a week, not consecutive, use List 1 entirely
    (b) The remaining days add foods from List 2 and 3 as indicated
    (c) Avoid List 4 entirely
3. Keep diet moderately low in fat.

Typical meal pattern

Breakfast	*Lunch*	*Dinner*
Fruit	Egg or cheese dish	Egg or cheese dish
Refined cereal and/or egg	Vegetables, as allowed	Cream of vegetable soup,
White toast	(cooked or salad)	if desired
Butter, 1 tsp.	Potato or substitute	Starch (potato or substitute)
Sugar	White bread	Colored vegetable, as allowed
Coffee	Butter, 1 tsp.	White bread, butter, 1 tsp.
Milk, if desired	Fruit or simple dessert	(if desired)
	Milk	Salad, as allowed
		Fruit or simple dessert
		Milk

Food list 1—These foods contain an insignificant amount of purines and may be used as desired

Beverages
  carbonated
  chocolate
  cocoa
  coffee
  fruit juices
  postum
  tea
Butter*
Breads—white and crackers, corn bread
Cereals and cereal products
  corn
  rice
  tapioca
  refined wheat
  macaroni
  noodles
Cheese of all kinds*
Eggs
Fats of all kinds* (moderation)
Fruits of all kinds
Gelatin, Jell-o
Milk—buttermilk, evaporated, malted, sweet
Nuts of all kinds*
  Peanut butter*
Pies* (except mince-meat)
Sugar and sweets
Vegetables
  artichokes
  beets
  beet greens

*High in fat.

Low purine diet (approximately 125 mg. purine)—cont'd

Vegetables—cont'd
  broccoli
  brussels sprouts
  cabbage
  carrots
  celery
  corn
  cucumber
  eggplant
  endive
  kohlrabi
  lettuce
  okra
  parsnips
  potato—white and sweet
  pumpkin
  rutabagas
  sauerkraut
  string beans
  summer squash
  swiss chard
  tomato
  turnips

Food list 2—one item 4 times a week; foods which contain a moderate amount (up to 75 mg.) of purine bodies in 100 gm. serving

Asparagus	Herring	Oysters
Bluefish	Kidney beans	Peas
Bouillon	Lima beans	Salmon
Cauliflower	Lobster	Shad
Chicken	Mushrooms	Spinach
Crab	Mutton	Tripe
Finnon haddie	Navy beans	Tuna fish
Ham	Oatmeal	Whitefish

Food list 3—one item once a week; foods which contain a large amount (75-150 mg.) of purine bodies in 100 gm. serving:

Bacon	Lentils	Quail
Beef	Liver sausage	Rabbit
Calf tongue	Meat soups	Sheep
Carp	Partridge	Shellfish
Chicken soup	Perch	Squab
Codfish	Pheasant	Trout
Duck	Pigeon	Turkey
Goose	Pike	Veal
Halibut	Pork	Venison

Food list 4—avoid entirely; foods which contain very large amounts (150 to 1000 mg.) of purine bodies in 100 gm. serving:

Sweetbreads	825 mg.
Anchovies	363 mg.
Sardines (in oil)	295 mg.
Liver (calf, beef)	233 mg.
Kidneys (beef)	200 mg.
Brains	195 mg.
Meat extracts	160 to 400 mg.
Gravies	variable

°High in fat.

Low methionine diet[*]

	Foods allowed	*Foods not allowed*
Soups	Any soup made without meat stock or addition of milk	Rich meat soups, broths, canned soups made with meat broth
Meat or meat substitute	Peanut butter sandwich, spaghetti or macaroni dish made without addition of meat, cheese or milk; one serving per day: chicken, lamb, veal, beef, pork, crab, or bacon (3)	Fish and those not listed above
Beverages	Soy milk, tea, coffee	Milk in any form
Vegetables	Asparagus, artichoke, beans, beets, carrots, chicory, cucumber, eggplant, escarole, lettuce, onions, parsnips, potato, pumpkin, rhubarb, tomatoes, turnips	Those not listed as allowed
Fruits	Apples, apricots, banana, berries, cherries, fruit cocktail, grapefruit, grapes, lemon juice, nectarines, oranges, peaches, pears, pineapple, plums, tangerines, watermelon, canteloupe	Those not listed as allowed
Salads	Raw or cooked vegetable or fruit salad	
Cereals	Macaroni, spaghetti, noodles	
Breads	Whole wheat, rye, white	
Nuts	Peanuts	
Desserts	Fresh or cooked fruit, ices, fruit pies	
Eggs		In any form
Cheese		All varieties
Concentrated sweets	Sugar, jams, jellies, syrup, honey, hard candy	
Concentrated fats	Butter, margarine, cream	
Miscellaneous	Pepper, mustard, vinegar, garlic, oil, herbs, spices	

Meal pattern

Breakfast	*Lunch*	*Dinner*
1 cup fruit juice	1 serving soup	2 oz. meat
½ cup fruit	1 serving sandwich	1 med. starch
1 slice toast	1 cup fruit	½ cup vegetable
1½ pats butter	8 oz. soy milk[†]	1 serving salad
2 tsp. jelly	3 tsp. sugar	1 T. dressing
1 T. sugar	1 T. cream	1 slice bread
beverage	beverage	1 serving dessert
1 T. cream		1 T. sugar
		1 T. cream
		1½ pats butter
		beverage

[*]Smith, D. R., Kolb, F. O., and Harper, H. A.: The Management of Cystinuria and Cystine-Stone Disease, J. Urol, 81:61, 1959.
[†]Optional; use in children to include protein intake. Omit if urine calcium is elevated in adults.

Low methionine diet*—cont'd

Sample menu

Breakfast	Lunch	Dinner
Orange juice	Vegetable soup, vegetarian	Chicken, roast
applesauce	peanut butter sandwich	baked potato
whole wheat toast	canned peaches	artichoke
butter	soy milk†	sliced tomatoes
jelly	sugar	French dressing
sugar	cream	whole wheat bread
coffee	coffee or tea	fruit ice
cream		sugar
		cream
		butter
		coffee or tea

*Smith, D. R., Kolb, F. O., and Harper, H. A.: The management of cystinuria and cystine-stone disease, J. Urol. 81:61, 1959.
†Optional; use in children to include protein intake. Omit if urine calcium is elevated in adults.

Summary of diet therapy principles in renal stone disease

Stone chemistry	Nutrient modification	Diet ash (urinary pH)
Calcium	Low calcium (400 mg.)	Acid ash
phosphate	Low phosphorus (1,000 to 1,200 mg.)	
oxalate	Low oxalate	
Uric acid	Low purine	Alkaline ash
Cystine	Low methionine	Alkaline ash

calcium and 1,200 mg. of phosphorus), to be used with aluminum hydroxide gels in the management of calcium-phosphate stones. A test diet of 200 mg. of calcium may be used also to rule out hyperparathyroidism as an etiologic factor. Such a test diet is given on p. 560.

Since calcium stones have an alkaline chemistry, an acid ash diet may also be used to create a urinary environment less conducive to precipitation of the basic stone elements. On p. 560 the classification of food groups is given according to pH of the metabolic ash produced. An acid ash diet would increase the amounts of meat, grains, egg and cheese used, and limit the amounts of vegetable, milk and fruit. An alkaline ash diet would outline the opposite use of these foods. An acid ash diet pattern applying these classifications is shown on p. 561. Cranberry juice seems to have a strong urinary acidifying effect or bacteriostatic value and is frequently used as a dietary adjunct.

Uric acid stones. About 4% of the total incidence of renal calculi are uric acid stones. Since uric acid is a metabolic product of purines, dietary control of this precursor is indicated. Purines are nucleoproteins (p. 44) found in active tissue such as glandular meat, other lean meat, meat extractives, and in lesser amounts in plant sources such as whole grains and legumes. A low purine diet is outlined on pp. 562-563. An effort to produce an alkaline ash would be made.

Cystine stones. About 1% of the total stones produced are cystine. Its occurrence is relatively rare. Cystine is a nonessential amino acid produced from the essential amino acid methionine. A diet low in methionine has been successfully used by Smith, Kolb and Harper[17] at the University of California Medical Center in San Francisco as part of their program for managing cystinuria and cystine-stone disease. The low methionine diet is outlined on pp. 564-565. It is used extensively with high-fluid and alkali therapy.

A summary of the diet therapy principles in renal stone disease is outlined on p. 565.

References
Specific

1. Illingsworth, and others: A controlled investigation of the effect of diet in acute nephritis, Arch. Dis. Child **29**:551, 1954.
2. Kark, R. M., and others: The nephrotic syndrome in adults: a common disorder with many causes, Ann. Int. Med. **49**:751, 1958.
3. Kark, R. M.: Some aspects of nutrition and the kidney. In Wohl, M., and Goodhart, R., editors: Modern nutrition in health and disease, Philadelphia, 1964, Lea & Febiger.
4. Borst, J. C. G.: Protein katabolism in uraemia, effects of protein-free diets, infections, and blood transfusions, Lancet **1**:824, 1948.
5. Jordan, W., Cimino, J., and others: Basic pattern for a controlled protein, sodium, and potassium diet, J. Amer. Diet. Ass. **50**:137, 1967.
6. Bakke, J., and others: Sodium-restricted diets for dialysis patients, Hospitals **40**:76, 1966.
7. Mitchell,, M. C., and Smith, E. J.: Dietary care of the patient with chronic oliguria, Amer. J. Clin. Nutr. **19**:163, 1966.
8. Merrill, A. J.: Nutrition in chronic renal failure, J.A.M.A. **173**:905, 1960.
9. Steele, B. F., and others: A yeast-leavened, low-protein bread for research diets, J. Amer. Diet. Ass. **47**:405, 1965.
10. Giordano, C.: Use of exogenous and endogenous urea for protein synthesis in normal and uremic subjects, J. Lab. Clin. Med. August, 1963.
11. Giovannetti, S., and Maggior, Q.: A Low-Nitrogen diet with proteins of high biological value for severe chronic uraemia, Lancet, **1**:1000, 1964.
12. Berlyne, G. M., and Shaw, A. B.: Giordano-Giovannetti diet in terminal renal failure, Lancet **2**:7, 1965.
13. Berlyne, G. M., Shaw, A. B., and Nilwarangkur, S.: Dietary treatment of chronic renal failure: experiences with a modified Giovannetti diet, Nephron **2**:129, 1965.
14. Shaw, A. B., and others: The treatment of chronic renal failure by a modified Giovannetti diet, Quart. J. Med. **34**(N.S.):237, 1965.
15. Schloerb, P. R.: Essential L-amino acid administration in uremia, Amer. J. Med. Sci. December, 1966.
16. Shorr, E.: Aluminum hydroxide gels in the management of renal stone, J. Urol. **53**:507, 1945.
17. Smith, D. R., Kolb, F. O., and Harper, H. A.: The management of cystinuria and cystine-stone disease, J. Urol. **81**:61, 1959.

General

Ackerman G., et al.: Reversible insufficiency in chronic renal disease, J.A.M.A. **197**:749, 1966.

Ansell, J. S., and Taufic, M. R.: Nephrectomy and nephrostomy and nursing the patient after nephrectomy, Amer. J. Nurs. **58**:1394, 1958.

Arneil, G. C.: Nephritis. 1. Acute hemorrhagic nephritis, Nurs. Times **57**:586, 1961.

Arneil, G. C.: Nephritis. 2. The nephrotic syndrome, Nurs. Times **57**:622, 1961.

Boyce, W. H.: Nutrition and the formation of urinary calculi, Borden's Review **21**:27, 1960.

Boyce, W. H., and others: Abnormalities of calcium metabolism in patients with "idiopathic" urinary calculi. Effect of oral administration of sodium phytate, J.A.M.A. **166**:1577, 1958.

Catlow, C. E.: The treatment of acute traumatic renal insufficiency, J. Urol. **73**:913, 1955.

Comty, C. M.: Long-term dietary management of dialysis patients, J. Amer. Diet. Ass. **53**:439, 1968.

Corcoran, A. C.: Renal failure, Amer. J. Nurs. **56**:768, 1956.

Dahl, L. K.: Possible role of salt intake in the development of essential hypertension. In M. Bock, K. D., and Cottier, P. T., editors: Essential hypertension, Berlin 1960, Springer-Verlag, p. 53.

Danowski, T. S.: Low-sodium diets, physiological adaptation and clinical usefulness, J.A.M.A. **168**:1886, 1958.

Danowski, T. S., and Mateer, F. M.: Therapy of acute and chronic glomerulonephritis, J. Chron. Dis. **5**:122, 1957.

DeTar, W. T., et al.: Hyperparathyroidism and renal lithiasis, J. Urol. **86**:24, 1961.

Elkinton, J. R.: Moral problems in the use of borrowed organs, artificial and transplanted, Ann. Int. Med. **60**:309, 1964.

Harlan, W. R., and others: Proteinuria and nephrotic syndrome associated with chronic rejection of kidney transplants, New Eng. J. Med. **277**:769, 1967.

Heckel, N. J.: Kidney stones—their etiology and treatment, Am. J. Nurs. **55**:194, 1955.

Higgins, C. C.: Etiology and prevention of renal calculi, J. Urol. **68**:117, 1952.

Hughes, J., and others: Oxalate urinary tract stones, J.A.M.A. **172**:774, 1960.

Keitzer, W. A.: Treatment of uremia, J. Urol. **73**:921, 1955.

Koeff, W. J.: Treatment of uremia with forced high calorie-low protein diet, Nutr. Rev. **11**:193, 1953.

Kushner, D. S.: Calcium and the kidney, Am. J. Clin. Nutr. **4**:561, 1956.

Levin, D. M., and Cade, R.: Influence of dietary sodium, Ann. Int. Med. **62**:231, 1965.

Levin, S., and Winkelstein, J. A.: Diet and infrequent peritoneal dialysis in chronic anuric uremia, New Eng. J. Med. **277**:619, 1967.

Lowe, K. G., and Valtin, H.: Dietary treatment in acute anuria, Am. J. Clin. Nutr. **4**:486, 1956.

Maclean, M. M., et al.: Hemodialysis and the artificial kidney, Amer. J. Nurs. **58**:1672, 1958.

McCracken, B. H., and others: Dietary protein and renal failure, New Eng. J. Med. **272**:1050, 1965.

McDonald, D. F.: Medical management of recurrent urinary calculi, New York J. Med. **59**:4212, 1959.

Merrill, A. J.: Nutrition in chronic renal failure, Amer. J. Clin. Nutr. **4**:497, 1956.

Merrill, J. P.: Treatment of renal failure, New York, 1955, Grune and Stratton, Inc.

Overly, V. A., and Greenwood, M. L.: Developing wafers and biscuits of varying protein content, J. Amer. Diet. Ass., **45**:342, 1964.

Rantz, L. A.: Current status of therapy in glomerulonephritis, J.A.M.A. **170**:948, 1959.

Sawyer, J. R.: Nursing care of patients with urologic diseases, St. Louis, 1963, The C. V. Mosby Co.

Schreiner, G. E., and Maher, J. F.: Hemodialysis for chronic renal failure. III. Medical, moral and ethical, and socio-economic problems, Ann. Int. Med. **62**:551, 1965.

Smith, H. W.: Kidney, structure and function in health and disease, New York, 1951, Oxford University Press.

Sobel, J., and Seifter, E.: Sweating in the treatment of chronic uremia, Lancet **2**:760, 1964.

Squire, J. R.: Nutrition and the nephrotic syndrome in adults, Amer. J. Clin. Nutr. **4**:509, 1956.

Trusk, C. W.: Hemodialysis for acute renal failure, Amer. J. Nurs. **65**:80, 1965.

Twiss, M. R., and Maxwell, M. H.: Peritoneal dialysis, Amer. J. Nurs. **59**:1560, 1959.

Winer, J. H.: Practical value of analysis of urinary calculi, J.A.M.A. **169**:1715, 1959.

Winter, C. G., and others: Urinary calculi, Amer. J. Nurs. **63**:72, 1963.

Winters, R. W.: Nutrition and renal disease, Borden's Review **19**:75, 1958.

Zimmerman, H. J.: Nutritional aspects of acute glomerulonephritis, Amer. J. Clin. Nutr. **4**:482, 1956.

CHAPTER 30

Care of the surgery patient

The physiologic stress of surgery places added nutritional demands upon the patient. Deficiencies can accrue easily and sooner or later may lead to serious clinical manifestations. Careful attention to preoperative preparation of the patient and to his postoperative therapeutic needs reduces complications and provides resources for better wound healing and a more rapid recovery period.

PREOPERATIVE NUTRITION

Nutrient stores. When time permits, nutritional preparation of the patient for surgery should correct any nutrient deficiencies and provide optimum reserves for the period of surgery itself and the time following until oral feedings can be resumed.

Protein. The most common nutritional deficiency related to surgery is that of protein. Tissue and plasma reserves are imperative to fortify the patient for blood losses during surgery and tissue catabolism in the immediate postoperative period.

Calories. Sufficient calories should be provided to build up any weight deficit. Carbohydrate is needed for glycogen stores and to spare protein for tissue synthesis. If the patient is overweight, some weight reduction is indicated to reduce surgical risks.

Vitamins and minerals. Tissue stores of vitamins are needed for metabolism of carbohydrate and protein. Any deficiency state, such as anemia, should be corrected. Electrolytes and fluid should be in balance, with any dehydration, acidosis or alkalosis corrected.

Immediate preoperative period. Nothing is given by mouth for at least eight hours prior to surgery, so that the stomach will have no retained food at the time of the operation. Food in the stomach may be vomited and aspirated during anesthesia or recovery from anesthesia. Also, any food present may increase the possibility of postoperative gastric retention, gastric dilatation, or interfere with the surgical procedure itself.

Minimum residue. Prior to gastrointestinal surgery, a low residue (p. 507) or residue-free diet (p. 569) may be followed for two to three days to clear the operative site of any fecal residue.

POSTOPERATIVE NUTRITION
Therapeutic nutritional needs

In health, the body tissues undergo continuous turnover, with small physiologic losses being constantly replenished with nutrients in food eaten. In disease, however, especially surgical disease, losses are greatly increased while at the same time replacement from food is diminished or even absent for a period of time. Therapeutic nutrition becomes all the more significant as a means of aiding recovery.

Protein. Adequate protein intake in the postoperative recovery period is of primary therapeutic concern to replace losses and supply increased needs.

Progressively increasing protein deficiency is common in surgical patients. Negative nitrogen balances of as much as 20 gm. per day may occur. This amount of nitrogen loss represents an actual loss of tissue protein of over a pound a day.

Nonresidue diet

General description:

1. This diet includes only those foods free from fiber, seeds, and skins, and with the minimum amount of residue.
2. Fruits and vegetables are omitted except for strained fruit juices.
3. Milk is omitted.
4. The diet is adequate in protein and calories, containing approximately 75 gm. protein, 110 gm. fat, 250 gm. carbohydrate, and 2,260 calories. It is likely to be inadequate in vitamin A, calcium, riboflavin.
5. If patients are to remain for a long length of time on this diet, supplementary vitamins and minerals should be given.

	Allowed	*Not allowed*
Beverages	Carbonated beverages, coffee, tea	Milk and milk drinks
Bread	Crackers, melba or rusks	Whole grain bread
Cereals	Refined as cream of wheat, Farina, fine cornmeal, Malt-o-Meal, pablum, rice, strained oatmeal, corn flakes, puffed rice, Rice Krispies	Whole grain and other cereals
Cheese		None allowed
Desserts	Plain cakes and cookies, gelatin desserts, water ices, angel food cake, Arrowroot cookies, tapioca puddings made with fruit juice only	Pastries and all others
Eggs	As desired, preferably hard cooked	Fried eggs
Fats	Butter or substitute, small amount cream	None
Fruits	Strained fruit juices	All others
Meat, fish, poultry	Tender beef, chicken, fish, lamb, liver, veal, and crisp bacon	Fried or tough meat, pork.
Potatoes or substitute:	Only macaroni, noodles, spaghetti, refined rice	Potatoes, corn, hominy, unrefined rice.
Soups	Bouillon and broth only	All others.
Sweets	Hard candy, fondant, gumdrops, jelly, marshmallows, sugar, syrup and honey	Other candy, jam, marmalade
Vegetables	Tomato juice	All others
Miscellaneous	Salt	Pepper

Note: Fruit juices and hard candies may be taken between meals to increase caloric intake.

Postsurgical nonresidue diet

General description:

1. This diet is slightly higher in residue, but has greater variety, including potatoes, white bread products, processed cheese, sauces, and desserts made with milk, and cream for coffee and cereal.
2. The average daily menu will contain 85 grams protein, 2300 calories, and is slightly higher in vitamins and minerals.

Selection of foods

To the above add:

Cheese:	Processed cheese, mild cream cheeses
Potatoes:	Prepared any way, no skin
Bread:	Any kind without bran, white bread, rolls, pancakes, waffles
Fats:	Two ounces of cream or half and half per meal, cream sauce, cream gravy
Desserts:	All desserts except those containing fruit and nuts
Condiments:	As desired

In addition to protein losses from tissue catabolism, there is loss of plasma proteins through hemorrhage, wound bleeding, and exudates. Increased metabolic losses result also from extensive tissue inflammation, or from infection and trauma. If any degree of prior malnutrition or chronic infection existed, the patient's protein deficit may become severe and cause serious complications to develop. The following are the body's protein needs:

1. *Tissue synthesis in wound healing.* Tissue proteins can only be synthesized by amino acids brought to the tissue by the circulating blood (p. 53). These necessary amino acids must come either from ingested protein or by intravenous injection. Tissue protein deficiencies are best met by oral feedings. When appetite is poor, often palatable concentrated liquid drinks are useful. Examples of oral nutrient feedings and high protein beverages are given in Table 27-1 (p. 516). During early feeding periods, or with the extremely malnourished patient, a daily intake of 50 to 75 gm. of protein may be all that can be tolerated. However, this amount should be increased as early as possible to achieve the 100 to 200 gm. daily that is needed to restore lost protein tissues and synthesize new tissue at the wound site. Although tissue protein is broken down more rapidly during stress, it is also built up more rapidly—provided sufficient amino acids are present to supply the demand.

2. *Avoidance of shock.* A reduction in blood volume, a loss of plasma proteins, and a decrease in circulating red blood cell volume contribute to the potential danger of shock. Where protein deficiencies exist, this danger is enhanced.

3. *Control of edema.* When the serum protein level is low, edema develops due to loss of colloidal osmotic pressure to maintain the normal shift of fluid between capillaries and surrounding interstitial tissues (p. 162). Considerable excess fluid may collect in the interstitial spaces before clinical edema is evident, and may affect heart and lung action. Local edema at the surgical site also delays closure of the wound and hinders the normal healing process.

4. *Bone healing.* In orthopedic surgery, where extensive bone healing is involved, protein is also essential for proper callus formation and calcification. A sound protein matrix must be present for the anchoring of mineral matter in the bone.

5. *Resistance to infection.* Amino acids are necessary constituents of the proteins involved in body defense mechanisms—antigens, antibodies, blood cells, hormones, enzymes. Tissue integrity itself is a bulwark against infection.

6. *Lipid transport.* Proteins are necessary for the transportation of lipids in the body, and therefore for the protection of the liver, a main site of fat metabolism, from damage by fatty infiltration. Protein provides essential lipotropic agents to form lipoproteins, the transport form of fat in the body (p. 38).

Effect of inadequate protein. It is evident, therefore, that multiple clinical problems may easily develop where protein deficiencies exist. There may be poor wound healing and dehiscence, delayed healing of fractures, anemia, failure of gastrointestinal stomas to function, depressed pulmonary and cardiac function, reduced resistance to infection, extensive weight loss, liver damage, and increased mortality risks.

Calories. Carbohydrate must be supplied in adequate quantities to ensure the use of protein for necessary tissue protein synthesis and to supply the energy required for increased metabolic demands. As protein is increased, the total calories must be increased also. The studies of Calloway and Spector[1] have indicated that a minimum of 2,800 calories per day must be provided before protein can be used for tissue repair and not be converted in part to provide energy. In acute stress, as in extensive radical surgery or burns, where protein needs are as high as 250 gm. daily, 4,000 to 6,000 calories are required. In addition to its protein-sparing action, carbohydrate also helps to avoid liver damage from depletion of glycogen reserves.

Fat calories must be adequate but not excessive. Excessive body fat is to be avoided as fatty tissue heals poorly and is more susceptible to infections, hematomas, and serum collections.

Fluid. Adequate fluid therapy is of paramount importance to ensure the patient against dehydration. During the postoperative period there may be large fluid losses from vomiting, hemorrhage, exudates, diuresis, or fever. Where drainage is involved more fluid loss is incurred. Table 30-1 indicates the magnitude of water requirements for surgical patients. Intravenous therapy will supply initial needs, but oral intake should begin as soon as possible and be maintained in sufficient quantity.

Minerals. Replacement of mineral deficiencies and insurance of continued adequacy is essential. In tissue catabolism, potassium and phosphorus are lost. Electrolyte imbalances in sodium and chloride result from fluid losses. Iron deficiency anemia may develop from blood loss or from faulty iron absorption.

Vitamins. Vitamin C is imperative for wound healing. Its presence is necessary for formation of cementing material in the ground substance of connective tissue, in capillary walls, and the building up of new tissue (p. 110). Extensive tissue regeneration as in burns or mastectomy may require as much as 1 gm. daily, about fifteen to twenty times the normal requirement. As calories and protein are increased, the B vitamins—thiamine, riboflavin, and niacin—must also be increased to provide essential coenzyme factors to metabolize carbohydrate and protein. Other B-complex vitamins—folic acid, B_{12}, pyridoxine, pantothenic acid—also have important metabolic roles in stress situations. Vitamin K is essential to the blood-clotting mechanism (p. 83).

Table 30-1. Daily water requirements of the surgical patient*

Type of case and fluid needs	Average fluid required ml.
Uncomplicated cases:	
For vaporizations	1,000 to 1,500
For urine	1,000 to 1,500
	2,000 to 3,000 total
Complicated cases (sepsis, elevation of temperature, humid weather, renal damage)	
For vaporization	2,000 to 2,500
For urine	1,000 to 1,500
	3,000 to 4,000 total
Seriously ill patients with drainage:	
For vaporization	2,000
For urine	1,000
For replacement of body fluid losses:	
1,000 ml. bile drainage	1,000
3,000 ml. Wangensteen drainage	3,000
	7,000 total

*Adapted from Zintel, H. A.: Nutrition in the care of the surgical patient. In Wohl, M., and Goodhart, R., editors: Modern nutrition in health and disease, ed. 3, Philadelphia, 1964, Lea and Febiger, p. 1055.

The occasions for therapeutic increases in vitamin intake have been well defined by the National Research Council in the pamphlet *Therapeutic Nutrition:*

1. A healthy person having a minor surgery or illness expected to last less than ten days, who is ambulatory and eating well and has no history of previous malnutrition, has no need for special consideration to vitamin therapy.
2. If the qualifications above are not met, the patient needs one to two times the normal daily requirement of vitamins.
3. If the patient is being fed entirely by the intravenous route, he should receive one to two times the minimum requirement for parenteral injection together with additional amounts of vitamin C.
4. If serious illness or severe trauma or burn is present, the vitamin requirement for the first few days is five to ten times the usual daily requirement. Thereafter, the patient will require two to three times the basic need until recovery is complete.

Dietary management

Oral vs. parenteral feeding. In a few patients the gastrointestinal tract cannot be used and parenteral feeding is the only way to sustain the patient. In such cases solutions of hydrolyzed proteins (amino acids and polypeptides) are used. Some fat emulsions are available for intravenous therapy but are more difficult to use.

However, the majority of patients can and should progress to oral feeding as soon as possible to provide adequate nutrition. One liter of a 5% dextrose solution contains 50 gm. of sugar with an energy value of 200 calories. Therefore, three liters a day at best can supply only 600 calories, and the *basal* energy requirement is about 700 calories, to say nothing of the increased metabolic demands of the stress of surgical illness. Ordinary intravenous feeding, therefore, cannot supply nutrient needs or

compete with oral feedings; *it can only compete with starvation!* Therefore a rapid return to regular eating should be encouraged and maintained.

Postoperative diets

Clear liquids. As soon as intestinal peristalsis returns, water and clear liquids—tea, coffee, broth, Jell-o, juice—are given to help supply important fluids and some sodium and chloride. These liquids also help stimulate normal gastrointestinal function and early return to a full diet.

Full liquids. Since clear liquids have little other nutrient value, progression to full liquids should soon follow. Milk and milk products—puddings, cream soups, high protein beverages, ice cream—supply much vital protein and carbohydrate.

Soft to regular diet. Each patient will progress to solid foods according to his individual tolerance, but encouragement and help should be supplied to enable him to eat as soon as possible. The usual diet pattern of postoperative feeding is outlined in Table 23-1, p. 471.

NUTRITIONAL CARE OF THE PATIENT WITH GASTROINTESTINAL SURGERY
Mouth, throat, or neck surgery

Surgery involving the mouth, throat, or neck will require modification in manner of feeding, as the patient usually cannot chew or swallow in the normal way.

Oral liquid feedings. Concentrated feedings in liquid form will need to be planned, using protein hydrolysates and added carbohydrate. Milk based beverages, soups, fruit juices with lactose or other sugar, and eggnogs can supply frequent reinforced nourishment. A milkshake formula, for example, supplemented with skimmed milk powder or a protein concentrate such as Casec, can supply 20 gm. of protein and 400 calories (p. 516).

Tube feedings. If a patient is comatose, severely debilitated, or has undergone radical neck or facial surgery, he may require tube feeding. Usually a nasogastric tube is used. However, in cases of esophagus obstruction, the tube is inserted into an opening made in the abdominal wall—a gastrostomy. The formula will be prescribed according to the need and tolerance of the individual patient. Small amounts are started and gradually increased. Usually two liters of formula are sufficient for a twenty-four-hour period, and the feeding should not exceed 8 to 12 oz. in each 3 to 4 hour interval. Two general types of formula may be used:

1. Nutrient preparations in powdered form, such as Sustagen, a protein hydrolysate, or Lonolac, a low sodium product can be used. These preparations, mixed with water in the desired proportions, are simple to prepare. However, in the higher calorie formula requirements, the amount of the nutrient material needed to fill the calorie requirement renders too concentrated an amount of carbohydrate and diarrhea results. In such cases, a planned formula of balanced ingredients would achieve a more desirable ratio of nutrients. For example, a 3,000 calorie formula using Sustagen alone would require about 5 cups to 2,500 ml. of water, and render a nutrient ratio of 180 gm. protein, 500 gm. carbohydrate, and 30 gm. fat. A planned food formula used instead, such as the example given in Table 30-2, would give a more

balanced ratio and probably be better tolerated. This formula may be compared with other sample mixtures given in Table 30-3.

2. Blenderized food mixtures are preferred by many patients because they feel they are getting regular food. Any foods that will liquify in a high-speed blender can be used, or strained baby food may be used to simplify the mixing. Usual ingredients include a milk base, with additions of egg, strained meat, vegetable, fruit, fruit juices, nonfat dry milk, cream, brewer's yeast, and ascorbic acid.

Gastric resection

A number of nutritional problems may develop following gastric surgery, depending upon the type of surgical procedure and the patient's individual response. A partial gastrectomy may create little postoperative difficulty. However, a total gastrectomy, in which there is complete excision of the stomach and establishment of an anastomosis between the jejunum and the remaining portion of the esophagus, may without care in planning the diet, produce serious nutritional deficits. When a vagotomy is performed there may be increased gastric fullness and distention. The stomach becomes atonic and empties poorly, so that food fermentation follows,

Table 30-2. Sample tube feeding formula (2,500 ml., 3,000 calories)

Ingredients	Amount	Protein	Fat	Carbohydrate
Homogenized milk	1 quart	32	40	48
Eggs	3	21	16	
Apple juice	400 ml.			55
Vegetable oil	30 ml.		30	
Strained baby food (4 oz. jars)				
Beef liver	4 cans	56	12	14
Beets	2 cans	3		20
Peaches	2 cans	1	1	59
Sustagen	1½ cups (225 gm.)	52	7	150
(Water as needed to total 2,500 ml.)				
	Totals	165	106	346
	Total calories		2,998	

Table 30-3. Types of tube feedings

Ingredients	Calories	Protein gm.	Fat gm.	Carbohydrate gm.
Regular tube feeding				
6 eggs	452	36.6	33.0	—
1 qt. homogenized milk	666	34.2	38.1	47.8
1 C. nonfat milk solids	434	42.7	1.2	121.3
½ C. Karo syrup				
1 tablet brewers yeast				
75 mg. ascorbic acid				
¼ tsp. salt				
1,500 ml.				
	2,021	113.5	72.3	231.5
Sustagen				
3 C. Sustagen	1,755	105.0	15.0	300.0
4 C. water				
1,200 ml.				
600 gm. Sustagen				
(4 C.)	2,300	140.0	20.0	400.0
1,200 ml. water				
1,400 ml.				
Add for banana Sustagen:				
2 tsp. banana flakes				
or	88	1.2	—	23.0
1 mashed banana				
Low calcium tube feeding				
6 cn. strained meat	540	80.4	25.2	0
1 qt. fruit juice	432	0	2.0	108.0
Karo syrup ¼ c.	234			61.0
ascorbic acid				
brewers yeast				
1,800 cc.				
	1,206	80.4	27.2	169.0
Low sodium tube feeding				
1 qt. low sodium milk	666	34.2	38.1	47.8
Casec 90 gm.—3 oz.	306	75.0		
18 Tbsp.				
Karo syrup ¼ c.	234			61.0
1,000 cc.				
	1,206	109.2	38.1	108.8

producing flatus and diarrhea. Following gastric surgery, about 50% of the patients fail to regain weight to optimum levels.

By and large, the nutritional care of patients who have had gastric surgery falls into two areas:

The immediate postoperative period. Following surgery, there is a very gradual resumption of oral feedings, according to the individual patient's tolerances. A typical pattern of dietary progression will cover about a two week period:

Gastrectomy diets

No. 1	No. 2	No. 3	No. 4
Breakfast	*Breakfast*	*Breakfast*	*Breakfast*
Soft Cooked egg Salt Sugar	Soft Cooked egg or poached egg Butter White toast Strained cereal Cream	Same as No. 2	Egg, not fried Cereal Toast Butter Canned fruit Cream
10:00 a.m.	*10:00 a.m.*	*10:00 a.m.*	*10:00 a.m.*
Jell-o with cream	Same as No. 1	Same as No. 1	Same as No. 1
Luncheon	*Luncheon*	*Luncheon*	*Luncheon*

Mashed potato
  with butter
Salt
Sugar
	Sliced turkey or
	  plain tender meat
	Baked potato with
	  butter
	Salt, sugar
		Roast beef
		Mashed potatoes
		Pureed vegetable
		White bread
		Butter
		Plain pudding
			Tender meat
			Potato or substitute
			Whole vegetables
			Bread, butter
			Dessert (no fresh fruit)

2:00 p.m.	*2:00 p.m.*	*2:00 p.m.*	*2:00 p.m.*
Baked custard	Same as No. 1	Same as No. 1	Same as No. 1
Dinner	*Dinner*	*Dinner*	*Dinner*
Baked potato	Small tender steak Baked potato with butter White toast Butter	Small tender steak Baked potato Pureed vegetable White bread Butter Vanilla ice cream	Tender meat Potato or substitute Whole vegetables Bread, butter Dessert (no fresh fruit)
8:00 p.m.	*8:00 p.m.*	*8:00 p.m.*	*8:00 p.m.*
Plain pudding	Same as No. 1	Plain pudding with cookie	Same as No. 3

Note: All meals are small in portions. Fluids, such as soup, milk, fruit juices and other beverages, should be taken in moderation.

First 24 to 48 hours	Nothing by mouth; intravenous therapy	Day 7	Same feedings—increase to 4 oz. each
Days 2 to 4	Ice chips, sips of water (temperature adjusted to patient response; some tolerate warm water better)	Day 8	Same feedings—add a soft egg at 8:00 a.m. and 6:00 p.m. feedings
Day 5	1 to 2 oz. water every even hour, and 1 to 2 oz. milk each odd hour between	Day 9 to 16	Water as desired; progress to a six-feeding ulcer-type diet
Day 6	Same feedings—increase to 3 oz. each	Day 16	Full bland diet; small meals with interval snacks

Principles of diet therapy. The basic principles of diet therapy for the postgastrectomy period are: (1) size of meals —small, frequent, and (2) type of food— simple, easily digested, mild, and low in bulk. A progressive gastrectomy diet in four stages is outlined on p. 575.

The later "dumping syndrome." After the patient has recovered from the surgery and begins to eat food in greater volume and variety, he may begin to experience increasing discomfort following meals. About ten to fifteen minutes after he has eaten, he has a cramping full feeling. His pulse is rapid, he feels a wave of weakness, cold sweating, and dizziness. Frequently he becomes nauseated and vomits. Such distressing reactions to food intake increase his anxiety and he eats less and less. He continues to lose weight and becomes increasingly malnourished.

This postgastrectomy complex of symptoms is commonly called the "dumping" syndrome, although the more precise term used by Lieber[2] is the *jejunal hyperosmolic syndrome.* This difficulty is more likely to occur in patients who have had total gastrectomies. The symptoms of shock result when a meal containing a high proportion of readily hydrolyzed carbohydrate rapidly enters the jejunum. This entering food mass is a concentrated hyperosmolar solution in relation to the surrounding extracellular fluid. To achieve an osmotic balance, water is drawn from the blood into the intestine, causing a rapid decrease in the vascular fluid compartment. The blood pressure drops, and signs of cardiac insufficiency appear—rapid pulse, sweating, weakness, and tremors.

A second sequence of events may follow about two hours later. The concentrated solution of carbohydrate is rapidly digested and absorbed, causing a postparandial rise in the blood glucose. The glucose load stimulates an overproduction of insulin which in turn leads to an eventual drop in the blood sugar below normal fasting levels. Symptoms of mild hypoglycemia result.

Principles of diet therapy. Careful control of the diet often brings dramatic relief of the distressing symptoms and leads to a gradual regaining of lost weight. Carbohydrate intake, especially simple sugars, is kept to a minimum to prevent rapid passage of food and formation of a concentrated, hyperosmolar solution. Protein and fat are increased to provide tissue building material and retard emptying of the food mass into the intestine. Meals are small, frequent, and dry, with fluid only between meals. There is less bulk to stimulate motility and less water to form rapid nutrient solutions. A summary of the dietary regimen is given on p. 577. Several follow-up studies of postgastrectomy patients on this regimen have indicated a good recovery of lost weight and correction of nutritional deficiencies.[3,4]

Cholecystectomy

For patients suffering from acute cholecystitis and cholelithiasis, the treatment is usually surgical removal of the gallbladder. The discussion of gallbladder disease in Chapter 27, p. 519 should be reviewed.

Following the surgery, control of fat in the diet remains essential to wound healing and comfort. The presence of fat in the duodenum continues to stimulate the cholecystokinin mechanism, which causes contraction and pain in the surgical area. There is also a period of adjustment to the more aqueous supply of liver bile for the preparation of fats for digestion. Depending upon individual toleration and response, a relatively low fat diet may need to be followed for as long as a month with moderate habits of fat use thereafter. The low fat regimen outlined on p. 520 for gallbladder disease may serve as a guide.

Ileostomy and colostomy

In cases of intestinal lesion or obstruction, or when chronic ulcerative colitis involves the entire colon, the treatment of choice is usually resection of the intestine and establishment of a permanent *ileostomy,* with removal of the diseased colon. The end of the remaining small intestine, the ileum, is attached to an opening in the

Diet for postoperative gastric dumping syndrome

General description:

1. Five or six small meals daily.
2. Relatively high fat content, to retard passage of food and help maintain weight.
3. High protein content (meat, egg, cheese) to rebuild tissue and maintain weight.
4. Relatively low carbohydrate content to prevent rapid passage of quickly utilized foods.
5. No milk; no sugar, sweets, or desserts; no alcohol or sweet carbonated beverages.
6. Liquids between meals only; avoid fluids for at least one hour before and after meals.
7. Relatively low roughage foods. Raw foods as tolerated.

Meal pattern:

Breakfast	2 scrambled eggs with 1 or 2 tablespoons butter or margarine
	½ to 1 slice bread or small serving cereal with butter or margarine
	2 crisp bacon
	1 serving solid fruit*
Mid-morning sandwich of:	1 slice bread
	butter or margarine
	2 oz. lean meat
Lunch	4 oz. lean meat with 1 or 2 T. butter or margarine
	Green or colored vegetable* with butter or margarine
	½—1 slice bread with butter or margarine
	½ banana or other solid fruit*
Mid-afternoon	Same snack as mid-morning
Dinner	4 oz. lean meat with 1 or 2 tbsp. butter or margarine
	green or colored vegetable† with butter or margarine
	½ to 1 slice bread with butter or margarine (or small serving starchy vegetable substitute)
	1 serving solid fruit*
Bedtime	2 oz. meat or 2 eggs or 2 oz. cheese or cottage cheese
	1 slice bread or 5 crackers
	butter or margarine

*Fruit choice: Applesauce, baked apple, canned fruit (drained), banana, orange or grapefruit sections
†Vegetable choice: Asparagus, spinach, green beans, squash, beets, carrots, green peas

abdominal wall and a stoma is formed to provide for discharge of intestinal contents. In a *colostomy,* the left side of the colon is resected and a stoma is made with the proximal sigmoid or descending colon.

Therefore, an ileostomy and a colostomy produce different problems in management. The intestinal contents at the point of the ileus are unformed, irritating, even erosive to the skin. The ileostomy drains freely, almost continuously, and should never be irrigated. Thus, establishment of controlled functioning is difficult, although many patients do develop a reasonable de-gree of regularity in relation to meals. Some sort of appliance is necessary to hold the discharge.

A colostomy is more manageable. The normal contents of the intestine at this point in the colon are solid, or semisolid, because of absorption of water and electrolytes by the proximal colon. The consistency of the discharge and its less irritating nature create fewer control problems. Often the sigmoid colostomy can be adequately controlled by simple dietary measures and periodic irrigation, so that in many cases no protective appliance is required.

A low residue diet (p. 507) is usually used in the immediate postoperative period. However, as soon as possible the diet should be advanced to a regular pattern of food to: (1) provide optimum nutrition and physical rehabilitation, and (2) provide an additional means of psychological support. Diet counseling with the patient and his family will help to establish the most successful pattern of meals for him and avoid those few foods which may cause individual discomfort.

Rectal surgery

For a brief period following rectal surgery (hemorrhoidectomy) a clear fluid or nonresidue diet may be indicated to delay initial bowel movement until healing has begun. The basic foods used are almost completely digested and absorbed in the small intestine leaving minimal residue for elimination by the colon. An outline of foods allowed is given on p. 569.

NUTRITIONAL CARE OF THE PATIENT WITH BURNS

A major aspect of therapy for the patient with extensive burns is rigorous nutritional care. Tremendous loss of tissue results from the burn itself, and in the catabolic period following, additional tissue destruction and nitrogen loss continues. Artz[5] describes studies in eight burned patients in whom the average daily portein loss for a catabolic period of one month was 166 gm. Fluid and electrolyte imbalances create management problems.

The nutritional care of the burned patient is adjusted to the individual patient's needs and responses over three distinct periods following the injury.

Immediate shock period—days 1 to 3 (4 or 5)

Initial fluid and electrolyte problems (day 1 to 2). A massive flooding edema occurs at the burn site during the first hours to about the second day. Loss of enveloping skin surface and exposure of extracellular fluids leads to immediate loss of interstitial water and electrolytes, mainly sodium, and large protein depletion. In an effort to balance the loss, water shifts from extracellular spaces in other parts of the body, only to add to the continuous loss at the burn site.

As a result of the initial shifts and losses, vascular fluid is decreased in volume and pressure, and there is hemoconcentration and diminished urine output. Cellular (hypertonic) dehydration (p. 161) follows as intracellular water is drawn out to balance extracellular fluid losses. Cell potassium is also withdrawn and circulating serum potassium levels rise.

Fluid therapy. Immediate intravenous fluid therapy seeks to replace:
1. Colloid (protein) through blood or plasma transfusion or by use of plasma expanders—Dextran
2. Electrolytes sodium and chlorine by use of a saline solution—lactated Ringer's solution
3. Water (dextrose solution) to cover additional insensible losses.

The amount of fluid given is calculated by the "rule of nines" and the Brooke formula,[6] or by a formula such as that of Evans[7] (1 ml. colloid plus 1 ml. electrolyte solution for each 1% of surface burned and each kilogram of body weight). The rate of flow should be carefully controlled. Half of the calculated fluid and electrolyte needs should be given during the first eight hours, ¼ during the second eight hours, and ¼ during the third eight hours. During the second twenty-four-hour period, the patient will require about half the amount of fluid given the first twenty-four hours. Throughout, there must be constant individual checks and adjustments.

Recovery period—days 3 to 5

As the fluid and electrolytes are gradually reabsorbed into the general circulation, balance is reestablished and the pattern of massive tissue loss is reversed. At this point there is a sudden diuresis. Intravenous therapy may be discontinued and oral solutions such as Holdrane's used:

Holdrane's solution (oral fluid and electrolyte replacement)
3 to 4 gm. (½ tsp.) salt
1.5 to 2 gm (1½ tsp.) sodium bicarbonate
  (baking soda)
1,000 ml. (1 qt.) water
Flavor with lemon juice and chill.
A careful check of fluid intake and output
is essential, with constant checks for signs
of dehydration or overhydration.

Secondary feeding period—days 6 to 15

*Factors demanding optimum nutritional
therapy.* Despite the patient's depression
and anorexia his life may well depend upon
rigorous nutritional therapy during the
secondary feeding period. Several factors
necessitate this increased intake.
1. Tissue destruction by the burn with
   large losses of protein and electrolytes
2. Tissue catabolism following with continuing nitrogen losses
3. Increased metabolic demands of *infection* or *fever* make extra calories
   necessary; for energy, extra carbohydrate and B vitamins are needed;
   tremendously increased basal needs
   as body resources are mobilized; *tissue regeneration* requires extra protein and vitamin C
4. Optimum tissue health necessary for
   subsequent grafting to be successful

Principles of diet therapy

High protein. Individual needs will vary
from 150 gm. to as high as 400 gm. Concentrated protein foods must be planned with
follow-through support to see that they
are consumed.

High calories. From 3,500 to 5,000 calories with a high percentage of carbohydrate is necessary to spare protein essential for tissue regeneration, and to supply
the greatly increased metabolic demands
for energy.

High vitamins. From 1 to 2 gm. of vitamin C are needed for tissue regeneration.
Increased thiamine, riboflavin, and niacin

are necessary to supply oxidative enzyme
systems to metabolize extra carbohydrate
and protein.

Intake record. Since the nutritional
needs are so vital, a careful record of protein and calorie value in the amount of
food consumed is a necessary tool for
planning care.

Dietary management

1. Initial tube feeding may be required
to ensure adequate intake. Formulas such
as those in Tables 30-2 and 30-3, pp. 573
and 574 may be used.
2. Concentrated oral liquids must be
given using protein hydrolysates to ensure
adequate intake. Milkshakes such as those
on p. 516 supply large amounts of nourishment.
3. Soft to regular diet will probably be
taken by the second week or so.
4. Individual support and care. Continuous support and encouragement are necessary to help the patient eat the food he
requires. Every effort should be made to
make the foods as attractive and appetizing
as possible, supplying items particularly
liked and respecting disliked foods.

Follow-up reconstruction period—weeks 2 to 5 and following

Grafting and plastic surgery. Continued
optimum nutrition is essential to maintain
tissue integrity for successful skin grafting
or plastic reconstructive surgery.

Rehabilitation. The principles of rehabilitation nursing discussed in Chapter 21
apply here. The patient will not only need
physical rebuilding of his body's resources,
but he will also need much emotional and
social support to rebuild his spirit and his
will. There may be disfigurement and disability. Health team members can do much
to help instill the courage and confidence
the patient must have to face the future
again. Whatever his future demands, however, optimum physical stamina gained
through persistent, supportive care—medical, nutritional, and nursing—will give him
the personal resources to cope.

References
Specific

1. Calloway, D., and Spector, H.: Nitrogen balance as related to caloric and protein intake in active young men, Amer. J. Clin. Nutr. **2:** 405, 1954.
2. Lieber, H.: The jejunal hyperosmolic syndrome (dumping) and its prophylaxis, J.A.M.A. **176:** 208, 1961.
3. Pittman, A. C., and Robinson, F. W.: Dumping syndrome—control by diet, J. Amer. Diet. Ass. **34:**596, 1958.
4. Pittman, A. C., and Robinson, F. W.: Dietary management of the "dumping" syndrome, J. Amer. Diet. Ass. **40:**108, 1962.
5. Artz, C. P., and others: Some recent developments in oral feedings for optimal nutrition in burns, Amer. J. Clin. Nutr. **4:**642, 1956.
6. Callentine, G. E., Jr.: How to calculate fluids for burned patients, Amer. J. Nurs. **62:**77, 1962.
7. Evans, I. E.: The early management of the severely burned patient, Surg. Gyn. Obstet. **94:**273, 1952.

General

Alexander E. L., and others: Care of the patient in surgery, ed. 4, St. Louis, 1967, The C. V. Mosby Co.
Artz, C. P.: Recent developments in burns, Amer. J. Surg. **108:**649, 1964.
Barron, J., and Fallis, L. S.: Tube feeding with natural foods in elderly patients, J. Amer. Geriat. Soc. **4:**400, 1956.
Barron, J., Prendergast, J. J., and Jocz, M. W.: Food pump: new approach to tube feeding, J.A.M.A. **161:**621, 1956.
Benjamin, H. B., and others: The surgical patient: oral bouillon feedings, J. Int. Coll. Surg. **30:**405, 1958.
Biggar, B. L., and others: Nutrition following gastric resection, J. Amer. Diet. Ass. **37:**344, 1960.
Blocker, T. G., Jr., and others: The care of patients with burns, Nurs. Outlook **6:**382, 1958.
Blocker, T. G., Jr., and others: Nutrition studies in the severely burned, Ann. Surg. **141:**589, 1955.
Brooke, C. E., and Anast, C. S.: Oral fluid and electrolytes, J.A.M.A. **179:**792, 1962.
Crandon, J. H.: Nutrition in surgical patients, J.A.M.A. **158:**264, 1955.
Davenport, R. R.: Tube feeding for long-term patients, Amer. J. Nurs. **64:**121, 1964.
Dericks, V. C.: Rehabilitation of patients with ileostomy, Amer. J. Nurs. **61:**48, 1961.
Editorial: Nutrition in the surgical patient, J.A.M.A. **165:**1830, 1957.
Elman, R.: Protein needs in surgical patients, J. Amer. Diet. Ass. **32:**524, 1956.

Fason, M. F.: Controlling bacterial growth in tube feedings, Amer. J. Nurs. **67:**1246, 1967.
Fisher, J. A.: The dumping syndrome, Amer. J. Nurs. **58:**1126, 1958.
Fisk, J. E.: Nursing care of the patient with surgery of the biliary tract, Amer. J. Nurs. **60:**53, 1960.
Glenn, F.: Surgical treatment of biliary tract disease, Amer. J. Nurs. **64:**88, 1964.
Hallburg, J. C.: The patient with surgery of the colon, Amer. J. Nurs. **61:**64, 1961.
Hayes, M. A.: Postoperative diet therapy, J. Amer. Diet. Ass. **35:**17, 1959.
Henderson, L. M.: Nursing care in acute cholecystitis, Amer. J. Nurs. **64:**93, 1964.
Holm, I., and others: Fat emulsion for complete intravenous nutrition; clinical studies, part 2, Postgrad. Med. **42:**A-99, 1967.
Jones, R. J.: Present knowledge of intravenous fat emulsions, Nutr. Rev. **24:**225, 1966.
Jordan, G. L., Jr.: Treatment of the dumping syndrome, J.A.M.A. **167:**1062, 1958.
Klug, T. J., and others: Gastric resection, Amer. J. Nurs. **61:**73, 1961.
Krehl, W. A.: Tube feeding, J.A.M.A. **169:**1153, 1959.
Kurihara, M.: The patient with an intestinal prosthesis, Amer. J. Nurs. **60:**852, 1960.
Larsen, R. B.: Dietary needs of patients following general surgery, Hospitals **39:**133, 1965.
Lehr, H. B., and others: The use of intravenous fat emulsions in surgical patients, J.A.M.A. **181:** 745, 1962.
Levey, S.: Reduction of nitrogen deficits in surgical patients maintained by intravenous ailmentation, Nutr. Rev. **24:**193, 1966.
Lewis, M. N., Murray, M. A., and Zollinger, R. M.: Dietary regimen following partial gastric resection, J. Amer. Diet. Ass. **30:**852, 1954.
Lewis, M. N., and others: Nutrition following gastric resection. I. The immediate postoperative period, J. Amer. Diet. Ass. **34:**1195, 1958.
Luschen, M.: Technique and temperament made the difference, Amer. J. Nurs. **64:**103, 1964.
Machella, T. E.: Postsurgical problems of the gastrointestinal tract, J.A.M.A. **174:**2111, 1960.
Machella, T. E., and Ravdin, R. G.: Jejunal feeding, Amer. J. Clin. Nutr. **3:**481, 1955.
McKittrick, J. B., and Shotkin, J. M.: Ulcerative colitis, Amer. J. Nurs. **62:**60, 1962.
Milner, C. W.: Nursing care of severely burned patients, Amer. J. Nurs. **54:**456, 1954.
Moore, F. D.: The treatment of severe burns, Amer. J. Nurs. **54:**454, 1954.
Pareira, M. D., and others: Therapeutic nutrition with tube feeding, J.A.M.A. **146:**810, 1954.
Pearson, E., and others: Metabolic derangements in burns, J. Amer. Diet. Ass. **32:**223, 1965.
Postoperative distention and fruit juices, questions and answers, J.A.M.A. **194:**476, 1965.

Quinlan, E.: Dietary treatment in burns, Canad. Nurse, Vol. 61, No. 5, 1965.

Rosenberg, S. A., and others: The syndrome of dehydration, coma, and severe hyperglycemia without ketosis in patients convalescing from burns, New Eng. J. Med. 272:931, 1965.

Secor, S. M.: Colostomy care—1964, Amer. J. Nurs. 64:127, 1964.

Sister Jeannette Marie: The 'ostomies': current concepts in dietary management, Hospitals, 38:88, 1964.

Smith, A. V.: Nasogastric tube feeding, Amer. J. Nurs. 57:1451, 1957.

Therapeutic nutrition, National Academy of Sciences, National Research Council, Washington, D. C., 1951.

White, D. R.: I have an ileostomy, Amer. J. Nurs. 61:51, 1961.

Willis, M. T., and Postlewait, R. W.: Dietary problems after gastric resection, J. Amer. Diet. Ass. 40:111, 1962.

Wolfman, E. F., and Flotte, C. T.: Carcinoma of the colon and rectum, Amer. J. Nurs. 61:60, 1961.

Zintel, H. A.: Nutrition in the care of the surgical patient. In Wohl, M., and Goodhart, R., editors: Modern nutrition in health and disease, Philadelphia, 1964, Lea and Febiger.

Zollinger, R. M., and Ellison, E. H.: Nutrition after gastric operations, J.A.M.A. 154:811, 1954.

Zollinger, R. M., and Stewart, W. R. C.: Surgical management of gastric ulcer, J.A.M.A. 171:2056, 1959.

APPENDIXES

Nutritive values of the edible part of foods[1]

Food, approximate measure, and weight (in grams)			Food energy	Protein	Fat (total lipid)	Fatty acids			Carbohydrate	Calcium	Iron	Vitamin A value	Thiamine	Riboflavin	Niacin	Ascorbic acid
						Saturated (total)	Unsaturated									
							Oleic	Linoleic								
		gm.	(Calories)	(gm.)	(gm.)	(gm.)	(gm.)	(gm.)	(gm.)	(mg.)	(mg.)	(I.U.)	(mg.)	(mg.)	(mg.)	(mg.)
Milk, cream, cheese (related products)																
Milk, cow's																
Fluid, whole (3.5% fat)	1 cup	244	160	9	9	5	3	Trace	12	288	0.1	350	0.08	0.42	0.1	2
Fluid, nonfat (skim)	1 cup	246	90	9	Trace	—	—	—	13	298	.1	10	.10	.44	.2	2
Buttermilk, cultured, from skim milk	1 cup	246	90	9	Trace	—	—	—	13	298	.1	10	.09	.44	.2	2
Evaporated, unsweetened, undiluted	1 cup	252	345	18	20	11	7	1	24	635	.3	820	.10	.84	.5	3
Condensed, sweetened, undiluted	1 cup	306	980	25	27	15	9	1	166	802	.3	1,090	.23	1.17	.5	3
Dry, whole	1 cup	103	515	27	28	16	9	1	39	936	.5	1,160	.30	1.50	.7	6
Dry, nonfat, instant	1 cup	70	250	25	Trace	—	—	—	36	905	.4	20	.24	1.25	.6	5
Milk, goat's																
Fluid, whole	1 cup	244	165	8	10	6	2	Trace	11	315	.2	390	.10	.27	.7	2
Cream																
Half-and-half (cream and milk)	1 cup	242	325	8	28	16	9	1	11	261	.1	1,160	.08	.38	.1	2
	1 tbsp.	15	20	Trace	2	1	1	Trace	1	16	Trace	70	Trace	.02	Trace	Trace
Light, coffee or table	1 cup	240	505	7	49	27	16	1	10	245	.1	2,030	.07	.36	.1	2
	1 tbsp.	15	30	Trace	3	2	1	Trace	1	15	Trace	130	Trace	.02	Trace	Trace
Whipping, unwhipped (volume about double when whipped)																
Light	1 cup	239	715	6	75	41	25	2	9	203	.1	3,070	.06	.30	.1	2
	1 tbsp.	15	45	Trace	5	3	2	Trace	1	13	Trace	190	Trace	.02	Trace	Trace
Heavy	1 cup	238	840	5	89	49	29	3	7	178	.1	3,670	.05	.26	.1	2

Cheese

Food	Measure														
Blue or Roquefort type	1 oz.	28	105	6	9	5	3	Trace	1	89	.1	350	.01	.17	.1	0
Cheddar or American Ungrated	1 inch cube	17	70	4	5	3	2	Trace	Trace	128	.2	220	Trace	.08	Trace	0
Grated	1 cup	112	445	28	36	20	12	1	2	840	1.1	1,470	.03	.51	.1	0
	1 tbsp.	7	30	2	2	1	1	Trace	Trace	52	.1	90	Trace	.03	Trace	0
Cheddar, process	1 oz.	28	105	7	9	5	3	Trace	1	219	.3	350	Trace	.12	Trace	0
Cheese foods, Cheddar	1 oz.	28	90	6	7	4	2	Trace	2	162	.2	280	.01	.16	Trace	0
Cottage cheese, from skim milk Creamed	1 cup	225	240	31	9	5	3	Trace	7	212	0.7	380	0.07	0.56	0.2	0
	1 oz.	28	30	4	1	1	Trace	Trace	1	27	.1	50	.01	.07	Trace	0
Uncreamed	1 cup	225	195	38	1	Trace	Trace	Trace	6	202	.9	20	.07	.63	.2	0
	1 oz.	28	25	5	Trace	—	—	—	1	26	.1	Trace	.01	.08	Trace	0
Cream cheese	1 oz.	28	105	2	11	6	4	Trace	1	18	.1	440	Trace	.07	Trace	0
	1 tbsp.	15	55	1	6	3	2	Trace	Trace	9	Trace	230	Trace	.04	Trace	0
Swiss (domestic)	1 oz.	28	105	8	8	4	3	Trace	1	262	.3	320	Trace	.11	Trace	0
Milk beverages Cocoa	1 cup	242	235	9	11	6	4	Trace	26	286	.9	390	.09	.45	.4	2
Chocolate-flavored milk drink (made with skim milk)	1 cup	250	190	8	6	3	2	Trace	27	270	.4	210	.09	.41	.2	2
Malted milk	1 cup	270	280	13	12	—	—	—	32	364	.8	670	.17	.56	.2	2
Milk desserts Cornstarch pudding, plain (blanc mange)	1 cup	248	275	9	10	5	3	Trace	39	290	.1	390	.07	.40	.1	2
Custard, baked	1 cup	248	285	13	14	6	5	1	28	278	1.0	870	.10	.47	.2	1
Ice cream, plain, factory packed Slice or cut brick, 1/8 of quart brick	1 slice or cut brick	71	145	3	9	5	3	Trace	15	87	.1	370	.03	.13	.1	1
Container	3½ fld. oz.	62	130	2	8	4	3	Trace	13	76	.1	320	.03	.12	.1	1
Container	8 fld. ozs.	142	295	6	18	10	6	1	29	175	.1	740	.06	.27	.1	1
Ice milk	1 cup	187	285	9	10	6	3	Trace	42	292	.2	390	.09	.41	.2	2
Yogurt, from partially skimmed milk	1 cup	246	120	8	4	2	1	Trace	13	295	.1	170	.09	.43	.2	2

[1] Reprinted from Nutritive value of foods, U.S. Department of Agriculture, Home and Garden Bulletin No. 72.
Dashes show that no basis could be found for imputing a value although there was some reason to believe that a measurable amount of the constituent might be present.

Food, approximate measure, and weight (in grams)	gm.	Food energy (Calories)	Protein (gm.)	Fat (total lipid) (gm.)	Fatty acids Saturated (total) (gm.)	Fatty acids Unsaturated Oleic (gm.)	Fatty acids Unsaturated Linoleic (gm.)	Carbohydrate (gm.)	Calcium (mg.)	Iron (mg.)	Vitamin A value (I.U.)	Thiamine (mg.)	Riboflavin (mg.)	Niacin (mg.)	Ascorbic acid (mg.)
Eggs															
Eggs, large, 24 ounces per dozen															
Raw															
Whole, without shell 1 egg	50	80	6	6	2	3	Trace	Trace	27	1.1	590	.05	.15	Trace	0
White of egg 1 white	33	15	4	Trace	—	—	—	Trace	3	Trace	0	Trace	.09	Trace	0
Yolk of egg 1 yolk	17	60	3	5	2	2	Trace	Trace	24	.9	580	.04	.07	Trace	0
Cooked															
Boiled, shell removed 2 eggs	100	160	13	12	4	5	1	1	54	2.3	1,180	.09	.28	.1	0
Scrambled, with milk and fat 1 egg	64	110	7	8	3	3	Trace	1	51	1.1	690	.05	.18	Trace	0
Meat, poultry, fish, shellfish (related products)															
Bacon, broiled or fried, crisp 2 slices	16	100	5	8	3	4	1	1	2	.5	0	.08	.05	.8	—
Beef, trimmed to retail basis[2], cooked															
Cuts braised, simmered, or pot-roasted															
Lean and fat 3 oz.	85	245	23	16	8	7	Trace	0	10	2.9	30	.04	.18	3.5	—
Lean only 2.5 oz.	72	140	22	5	2	2	Trace	0	10	2.7	10	.04	.16	3.3	—
Hamburger (ground beef), broiled															
Lean 3 oz.	85	185	23	10	5	4	Trace	0	10	3.0	20	.08	.20	5.1	—
Regular 3 oz.	85	245	21	17	8	8	Trace	0	9	2.7	30	.07	.18	4.6	—
Roast, oven-cooked, no liquid added															
Relatively fat, such as rib															
Lean and fat 3 oz.	85	375	17	34	16	15	1	0	8	2.2	70	.05	.13	3.1	—
Lean only 1.8 oz.	51	125	14	7	3	3	Trace	0	6	1.8	10	.04	.11	2.6	—
Relatively lean, such as heel of round															
Lean and fat 3 oz.	85	165	25	7	3	3	Trace	0	11	3.2	10	.06	.19	4.5	—
Lean only 2.7 oz.	78	125	24	3	1	1	Trace	0	10	3.0	Trace	.06	.18	4.3	—
Steak, broiled															
Relatively fat, such as sirloin															
Lean and fat 3 oz.	85	330	20	27	13	12	1	0	9	2.5	50	.05	.16	4.0	—
Lean only 2.0 oz.	56	115	18	4	2	2	Trace	0	7	2.2	10	.05	.14	3.6	—
Relatively lean, such as round															
Lean and fat 3 oz.	85	220	24	13	6	6	Trace	0	10	3.0	20	.07	.19	4.8	—

Food	Amount															
Corned beef	3 oz.	85	185	22	10	5	4	Trace	0	17	3.7	20	.01	.20	2.9	—
Corned beef hash	3 oz.	85	155	7	10	5	4	Trace	9	11	1.7	—	.01	.08	1.8	—
Beef, dried or chipped	2 oz.	57	115	19	4	2	2	Trace	0	11	2.9	—	.04	.18	2.2	—
Beef and vegetable stew	1 cup	235	210	15	10	5	4	Trace	15	28	2.8	2,310	.13	.17	4.4	15
Beef potpie, baked: individual pie, 4¼-inch diameter, weight before baking about 8 oz.	1 pie	227	560	23	33	9	20	2	43	32	4.1	1,860	.25	.27	4.5	7
Chicken, cooked																
Flesh only, broiled	3 oz.	85	115	20	3	1	1	1	0	8	1.4	80	0.05	0.16	7.4	—
Breast, fried, ½ breast																
With bone	3.3 oz.	94	155	25	5	1	2	1	1	9	1.3	70	.04	.17	11.2	—
Flesh and skin only	2.7 oz.	76	155	25	5	1	2	1	1	9	1.3	70	.04	.17	11.2	—
Drumstick, fried																
With bone	2.1 oz.	59	90	12	4	1	2	1	Trace	6	.9	50	.03	.15	2.7	—
Flesh and skin only	1.3 oz.	38	90	12	4	1	2	1	Trace	6	.9	50	.03	.15	2.7	—
Chicken, canned, boneless	3 oz.	85	170	18	10	3	4	2	0	18	1.3	200	.03	.11	3.7	3
Chicken potpie—See Poultry potpie																
Chile con carne, canned																
With beans	1 cup	250	335	19	15	7	7	Trace	30	80	4.2	150	.08	.18	3.2	—
Without beans	1 cup	255	510	26	38	18	17	1	15	97	3.6	380	.05	.31	5.6	—
Heart, beef, lean, braised	3 oz.	85	160	27	5	—	—	—	1	5	5.0	20	.21	1.04	6.5	1
Lamb, trimmed to retail basis,[2] cooked																
Chop, thick, with bone, broiled	1 chop, 4.8 oz.	137	400	25	33	18	12	1	0	10	1.5	—	.14	.25	5.6	—
Lean and fat	4.0 oz.	112	400	25	33	18	12	1	0	10	1.5	—	.14	.25	5.6	—
Lean only	2.6 oz.	74	140	21	6	3	2	Trace	0	9	1.5	—	.11	.20	4.5	—
Leg, roasted																
Lean and fat	3 oz.	85	235	22	16	9	6	Trace	0	9	1.4	—	.13	.23	4.7	—
Lean only	2.5 oz.	71	130	20	5	3	2	Trace	0	9	1.4	—	.12	.21	4.4	—
Shoulder, roasted																
Lean and fat	3 oz.	85	285	18	23	13	8	1	0	9	1.0	—	.11	.20	4.0	—
Lean only	2.3 oz.	64	130	17	6	3	2	Trace	0	8	1.0	—	.10	.18	3.7	—
Liver, beef, fried	2 oz.	57	130	15	6	—	—	—	3	6	5.0	30,280	.15	2.37	9.4	15

[2]Outer layer of fat on the cut was removed to within approximately ½ inch of the lean. Deposits of fat within the cut were not removed.

Food, approximate measure, and weight (in grams)		gm.	Food energy (Calories)	Protein (gm.)	Fat (total lipid) (gm.)	Fatty acids Saturated (total) (gm.)	Fatty acids Unsaturated Oleic (gm.)	Fatty acids Unsaturated Linoleic (gm.)	Carbohydrate (gm.)	Calcium (mg.)	Iron (mg.)	Vitamin A value (I.U.)	Thiamine (mg.)	Riboflavin (mg.)	Niacin (mg.)	Ascorbic acid (mg.)
Pork, cured, cooked																
Ham, light cure, lean and fat, roasted	3 oz.	85	245	18	19	7	8	2	0	8	2.2	0	.40	.16	3.1	—
Luncheon meat																
Boiled ham, sliced	2 oz.	57	135	11	10	4	4	1	0	6	1.6	0	.25	.09	1.5	—
Canned, spiced or unspiced	2 oz.	57	165	8	14	5	6	1	1	5	1.2	0	.18	.12	1.6	—
Pork, fresh, trimmed to retail basis,[2] cooked																
Chop, thick, with bone	1 chop, 3.5 oz.	98	260	16	21	8	9	2	0	8	2.2	0	.63	.18	3.8	—
Lean and fat	2.3 oz.	66	260	16	21	8	9	2	0	8	2.2	0	.63	.18	3.8	—
Lean only	1.7 oz.	48	130	15	7	2	3	1	0	7	1.9	0	.54	.16	3.3	—
Roast, oven-cooked, no liquid added																
Lean and fat	3 oz.	85	310	21	24	9	10	2	0	9	2.7	0	.78	.22	4.7	—
Lean only	2.4 oz.	68	175	20	10	3	4	1	0	9	2.6	0	.73	.21	4.4	—
Cuts, simmered																
Lean and fat	3 oz.	85	320	20	26	9	11	2	0	8	2.5	0	.46	.21	4.1	—
Lean only	2.2 oz.	63	135	18	6	2	3	1	0	8	2.3	0	.42	.19	3.7	—
Poultry potpie (based on chicken potpie). Individual pie, 4¼-inch diameter, weigh before baking	1 pie	227	535	23	31	10	15	3	42	68	3.0	3,020	.25	.26	4.1	5
Sausage																
Bologna, slice, 4.1 by 0.1 inch	8 slices	227	690	27	62	—	—	—	2	16	4.1	—	.36	.49	6.0	—
Frankfurter, cooked	1	51	155	6	14	—	—	—	1	3	.8	—	.08	.10	1.3	—
Pork, links or patty, cooked	4 oz.	113	540	21	50	18	21	5	Trace	8	2.7	0	.89	.39	4.2	—
Tongue, beef, braised	3 oz.	85	210	18	14	—	—	—	Trace	6	1.9	—	.04	.25	3.0	—
Turkey potpie. See Poultry potpie																
Veal, cooked																
Cutlet, without bone, broiled	3 oz.	85	185	23	9	5	4	Trace	—	9	2.7	—	.06	.21	4.6	—
Roast, medium fat, me-	3 oz.	85	230	23	14	7	6	Trace	0	10	2.9	—	.11	.26	6.6	—

Food	Measure	Grams	Food energy	Protein	Fat	Saturated fatty acids	Oleic	Linoleic	Carbohydrate	Calcium	Iron	Vitamin A	Thiamine	Riboflavin	Niacin	Ascorbic acid
Bluefish, baked or broiled	3 oz.	85	135	22	4	—	—	—	0	25	.6	40	.09	.08	1.6	—
Clams																
Raw, meat only	3 oz.	85	65	11	1	—	—	—	2	59	5.2	90	.08	.15	1.1	8
Canned, solids and liquid	3 oz.	85	45	7	1	—	—	—	2	47	3.5	—	.01	.09	.9	—
Crabmeat, canned	3 oz.	85	85	15	2	—	—	—	1	38	.7	—	.07	.07	1.6	—
Fish sticks, breaded, cooked, frozen; stick 3.8 by 1.0 by 0.5 inch	10 sticks or 8 oz. package	227	400	38	20	5	4	10	15	25	.9	—	.09	.16	3.6	—
Haddock, fried	3 oz.	85	140	17	5	1	3		5	34	1.0	—	0.03	0.06	2.7	2
Mackerel																
Broiled, Atlantic	3 oz.	85	200	19	13	—	—	—	0	5	1.0	450	.13	.23	6.5	—
Canned, Pacific, solids and liquid[3]	3 oz.	85	155	18	9	—	—	—	0	221	1.9	20	.02	.28	7.4	—
Ocean perch, breaded (egg and breadcrumbs), fried	3 oz.	85	195	16	11	—	—	—	6	28	1.1	—	.08	.09	1.5	—
Oysters, meat only. Raw, 13-19 medium selects	1 cup	240	160	20	4	—	—	—	8	226	13.2	740	.33	.43	6.0	—
Oyster stew, 1 part oysters to 3 parts milk by volume, 3-4 oysters	1 cup	230	200	11	12	—	—	—	11	269	3.3	640	.13	.41	1.6	—
Salmon, pink, canned	3 oz.	85	120	17	5	1	1	Trace	0	[4]167	.7	60	.03	.16	6.8	—
Sardines, Atlantic, canned in oil, drained solids	3 oz.	85	175	20	9	—	—	—	0	372	2.5	190	.02	.17	4.6	—
Shad, baked	3 oz.	85	170	20	10	—	—	—	0	20	.5	20	.11	.22	7.3	—
Shrimp, canned, meat only	3 oz.	85	100	21	1	—	—	—	1	98	2.6	50	.01	.03	1.5	—
Swordfish, broiled with butter or margarine	3 oz.	85	150	24	5	—	—	—	0	23	1.1	1,780	.03	.04	9.3	—
Tuna, canned in oil, drained solids	3 oz.	85	170	24	7	—	—	—	0	7	1.6	70	.04	.10	10.1	—
Mature dry beans and peas, nuts, peanuts (related products)																
Almonds, shelled	1 cup	142	850	26	77	6	52	15	28	332	6.7	0	.34	1.31	5.0	Trace

[2] Outer layer of fat on the cut was removed to within approximately ½ inch of the lean. Deposits of fat within the cut were not removed.
[3] Vitamin values based on drained solids.
[4] Based on total contents of can. If bones are discarded, value will be greatly reduced.

Food, approximate measure, and weight (in grams)		Food energy	Protein	Fat (total lipid)	Fatty acids			Carbo-hydrate	Cal-cium	Iron	Vita-min A value	Thia-mine	Ribo-flavin	Niacin	Ascor-bic acid
					Satu-rated (total)	Unsaturated Oleic	Unsaturated Linoleic								
	gm.	(Calo-ries)	(gm.)	(gm.)	(gm.)	(gm.)	(gm.)	(gm.)	(mg.)	(mg.)	(I.U.)	(mg.)	(mg.)	(mg.)	(mg.)
Beans, dry															
Common varieties, such as Great Northern, navy, and others, canned:															
Red	1 cup	256	230	15	1	—	—	—	42	74	4.6	Trace	.13	.10	1.5	—
White, with tomato sauce															
With pork	1 cup	261	320	16	7	3	3	1	50	141	4.7	340	.20	.08	1.5	5
Without pork	1 cup	261	310	16	1	—	—	—	60	177	5.2	160	.18	.09	1.5	5
Lima, cooked	1 cup	192	260	16	1	—	—	—	48	56	5.6	Trace	.26	.12	1.3	Trace
Brazil nuts	1 cup	140	915	20	94	19	45	24	15	260	4.8	Trace	1.34	.17	2.2	—
Cashew nuts, roasted	1 cup	135	760	23	62	10	43	4	40	51	5.1	140	.58	.33	2.4	—
Coconut															
Fresh, shredded	1 cup	97	335	3	34	29	2	Trace	9	13	1.6	0	.05	.02	.5	3
Dried, shredded, sweetened	1 cup	62	340	2	24	21	2	Trace	33	10	1.2	0	.02	.02	.2	0
Cowpeas or blackeye peas, dry, cooked	1 cup	248	190	13	1	—	—	—	34	42	3.2	20	.41	.11	1.1	Trace
Peanuts, roasted, salted															
Halves	1 cup	144	840	37	72	16	31	21	27	107	3.0	—	.46	.19	24.7	0
Chopped	1 tbsp.	9	55	2	4	1	2	1	2	7	.2	—	.03	.01	1.5	0
Peanut butter	1 tbsp.	16	95	4	8	2	4	2	3	9	.3	—	.02	.02	2.4	0
Peas, split, dry, cooked	1 cup	250	290	20	1	—	—	—	52	28	4.2	100	.37	.22	2.2	—
Pecans															
Halves	1 cup	108	740	10	77	5	48	15	16	79	2.6	140	.93	.14	1.0	2
Chopped	1 tbsp.	7.5	50	1	5	Trace	3	1	1	5	.2	10	.06	.01	.1	Trace
Walnuts, shelled															
Black or native, chopped	1 cup	126	790	26	75	4	26	36	19	Trace	7.6	380	.28	.14	.9	—
English or Persian															
Halves	1 cup	100	650	15	64	4	10	40	16	99	3.1	30	.33	.13	.9	3
Chopped	1 tbsp.	8	50	1	5	Trace	1	3	1	8	.2	Trace	.03	.01	.1	Trace
Vegetables and vegetable products															
Asparagus															
Cooked, cut spears	1 cup	175	35	4	Trace	—	—	—	6	37	1.0	1,580	.27	.32	2.4	46
Canned spears, medium															
Green	6 spears	96	20	2	Trace	—	—	—	3	18	1.8	770	.06	.10	.8	14
Bleached	6 spears	96	20	2	Trace	—	—	—	4	15	1.0	80	.05	.06	.7	14

Food	Measure															
Lima, immature, cooked	1 cup	160	180	12	1	—	—	—	32	75	4.0	450	.29	.16	2.0	28
Snap, green																
Cooked																
In small amount of water, short time	1 cup	125	30	2	Trace	—	—	—	7	62	.8	680	.08	.11	.6	16
In large amount of water, long time	1 cup	125	30	2	Trace	—	—	—	7	62	0.8	680	0.07	0.10	0.4	13
Canned																
Solids and liquid	1 cup	239	45	2	Trace	—	—	—	10	81	2.9	690	.08	.10	.7	9
Strained or chopped (baby food)	1 oz.	28	5	Trace	Trace	—	—	—	1	9	.3	110	.01	.02	.1	Trace
Bean sprouts. See Sprouts																
Beets, cooked, diced	1 cup	165	50	2	Trace	—	—	—	12	23	.8	40	.04	.07	.5	11
Broccoli spears, cooked	1 cup	150	40	5	Trace	—	—	—	7	132	1.2	3,750	.14	.29	1.2	135
Brussels sprouts, cooked	1 cup	130	45	5	1	—	—	—	8	42	1.4	680	.10	.18	1.1	113
Cabbage																
Raw																
Finely shredded	1 cup	100	25	1	Trace	—	—	—	5	49	.4	130	.05	.05	.3	47
Coleslaw	1 cup	120	120	1	9	2	2	5	9	52	.5	180	.06	.06	.3	35
Cooked																
In small amount of water, short time	1 cup	170	35	2	Trace	—	—	—	7	75	.5	220	.07	.07	.5	56
In large amount of water, long time	1 cup	170	30	2	Trace	—	—	—	7	71	.5	200	.04	.04	.2	40
Cabbage, celery or Chinese																
Raw, leaves and stalk, 1-inch pieces	1 cup	100	15	1	Trace	—	—	—	3	43	.6	150	.05	.04	.6	25
Cabbage, spoon (or pakchoy), cooked	1 cup	150	20	2	Trace	—	—	—	4	222	.9	4,650	.07	.12	1.1	23
Carrots																
Raw																
Whole, 5½ by 1 inch, (25 thin strips)	1	50	20	1	Trace	—	—	—	5	18	.4	5,500	.03	.03	.3	4
Grated	1 cup	110	45	1	Trace	—	—	—	11	41	.8	12,100	.06	.06	.7	9
Cooked, diced	1 cup	145	45	1	Trace	—	—	—	10	48	.9	15,220	.08	.07	.7	9
Canned, strained or chopped (baby food)	1 oz.	28	10	Trace	Trace	—	—	—	2	7	.1	3,690	.01	.01	.1	1
Cauliflower, cooked, flowerbuds	1 cup	120	25	3	Trace	—	—	—	5	25	.8	70	.11	.10	.7	66

Food, approximate measure, and weight (in grams)		Food energy	Protein	Fat (total lipid)	Fatty acids			Carbohydrate	Calcium	Iron	Vitamin A value	Thiamine	Riboflavin	Niacin	Ascorbic acid
					Saturated (total)	Unsaturated									
						Oleic	Linoleic								
	gm.	(Calories)	(gm.)	(gm.)	(gm.)	(gm.)	(gm.)	(gm.)	(mg.)	(mg.)	(I.U.)	(mg.)	(mg.)	(mg.)	(mg.)
Celery, raw — Stalk, large outer, 8 by 1½ inches, at root end	1 stalk	40	5	Trace	Trace	—	—	—	2	16	.1	100	.01	.01	.1	4
Pieces, diced	1 cup	100	15	1	Trace	—	—	—	4	39	.3	240	.03	.03	.3	9
Collards, cooked	1 cup	190	55	5	1	—	—	—	9	289	1.1	10,260	.27	.37	2.4	87
Corn, sweet — Cooked, ear 5 by 1¾ inches[5]	1 ear	140	70	3	1	—	—	—	16	2	.5	[6]310	.09	.08	1.0	7
Canned, solids and liquid	1 cup	256	170	5	2	—	—	—	40	10	1.0	[6]690	.07	.12	2.3	13
Cowpeas, cooked, immature seeds	1 cup	160	175	13	1	—	—	—	29	38	3.4	560	.49	.18	2.3	28
Cucumbers, 10 oz., 7½ by about 2 inches — Raw, pared	1	207	30	1	Trace	—	—	—	7	35	.6	Trace	.07	.09	.4	23
Raw, pared, center slice ⅛-inch thick	6 slices	50	5	Trace	Trace	—	—	—	2	8	.2	Trace	.02	.02	.1	6
Dandelion greens, cooked	1 cup	180	60	4	1	—	—	—	12	252	3.2	21,060	.24	.29	—	32
Endive, curly (including escarole)	2 oz.	57	10	1	Trace	—	—	—	2	46	1.0	1,870	.04	.08	.3	6
Kale, leaves including stems, cooked	1 cup	110	30	4	1	—	—	—	4	147	1.3	8,140	—	—	—	68
Lettuce, raw — Butterhead, as Boston types; head, 4-inch diameter	1 head	220	30	3	Trace	—	—	—	6	77	4.4	2,130	.14	.13	.6	18
Crisphead, as Iceberg; head, 4¾-inch diameter	1 head	454	60	4	Trace	—	—	—	13	91	2.3	1,500	.29	.27	1.3	29
Looseleaf, or bunching varieties, leaves	2 large	50	10	1	Trace	—	—	—	2	34	.7	950	.03	.04	.2	9
Mushrooms, canned, solids and liquid	1 cup	244	40	5	Trace	—	—	—	6	15	1.2	Trace	.04	.60	4.8	4
Mustard greens, cooked	1 cup	140	35	3	1	—	—	—	6	193	2.5	8,120	.11	.19	.9	68
Okra, cooked, pod 3 by	8 pods	85	25	3	Trace	—	—	—	5	78	.4	420	.11	.15	.8	17

Food	Measure	Weight (g)														
Mature																
Raw, onion 2½-inch diameter	1	110	40	2	Trace	—	—	—	10	30	0.6	40	0.04	0.04	0.2	11
Cooked	1 cup	210	60	3	Trace	—	—	—	14	50	.8	80	.06	.06	.4	14
Young green, small, without tops	6	50	20	1	Trace	—	—	—	5	20	.3	Trace	.02	.02	.2	12
Parsley, raw, chopped	1 tbsp.	3.5	1	Trace	Trace	—	—	—	Trace	7	.2	300	Trace	.01	Trace	6
Parsnips, cooked	1 cup	155	100	2	1	—	—	—	23	70	.9	50	.11	.13	.2	16
Peas, green																
Cooked	1 cup	160	115	9	1	—	—	—	19	37	2.9	860	.44	.17	3.7	33
Canned, solids and liquid	1 cup	249	165	9	1	—	—	—	31	50	4.2	1,120	.23	.13	2.2	22
Canned, strained (baby food)	1 oz.	28	15	1	Trace	—	—	—	3	3	.4	140	.02	.02	.4	3
Peppers, hot, red, without seeds, dried (ground chili powder, added seasonings)	1 tbsp.	15	50	2	2	—	—	—	8	40	2.3	9,750	.03	.17	1.3	2
Peppers, sweet																
Raw, medium, about 6 per pound																
Green pod without stem and seeds	1 pod	62	15	1	Trace	—	—	—	3	6	.4	260	.05	.05	.3	79
Red pod without stem and seeds	1 pod	60	20	1	Trace	—	—	—	4	8	.4	2,670	.05	.05	.3	122
Canned, pimentos, medium	1 pod	38	10	Trace	Trace	—	—	—	2	3	.6	870	.01	.02	.1	36
Potatoes, medium (about 3 per pound raw)																
Baked, peeled after baking	1	99	90	3	Trace	—	—	—	21	9	.7	Trace	.10	.04	1.7	20
Boiled																
Peeled after boiling	1	136	105	3	Trace	—	—	—	23	10	.8	Trace	.13	.05	2.0	22
Peeled before boiling	1	122	80	2	Trace	—	—	—	18	7	.6	Trace	.11	.04	1.4	20
French-fried, piece 2 by ½ by ½ inch																
Cooked in deep fat	10 pieces	57	155	2	7	2	2	4	20	9	.7	Trace	.07	.04	1.8	12
Frozen, heated	10 pieces	57	125	2	5	1	1	2	19	5	1.0	Trace	.08	.01	1.5	12
Mashed																
Milk added	1 cup	195	125	4	1	—	—	—	25	47	.8	50	.16	.10	2.0	19
Milk and butter added	1 cup	195	185	4	8	3	4	Trace	24	47	.8	330	.16	.10	1.9	18

[5]Measure and weight apply to entire vegetable or fruit including parts not usually eaten.
[6]Based on yellow varieties; white varieties contain only a trace of cryptoxanthin and carotenes, the pigments in corn that have biological activity.

Food, approximate measure, and weight (in grams)		gm.	Food energy (Calories)	Protein (gm.)	Fat (total lipid) (gm.)	Fatty acids			Carbohydrate (gm.)	Calcium (mg.)	Iron (mg.)	Vitamin A value (I.U.)	Thiamine (mg.)	Riboflavin (mg.)	Niacin (mg.)	Ascorbic acid (mg.)
						Saturated (total) (gm.)	Unsaturated Oleic (gm.)	Linoleic (gm.)								
Potato chips, medium, 2-inch diameter	10 chips	20	115	1	8	3	2	4	10	8	.4	Trace	.04	.01	1.0	3
Pumpkin, canned	1 cup	228	75	2	1	—	—	—	18	57	.9	14,590	.07	.12	1.3	12
Radishes, raw, small, without tops	4	40	5	Trace	Trace	—	—	—	1	12	.4	Trace	.01	.01	.1	10
Sauerkraut, canned, solids and liquid	1 cup	235	45	2	Trace	—	—	—	9	85	1.2	120	.07	.09	.4	33
Spinach																
Cooked	1 cup	180	40	5	1	—	—	—	6	167	4.0	14,580	.13	.25	1.0	50
Canned, drained solids	1 cup	180	45	5	1	—	—	—	6	212	4.7	14,400	.03	.21	.6	24
Canned, strained or chopped (baby food)	1 oz.	28	10	1	Trace	—	—	—	2	18	.2	1,420	.01	.04	.1	2
Sprouts, raw																
Mung bean	1 cup	83	30	3	Trace	—	—	—	6	17	1.2	20	.12	.12	.7	17
Soybean	1 cup	107	40	6	2	—	—	—	4	46	.7	90	.17	.16	.8	4
Squash																
Cooked																
Summer, diced	1 cup	210	30	2	Trace	—	—	—	7	52	.8	820	.10	.16	1.6	21
Winter, baked, mashed	1 cup	205	130	4	1	—	—	—	32	57	1.6	8,610	.10	.27	1.4	27
Canned, winter, strained and chopped (baby food)	1 oz.	28	10	Trace	Trace	—	—	—	2	7	.1	510	.01	.01	.1	1
Sweetpotatoes																
Cooked, medium, 5 by 2 inches, weight raw about 6 oz.																
Baked, peeled after baking	1	110	155	2	1	—	—	—	36	44	1.0	8,910	.10	.07	.7	24
Boiled, peeled after boiling	1	147	170	2	1	—	—	—	39	47	1.0	11,610	.13	.09	.9	25
Candied, 3½ by 2¼ inches	1	175	295	2	6	2	3	1	60	65	1.6	11,030	.10	.08	.8	17
Canned, vacuum or solid pack	1 cup	218	235	4	Trace	—	—	—	54	54	1.7	17,000	.10	.10	1.4	30

Tomatoes

Food	Measure	Weight (g)	Food energy	Protein	Fat	Saturated fatty acids	Unsaturated oleic	Unsaturated linoleic	Carbohydrate	Calcium	Iron	Vitamin A	Thiamine	Riboflavin	Niacin	Ascorbic acid
Raw, medium, 2 by 2½ inches, about 3 per pound	1	150	35	2	Trace	—	—	—	7	20	.8	1,350	.10	.06	1.0	34[7]
Canned	1 cup	242	50	2	Trace	—	—	—	10	15	1.2	2,180	.13	.07	1.7	40
Tomato juice, canned	1 cup	242	45	2	Trace	—	—	—	10	17	2.2	1,940	.13	.07	1.8	39
Tomato catsup	1 tbsp.	17	15	Trace	Trace	—	—	—	4	4	.1	240	.02	.01	.3	3
Turnips, cooked, diced	1 cup	155	35	1	Trace	—	—	—	8	54	.6	Trace	.06	.08	.5	33
Turnip greens, Cooked																
In small amount of water, short time	1 cup	145	30	3	Trace	—	—	—	5	267	1.6	9,140	.21	.36	.8	100
In large amount of water, long time	1 cup	145	25	3	Trace	—	—	—	5	252	1.4	8,260	.14	.33	.8	68
Canned, solids and liquid	1 cup	232	40	3	1	—	—	—	7	232	3.7	10,900	.04	.21	1.4	44
Fruits and fruit products																
Apples, raw, medium, 2½-inch diameter, about 3 per pound[5]	1	150	70	Trace	Trace	—	—	—	18	8	.4	50	.04	.02	.1	3
Apple brown betty	1 cup	230	345	4	8	4	3	Trace	68	41	1.4	230	.13	.10	.9	3
Apple juice, bottled or canned	1 cup	249	120	Trace	Trace	—	—	—	30	15	1.5	—	.01	.04	.2	2
Applesauce, canned, Sweetened	1 cup	254	230	1	Trace	—	—	—	60	10	1.3	100	.05	.03	.1	3
Unsweetened or artificially sweetened	1 cup	239	100	Trace	Trace	—	—	—	26	10	1.2	100	.04	.02	.1	2
Applesauce and apricots, canned, strained or junior (baby food)	1 oz.	28	25	Trace	Trace	—	—	—	6	1	.1	170	Trace	Trace	Trace	1
Apricots, Raw, about 12 per pound[5]	3 apricots	114	55	1	Trace	—	—	—	14	18	.5	2,890	.03	.04	.7	10
Canned in heavy syrup, Halves and syrup	1 cup	259	220	2	Trace	—	—	—	57	28	.8	4,510	.05	.06	.9	10
Halves (medium) and syrup	4 halves; 2 tbsp. syrup	122	105	1	Trace	—	—	—	27	13	.4	2,120	.02	.03	.4	5

5 Measure and weight apply to entire vegetable or fruit including parts not usually eaten.
7 Year-round average. Samples marketed from November through May average around 15 milligrams per 150-gram tomato; from June through October, around 39 milligrams.

Food, approximate measure, and weight (in grams)		gm.	Food energy (Calories)	Protein (gm.)	Fat (total lipid) (gm.)	Fatty acids			Carbohydrate (gm.)	Calcium (mg.)	Iron (mg.)	Vitamin A value (I.U.)	Thiamine (mg.)	Riboflavin (mg.)	Niacin (mg.)	Ascorbic acid (mg.)
						Saturated (total) (gm.)	Unsaturated Oleic (gm.)	Unsaturated Linoleic (gm.)								
Apricots—cont'd																
Dried																
Uncooked, 40 halves, small	1 cup	150	390	8	1	—	—	—	100	100	8.2	16,350	.02	.23	4.9	19
Cooked, unsweetened, fruit and liquid	1 cup	285	240	5	1	—	—	—	62	63	5.1	8,550	.01	.13	2.8	8
Apricot nectar, canned	1 cup	250	140	1	Trace	—	—	—	36	22	.5	2,380	.02	.02	.5	7
Avocados, raw																
California varieties, mainly Fuerte																
10-ounce avocado, about 3½ by 4¼ inches, peeled, pitted	½	108	185	2	18	4	8	2	6	11	.6	310	.12	.21	1.7	15
½-inch cubes	1 cup	152	260	3	26	5	12	3	9	15	.9	440	.16	.30	2.4	21
Florida varieties																
13 oz. avocado, about 4 by 3 inches, peeled, pitted	½	123	160	2	14	3	6	2	11	12	.7	360	.13	.24	2.0	17
½-inch cubes	1 cup	152	195	2	17	3	8	2	13	15	.9	440	.16	.30	2.4	21
Bananas, raw, 6 by 1½ inches, about 3 per pound[5]	1	150	85	1	Trace	—	—	—	23	8	.7	190	.05	.06	.7	10
Blackberries, raw	1 cup	144	85	2	1	—	—	—	19	46	1.3	290	.05	.06	.5	30
Blueberries, raw	1 cup	140	85	1	1	—	—	—	21	21	1.4	140	.04	.08	.6	20
Cantaloups, raw; medium, 5-inch diameter, about 1⅔ pounds[5]	½	385	60	1	Trace	—	—	—	14	27	.8	[8]6,540	.08	.06	1.2	63
Cherries																
Raw, sweet, with stems[5]	1 cup	130	80	2	Trace	—	—	—	20	26	.5	130	.06	.07	.5	12
Canned, red, sour, pitted, heavy syrup	1 cup	260	230	2	1	—	—	—	59	36	.8	1,680	.07	.06	.4	13
Cranberry juice cocktail, canned	1 cup	250	160	Trace	Trace	—	—	—	41	12	.8	Trace	.02	.02	.1	(?)

Food and description	Measure	Weight (g)	Food energy	Protein	Fat				Carbohydrate	Calcium	Iron	Vitamin A	Thiamine	Riboflavin	Niacin	Ascorbic acid
...ened, canned, strained																
Dates, domestic, natural and dry, pitted, cut	1 cup	178	490	4	1	—	—	—	130	105	5.3	90	.16	.17	3.9	0
Figs																
Raw, small, 1½-inch diameter, about 12 per pound	3 figs	114	90	1	Trace	—	—	—	23	40	.7	90	.07	.06	.5	2
Dried, large, 2 by 1 inch	1 fig	21	60	1	Trace	—	—	—	15	26	.6	20	.02	.02	.1	0
Fruit cocktail, canned in heavy syrup, solids and liquid	1 cup	256	195	1	1	—	—	—	50	23	1.0	360	.04	.03	1.1	5
Grapefruit																
Raw, medium, 4¼-inch diameter, size 64																
White[5]	½	285	55	1	Trace	—	—	—	14	22	.6	10	.05	.02	.2	52
Pink or red[5]	½	285	60	1	Trace	—	—	—	15	23	.6	640	.05	.02	.3	52
Raw sections, white	1 cup	194	75	1	Trace	—	—	—	20	31	.8	20	.07	.03	.3	72
Canned, white																
Syrup pack, solids and liquid	1 cup	249	175	1	Trace	—	—	—	44	32	.7	20	.07	.04	.5	75
Water pack, solids and liquid	1 cup	240	70	1	Trace	—	—	—	18	31	.7	20	.07	.04	.5	72
Grapefruit juice																
Fresh	1 cup	246	95	1	Trace	—	—	—	23	22	.5	(10)	.09	.04	.4	92
Canned, white																
Unsweetened	1 cup	247	100	1	Trace	—	—	—	24	20	1.0	20	.07	.04	.4	84
Sweetened	1 cup	250	130	1	Trace	—	—	—	32	20	1.0	20	.07	.04	.4	78
Frozen, concentrate, unsweetened																
Undiluted, can, 6 fluid oz.	1 can	207	300	4	1	—	—	—	72	70	.8	60	.29	.12	1.4	286
Diluted with 3 parts water, by volume	1 cup	247	100	1	Trace	—	—	—	24	25	.2	20	.10	.04	.5	96
Frozen, concentrate, sweetened																
Undiluted, can, 6 fluid oz.	1 can	211	350	3	1	—	—	—	85	59	.6	50	.24	.11	1.2	245
Diluted with 3 parts water, by volume	1 cup	249	115	1	Trace	—	—	—	28	20	.2	20	.08	.03	.4	82

[5]Measure and weight apply to entire vegetable or fruit including parts not usually eaten.

[8]Value based on varieties with orange-colored flesh, for green-fleshed varieties value is about 540 I.U. per ½ melon.

[9]About 5 milligrams per 8 fluid ounces is from cranberries. Ascorbic acid is usually added to approximately 100 milligrams per 8 fluid ounces.

[10]For white-fleshed varieties value is about 20 I.U. per cup; for red-fleshed varieties, 1,080 I.U. per cup.

Food, approximate measure, and weight (in grams)		gm.	Food energy (Calories)	Protein (gm.)	Fat (total lipid) (gm.)	Saturated (total) (gm.)	Unsaturated Oleic (gm.)	Unsaturated Linoleic (gm.)	Carbohydrate (gm.)	Calcium (mg.)	Iron (mg.)	Vitamin A value (I.U.)	Thiamine (mg.)	Riboflavin (mg.)	Niacin (mg.)	Ascorbic acid (mg.)
Grapefruit juice—cont'd																
Dehydrated																
Crystals, can, net weight 4 oz.	1 can	114	430	5	1	—	—	—	103	99	1.1	90	.41	.18	2.0	399
Prepared with water (1 pound yields about 1 gal.)	1 cup	247	100	1	Trace	—	—	—	24	22	.2	20	.10	.05	.5	92
Grapes, raw																
American type (slip skin), such as Concord, Delaware, Niagara, Catawba, and Scuppernong[5]	1 cup	153	65	1	1	—	—	—	15	15	.4	100	.05	.03	.2	3
European type (adherent skin), such as Malaga, Muscat, Thompson Seedless, Emperor, and Flame Tokay[5]	1 cup	160	95	1	Trace	—	—	—	25	17	.6	140	.07	.04	.4	6
Grape juice, bottled or canned	1 cup	254	165	1	Trace	—	—	—	42	28	.8	—	.10	.05	.6	Trace
Lemons, raw, medium, 2½-inch diameter, size 150[5]	1 lemon	106	20	1	Trace	—	—	—	6	18	.4	10	.03	.01	.1	38
Lemon juice																
Fresh	1 cup	246	60	1	Trace	—	—	—	20	17	.5	40	.08	.03	.2	113
	1 tbsp.	15	5	Trace	Trace	—	—	—	1	1	Trace	Trace	Trace	Trace	Trace	7
Canned, unsweetened	1 cup	245	55	1	Trace	—	—	—	19	17	.5	40	.07	.03	.2	102
Lemonade concentrate, frozen, sweetened																
Undiluted, can, 6 fluid oz.	1 can	220	430	Trace	Trace	—	—	—	112	9	.4	40	.05	.06	.7	66
Diluted with 4½ parts water, by volume	1 cup	248	110	Trace	Trace	—	—	—	28	2	.1	10	.01	.01	.2	17
Lime juice																
Fresh	1 cup	246	65	1	Trace	—	—	—	22	22	.5	30	.05	.03	.03	80
Canned	1 cup	246	65	1	Trace	—	—	—	22	22	.5	30	.05	.03	.3	52

Food	Measure															
Limeade concentrate, frozen, sweetened																
Undiluted, can, 6 fluid oz.	1 can	218	410	Trace	Trace	—	—	—	108	11	.2	Trace	.02	.02	.3	26
Diluted with 4⅓ parts water, by volume	1 cup	248	105	Trace	Trace	—	—	—	27	2	Trace	Trace	Trace	Trace	Trace	6
Oranges, raw																
California, Navel (winter), 2⅘-inch diameter, size 88[5]	1 orange	180	60	2	Trace	—	—	—	16	49	.5	240	.12	.05	.5	75
Florida, all varieties, 3-inch diameter[5]	1	210	75	1	Trace	—	—	—	19	67	.3	310	.16	.06	.6	70
Orange juice																
Fresh																
California, Valencia (summer)	1 cup	249	115	2	1	—	—	—	26	27	.7	500	.22	.06	.9	122
Florida varieties																
Early and mid-season	1 cup	247	100	1	Trace	—	—	—	23	25	.5	490	.22	.06	.9	127
Late season, Valencia	1 cup	248	110	1	Trace	—	—	—	26	25	.5	500	.22	.06	.9	92
Canned, unsweetened	1 cup	249	120	2	Trace	—	—	—	28	25	1.0	500	.17	.05	.6	100
Frozen concentrate																
Undiluted, can, 6 fluid oz.	1 can	210	330	5	Trace	—	—	—	80	69	.8	1,490	.63	.10	2.4	332
Diluted with 3 parts water, by volume	1 cup	248	110	2	Trace	—	—	—	27	22	.2	500	.21	.03	.8	112
Dehydrated																
Crystals, can, net weight 4 oz.	1 can	113	430	6	2	—	—	—	100	95	1.9	1,900	.76	.24	3.3	406
Prepared with water, 1 lb. yields about 1 gal.	1 cup	248	115	1	Trace	—	—	—	27	25	.5	500	.20	.06	.9	108
Orange and grapefruit juice																
Frozen concentrate																
Undiluted, can, 6 fluid oz.	1 can	209	325	4	1	—	—	—	78	61	.8	790	.47	.06	2.3	301
Diluted with 3 parts water, by volume	1 cup	248	110	1	Trace	—	—	—	26	20	.3	270	.16	.02	.8	102
Papayas, raw, ½-inch cubes	1 cup	182	70	1	Trace	—	—	—	18	36	.5	3,190	.07	.08	.5	102

[5]Measure and weight apply to entire vegetable or fruit including parts not usually eaten.

Food, approximate measure, and weight (in grams)		gm.	Food energy (Calories)	Protein (gm.)	Fat (total lipid) (gm.)	Fatty acids Saturated (total) (gm.)	Unsaturated Oleic (gm.)	Unsaturated Linoleic (gm.)	Carbohydrate (gm.)	Calcium (mg.)	Iron (mg.)	Vitamin A value (I.U.)	Thiamine (mg.)	Riboflavin (mg.)	Niacin (mg.)	Ascorbic acid (mg.)
Peaches																
Raw																
Whole, medium, 2-inch diameter, about 4 per pound[5]	1	114	35	1	Trace	—	—	—	10	9	.5	[11]1,320	.02	.05	1.0	7
Sliced	1 cup	168	65	1	Trace	—	—	—	16	15	.8	[11]2,230	.03	.08	1.6	12
Canned, yellow-fleshed, solids and liquid																
Syrup pack, heavy																
Halves or slices	1 cup	257	200	1	Trace	—	—	—	52	10	.8	1,100	.02	.06	1.4	7
Halves (medium) and 2 tbsp. syrup	2 halves and 2 tbsp. syrup	117	90	Trace	Trace	—	—	—	24	5	.4	500	.01	.03	.7	3
Water pack	1 cup	245	75	1	Trace	—	—	—	20	10	.7	1,100	.02	.06	1.4	7
Strained or chopped (baby food)	1 oz.	28	25	Trace	Trace	—	—	—	6	2	.1	140	Trace	.01	.2	1
Dried																
Uncooked	1 cup	160	420	5	1	—	—	—	109	77	9.6	6,240	.02	.31	8.5	28
Cooked, unsweetened, 10-12 halves and 6 tbsp. liquid	1 cup	270	220	3	1	—	—	—	58	41	5.1	3,290	.01	.15	4.2	6
Frozen																
Carton, 12 oz., not thawed	1 carton	340	300	1	Trace	—	—	—	77	14	1.7	2,210	.03	.14	2.4	[12]135
Can, 16 oz., not thawed	1 can	454	400	2	Trace	—	—	—	103	18	2.3	2,950	.05	.18	3.2	[12]181
Peach nectar, canned	1 cup	250	120	Trace	Trace	—	—	—	31	10	.5	1,080	.02	.05	1.0	1
Pears																
Raw, 3 by 2½-inch diameter[5]	1	182	100	1	1	—	—	—	25	13	.5	30	.04	.07	.2	7
Canned, solids and liquid																
Syrup pack, heavy																
Halves or slices	1 cup	255	195	1	1	—	—	—	50	13	.5	Trace	.03	.05	.3	4
Halves (medium) and 2 tbsp. syrup	2 halves and 2 tbsp.	117	90	Trace	Trace	—	—	—	23	6	.2	Trace	.01	.02	.2	2

Food	Measure	Weight (g)	Cal.	Prot.	Fat				Carb.	Calcium	Iron	Vit. A (I.U.)	Thiamine	Riboflavin	Niacin	Ascorbic acid
Strained or chopped (baby food)	1 oz.	28	20	Trace	Trace	—	—	—	5	2	.1	10	Trace	.01	.1	1
Pear nectar, canned	1 cup	250	130	1	Trace	—	—	—	33	8	.2	Trace	.01	.05	Trace	1
Persimmons, Japanese or kaki, raw, seedless, 2½-inch diameter[5]	1	125	75	1	Trace	—	—	—	20	6	.4	2,740	.01	.02	.1	11
Pineapple																
Raw, diced	1 cup	140	75	1	Trace	—	—	—	19	24	.7	100	.12	.04	.3	24
Canned, heavy syrup pack, solids and liquid																
Crushed	1 cup	260	195	1	Trace	—	—	—	50	29	.8	120	.20	.06	.5	17
Sliced, slices and juice	2 small or 1 large and 2 tbsp. juice	122	90	Trace	Trace	—	—	—	24	13	.4	50	.09	.03	.2	8
Pineapple juice, canned	1 cup	249	135	1	Trace	—	—	—	34	37	.7	120	.12	.04	.5	22
Plums, all except prunes																
Raw, 2-inch diameter, about 2 ounces[5]	1	60	25	Trace	Trace	—	—	—	7	7	.3	140	.02	.02	.3	3
Canned, syrup pack (Italian prunes)																
Plums (with pits) and juice[5]	1 cup	256	205	1	Trace	—	—	—	53	22	2.2	2,970	.05	.05	.9	4
Plums (without pits) and juice	3 plums and 2 tbsp. juice	122	100	Trace	Trace	—	—	—	26	11	1.1	1,470	.03	.02	.5	2
Prunes, dried, "softenized," medium																
Uncooked[5]	4	32	70	1	Trace	—	—	—	18	14	1.1	440	.02	.04	.4	1
Cooked, unsweetened, 17-18 prunes and ⅓ cup liquid[5]	1 cup	270	295	2	1	—	—	—	78	60	4.5	1,860	.08	.18	1.7	2
Prunes with tapioca, canned, strained or junior (baby food)	1 oz.	28	25	Trace	Trace	—	—	—	6	2	.3	110	.01	.02	.1	1
Prune juice, canned	1 cup	256	200	1	Trace	—	—	—	49	36	10.5	—	.02	.03	1.1	4
Raisin, dried	1 cup	160	460	4	Trace	—	—	—	124	99	5.6	30	.18	.13	.9	2

[5] Measure and weight apply to entire vegetable or fruit including parts not usually eaten.

[11] Based on yellow-fleshed varieties; for white-fleshed varieties value is about 50 I.U. per 114-gram peach and 80 I.U. per cup of sliced peaches.

[12] Average weighted in accordance with commercial freezing practices. For products without added ascorbic acid, value is about 37 milligrams per 12-ounce carton and 50 milligrams per 16-ounce can; for those with added ascorbic acid, 139 milligrams per 12 ounces and 186 milligrams per 16 ounces.

Food, approximate measure, and weight (in grams)		Food energy	Protein	Fat (total lipid)	Fatty acids			Carbohydrate	Calcium	Iron	Vitamin A value	Thiamine	Riboflavin	Niacin	Ascorbic acid
					Saturated (total)	Unsaturated Oleic	Unsaturated Linoleic								
	gm.	(Calories)	(gm.)	(gm.)	(gm.)	(gm.)	(gm.)	(gm.)	(mg.)	(mg.)	(I.U.)	(mg.)	(mg.)	(mg.)	(mg.)
Raspberries, red															
Raw — 1 cup	123	70	1	1	—	—	—	17	27	1.1	160	.04	.11	1.1	31
Frozen, 10 oz. carton, not thawed — 1 carton	284	275	2	1	—	—	—	70	37	1.7	200	.06	.17	1.7	59
Rhubarb, cooked, sugar added — 1 cup	272	385	1	Trace	—	—	—	98	212	1.6	220	.06	.15	.7	17
Strawberries															
Raw, capped — 1 cup	149	55	1	1	—	—	—	13	31	1.5	90	.04	.10	1.0	88
Frozen, 10-oz. carton, not thawed — 1 carton	284	310	1	1	—	—	—	79	40	2.0	90	.06	.17	1.5	150
Frozen, 16-ounce can, not thawed — 1 can	454	495	2	1	—	—	—	126	64	3.2	150	.09	.27	2.4	240
Tangerines, raw, medium, 2½-inch diameter, about 4 per pound[5] — 1	114	40	1	Trace	—	—	—	10	34	.3	350	.05	.02	.1	26
Tangerine juice															
Tangerine juice															
Canned, unsweetened — 1 cup	248	105	1	Trace	—	—	—	25	45	.5	1,040	.14	.04	.3	56
Frozen concentrate															
Undiluted, can, 6 fluid oz. — 1 can	210	340	4	1	—	—	—	80	130	1.5	3,070	.43	.12	.9	202
Diluted with 3 parts water, by volume — 1 cup	248	115	1	Trace	—	—	—	27	45	.5	1,020	.14	.04	.3	67
Watermelon, raw, wedge, 4 by 8 inches (1/16 of 10 by 16-inch melon, about 2 pounds with rind)[5] — 1 wedge	925	115	2	1	—	—	—	27	30	2.1	2,510	.13	.13	.7	30
Barley, pearled, light, uncooked — 1 cup	203	710	17	2	Trace	1	1	160	32	4.1	0	.25	.17	6.3	0
Biscuits, baking powder with enriched flour, 2½-inch diameter — 1	38	140	3	6	2	3	1	17	46	.6	Trace	.08	.08	.7	Trace
Bran flakes (40 percent bran) added thiamine — 1 oz.	28	85	3	1	—	—	—	23	20	1.2	0	.11	.05	1.7	0

Breads

Food	Measure	Weight (grams)	Food energy (calories)	Protein (grams)	Fat (grams)	Saturated fatty acids (grams)	Oleic (grams)	Linoleic (grams)	Carbohydrate (grams)	Calcium (mg)	Iron (mg)	Vitamin A (I.U.)	Thiamine (mg)	Riboflavin (mg)	Niacin (mg)	Ascorbic acid (mg)
Boston brown bread, slice, 3 by ¾ inch	1 slice	48	100	3	1	—	—	—	22	43	.9	0	.05	.03	.6	0
Cracked-wheat bread																
Loaf, 1-pound, 20 slices	1 loaf	454	1,190	39	10	2	5	2	236	399	5.0	Trace	.53	.42	5.8	Trace
Slice	1	23	60	2	1	—	—	—	12	20	.3	Trace	.03	.02	.3	Trace
French or Vienna bread																
Enriched, 1-pound loaf	1 loaf	454	1,315	41	14	3	8	2	251	195	10.0	Trace	1.26	.98	11.3	Trace
Unenriched, 1-pound loaf	1 loaf	454	1,315	41	14	3	8	2	251	195	3.2	Trace	.39	.39	3.6	Trace
Italian bread																
Enriched, 1-pound loaf	1 loaf	454	1,250	41	4	Trace	1	2	256	77	10.0	0	1.31	.93	11.7	0
Unenriched, 1-pound loaf	1 loaf	454	1,250	41	4	Trace	1	2	256	77	3.2	0	.39	.27	3.6	0
Raisin bread																
Loaf, 1-pound, 20 slices	1 loaf	454	1,190	30	13	3	8	2	243	322	5.9	Trace	.24	.42	3.0	Trace
Slice	1	23	60	2	1	—	—	—	12	16	.3	Trace	.01	.02	.2	Trace
Rye bread																
American, light (⅓ rye, ⅔ wheat)																
Loaf, 1-pound, 20 slices	1 loaf	454	1,100	41	5	—	—	—	236	340	7.3	0	.81	.33	6.4	0
Slice	1	23	55	2	Trace	—	—	—	12	17	.4	0	.04	.02	.3	0
Pumpernickel, loaf, 1 pound	1 loaf	454	1,115	41	5	—	—	—	241	381	10.9	0	1.05	.63	5.4	0
White bread, enriched																
1 to 2 percent nonfat dry milk																
Loaf, 1-pound, 20 slices	1 loaf	454	1,225	39	15	3	8	2	229	318	10.9	Trace	1.13	.77	10.4	Trace
Slice	1 slice	23	60	2	1	Trace	Trace	Trace	12	16	.6	Trace	.06	.04	.5	Trace
3 to 4 percent nonfat dry milk[13]																
Loaf, 1-pound	1	454	1,225	39	15	3	8	2	229	381	11.3	Trace	1.13	.95	10.8	Trace
Slice, 20 per loaf	1	23	60	2	1	Trace	Trace	Trace	12	19	.6	Trace	.06	.05	.6	Trace
Slice, toasted	1	20	60	2	1	Trace	Trace	Trace	12	19	.6	Trace	.05	.05	.6	Trace
Slice, 26 per loaf	1	17	45	1	1	Trace	Trace	Trace	9	14	.4	Trace	.04	.04	.4	Trace

[5] Measure and weight apply to entire vegetable or fruit including parts not usually eaten.

[13] When the amount of nonfat dry milk in commercial white bread is unknown, values for bread with 3 to 4% nonfat dry milk are suggested.

Food, approximate measure, and weight (in grams)		gm.	Food energy	Protein	Fat (total lipid)	Fatty acids Saturated (total)	Fatty acids Unsaturated Oleic	Fatty acids Unsaturated Linoleic	Carbohydrate	Calcium	Iron	Vitamin A value	Thiamine	Riboflavin	Niacin	Ascorbic acid
			(Calories)	(gm.)	(gm.)	(gm.)	(gm.)	(gm.)	(gm.)	(mg.)	(mg.)	(I.U.)	(mg.)	(mg.)	(mg.)	(mg.)
Bread—cont'd																
White bread, enriched—cont'd																
5 to 6 percent nonfat dry milk																
Loaf, 1-pound, 20 slices	1 loaf	454	1,245	41	17	4	10	2	228	435	11.3	Trace	1.22	.91	11.0	Trace
Slice	1	23	65	2	1	Trace	Trace	Trace	12	22	.6	Trace	.06	.05	.6	Trace
White bread, unenriched																
1 to 2 percent nonfat dry milk																
Loaf, 1-pound, 20 slices	1 loaf	454	1,225	39	15	3	8	2	229	318	3.2	Trace	.40	.36	5.6	Trace
Slice	1	23	60	2	1	Trace	Trace	Trace	12	16	.2	Trace	.02	.02	.3	Trace
3 to 4 percent nonfat dry milk[13]																
Loaf, 1-pound	1 loaf	454	1,225	39	15	3	8	—	229	381	3.2	Trace	.31	.39	5.0	Trace
Slice, 20 per loaf	1 slice	23	60	2	1	Trace	Trace	Trace	12	19	.2	Trace	.02	.02	.3	Trace
Slice, toasted	1	20	60	2	1	Trace	Trace	Trace	12	19	.2	Trace	.01	.02	.3	Trace
Slice, 26 per loaf	1 slice	17	45	1	1	Trace	Trace	Trace	9	14	.1	Trace	.01	.01	.2	Trace
5 to 6 percent nonfat dry milk																
Loaf, 1-pound, 20 slices	1 loaf	454	1,245	41	17	4	10	2	228	435	3.2	Trace	.32	.39	4.1	Trace
Slice	1	23	65	2	1	Trace	Trace	Trace	12	22	.2	Trace	.02	.03	.2	Trace
Whole-wheat bread, made with 2 percent nonfat dry milk																
Loaf, 1-pound, 20 slices	1 loaf	454	1,105	48	14	3	6	3	216	449	10.4	Trace	1.17	.56	12.9	Trace
Slice	1	23	55	2	1	Trace	Trace	Trace	11	23	.5	Trace	.06	.03	.7	Trace
Slice, toasted	1	19	55	2	1	Trace	Trace	Trace	11	22	.5	Trace	.05	.03	.6	Trace
Breadcrumbs, dry, grated	1 cup	88	345	11	4	1	2	1	65	107	3.2	Trace	.19	.26	3.1	Trace
Cakes[14]																
Angelfood cake; sector, 2-inch (1/12 of 8-inch-diameter cake)	1 sector	40	110	3	Trace	—	—	—	24	4	.1	0	Trace	.06	.1	0
Chocolate cake, chocolate icing; sector, 2-inch (1/16 of 10-inch-	1 sector	120	445	5	20	8	10	1	67	84	1.2	15190	.03	.12	.3	Trace

[fr]uitcake, dark (made with enriched flour); piece, 2 by 2 by ½ inch	1 piece															
Gingerbread (made with enriched flour); piece, 2 by 2 by 2 inches	1 piece	55	175	2	6	1	4	Trace	29	37	1.3	50	.06	.06	.5	0
Plain cake and cupcakes, without icing																
Piece, 3 by 2 by 1½ inches	1	55	200	2	8	2	5	1	31	35	.2	[15]90	.01	.05	.1	Trace
Cupcake, 2¾-inch diameter	1	40	145	2	6	1	3	Trace	22	26	.2	[15]70	.01	.03	.1	Trace
Plain cake and cupcakes, with chocolate icing																
Sector, 2-inch (1/16 of 10-inch-layer cake)	1	100	370	4	14	5	7	1	59	63	.6	[15]180	.02	.09	.2	Trace
Cupcake, 2¾-inch diameter	1	50	185	2	7	2	4	Trace	30	32	.3	[15]90	.01	.04	.1	Trace
Poundcake, old-fashioned (equal weights flour, sugar, fat, eggs); slice, 2¾ by 3 by ⅝ inch	1 slice	30	140	2	9	2	5	1	14	6	.2	[15]80	.01	.03	.1	0
Sponge cake; sector, 2-inch (1/12 of 8-inch-diameter cake)	1	40	120	3	2	1	1	Trace	22	12	.5	180	.02	.06	.1	Trace
Cookies																
Plain and assorted, 3-inch diameter	1 cooky	25	120	1	5	—	—	—	18	9	.2	20	.01	.01	.1	Trace
Fig bars, small	1	16	55	1	1	—	—	—	12	12	.2	20	.01	.01	.1	Trace
Corn, rice and wheat flakes, mixed, added nutrients	1 oz.	28	110	2	Trace	—	—	—	24	11	.5	0	.11	—	.9	0
Corn flakes, added nutrients																
Plain	1 oz.	28	110	2	Trace	—	—	—	24	5	.4	0	.12	.02	.6	0
Sugar-covered	1 oz.	28	110	1	Trace	—	—	—	26	3	.3	0	.12	.01	.5	0

[13] When the amount of nonfat dry milk in commercial white bread is unknown, values for bread with 3 to 4% nonfat dry milk are suggested.

[14] Unenriched cake flour and vegetable cooking fat used unless otherwise specified.

[15] If the fat used in the recipe is butter or fortified margarine, the vitamin A value for chocolate cake with chocolate icing will be 490 I.U. per 2-inch sector; 100 I.U. for fruitcake; for plain cake without icing, 300 I.U. per piece; 220 I.U. per cupcake; for plain cake with icing, 440 I.U. per 2-inch sector; 220 I.U. per cupcake; and 300 I.U. for poundcake.

Food, approximate measure, and weight (in grams)		Food energy	Protein	Fat (total lipid)	Fatty acids			Carbohydrate	Calcium	Iron	Vitamin A value	Thiamine	Riboflavin	Niacin	Ascorbic acid
					Saturated (total)	Unsaturated Oleic	Linoleic								
	gm.	(Calories)	(gm.)	(gm.)	(gm.)	(gm.)	(gm.)	(gm.)	(mg.)	(mg.)	(I.U.)	(mg.)	(mg.)	(mg.)	(mg.)
Corn grits, degermed, cooked															
Enriched 1 cup	242	120	3	Trace	—	—	—	27	2	[16].7	150	[16].10	[16].07	[16]1.0	0
Unenriched 1 cup	242	120	3	Trace	—	—	—	27	2	.2	150	.05	.02	.5	0
Cornmeal, white or yellow, dry															
Whole ground, unbolted 1 cup	118	420	11	5	1	2	2	87	24	2.8	600	.45	.13	2.4	0
Degermed, enriched 1 cup	145	525	11	2	Trace	1	1	114	9	[16]4.2	640	[16].64	[16].38	[16]5.1	0
Corn muffins, made with enriched degermed cornmeal and enriched flour; muffin, 2¾-inch diameter 1 muffin	48	150	3	5	2	2	Trace	23	50	.8	80	.09	.11	.8	Trace
Corn, puffed, pre-sweetened, added nutrients 1 oz.	28	110	1	Trace	—	—	—	26	3	.5	0	.12	.05	.6	0
Corn, shredded, added nutrients 1 oz.	28	110	2	Trace	—	—	—	25	1	.7	0	.12	.05	.6	0
Crackers															
Graham, plain 4 small or 2 medium	14	55	1	1	—	—	—	10	6	.2	0	.01	.03	.2	0
Saltines, 2 inches squares 2 crackers	8	35	1	1	—	—	—	6	2	.1	0	Trace	Trace	.1	0
Soda															
Cracker, 2½ inches square 2 crackers	11	50	1	1	Trace	1	Trace	8	2	.2	0	Trace	Trace	.1	0
Oyster crackers 10 crackers	10	45	1	1	Trace	1	Trace	7	2	.2	0	Trace	Trace	.1	0
Cracker meal 1 tbsp.	10	45	1	1	Trace	1	Trace	7	2	.1	0	.01	Trace	.1	0
Doughnuts, cake type 1 doughnut	32	125	1	6	1	4	Trace	16	13	[19].4	30	[19].05	[19].05	[19].4	Trace
Farina, regular, enriched, cooked 1 cup	238	100	3	Trace	—	—	—	21	10	[16].7	0	[16].11	[16].07	[16]1.0	0
Macaroni, cooked															
Enriched Cooked, firm stage (8 to 10 minutes; undergoes additional cooking in a food mixture) 1 cup	130	190	6	1	—	—	—	39	14	[16]1.4	0	[16].23	[16].14	[16]1.9	0

Food	Measure	Weight (g)	Food energy (Cal.)	Protein (g)	Fat (g)	Saturated (g)	Oleic (g)	Linoleic (g)	Carbohydrate (g)	Calcium (mg)	Iron (mg)	Vitamin A (I.U.)	Thiamine (mg)	Riboflavin (mg)	Niacin (mg)	Ascorbic acid (mg)
Cooked until tender, Unenriched	1 cup	140	155	5	1	—	—	—	32	11	[16]1.3	0	[16].19	[16].11	[16]1.5	0
Cooked, firm stage (8 to 10 minutes; undergoes additional cooking in a food mixture)	1 cup	130	190	6	1	—	—	—	39	14	.6	0	.02	.02	.5	0
Cooked until tender	1 cup	140	155	5	1	—	—	—	32	11	.6	0	.02	.02	.4	0
Macaroni (enriched) and cheese, baked	1 cup	220	470	18	24	11	10	1	44	398	2.0	950	.22	.44	2.0	Trace
Muffins, with enriched white flour; muffin, 2¾-inch diameter	1	48	140	4	5	1	3	Trace	20	50	.8	50	.08	.11	.7	Trace
Noodles (egg noodles), cooked																
Enriched	1 cup	160	200	7	2	1	1	Trace	37	16	[16]1.4	110	[16].23	[16].14	[16]1.8	0
Unenriched	1 cup	160	200	7	2	1	1	Trace	37	16	1.0	110	.04	.03	.7	0
Oats (with or without corn) puffed, added nutrients	1 oz.	28	115	3	2	Trace	1	1	21	50	1.3	0	.28	.05	.5	0
Oatmeal or rolled oats, regular or quick-cooking, cooked	1 cup	236	130	5	2	Trace	1	1	23	21	1.4	0	.19	.05	.3	0
Pancakes (griddlecakes), 4-inch diameter																
Wheat, enriched flour (home recipe)	1 cake	27	60	2	2	Trace	1	Trace	9	27	.4	30	.05	.06	.3	Trace
Buckwheat (buckwheat pancake mix, made with egg and milk)	1 cake	27	55	2	2	1	1	Trace	6	59	.4	60	.03	.04	.2	Trace
Piecrust, plain, baked. Enriched flour																
Lower crust, 9-inch shell	1	135	675	8	45	10	29	3	59	19	2.3	0	.27	.19	2.4	0
Double crust, 9-inch pie	1	270	1,350	16	90	21	58	7	118	38	4.6	0	.55	.39	4.9	0

[16] Iron, thiamine, riboflavin, and niacin are based on the minimum levels of enrichment specified in standards of identity promulgated under the Federal Food, Drug, and Cosmetic Act.

[17] Vitamin A value based on yellow product. White product contains only a trace.

[18] Based on recipe using white cornmeal; if yellow cornmeal is used, the vitamin A value is 140 I.U. per muffin.

[19] Based on product made with enriched flour. With unenriched flour, approximate values per doughnut are: Iron, 0.2 milligram; thiamine, 0.01 milligram; riboflavin, 0.03 milligram; niacin, 0.2 milligram.

Food, approximate measure, and weight (in grams)		gm.	Food energy (Calories)	Protein (gm.)	Fat (total lipid) (gm.)	Fatty acids Saturated (total) (gm.)	Fatty acids Unsaturated Oleic (gm.)	Fatty acids Unsaturated Linoleic (gm.)	Carbohydrate (gm.)	Calcium (mg.)	Iron (mg.)	Vitamin A value (I.U.)	Thiamine (mg.)	Riboflavin (mg.)	Niacin (mg.)	Ascorbic acid (mg.)
Piecrust, plain, baked—cont'd																
Unenriched flour																
Lower crust, 9-inch shell	1	135	675	8	45	10	29	3	59	19	.7	0	.04	.04	.6	0
Double crust, 9-inch pie	1	270	1,350	16	90	21	58	7	118	38	1.4	0	.08	.07	1.3	0
Pies (piecrust made with unenriched flour); sector, 4-inch, 1/7 of 9-inch-diameter pie																
Apple	1 sector	135	345	3	15	4	9	1	51	11	.4	40	.03	.02	.5	1
Cherry	1 sector	135	355	4	15	4	10	1	52	19	.4	590	.03	.03	.6	1
Custard	1 sector	130	280	8	14	5	8	1	30	125	.8	300	.07	.21	.4	0
Lemon meringue	1 sector	120	305	4	12	4	7	1	45	17	.6	200	.04	.10	.2	4
Mince	1 sector	135	365	3	16	4	10	1	56	38	1.4	Trace	.09	.05	.5	1
Pumpkin	1 sector	130	275	5	15	5	7	1	32	66	.6	3,210	.04	.13	.6	Trace
Pizza (cheese); 5½-inch sector; 1/8 of 14-inch-diameter pie	1 sector	75	185	7	6	2	3	Trace	27	107	.7	290	.04	.12	.7	4
Popcorn, popped, with added oil and salt	1 cup	14	65	1	3	2	Trace	Trace	8	1	.3	0	—	.01	.2	0
Pretzels, small stick	5 sticks	5	20	Trace	Trace	—	—	—	4	1	0	0	Trace	Trace	Trace	0
Rice, white (fully milled or polished), enriched, cooked																
Common commercial varieties, all types	1 cup	168	185	3	Trace	—	—	—	41	17	[20] 1.5	0	[20] .19	[20] .01	[20] 1.6	0
Long grain, parboiled	1 cup	176	185	4	Trace	—	—	—	41	33	[20] 1.4	0	[20] .19	[20] .02	[20] 2.0	0
Rice, puffed, added nutrients (without salt)	1 cup	14	55	1	Trace	—	—	—	13	3	.3	0	.06	.01	.6	0
Rice flakes, added nutrients	1 cup	30	115	2	Trace	—	—	—	26	9	.5	0	.10	.02	1.6	0
Rolls																
Plain, pan; 12 per 16 ounces																
Enriched	1 roll	38	115	3	2	Trace	1	Trace	20	28	.7	Trace	.11	.07	.8	Trace
Unenriched	1 roll	38	115	3	2	Trace	1	Trace	20	28	.3	Trace	.02	.03	.3	Trace
Hard, round; 12 per 22 oz.	1 roll	52	160	5	2	Trace	1	Trace	31	24	.4	Trace	.03	.05	.4	Trace
Sweet, pan; 12 per 18 oz.	1 roll	43	135	4	4	1	2	Trace	21	37	.3	30	.03	.06	.4	Trace

Food	Measure	Grams	Calories	Protein	Fat	Sat.	Unsat.	Unsat.	Carb.	Calcium	Iron	Vit. A	Thiamine	Riboflavin	Niacin	Ascorbic
Rye wafers, whole-grain, 1⅞ by 3½ inches	2 wafers	13	45	2	Trace	—	—	—	10	7	.5	0	.04	.03	.2	0
Spaghetti																
Cooked, tender stage (14 to 20 minutes)																
Enriched	1 cup	140	155	5	1	—	—	—	32	11	[16]1.3	0	[16].19	[16].11	[16]1.5	0
Unenriched	1 cup	140	155	5	1	—	—	—	32	11	.6	0	.02	.02	.4	0
Spaghetti with meat balls in tomato sauce (home recipe)	1 cup	250	335	19	12	4	6	1	39	125	3.8	1,600	.26	.30	4.0	22
Spaghetti in tomato sauce with cheese (home recipe)	1 cup	250	260	9	9	2	5	1	37	80	2.2	1,080	.24	.18	2.4	14
Waffles, with enriched flour, ½ by 4½ by 5½ inches	1	75	210	7	7	2	4	1	28	85	1.3	250	.13	.19	1.0	Trace
Wheat, puffed																
With added nutrients (without salt)	1 oz.	28	105	4	Trace	—	—	—	22	8	1.2	0	.15	.07	2.2	0
With added nutrients, with sugar and honey	1 oz.	28	105	2	1	—	—	—	25	7	.9	0	.14	.05	1.8	0
Wheat, rolled; cooked	1 cup	236	175	5	1	—	—	—	40	19	1.7	0	.17	.06	2.1	0
Wheat, shredded, plain (long, round, or bite-size)	1 oz.	28	100	3	1	—	—	—	23	12	1.0	0	.06	.03	1.2	0
Wheat and malted barley flakes, with added nutrients	1 oz.	28	110	2	Trace	—	—	—	24	14	.7	0	.13	.03	1.1	0
Wheat flakes, with added nutrients	1 oz.	28	100	3	Trace	—	—	—	23	12	1.2	0	.18	.04	1.4	0
Wheat flours																
Whole-wheat, from hard wheats, stirred	1 cup	120	400	16	2	Trace	1	1	85	49	4.0	0	.66	.14	5.2	0
All-purpose or family flour																
Enriched, sifted	1 cup	110	400	12	1	Trace	Trace	Trace	84	18	[16]3.2	0	[16].48	[16].29	[16]3.8	0
Unenriched, sifted	1 cup	110	400	12	1	Trace	Trace	Trace	84	18	.9	0	.07	.05	1.0	0
Self-rising, enriched	1 cup	110	385	10	1	Trace	Trace	Trace	82	292	[16]3.2	0	[16].49	[16].29	[16]3.9	0
Cake or pastry flour, sifted	1 cup	100	365	8	1	Trace	Trace	Trace	79	17	.5	0	.03	.03	.7	0
Wheat germ, crude, commercially milled	1 cup	68	245	18	7	1	2	4	32	49	6.4	0	1.36	.46	2.9	0

[16]Iron, thiamine, riboflavin, and niacin are based on the minimum levels of enrichment specified in standards of identity promulgated under the Federal Food, Drug, and Cosmetic Act.

[20]Iron, thiamine, and niacin are based on the minimum levels of enrichment specified in standards of identity promulgated under the Federal Food, Drug, and Cosmetic Act. Riboflavin is based on unenriched rice. When the minimum level of enrichment for riboflavin specified in the standards of identity becomes effective the value will be 0.12 milligram per cup of parboiled rice and of white rice.

Food, approximate measure, and weight (in grams)	Food energy (Calories)	Protein (gm.)	Fat (total lipid) (gm.)	Fatty acids Saturated (total) (gm.)	Fatty acids Unsaturated Oleic (gm.)	Fatty acids Unsaturated Linoleic (gm.)	Carbohydrate (gm.)	Calcium (mg.)	Iron (mg.)	Vitamin A value (I.U.)	Thiamine (mg.)	Riboflavin (mg.)	Niacin (mg.)	Ascorbic acid (mg.)
Fats, oils														
Butter, 4 sticks per pound														
Sticks, 2 — 1 cup — 227 gm.	1,625	1	184	101	61	6	1	45	0	[21]7,500	—	—	—	0
Stick, 1/8 — 1 tbsp. — 14	100	Trace	11	6	4	Trace	Trace	3	0	[21]460	—	—	—	0
Pat or square (64 per pound) — 1 — 7	50	Trace	6	3	2	Trace	Trace	1	0	[21]230	—	—	—	0
Fats, cooking														
Lard — 1 cup — 220	1,985	0	220	84	101	22	0	0	0	0	0	0	0	0
Lard — 1 tbsp. — 14	125	0	14	5	6	1	0	0	0	0	0	0	0	0
Vegetable fats — 1 cup — 200	1,770	0	200	46	130	14	0	0	0	—	0	0	0	0
Vegetable fats — 1 tbsp. — 12.5	110	0	12	3	8	1	0	0	0	—	0	0	0	0
Margarine, 4 sticks per pound														
Sticks, 2 — 1 cup — 227	1,635	1	184	37	105	33	1	45	0	[22]7,500	—	—	—	0
Stick, 1/8 — 1 tbsp. — 14	100	Trace	11	2	6	2	Trace	3	0	[22]460	—	—	—	0
Pat or square (64 per pound) — 1 pat — 7	50	Trace	6	1	3	1	Trace	1	0	[22]230	—	—	—	0
Oils, salad or cooking														
Corn — 1 tbsp. — 14	125	0	14	1	4	7	0	0	0	—	0	0	0	0
Cottonseed — 1 tbsp. — 14	125	0	14	4	3	7	0	0	0	—	0	0	0	0
Olive — 1 tbsp. — 14	125	0	14	2	11	1	0	0	0	—	0	0	0	0
Soybean — 1 tbsp. — 14	125	0	14	2	3	7	0	0	0	—	0	0	0	0
Salad dressings														
Blue cheese — 1 tbsp. — 16	80	1	8	2	2	4	1	13	Trace	30	Trace	.02	Trace	Trace
Commercial, mayonnaise type — 1 tbsp. — 15	65	Trace	6	1	1	3	2	2	Trace	30	Trace	Trace	Trace	—
French — 1 tbsp. — 15	60	Trace	6	1	1	3	3	2	.1	—	—	—	—	—
Home cooked, boiled — 1 tbsp. — 17	30	1	2	1	1	Trace	3	15	.1	80	.01	.03	—	—
Mayonnaise — 1 tbsp. — 15	110	Trace	12	2	3	6	Trace	3	.1	40	Trace	.01	Trace	Trace
Thousand island — 1 tbsp. — 15	75	Trace	8	1	2	4	2	2	.1	50	Trace	Trace	Trace	Trace
Sugars, sweets														
Candy														
Caramels — 1 oz. — 28	115	1	3	2	1	Trace	22	42	.4	Trace	.01	.05	Trace	Trace
Chocolate, milk, plain — 1 oz. — 28	150	2	9	5	3	Trace	16	65	.3	80	.02	.09	.1	Trace
Fudge, plain — 1 oz. — 28	115	1	3	2	1	Trace	21	22	.3	Trace	.01	.03	.1	Trace

Food	Measure															
Hard candy	1 oz.	28	110	0	Trace	—	—	—	28	6	.5	0	0	0	0	0
Marshmallows	1 oz.	28	90	1	Trace	—	—	—	23	5	.5	0	0	Trace	Trace	0
Chocolate sirup, thin type	1 tbsp.	20	50	Trace	Trace	—	—	—	13	3	.3	—	Trace	.01	.1	0
Honey, strained or extracted	1 tbsp.	21	65	Trace	0	—	—	—	17	1	.1	0	Trace	.01	.1	Trace
Jams and preserves	1 tbsp.	20	55	Trace	Trace	—	—	—	14	4	.2	Trace	Trace	.01	Trace	Trace
Jellies	1 tbsp.	20	55	Trace	Trace	—	—	—	14	4	.3	Trace	Trace	.01	Trace	1
Molasses, cane																
Light (first extraction)	1 tbsp.	20	50	—	—	—	—	—	13	33	.9	—	.01	.01	Trace	—
Blackstrap (third extraction)	1 tbsp.	20	45	—	—	—	—	—	11	137	3.2	—	.02	.04	.4	—
Sirup, table blends (chiefly corn, light and dark)	1 tbsp.	20	60	0	0	—	—	—	15	9	.8	0	0	0	0	0
Sugars (cane or beet)																
Granulated	1 cup	200	770	0	0	—	—	—	199	0	.2	0	0	0	0	0
	1 tbsp.	12	45	0	0	—	—	—	12	0	Trace	0	0	0	0	0
Lump, 1⅛ by ¾ by ⅜	1 lump	6	25	0	0	—	—	—	6	0	Trace	0	0	0	0	0
Powdered, stirred before measuring	1 cup	128	495	0	0	—	—	—	127	0	.1	0	0	0	0	0
	1 tbsp.	8	30	0	0	—	—	—	8	0	Trace	0	0	0	0	0
Brown, firm-packed	1 cup	220	820	0	0	—	—	—	212	187	7.5	0	.02	.07	.4	0
	1 tbsp.	14	50	0	0	—	—	—	13	12	.5	0	Trace	Trace	Trace	0
Miscellaneous items																
Beer (average 3.6 percent alcohol by weight)	1 cup	240	100	1	0	—	—	—	9	12	Trace	—	.01	.07	1.6	—
Beverages, carbonated																
Cola type	1 cup	240	95	0	0	—	—	—	24	—	—	0	0	0	0	0
Ginger ale	1 cup	230	70	0	0	—	—	—	18	—	—	0	0	0	0	0
Bouillon cube, ⅝ inch	1 cube	4	5	1	Trace	—	—	—	Trace	—	—	—	—	—	—	—
Chili powder. See Vegetables, peppers																
Chili sauce (mainly tomatoes)	1 tbsp.	17	20	Trace	Trace	—	—	—	4	3	.1	240	.02	.01	.3	3
Chocolate																
Bitter or baking	1 oz.	28	145	3	15	8	6	Trace	8	22	1.9	20	.01	.07	.4	0
Sweet	1 oz.	28	150	1	10	6	4	Trace	16	27	.4	Trace	.01	.04	.1	Trace
Cider. See Fruits, apple juice																

[21] Year-round average.

[22] Based on the average vitamin A content of fortified margarine. Federal specifications for fortified margarine require a minimum of 15,000 I.U. of vitamin A per pound.

Food, approximate measure, and weight (in grams)		gm.	Food energy (Calories)	Protein (gm.)	Fat (total lipid) (gm.)	Fatty acids Saturated (total) (gm.)	Fatty acids Unsaturated Oleic (gm.)	Fatty acids Unsaturated Linoleic (gm.)	Carbohydrate (gm.)	Calcium (mg.)	Iron (mg.)	Vitamin A value (I.U.)	Thiamine (mg.)	Riboflavin (mg.)	Niacin (mg.)	Ascorbic acid (mg.)
Gelatin, dry																
Plain	1 tbsp.	10	35	9	Trace	—	—	—	—	—	—	—	—	—	—	—
Dessert powder, 3-oz. package	½ cup	85	315	8	0	—	—	—	75	—	—	—	—	—	—	—
Gelatin dessert, ready-to-eat																
Plain	1 cup	239	140	4	0	—	—	—	34	—	—	—	—	—	—	—
With fruit	1 cup	241	160	3	Trace	—	—	—	40	—	—	—	—	—	—	—
Olives, pickled																
Green	4 medium or 3 extra large or 2 giant	16	15	Trace	2	Trace	2	Trace	Trace	8	.2	40	—	—	—	—
Ripe: Mission	3 small or 2 large	10	15	Trace	2	Trace	2	Trace	Trace	9	.1	10	Trace	Trace	—	—
Pickles, cucumber																
Dill, large, 4 by 1¾ inches	1	135	15	1	Trace	—	—	—	3	35	1.4	140	Trace	.03	Trace	8
Sweet, 2¾ by ¾ inches	1	20	30	Trace	Trace	—	—	—	7	2	.2	20	Trace	Trace	Trace	1
Popcorn. See Grain products																
Sherbet, orange	1 cup	193	260	2	2	—	—	—	59	31	Trace	110	.02	.06	Trace	4
Soups, canned; ready-to-serve (prepared with equal volume of water)																
Bean with pork	1 cup	250	170	8	6	1	2	2	22	62	2.2	650	.14	.07	1.0	2
Beef noodle	1 cup	250	70	4	3	1	1	1	7	8	1.0	50	.05	.06	1.1	Trace
Beef bouillon, broth, consomme	1 cup	240	30	5	0	0	0	0	3	Trace	.5	Trace	Trace	.02	1.2	—
Chicken noodle	1 cup	250	65	4	2	Trace	1	1	8	10	.5	50	.02	.02	.8	Trace
Clam chowder	1 cup	255	85	2	3	—	—	—	13	36	1.0	920	.03	.03	1.0	—
Cream soup (mushroom)	1 cup	240	135	2	10	1	3	5	10	41	.5	70	.02	.12	.7	Trace
Minestrone	1 cup	245	105	5	3	1	1	—	14	37	1.0	2,350	.07	.05	1.0	—
Pea, green	1 cup	245	130	6	2	1	1	Trace	23	44	1.0	340	.05	.05	1.0	7
Tomato	1 cup	245	90	2	2	Trace	1	1	16	15	.7	1,000	.06	.05	1.1	12
Vegetable with beef broth	1 cup	250	80	3	2	—	—	—	14	20	.8	3,250	.05	.02	1.2	—

Food	Measure															
Starch (cornstarch)	1 cup	128	465	Trace	Trace	—	—	—	112	0	0	0	0	0	0	0
	1 tbsp.	8	30	Trace	Trace	—	—	—	7	0	0	0	0	0	0	0
Tapioca, quick-cooking granulated, dry, stirred before measuring	1 cup	152	535	1	Trace	—	—	—	131	15	.6	0	0	0	0	0
	1 tbsp.	10	35	Trace	Trace	—	—	—	9	1	Trace	0	0	0	0	0
Vinegar	1 tbsp.	15	2	0	0	—	—	—	1	1	.1	—	—	—	—	—
White sauce, medium	1 cup	265	430	10	33	18	11	1	23	305	.5	1,220	.12	.44	.6	Trace
Yeast																
Baker's Compressed	1 oz.	28	25	3	Trace	—	—	—	3	4	1.4	Trace	.20	.47	3.2	Trace
Dry active	1 oz.	28	80	10	Trace	—	—	—	11	12	4.6	Trace	.66	1.53	10.4	Trace
Brewer's, dry, debittered	1 tbsp.	8	25	3	Trace	—	—	—	3	17	1.4	Trace	1.25	.34	3.0	Trace
Yogurt. See Milk, cream, cheese; related products																

APPENDIX B

Amino acid content of foods, 100 grams, edible portion[1]

Protein content, and nitrogen conversion factor	Trypto-phan (gm.)	Threo-nine (gm.)	Iso-leucine (gm.)	Leucine (gm.)	Lysine (gm.)	Methi-onine (gm.)	Cystine (gm.)	Phenyl-alanine (gm.)	Tyro-sine (gm.)	Valine (gm.)	Argi-nine (gm.)	Histi-dine (gm.)
Milk; milk products												
Milk (Protein, N × 6.38)												
Cow												
fluid, whole and non-fat (3.5% protein)	0.049	0.161	0.223	0.344	0.272	0.086	0.031	0.170	0.178	0.240	0.128	0.092
canned												
evaporated, unsweetened (7.0% protein)	0.099	0.323	0.447	0.688	0.545	0.171	0.063	0.340	0.357	0.481	0.256	0.185
condensed, sweetened (8.1% protein)	0.114	0.374	0.518	0.796	0.631	0.198	0.072	0.393	0.413	0.557	0.296	0.214
dried												
whole (25.8% protein)	0.364	1.191	1.648	2.535	2.009	0.632	0.231	1.251	1.316	1.774	0.944	0.680
nonfat (35.6% protein)	0.502	1.641	2.271	3.493	2.768	0.870	0.318	1.724	1.814	2.444	1.300	0.937
Goat (3.3% protein)	0.039	0.217	0.087	0.278	0.312	0.065	—	0.121	—	0.139	0.174	0.068
Human (1.4% protein)	0.023	0.062	0.075	0.124	0.090	0.028	0.027	0.060	0.071	0.086	0.055	0.030
Indian buffalo (4.2% protein)	0.059	0.212	0.204	0.420	0.331	0.112	0.058	0.177	—	0.255	0.136	0.086
Milk products												
Buttermilk (3.5% protein, N × 6.38)	0.038	0.165	0.219	0.348	0.291	0.082	0.032	0.186	0.137	0.262	0.168	0.099
Casein (100% protein, N × 6.29)	1.335	4.277	6.550	10.048	8.013	3.084	0.382	5.389	5.819	7.393	4.070	3.021
Cheese (protein, N × 6.38)												
blue mold (21.5% protein)	0.293	0.799	1.449	2.096	1.577	0.559	0.121	1.153	1.028	1.543	0.785	0.701
Camembert (17.5% protein)	0.239	0.650	1.179	1.706	1.284	0.455	0.099	0.938	0.837	1.256	0.639	0.571
Cheddar (25.0% protein)	0.341	0.929	1.685	2.437	1.834	0.650	0.141	1.340	1.195	1.794	0.913	0.815
Cheddar processed (23.2% protein)	0.316	0.862	1.563	2.262	1.702	0.604	0.131	1.244	1.109	1.665	0.847	0.756
cheese foods, Cheddar (20.5% protein)	0.280	0.761	1.382	1.998	1.504	0.533	0.116	1.099	0.980	1.472	0.749	0.668
cottage (17.0% protein)	0.179	0.794	0.989	1.826	1.428	0.469	0.147	0.917	0.917	0.978	0.802	0.549
cream cheese (9.0% protein)	0.080	0.408	0.519	0.923	0.721	0.229	0.085	0.547	0.408	0.538	0.313	0.278
Limburger (21.2% protein)	0.289	0.788	1.429	2.067	1.555	0.552	0.120	1.136	1.014	1.522	0.774	0.691
Parmesan (36.0% protein)	0.491	1.337	2.426	3.510	2.641	0.937	0.203	1.930	1.721	2.584	1.315	1.174

Food												
Swiss (27.5% protein)	0.373	1.021	1.855	2.061	2.011		0.130	1.414	1.575	1.774	0.964	0.870
Swiss processed (26.4% protein)	0.360	0.981	1.779	2.574	1.937	0.687	0.149	1.415	1.262	1.895	0.964	0.861
Lactalbumin (100% protein, N × 6.49)	2.203	5.239	6.209	12.342	9.060	2.250	3.405	4.360	3.806	5.686	3.498	1.911
Whey (protein, N × 6.49)												
fluid (0.9% protein)	0.010	0.048	0.052	0.074	0.055	0.013	0.018	0.023	0.009	0.045	0.017	0.011
dried (12.7% protein)	0.147	0.677	0.734	1.043	0.769	0.188	0.250	0.323	0.131	0.640	0.235	0.159
Eggs, chicken (protein, N × 6.25)												
Fresh or stored												
whole (12.8% protein)	0.211	0.637	0.850	1.126	0.819	0.401	0.299	0.739	0.551	0.950	0.840	0.307
whites (10.8% protein)	0.164	0.477	0.698	0.950	0.648	0.420	0.263	0.689	0.449	0.842	0.634	0.233
yolks (16.3% protein)	0.235	0.827	0.996	1.372	1.074	0.417	0.274	0.717	0.756	1.121	1.132	0.368
Dried												
whole (46.8% protein)	0.771	2.329	3.108	4.118	2.995	1.468	1.093	2.703	2.014	3.474	3.070	1.123
whites (85.9% protein)	1.306	3.793	5.553	7.559	5.154	3.340	3.089	5.484	3.573	6.693	5.044	1.855
yolks (31.2% protein)	0.449	1.582	1.907	2.626	2.057	0.799	0.524	1.373	1.448	2.147	2.167	0.704
Meat; poultry; fish and shellfish (their products)												
Meat (protein, N × 6.25)												
Beef carcass or side												
thin (18.8% protein)	0.220	0.830	0.984	1.540	1.642	0.466	0.238	0.773	0.638	1.044	1.212	0.653
medium fat (17.5% protein)	0.204	0.773	0.916	1.434	1.529	0.434	0.221	0.720	0.594	0.972	1.128	0.608
fat (16.3% protein)	0.190	0.720	0.853	1.335	1.424	0.404	0.206	0.670	0.553	0.905	1.051	0.566
very fat (13.7% protein)	0.160	0.605	0.717	1.122	1.197	0.340	0.173	0.563	0.465	0.761	0.883	0.476
medium fat, trimmed to retail basis (18.2% protein)	0.213	0.804	0.952	1.491	1.590	0.451	0.230	0.748	0.617	1.010	1.174	0.632
Beef cuts, medium fat												
chuck (18.6% protein)	0.217	0.821	0.973	1.524	1.625	0.461	0.235	0.765	0.631	1.033	1.199	0.646
flank (19.9% protein)	0.232	0.879	1.041	1.630	1.738	0.494	0.252	0.818	0.675	1.105	1.283	0.691
hamburger (16.0% protein)	0.187	0.707	0.837	1.311	1.398	0.397	0.202	0.658	0.543	0.888	1.032	0.556
porterhouse (16.4% protein)	0.192	0.724	0.858	1.343	1.433	0.407	0.220	0.674	0.556	0.911	1.057	0.569
rib roast (17.4% protein)	0.203	0.768	0.910	1.425	1.520	0.432	0.246	0.715	0.590	0.966	1.122	0.604
round (19.5% protein)	0.228	0.861	1.020	1.597	1.704	0.484	0.205	0.802	0.661	1.083	1.257	0.677
rump (16.2% protein)	0.189	0.715	0.848	1.327	1.415	0.402	0.219	0.666	0.550	0.899	1.045	0.562
sirloin (17.3% protein)	0.202	0.764	0.905	1.417	1.511	0.429		0.711	0.587	0.960	1.116	0.601
Beef, canned (25.0% protein)	0.292	1.104	1.308	2.048	2.184	0.620	0.316	1.028	0.848	1.388	1.612	0.868
Beef, dried or chipped (34.3% protein)	0.401	1.515	1.795	2.810	2.996	0.851	0.434	1.410	1.163	1.904	2.212	1.191

[1] Courtesy Orr, M. L., and Watt, B. K.: Amino acid content of foods, Home Economics Research Report No. 4, U. S. Department of Agriculture, 1966. This selected listing reprinted here is taken from the original report of the Agricultural Research Service which contains data on 18 amino acids in 202 food items.

Protein content, and nitrogen conversion factor	Trypto-phan (gm.)	Threo-nine (gm.)	Iso-leucine (gm.)	Leucine (gm.)	Lysine (gm.)	Methi-onine (gm.)	Cystine (gm.)	Phenyl-alanine (gm.)	Tyro-sine (gm.)	Valine (gm.)	Argi-nine (gm.)	Histi-dine (gm.)
Lamb carcass or side												
thin (17.1% protein)	0.222	0.782	0.886	1.324	1.384	0.410	0.224	0.695	0.594	0.843	1.114	0.476
medium fat (15.7% protein)	0.203	0.718	0.814	1.216	1.271	0.377	0.206	0.638	0.545	0.774	1.022	0.437
fat (13.0% protein)	0.168	0.595	0.674	1.007	1.052	0.312	0.171	0.528	0.451	0.641	0.847	0.362
Lamb cuts, medium fat												
leg (18.0% protein)	0.233	0.824	0.933	1.394	1.457	0.432	0.236	0.732	0.625	0.887	1.172	0.501
rib (14.9% protein)	0.193	0.682	0.772	1.154	1.206	0.358	0.195	0.606	0.517	0.734	0.970	0.415
shoulder (15.6% protein)	0.202	0.714	0.809	1.208	1.263	0.374	0.205	0.634	0.542	0.769	1.016	0.434
Pork, packer's carcass or side												
thin (14.1% protein)	0.183	0.654	0.724	1.038	1.157	0.352	0.165	0.555	0.503	0.733	0.864	0.487
medium fat (11.9% protein)	0.154	0.552	0.611	0.876	0.977	0.297	0.139	0.468	0.425	0.619	0.729	0.411
Fat (9.8% protein)	0.127	0.455	0.503	0.721	0.804	0.245	0.114	0.386	0.350	0.510	0.601	0.339
Pork cuts, medium fat, fresh												
ham (15.2% protein)	0.197	0.705	0.781	1.119	1.248	0.379	0.178	0.598	0.542	0.790	0.931	0.525
loin (16.4% protein)	0.213	0.761	0.842	1.207	1.346	0.409	0.192	0.646	0.585	0.853	1.005	0.567
miscellaneous lean cuts (14.5% protein)	0.188	0.673	0.745	1.067	1.190	0.362	0.169	0.571	0.517	0.754	0.889	0.501
Pork, cured												
bacon, medium fat (9.1% protein)	0.095	0.306	0.399	0.728	0.587	0.141	0.106	0.434	0.234	0.434	0.622	0.246
fat back or salt pork (3.9% protein)	0.006	0.141	0.110	0.367	0.317	0.055	0.043	0.157	0.052	0.168	0.379	0.035
ham (16.9% protein)	0.162	0.692	0.841	1.306	1.420	0.411	0.273	0.646	0.652	0.879	1.068	0.544
luncheon meat												
boiled ham (22.8% protein)	0.219	0.934	1.135	1.762	1.915	0.554	0.368	0.872	0.879	1.186	1.441	0.733
canned, spiced (14.9% protein)	0.143	0.610	0.741	1.161	1.252	0.362	0.241	0.570	0.575	0.775	0.942	0.479
Rabbit, domesticated, flesh only (21.9% protein)	—	1.021	1.082	1.636	1.818	0.541	—	0.793	—	1.021	1.176	0.474
Veal, carcass or side												
thin (19.7% protein)	0.258	0.854	1.040	1.444	1.645	0.451	0.233	0.801	0.709	1.018	1.283	0.634
medium fat (19.1% protein)	0.251	0.828	1.008	1.400	1.595	0.437	0.226	0.776	0.688	0.987	1.244	0.614
Fat (18.5% protein)	0.243	0.802	0.977	1.356	1.545	0.423	0.219	0.752	0.666	0.956	1.205	0.595
Veal cuts, medium fat												
round (19.5% protein)	0.256	0.846	1.030	1.429	1.629	0.446	0.231	0.792	0.702	1.008	1.270	0.627
shoulder (19.4% protein)	0.255	0.841	1.024	1.422	1.620	0.444	0.230	0.788	0.698	1.003	1.263	0.624
stew meat (18.3% protein)	0.240	0.793	0.966	1.341	1.528	0.419	0.217	0.744	0.659	0.946	1.192	0.589
Poultry (protein, N × 6.25)												
Chicken, flesh only												
broilers or fryers (20.6% protein)	0.250	0.877	1.088	1.490	1.810	0.537	0.277	0.811	0.725	1.012	1.302	0.593
hens (21.3% protein)	0.259	0.907	1.125	1.540	1.871	0.556	0.286	0.838	0.750	1.046	1.346	0.613

protein)	—	0.935	1.109	1.657	1.842	0.531	—	0.842	—	1.027	1.301	0.486
Turkey, flesh only (24.0% protein)	—	1.014	1.260	1.836	2.173	0.664	0.330	0.960	—	1.187	1.513	0.649
Fish and shellfish (protein, N× 6.25)												
Bluefish (20.5% protein)	0.203	0.889	1.040	1.548	1.797	0.597	0.276	0.761	0.554	1.092	1.155	—
Cod												
fresh (16.5% protein)	0.164	0.715	0.837	1.246	1.447	0.480	0.222	0.612	0.446	0.879	0.929	—
dried (81.8% protein)	0.811	3.547	4.149	6.178	7.172	2.382	1.099	3.036	2.212	4.358	4.607	—
Croaker (17.8% protein)	0.177	0.772	0.903	1.344	1.561	0.518	0.239	0.661	0.481	0.948	1.002	—
Eel (18.6% protein)	0.185	0.806	0.943	1.405	1.631	0.542	0.250	0.690	0.503	0.991	1.048	—
Flounder (14.9% protein)	0.148	0.646	0.756	1.125	1.306	0.434	0.200	0.553	0.403	0.794	0.839	—
Haddock (18.2% protein)	0.181	0.789	0.923	1.374	1.596	0.530	0.245	0.676	0.492	0.970	1.025	—
Halibut (18.6% protein)	0.185	0.806	0.943	1.405	1.631	0.542	0.250	0.690	0.503	0.991	1.048	—
Herring												
Atlantic (18.3% protein)	0.182	0.793	0.928	1.382	1.605	0.533	0.246	0.679	0.495	0.975	1.031	—
lake (18.5% protein)	0.184	0.802	0.938	1.397	1.622	0.539	0.249	0.687	0.500	0.986	1.042	—
Pacific (16.6% protein)	0.165	0.720	0.842	1.254	1.455	0.483	0.223	0.616	0.449	0.884	0.935	—
Mackerels												
raw, common Atlantic (18.7% protein)	0.186	0.811	0.948	1.412	1.640	0.545	0.251	0.694	0.506	0.996	1.053	—
canned, solids and liquid												
Atlantic (19.3% protein)	0.191	0.837	0.979	1.458	1.692	0.562	0.259	0.716	0.522	1.028	1.087	—
Pacific (21.1% protein)	0.209	0.915	1.070	1.593	1.850	0.614	0.284	0.783	0.571	1.124	1.188	—
Salmon												
raw, Pacific (Chinook or King) (17.4% protein)	0.173	0.754	0.883	1.314	1.526	0.507	0.234	0.646	0.470	0.927	0.980	—
canned, solids and liquid (sockeye or red) (20.2% protein)	0.200	0.876	1.025	1.526	1.771	0.588	0.271	0.750	0.546	1.076	1.138	—
Sardines, canned, solids and liquid												
Atlantic type (21.1% protein)	0.209	0.915	1.070	1.593	1.850	0.614	0.284	0.783	0.571	1.124	1.188	—
Pacific type (17.7% protein)	0.176	0.767	0.898	1.337	1.552	0.515	0.238	0.657	0.479	0.943	0.997	—
Shrimp, canned, solids and liquid (18.7% protein)	0.186	0.811	0.948	1.412	1.640	0.545	0.251	0.694	0.506	0.996	1.053	—
Products from meat, poultry, and fish (protein, N× 6.25)												
Brains (10.4% protein)	0.138	0.494	0.504	0.845	0.760	0.220	0.145	0.506	0.433	0.536	0.614	0.278
Chitterlings (8.6% protein)	0.094	0.398	0.308	0.457	0.670	0.193	0.109	0.359	0.228	0.462	1.406	0.169
Fish flour (76.0% protein)	0.754	4.378	4.232	6.189	7.381	2.019	—	2.845	—	3.916	5.204	1.289
Gelatin (85.6% protein, N× 5.55)	0.006	1.912	1.357	2.930	4.226	0.787	0.077	2.036	0.401	2.421	7.866	0.771
Gizzard, chicken (23.1% protein)	0.207	1.072	1.094	1.689	1.567	0.554	0.218	0.968	0.680	1.116	1.741	0.480

Protein content, and nitrogen conversion factor	Trypto-phan (gm.)	Threo-nine (gm.)	Iso-leucine (gm.)	Leucine (gm.)	Lysine (gm.)	Methi-onine (gm.)	Cystine (gm.)	Phenyl-alanine (gm.)	Tyro-sine (gm.)	Valine (gm.)	Argi-nine (gm.)	Histi-dine (gm.)
Products from meat, poultry and fish—cont'd												
Heart												
beef or pork (16.9% protein)	0.219	0.776	0.857	1.509	1.387	0.403	0.168	0.765	0.627	0.973	1.068	0.433
chicken (20.5% protein)	0.266	0.941	1.040	1.830	1.683	0.489	0.203	0.928	0.761	1.181	1.296	0.525
Kidney												
beef (15.0% protein)	0.221	0.665	0.730	1.301	1.087	0.307	0.182	0.706	0.557	0.876	0.934	0.377
pork (16.3% protein)	0.240	0.722	0.793	1.414	1.181	0.334	0.198	0.767	0.605	0.952	1.015	0.409
sheep (16.6% protein)	0.244	0.736	0.807	1.440	1.203	0.340	0.202	0.781	0.616	0.969	1.033	0.417
Liver												
beef or pork (19.7% protein)	0.296	0.936	1.031	1.819	1.475	0.463	0.243	0.993	0.738	1.239	1.201	0.523
calf (19.0% protein)	0.286	0.903	0.994	1.754	1.423	0.447	0.234	0.958	0.711	1.195	1.158	0.505
chicken (22.1% protein)	0.332	1.050	1.156	2.040	1.655	0.520	0.272	1.114	0.827	1.390	1.347	0.587
sheep or lamb (21.0% protein)	0.316	0.998	1.099	1.939	1.572	0.494	0.259	1.058	0.786	1.320	1.280	0.558
Pancreas												
beef (13.5% protein)	0.175	0.626	0.683	1.054	0.996	0.244	—	0.562	0.590	0.724	0.771	0.266
pork (14.5% protein)	0.188	0.673	0.733	1.132	1.070	0.262	—	0.603	0.633	0.777	0.828	0.285
Pork or beef, canned (14.3% protein)	0.151	0.618	0.730	1.190	1.345	0.327	0.261	0.579	0.570	0.810	1.050	0.460
Potted meat (16.1% protein)	0.149	0.662	0.641	1.203	1.061	0.361	—	0.641	—	0.943	1.002	0.322
Sausage												
Bologna (14.8% protein)	0.126	0.606	0.718	1.061	1.191	0.313	0.185	0.540	0.481	0.744	1.028	0.398
Braunschweiger (15.4% protein)	0.172	0.668	0.754	1.291	1.200	0.320	0.187	0.700	0.471	0.956	0.954	0.458
frankfurters (14.2% protein)	0.120	0.582	0.688	1.018	1.143	0.300	0.177	0.518	0.461	0.713	0.986	0.382
head cheese (15.0% protein)	0.079	0.418	0.509	0.946	0.907	0.250	0.209	0.569	0.569	0.617	1.075	0.278
liverwurst (16.7% protein)	0.187	0.724	0.818	1.400	1.301	0.347	0.203	0.759	0.510	1.037	1.034	0.497
pork, links or bulk, raw (10.8% protein)	0.092	0.442	0.524	0.774	0.869	0.228	0.135	0.394	0.351	0.543	0.750	0.290
pork, bulk, canned (15.4% protein)	0.131	0.631	0.747	1.104	1.239	0.325	0.192	0.562	0.500	0.774	1.069	0.414
salami (23.9% protein)	0.203	0.979	1.159	1.713	1.923	0.505	0.298	0.872	0.776	1.201	1.660	0.642
Vienna sausage, canned (15.8% protein)	0.134	0.647	0.766	1.133	1.272	0.334	0.197	0.576	0.513	0.794	1.097	0.425
Tongue												
beef (16.4% protein)	0.197	0.708	0.792	1.286	1.364	0.357	0.207	0.661	0.548	0.840	1.065	0.412
pork (16.8% protein)	0.202	0.726	0.812	1.317	1.398	0.366	0.212	0.677	0.562	0.860	1.091	0.422
Veal and pork loaf, canned (17.2% protein)	0.198	0.627	0.859	1.236	1.258	0.418	0.209	0.619	0.468	0.958	0.916	0.388

Legumes (dry seed), common nuts, other nuts and dry seeds (their products)

Legume seeds and their products

Food												
Beans (*Phaseolus vulgaris*) (N× 6.25)												
pinto and red Mexican (23.0% protein)	0.213	0.997	1.306	1.976	1.708	0.232	0.228	1.270	0.887	1.395	1.384	0.655
red kidney												
raw (23.1% protein)	0.214	1.002	1.312	1.985	1.715	0.233	0.229	1.275	0.891	1.401	1.390	0.658
canned, solids and liquid (5.7% protein)	0.053	0.247	0.324	0.490	0.423	0.057	0.057	0.315	0.220	0.346	0.343	0.162
other common beans including navy, pea-bean, white marrow												
raw (21.4% protein)	0.199	0.928	1.216	1.839	1.589	0.216	0.212	1.181	0.825	1.298	1.287	0.609
baked with pork, canned (5.8% protein)	0.057	0.274	0.291	0.486	0.354	0.059	0.018	0.333	0.165	0.312	0.251	0.186
Black gram, raw (23.6% protein, N× 6.25)	0.242	0.801	1.390	2.062	1.510	0.332	0.287	1.242	0.551	1.450	1.552	0.559
Broadbeans, raw (25.4% protein, N× 6.25)	0.236	0.829	1.593	2.211	1.426	0.106	0.179	1.057	0.687	1.276	1.780	0.748
Chickpeas (20.8% protein, N + 6.25)	0.170	0.739	1.195	1.538	1.434	0.276	0.296	1.012	0.692	1.025	1.551	0.559
Cowpeas (22.9% protein, N× 6.25)	0.220	0.901	1.110	1.715	1.491	0.352	0.297	1.198	0.678	1.293	1.473	0.692
Dolichos, twinflower (21.6% protein, N× 6.25)	0.221	0.836	1.448	1.707	1.700	0.294	0.480	1.486	0.560	1.286	1.230	0.650
Lentils, whole (25.0% protein, N× 6.25)	0.216	0.896	1.316	1.760	1.528	0.180	0.294	1.104	0.664	1.360	1.908	0.548
Lima beans (20.7% protein, N× 6.25)	0.195	0.980	1.199	1.722	1.378	0.331	0.311	1.222	0.543	1.298	1.315	0.669
Lupine (32.3% protein, N× 6.25)	—	1.101	1.618	1.964	1.447	0.114	—	1.271	—	1.328	2.718	0.811
Moth beans (24.4% protein, N× 6.25)	0.164	—	1.093	1.484	1.202	0.191	0.109	1.003	1.245	0.695	—	0.722
Mung beans (24.4% protein, 6.25)	0.180	0.765	1.351	2.202	1.667	0.265	0.152	1.167	0.390	1.444	1.370	0.543
Peanuts (26.9% protein, N× 5.46)	0.340	0.828	1.266	1.872	1.099	0.271	0.463	1.557	1.104	1.532	3.296	0.749
Peanut flour (51.2% protein, N× 5.46)	0.647	1.575	2.410	3.563	2.091	0.516	0.881	2.963	2.100	2.916	6.273	1.425
Peanut butter (26.1% protein, N× 5.46)	0.330	0.803	1.228	1.816	1.066	0.263	0.449	1.510	1.071	1.487	3.198	0.727
Peas (*Pisum sativum*) (N× 6.25)												
entire seeds (23.8% protein)	0.251	0.918	1.340	1.969	1.744	0.286	0.308	1.200	0.960	1.333	2.102	0.651
split (24.5% protein)	0.259	0.945	1.380	2.027	1.795	0.294	0.318	1.235	0.988	1.372	2.164	0.670
Pigeonpeas, without seed coat (21.9% protein, N× 6.25)	0.119	0.834	1.346	1.717	1.580	0.256	0.308	1.875	0.725	1.153	1.489	0.617
Soybeans, whole (34.9% protein, N× 5.71)	0.526	1.504	2.054	2.946	2.414	0.513	0.678	1.889	1.216	2.005	2.763	0.911
Soybean flour, flakes, and grits (protein, N× 5.71)												
low fat (44.7% protein)	0.673	1.926	2.630	3.773	3.092	0.658	0.869	2.419	1.558	2.568	3.538	1.166
medium fat (42.5% protein)	0.640	1.831	2.501	3.588	2.940	0.625	0.826	2.300	1.481	2.441	3.364	1.109
full fat (35.9% protein)	0.541	1.547	2.112	3.030	2.483	0.528	0.698	1.943	1.251	2.062	2.842	0.937
Soybean curd (7.0% protein, N× 5.71)	—	—	—	—	—	0.081	0.091	—	—	—	—	—
Soybean milk (3.4% protein, N× 5.71)	0.051	0.176	0.175	0.305	0.269	0.054	0.071	0.195	0.193	0.186	0.302	0.121
Vetch (28.8% protein, N× 6.25)	0.203	0.899	2.198	2.290	1.898	0.346	0.336	1.014	0.369	1.442	2.249	0.659

Protein content, and nitrogen conversion factor	Trypto-phan (gm.)	Threo-nine (gm.)	Iso-leucine (gm.)	Leucine (gm.)	Lysine (gm.)	Methi-onine (gm.)	Cystine (gm.)	Phenyl-alanine (gm.)	Tyro-sine (gm.)	Valine (gm.)	Argi-nine (gm.)	Histi-dine (gm.)
Common nuts and their products												
Almonds (18.6% protein, N× 5.18)	0.176	0.610	0.873	1.454	0.582	0.259	0.377	1.146	0.618	1.124	2.729	0.517
Brazil nuts (14.4% protein, N× 5.46)	0.187	0.422	0.593	1.129	0.443	0.941	0.504	0.617	0.483	0.823	2.247	0.367
Cashews (18.5% protein, N× 5.30)	0.471	0.737	1.222	1.522	0.792	0.353	0.527	0.946	0.712	1.592	2.098	0.415
Coconut (3.4% protein, N× 5.30)	0.033	0.129	0.180	0.269	0.152	0.071	0.062	0.174	0.101	0.212	0.486	0.069
Coconut meal (20.3% protein, N× 5.30)	0.199	0.770	1.076	1.605	0.908	0.421	0.372	1.038	0.605	1.268	2.899	0.414
Filberts (12.7% protein, N× 5.30)	0.211	0.415	0.853	0.939	0.417	0.139	0.165	0.537	0.434	0.934	2.171	0.288
Peanuts. See Legumes.												
Pecans (9.4% protein, N× 5.30)	0.138	0.389	0.553	0.773	0.435	0.153	0.216	0.564	0.316	0.525	1.185	0.273
Walnuts (English or Persian) (15.0% protein, N× 5.30)	0.175	0.589	0.767	1.228	0.441	0.306	0.320	0.767	0.583	0.974	2.287	0.405
Other nuts and seeds and their products (protein N× 5.30)												
Acorns (10.4% protein)	0.126	0.434	0.561	0.808	0.636	0.139	0.184	0.473	—	0.718	0.722	0.251
Amaranth (14.6% protein)	0.149	0.832	0.882	1.209	1.074	0.372	0.521	1.141	—	0.849	1.747	0.441
Balsam pear seed meal (41.9% protein)	—	—	—	—	1.265	—	—	2.609	0.617	—	5.914	0.917
Breadnut tree, Ramon (9.6% protein)	0.261	0.373	0.543	1.041	0.418	0.056	—	0.453	—	0.927	0.884	0.147
Chinese tallow tree-nut flour (57.6% protein)	0.837	2.174	3.510	4.347	1.587	0.924	0.696	2.847	2.011	4.510	10.031	1.587
Chocolate tree, Nicaragua (38.5% protein)	0.588	1.496	2.092	3.952	2.223	0.276	—	2.630	—	2.404	4.220	0.683
Cottonseed flour and meal (42.3% protein)	0.591	1.764	1.884	2.945	2.139	0.686	0.814	2.610	1.365	2.458	5.603	1.325
Earpod tree, Guanacaste (34.1% protein)	0.444	1.165	2.213	4.581	1.930	0.360	—	1.325	—	1.570	2.857	1.004
Lead tree (24.1% protein)	0.191	0.828	1.651	1.787	1.164	0.055	—	0.855	—	0.864	2.410	0.564
Pumpkin seed (30.9% protein)	0.560	0.933	1.737	2.437	1.411	0.577	—	1.749	—	1.679	4.810	0.711
Safflower seed meal (42.1% protein)	0.675	1.462	1.914	2.740	1.525	0.731	—	2.605	—	2.446	4.623	0.985
Sesame												
seed (19.3% protein)	0.331	0.707	0.951	1.679	0.583	0.637	0.495	1.457	0.951	0.885	1.992	0.441
meal (33.4% protein)	0.573	1.223	1.645	2.905	1.008	1.103	0.857	2.521	1.645	1.531	3.447	0.763
Sunflower												
kernel (23.0% protein)	0.343	0.911	1.276	1.736	0.868	0.443	0.464	1.220	0.647	1.354	2.370	0.586
meal (39.5% protein)	0.589	1.565	2.191	2.981	1.491	0.760	0.797	2.094	1.110	2.325	4.069	1.006
Grains and their products												
Barley (12.8% protein, N× 5.83)	0.160	0.433	0.545	0.889	0.433	0.184	0.257	0.661	0.466	0.643	0.659	0.239
Bread, white (4% non-fat dry milk, flour basis) (8.5% protein, N× 5.70)	0.091	0.282	0.429	0.668	0.225	0.142	0.200	0.465	0.243	0.435	0.340	0.192

Buckwheat flour												
dark (11.7% protein, N × 6.25)	0.165	0.461	0.440	0.683	0.687	0.206	0.228	0.442	0.240	0.607	0.930	0.256
light (6.4% protein, N × 6.25)	0.090	0.252	0.241	0.374	0.376	0.113	0.125	0.242	0.131	0.332	0.509	0.140
Canihua (14.7% protein, N × 6.25)	0.118	0.706	1.000	0.851	0.882	0.263	0.162	0.529	0.294	0.677	1.162	0.367
Cereal combinations												
corn and soy grits (18.0% protein, N × 6.25)	0.161	0.792	0.841	1.656	0.772	0.271	0.311	0.832	0.562	1.054	0.982	0.472
infant food, precooked, mixed cereals with non-fat dry milk and yeast (19.4% protein, N × 6.25)	0.118	—	—	—	0.273	0.310	0.137	0.543	0.447	—	0.447	0.233
oat-corn-rye mixture, puffed (14.5% protein, N × 5.83)	0.172	0.545	0.841	1.368	0.343	0.388	0.234	0.933	0.622	0.900	0.776	0.326
Corn, field (10.0% protein, N × 6.25)	0.061	0.398	0.462	1.296	0.288	0.186	0.130	0.454	0.611	0.510	0.352	0.206
Corn flour (7.8% protein, N × 6.25)	0.047	0.311	0.361	1.011	0.225	0.145	0.101	0.354	0.477	0.398	0.275	0.161
Corn grits (8.7% protein, N × 6.25)	0.053	0.347	0.402	1.128	0.251	0.161	0.113	0.395	0.532	0.444	0.306	0.180
Cornmeal												
whole ground (9.2% protein, N × 6.25)	0.056	0.367	0.425	1.192	0.265	0.171	0.119	0.418	0.562	0.470	0.324	0.190
de-germed (7.9% protein, N × 6.25)	0.048	0.315	0.365	1.024	0.228	0.147	0.102	0.359	0.483	0.403	0.278	0.163
Corn products												
flakes (8.1% protein, N × 6.25)	0.052	0.275	0.306	1.047	0.154	0.135	0.152	0.354	0.283	0.386	0.231	0.226
germ (14.5% protein, N × 6.25)	0.144	0.622	0.578	1.030	0.791	0.232	0.130	0.483	0.343	0.789	1.134	0.464
gluten (10.0% protein, N × 6.25)	0.059	0.344	0.443	1.563	0.179	0.282	0.141	0.558	0.582	0.512	0.322	0.200
hominy (8.7% protein, N × 6.25)	0.084	0.316	0.349	0.810	0.358	0.099	—	0.333	0.331	0.398	0.444	0.203
masa (2.8% protein, N × 6.25)	0.010	—	—	—	0.103	0.108	0.030	—	—	—	—	—
pozol (5.9% protein, N × 6.25)	0.042	0.336	0.304	0.591	0.234	0.087	—	0.254	—	0.267	0.197	0.122
tortilla (5.8% protein, N × 6.25)	0.031	0.235	0.345	0.939	0.145	0.111	—	0.252	—	0.304	0.223	0.128
zein (16.1% protein, N × 6.25)	0.010	0.495	0.822	3.184	—	0.281	0.162	1.664	0.981	0.654	0.286	0.216
Job's tears (13.8% protein, N × 5.83)	0.066	0.620	1.065	3.506	0.362	0.459	0.265	0.703	—	—	0.518	0.317
Millets												
foxtail millet (9.7% protein, N × 5.83)	0.103	0.323	0.790	1.737	0.218	0.291	—	0.697	—	0.717	0.374	0.218
little millet (7.2% protein, N × 5.83)	0.047	0.262	0.517	0.841	0.138	0.178	—	0.370	—	0.471	0.363	0.147
pearl millet (11.4% protein, N × 5.83)	0.248	0.456	0.635	1.746	0.383	0.270	0.152	0.506	—	0.682	0.524	0.240
ragimillet (6.2% protein, N × 5.83)	0.085	0.270	0.398	0.620	0.202	0.270	0.187	0.263	—	0.473	0.100	0.079
Oatmeal and rolled oats (14.2% protein, N × 5.83)	0.183	0.470	0.733	1.065	0.521	0.209	0.309	0.758	0.524	0.845	0.935	0.261
Quinoa (11.0% protein, N × 6.25)	0.120	0.523	0.722	0.781	0.729	0.278	0.107	0.394	0.253	0.447	0.820	0.297
Rice												
brown (7.5% protein, N × 5.95)	0.081	0.294	0.352	0.646	0.296	0.135	0.102	0.377	0.343	0.524	0.432	0.126
white and converted (7.6% protein, N × 5.95)	0.082	0.298	0.356	0.655	0.300	0.137	0.103	0.382	0.347	0.531	0.438	0.128

Protein content, and nitrogen conversion factor	Trypto-phan (gm.)	Threo-nine (gm.)	Iso-leucine (gm.)	Leucine (gm.)	Lysine (gm.)	Methi-onine (gm.)	Cystine (gm.)	Phenyl-alanine (gm.)	Tyro-sine (gm.)	Valine (gm.)	Argi-nine (gm.)	Histi-dine (gm.)
Rice products												
flakes or puffed (5.9% protein, N × 5.95)	0.046	—	—	—	0.056	—	0.044	0.286	0.124	—	0.137	0.137
germ (14.2% protein, N × 5.95)	0.270	2.177	0.630	0.838	1.707	0.420	0.169	0.750	0.929	0.938	1.559	0.430
Rye (12.1% protein, N × 5.83)	0.137	0.448	0.515	0.813	0.494	0.191	0.241	0.571	0.390	0.631	0.591	0.276
Rye flour												
light (9.4% protein, N × 5.83)	0.106	0.348	0.400	0.632	0.384	0.148	0.187	0.443	0.303	0.490	0.459	0.214
medium (11.4% protein, N × 5.83)	0.129	0.422	0.485	0.766	0.465	0.180	0.227	0.538	0.368	0.594	0.557	0.260
Sorghum (11.0% protein, N × 6.25)	0.123	0.394	0.598	1.767	0.299	0.190	0.183	0.547	0.303	0.628	0.417	0.211
Teosinte (22.0% protein, N × 6.25)	0.049	—	—	—	0.348	0.496	—	—	—	—	—	—
Wheat, whole grain												
hard red spring (14.0% protein, N × 5.83)	0.173	0.403	0.607	0.939	0.384	0.214	0.307	0.691	0.523	0.648	0.670	0.286
hard red winter (12.3% protein, N × 5.83)	0.152	0.354	0.534	0.825	0.338	0.188	0.270	0.608	0.460	0.570	0.589	0.251
soft red winter (10.2% protein, N × 5.83)	0.126	0.294	0.443	0.684	0.280	0.156	0.224	0.504	0.382	0.472	0.488	0.208
white (9.4% protein, N × 5.83)	0.116	0.271	0.408	0.630	0.258	0.143	0.206	0.464	0.351	0.435	0.450	0.192
durum (12.7% protein, N × 5.83)	0.157	0.366	0.551	0.852	0.348	0.194	0.279	0.627	0.475	0.588	0.608	0.259
Wheat flour												
whole grain (13.3% protein, N × 5.83)	0.164	0.383	0.577	0.892	0.365	0.203	0.292	0.657	0.497	0.616	0.636	0.271
intermediate extraction (12.0% protein, N × 5.70)	—	0.392	0.619	0.924	0.356	0.198	0.320	0.732	0.335	0.583	0.549	0.286
white (10.5% protein, N × 5.70)	0.129	0.302	0.483	0.809	0.239	0.138	0.210	0.577	0.539	0.453	0.466	0.210
Wheat products												
bran (12.0% protein, N × 6.31)	0.196	0.342	0.485	0.717	0.491	0.145	0.270	0.434	0.259	0.552	0.742	0.280
burghul (12.4% protein, N × 5.83)	0.070	—	—	—	0.430	0.300	0.319	—	0.447	—	0.424	0.268
farina (10.9% protein, N × 5.70)	0.124	—	—	—	0.199	0.143	0.184	0.579	0.311	—	0.559	0.231
flakes (10.8% protein, N × 5.70)	0.121	0.356	0.496	0.891	0.360	0.127	0.191	0.478	—	0.572	—	—
germ (25.2% protein, N × 5.80)	0.265	1.343	1.177	1.708	1.534	0.404	0.287	0.908	0.882	1.364	1.825	0.687
gluten, commercial (80.0% protein, N × 5.70)	0.856	2.119	3.677	5.993	1.530	1.389	1.726	4.351	2.596	3.789	3.481	1.825
gluten flour (41.4% protein, N × 5.70)	0.443	1.097	1.903	3.101	0.792	0.719	0.893	2.252	1.344	1.961	1.801	0.944
macaroni or spaghetti (12.8% protein, N × 5.70)	0.150	0.499	0.642	0.849	0.413	0.193	0.243	0.669	0.422	0.728	0.582	0.303
noodles, containing egg solids (12.6% protein, N × 5.70)	0.133	0.533	0.621	0.834	0.411	0.212	0.245	0.610	0.312	0.745	0.621	0.301
Shredded Wheat (10.1% protein, N × 5.83)	0.085	0.405	0.449	0.684	0.331	0.139	0.204	0.481	0.236	0.577	0.523	0.236
whole wheat with added germ (12.8% protein, N × 5.82)	0.126											

Fruits (protein, N × 6.25)

	1	2	3	4	5	6	7	8	9	10	11	12
Abiu (1.7% protein)	0.028	—	—	—	0.085	0.013	—	—	—	—	—	—
Avocados (1.3% protein)	0.014	—	—	—	0.074	0.012	—	—	—	—	—	—
Bananas, ripe												
common (1.2% protein)	0.018	—	—	—	0.055	0.011	—	—	0.031	—	—	—
dwarf (1.2% protein)	0.012	—	—	0.077	0.049	0.004	—	—	—	0.094	0.049	0.049
Dates (2.2% protein)	0.061	0.061	0.074	—	0.065	0.027	—	0.063	—	—	—	—
Grapefruit (0.5% protein)	0.001	—	—	—	0.006	0.000	—	—	—	—	—	—
Guavas, common (1.0% protein)	0.010	—	—	—	0.030	0.010	—	—	—	—	—	—
Limes (0.8% protein)	0.003	—	—	—	0.015	0.002	—	—	—	—	—	—
Mamey (0.5% protein)	0.006	—	—	—	0.040	0.007	—	—	—	—	—	—
Mangos (0.7% protein)	0.014	—	—	—	0.093	0.008	—	—	—	—	—	—
Muskmelons (0.6% protein)	0.001	—	—	—	0.015	0.002	—	—	—	—	—	—
Oranges, sweet (0.9% protein)	0.003	—	—	—	0.024	0.003	—	—	—	—	—	—
Orange juice (0.8% protein)	0.003	—	—	—	0.021	0.002	—	—	—	—	—	—
Oranges, mandarin, including tangerines (0.8% protein)	0.003	—	—	—	0.028	0.004	—	—	—	—	—	—
Papayas (0.6% protein)	0.005	—	—	—	0.038	0.002	—	—	—	—	—	—
Pineapple (0.4% protein)	0.012	—	—	—	0.009	0.001	—	—	—	—	—	—
Plantain or baking banana (1.1% protein)	0.005	0.027	0.056	0.059	0.050	0.005	0.016	0.049	—	0.065	0.045	—
Soursop (1.0% protein)	0.010	—	—	—	0.060	0.007	—	—	—	—	—	—
Sugarapple (1.8% protein)	0.011	—	—	—	0.071	0.008	—	—	—	—	—	—

Vegetables

Immature seeds (protein, N × 6.25)

	1	2	3	4	5	6	7	8	9	10	11	12
Corn, sweet, white or yellow												
raw (3.7% protein)	0.023	0.151	0.137	0.407	0.137	0.072	0.062	0.207	0.124	0.231	0.174	0.095
canned, solids and liquid (2.0% protein)	0.012	0.082	0.074	0.220	0.074	0.039	0.033	0.112	0.067	0.125	0.094	0.052
Cowpeas (9.4% protein)	0.099	0.353	0.465	0.653	0.617	0.131	—	0.523	—	0.513	0.615	0.310
Lima beans												
raw (7.5% protein)	0.097	0.338	0.460	0.605	0.474	0.080	0.083	0.389	0.259	0.485	0.454	0.247
canned, solids and liquid (3.8% protein)	0.049	0.171	0.233	0.306	0.240	0.041	0.042	0.197	0.131	0.246	0.230	0.125
Peas												
raw (6.7% protein)	0.056	0.245	0.308	0.418	0.316	0.054	0.073	0.257	0.163	0.274	0.595	0.109
canned solids and liquid (3.4% protein)	0.028	0.125	0.156	0.212	0.160	0.027	0.037	0.131	0.083	0.139	0.302	0.055
Leafy vegetables, raw (protein, N × 6.25)												
Amaranth (3.5% protein)	0.038	0.056	0.164	0.206	0.141	0.025	0.024	0.096	0.105	0.136	0.134	0.069
Beet greens (2.0% protein)	0.024	0.076	0.084	0.129	0.108	0.034	—	0.116	—	0.101	0.083	0.026
Brussels sprouts (4.4% protein)	0.044	0.153	0.186	0.194	0.197	0.046	—	0.148	—	0.193	0.279	0.106
Cabbage (1.4% protein)	0.011	0.039	0.040	0.057	0.066	0.013	0.028	0.030	0.030	0.043	0.105	0.025
Chard (1.4% protein)	0.014	0.058	0.060	0.076	0.055	0.004	—	0.046	—	0.055	0.035	0.018

Protein content, and nitrogen conversion factor	Trypto-phan (gm.)	Threo-nine (gm.)	Iso-leucine (gm.)	Leucine (gm.)	Lysine (gm.)	Methi-onine (gm.)	Cystine (gm.)	Phenyl-alanine (gm.)	Tyro-sine (gm.)	Valine (gm.)	Argi-nine (gm.)	Histi-dine (gm.)
Leafy vegetables, raw (protein, N × 6.25)—cont'd												
Chicory (1.6% protein)	0.024	—	—	—	0.052	0.016	0.006	—	0.040	—	—	0.024
Collards (3.9% protein)	0.055	0.114	0.121	0.218	0.202	0.046	0.059	0.124	0.151	0.195	0.258	0.087
Kale (3.9% protein)	0.042	0.139	0.133	0.252	0.121	0.035	0.036	0.158	—	0.184	0.202	0.062
Lettuce (1.2% protein)	0.012	—	—	—	0.070	0.004	0.035	—	—	—	—	—
Mustard greens (2.3% protein)	0.037	0.060	0.075	0.062	0.111	0.024	—	0.074	0.121	0.108	0.167	0.041
Parsley, curly garden (2.5% protein)	0.050	—	—	—	0.160	0.012	—	—	—	—	—	—
Spinach (2.3% protein)	0.037	0.102	0.107	0.176	0.142	0.039	0.046	0.099	0.073	0.126	0.116	0.049
Turnip greens (2.9% protein)	0.045	0.125	0.107	0.207	0.129	0.052	0.045	0.146	0.105	0.149	0.167	0.051
Watercress (1.7% protein)	0.028	0.084	0.076	0.131	0.091	0.010	—	0.062	0.036	0.084	0.053	0.034
Starchy roots and tubers (protein, N × 6.25)												
Apio arracacia (1.2% protein)	0.008	—	—	—	0.042	0.003	—	—	—	—	—	—
Cassava												
flour (1.6% protein)	0.021	0.044	0.045	0.066	0.066	0.010	0.018	0.045	0.030	0.049	0.159	0.025
root (1.1% protein)	0.014	0.030	0.031	0.045	0.045	0.007	0.012	0.031	0.021	0.033	0.110	0.017
Potatoes												
raw (2.0% protein)	0.021	0.079	0.088	0.100	0.107	0.025	0.019	0.088	0.036	0.107	0.099	0.029
canned, solids and liquid (1.7% protein)	0.018	0.067	0.075	0.085	0.091	0.021	0.016	0.075	0.030	0.091	0.084	0.024
flour (7.1% protein)	0.076	0.279	0.311	0.353	0.378	0.089	0.068	0.314	0.127	0.379	0.350	0.102
Sweet potatoes (Ipomaea batatas)												
raw (1.8% protein)	0.031	0.085	0.087	0.103	0.085	0.033	0.029	0.100	0.081	0.135	0.094	0.036
dehydrated (5.0% protein)	0.087	0.235	0.241	0.286	0.236	0.093	0.080	0.278	0.225	0.374	0.261	0.099
Taro (1.9% protein)	0.035	0.089	0.099	0.169	0.110	0.021	—	0.099	—	0.114	0.118	0.032
Yam (Dioscorea spp.) (2.1% protein)	0.035	—	—	—	0.110	0.034	—	—	—	—	—	—
Yautia malanga (1.7% protein)	0.023	—	—	—	0.067	0.016	—	—	—	—	—	—
Other vegetables (protein, N × 6.25)												
Asparagus												
raw (2.2% protein)	0.027	0.066	0.080	0.096	0.103	0.032	—	0.069	—	0.106	0.123	0.036
canned, solids and liquid (1.9% protein)	0.023	0.057	0.069	0.083	0.089	0.027	—	0.060	—	0.092	0.106	0.031
Beans, snap												
raw (2.4% protein)	0.033	0.091	0.109	0.139	0.126	0.035	0.024	0.057	0.050	0.115	0.101	0.045
canned, solids and liquid (1.0% protein)	0.014	0.038	0.045	0.058	0.052	0.014	0.010	0.024	0.021	0.048	0.042	0.019
Beets												
raw (1.6% protein)	0.014	0.034	0.051	0.055	0.086	0.006	—	0.027	—	0.049	0.028	0.022
canned, solids and liquid (0.9% protein)	0.008	0.019	0.029	0.031	0.048	0.003	—	0.015	—	0.028	0.016	0.012

Food item												
Carrots												
raw (1.2% protein)	0.010	0.043	0.046	0.065	0.052	0.010	0.029	0.042	0.020	0.056	0.041	0.017
canned, solids and liquid (0.5% protein)	0.004	0.018	0.019	0.027	0.022	0.004	0.012	0.018	0.008	0.023	0.017	0.007
Cauliflower (2.4% protein)	0.033	0.102	0.104	0.162	0.134	0.047	—	0.075	0.034	0.144	0.110	0.048
Celery (1.3% protein)	0.012	—	—	—	0.021	0.015	0.006	—	0.016	—	—	—
Chayote (0.6% protein)	0.008	—	—	—	0.038	0.001	—	—	—	—	—	—
Cowpeas, yardlong, immature pod (3.4% protein)	0.034	—	—	—	0.203	0.021	—	—	—	—	—	—
Cucumbers (0.7% protein)	0.005	0.019	0.022	0.030	0.031	0.007	—	0.016	—	0.024	0.053	0.001
Cushaw (1.5% protein)	0.014	—	—	—	0.044	0.008	—	—	—	—	—	—
Eggplant (1.1% protein)	0.010	0.038	0.056	0.068	0.030	0.006	—	0.048	—	0.065	0.037	0.019
Mallow (3.7% protein)	0.144	0.155	—	0.259	0.155	0.030	—	0.166	—	0.181	0.189	0.063
Mushrooms (Agaricus campestris)[2]	0.006	0.156	0.532	0.281	0.088	0.167	—	0.018	—	0.378	0.235	00.27
(Lactarius spp.)[3]	0.006	0.201	0.201	0.139	0.021	0.021	—	0.065	—	0.116	0.021	0.030
Okra (1.8% protein)	0.018	0.066	0.069	0.101	0.076	0.022	0.017	0.039	0.079	0.091	0.093	0.030
Onions, mature (1.4% protein)	0.021	0.022	0.021	0.037	0.064	0.013	—	0.055	0.046	0.031	0.180	0.014
Peppers (1.2% protein)	0.009	0.050	0.046	0.046	0.051	0.016	—	0.059	—	0.033	0.024	0.014
Prickly pears (1.1% protein)	0.009	0.053	0.057	0.057	0.044	0.008	—	0.032	—	0.041	0.032	0.016
Pumpkin (1.2% protein)	0.016	0.028	0.044	0.063	0.058	0.011	—	—	0.016	0.045	0.043	0.019
Radishes (1.2% protein)	0.005	0.059	—	—	0.034	0.002	—	0.116	—	0.030	—	—
Seepweed (2.6% protein)	0.027	0.089	0.113	0.152	0.089	0.013	—	0.186	—	0.091	0.062	0.036
Soybean sprouts (6.2% protein)	—	0.159	0.225	0.265	0.211	0.045	—	0.016	—	0.225	0.225	0.133
Squash, summer (0.6% protein)	0.005	0.014	0.019	0.027	0.023	0.008	—	0.028	0.014	0.022	0.027	0.009
Tomatoes and cherry tomatoes (1.0% protein)	0.009	0.033	0.029	0.041	0.042	0.007	—	0.020	0.029	0.028	0.029	0.015
Turnips (1.1% protein)	—	—	0.020	—	0.057	0.012	—	—	—	—	—	—
Waxgourd, Chinese (0.4% protein)	0.002	—	—	—	0.009	0.003	—	—	—	—	—	—
Miscellaneous food items												
Vegetable patty or steak (principally wheat protein) (15% protein, N × 5.70)	0.142	0.411	0.884	1.079	0.321	0.253	—	0.811	—	0.705	0.597	0.321
Yeast												
baker's, compressed[4] (N × 6.25)	0.122	0.655	0.655	1.151	0.914	0.248	0.120	0.607	0.580	0.840	0.536	0.353
brewer's, dried[5] (N × 6.25)	0.710	2.353	2.398	3.226	3.300	0.836	0.548	1.902	1.902	2.723	2.250	1.251
primary, dried (Saccharomyces cerevisiae)[5] (N × 6.25)	0.636	2.353	2.708	3.300	3.337	0.851	0.444	1.813	2.472	2.553	1.931	1.103
(Torulopsis utilis)[5] (N × 6.25)	0.636	2.331	3.323	3.707	3.648	0.710	0.422	2.361	2.464	2.901	3.337	1.251

[2] Total nitrogen is 0.58%. This is equivalent to 2.4% protein on the basis that two-thirds of the nitrogen is protein nitrogen. If total nitrogen is used for the calculation, the protein content is 3.6%.

[3] Total nitrogen is 0.69%. This is equivalent to 2.9% protein on the basis that two-thirds of the nitrogen is protein nitrogen. If total nitrogen is used for the calculation, the protein content is 4.3%.

[4] Total nitrogen is 2.1%. This is equivalent to 10.6% protein on the basis that four-fifths of the nitrogen is protein nitrogen. If total nitrogen is used for the calculation, the protein content is 13.1%.

[5] Total nitrogen is 7.4%. This is equivalent to 36.9% protein on the basis that four-fifths of the nitrogen is protein nitrogen. If total nitrogen is used for the calculation, the protein content is 46.1%.

Sodium and potassium content of foods, 100 grams, edible portion[1]

Food and description	Sodium (mg.)	Potassium (mg.)
Almonds		
dried	4	773
roasted and salted	198	773
Apples		
raw, pared	1	110
frozen, sliced, sweetened	14	68
Apple brown betty	153	100
Apple butter	2	252
Apple juice, canned or bottled	1	101
Applesauce, canned, sweetened	2	65
Apricots		
raw	1	281
canned, syrup pack, light	1	239
dried, sulfured, cooked, fruit, and liquid	8	318
Apricot nectar, canned (approx. 40% fruit)	Trace	151
Asparagus		
cooked spears, boiled, drained	1	183
canned spears, green		
regular pack, solids and liquid	236[2]	166
special dietary pack (low-sodium), solids and liquids	3	166
frozen		
cuts and tips, cooked, boiled, drained	1	220
spears, cooked, boiled, drained	1	238
Avocados, raw, all commercial varieties	4	604
Bacon, cured, cooked, broiled or fried, drained	1,021	236
Bacon, Canadian, cooked, broiled or fried, drained	2,555	432
Baking powders		
home use		
straight phosphate	8,220	170
special low-sodium preparations	6	10,948
Bananas, raw, common	1	370
Barbecue sauce	815	174
Bass, black sea, raw	68	256

[1]Numbers in parentheses denote values inputed—usually from another form of the food or from a similar food. Dashes denote lack of reliable data for a constituent believed to be present in measurable amount. Values are selected from Watt, B. K., and Merrill, A. L.: Composition of foods—raw, processed, prepared, U. S. Department of Agriculture, Agriculture Handbook No. 8, December, 1963.
[2]Estimated average based on addition of salt in the amount of 0.6% of the finished product.

Food and description	Sodium (mg.)	Potassium (mg.)
Beans, common, mature seeds, dry		
white		
cooked	7	416
canned, solids and liquid, with pork and tomato sauce	463	210
red, cooked	3	340
Beans, lima		
immature seeds		
cooked, boiled, drained	1	422
canned		
regular pack, solids and liquid	236[2]	222
special dietary pack (low-sodium), solids and liquid	4	222
frozen, thin-seeded types, commonly called baby limas, cooked,		
boiled, drained	129	394
mature seeds, dry, cooked	2	612
Beans, mung, sprouted seeds, cooked, boiled, drained	4	156
Beans, snap		
green		
cooked, boiled, drained	4	151
canned		
regular pack, solids and liquid	236[2]	95
special dietary pack (low sodium), solids and liquid	2	95
frozen, cut, cooked, boiled, drained	1	152
yellow or wax		
cooked, boiled, drained	3	151
canned		
regular pack, solids and liquid	236[2]	95
special dietary pack (low-sodium), solids and liquid	2	95
frozen, cut, cooked, boiled, drained	1	164
Beans and frankfurters, canned	539	262
Beef		
retail cuts, trimmed to retail level		
round	60	370
rump	60	370
hamburger, regular ground, cooked	47	450
Beef and vegetable stew, canned	411	174
Beef, corned, boneless		
cooked, medium-fat	1,740	150
canned corned-beef hash (with potato)	540	200
Beef, dried, cooked, creamed	716	153
Beef potpie, commercial, frozen, unheated	366	93
Beets, common, red		
canned		
regular pack, solids and liquid	236[2]	167
special dietary pack (low-sodium), solids and liquid	46	167
Beet greens, common, cooked, boiled, drained	76	332
Beverages, alcoholic		
beer, alcohol 4.5% by volume (3.6% by weight)	7	25
gin, rum, vodka, whisky		
80-proof (33.4% alcohol by weight)	1	2
86-proof (36.0% alcohol by weight)	1	2
90-proof (37.9% alcohol by weight)	1	2
94-proof (39.7% alcohol by weight)	1	2
100-proof (42.5% alcohol by weight)	1	2
wines		
dessert, alcohol 18.8% by volume (15.3% by weight)	4	75
table, alcohol 12.2% by volume (9.9% by weight)	5	92

[2]Estimated average based on addition of salt in the amount of 0.6% of the finished product.

Food and description	Sodium (mg.)	Potassium (mg.)
Biscuits, baking powder, made with enriched flour	626	117
Biscuit dough, commercial, frozen	910	86
Biscuit mix, with enriched flour, and biscuits baked from mix		
mix, dry form	1,300	80
biscuits, made with milk	973	116
Blackberries, including dewberries, boysenberries, and young-berries, raw	1	170
Blackberries, canned, solids and liquid		
water pack, with or without artificial sweetener	1	115
syrup pack, heavy	1	109
Blueberries		
raw	1	81
frozen, not thawed, sweetened	1	66
Bluefish, cooked		
baked or broiled	104	—
fried	146	—
Boston brown bread	251	292
Bouillon cubes or powder	24,000	100
Boysenberries, frozen, not thawed, sweetened	1	105
Bran, added sugar and malt extract	1,060	1,070
Bran flakes (40% bran), added thiamine	925	—
Bran flakes with raisins, added thiamine	800	—
Brazil nuts	1	715
Breads		
cracked-wheat	529	134
French or vienna, enriched	580	90
Italian, enriched	585	74
raisin	365	233
rye, American (1/3 rye, 2/3 clear flour)	557	145
white, enriched, made with 3%-4% non-fat dry milk	507	105
whole-wheat, made with 2% non-fat dry milk	527	273
Bread crumbs, dry, grated	736	152
Bread stuffing mix and stuffings prepared from mix		
mix, dry form	1,331	172
Broccoli		
cooked spears, boiled, drained	10	267
frozen, spears, cooked, boiled, drained	12	220
Brussels sprouts, frozen, cooked, boiled, drained	14	295
Buffalo fish, raw	52	293
Bulgur (parboiled wheat)		
canned, made from hard red winter wheat		
unseasoned[3]	599	87
seasoned[4]	460	112
Butter[5]	987	23
Buttermilk, fluid, cultured (made from skim milk)	130	140
Cabbage		
common varieties (Danish, domestic, and pointed types)		
raw	20	233
cooked, boiled until tender, drained, shredded, cooked in small amount of water	14	163
red, raw	26	268

[3]Processed, partially debranned, whole-kernel wheat with salt added.
[4]Processed, partially debranned, whole-kernel wheat with chicken fat, chicken stock base, dehydrated onion flakes, salt, monosodium glutamate, and herbs.
[5]Values apply to salted butter. Unsalted butter contains less than 10 mg. of either sodium or potassium per 100 grams. Value for vitamin A is the year-round average.

Food and description	Sodium (mg.)	Potassium (mg.)
Cabbage, Chinese (also called celery cabbage or petsai)	23	253
Cakes		
baked from home recipes		
angelfood	283	88
fruitcake, made with enriched flour, dark	158	496
gingerbread, made with enriched flour	237	454
plain cake or cupcake, without icing	300	79
pound, modified	178	78
frozen, commercial, devil's food, with chocolate icing	420	119
Candy		
caramels, plain or chocolate	226	192
chocolate, sweet	33	269
chocolate-coated, chocolate fudge	228	193
gum drops, starch jelly pieces	35	5
hard	32	4
marshmallows	39	6
peanut bars	10	448
Carp, raw	50	286
Carrots		
raw	47	341
canned		
regular pack, solids and liquid	236[2]	120
special dietary pack (low-sodium), solids and liquid	39	120
Cashew nuts	15[6]	464
Catfish, freshwater, raw	60	330
Cauliflower		
cooked, boiled, drained	9	206
frozen, cooked, boiled, drained	10	207
Caviar, sturgeon, granular	2,200	180
Celery, all, including green and yellow varieties		
raw	126	341
cooked, boiled, drained	88	239
Chard, Swiss, cooked, boiled, drained	86	321
Cheese straws	721	63
Cheeses		
natural cheeses		
cheddar (domestic type, commonly called American)	700	82
cottage (large or small curd)		
creamed	229	85
uncreamed	290	72
cream	250	74
parmesan	734	149
Swiss (domestic)	710	104
pasteurized process cheese, American	1,136[7]	80
pasteurized process cheese spread, American	1,625[7]	240

[2]Estimated average based on addition of salt in the amount of 0.6% of the finished product.
[6]Applies to unsalted nuts. For salted nuts, value is approximately 200 mg. per 100 grams.
[7]Values for phosphorus and sodium are based on use of 1.5% anhydrous disodium phosphate as the emulsifying agent. If emulsifying agent does not contain either phosphorus or sodium, the content of these two nutrients in milligrams per 100 grams is as follows:

	P	Na
American process cheese	444	650
Swiss process cheese	540	681
American cheese food	427	—
American cheese spread	548	1,139

Food and description	Sodium (mg.)	Potassium (mg.)
Cherries		
raw, sweet	2	191
canned		
sour, red, solids and liquid, water pack	2	130
sweet, solids and liquid, syrup pack, light	1	128
frozen, not thawed, sweetened	2	130
Chicken		
all classes		
light meat without skin, cooked, roasted	64	411
dark meat without skin, cooked, roasted	86	321
Chicken potpie, commercial, frozen, unheated	411	153
Chicory, Witloof (also called French or Belgian endive), bleached head (forced), raw	7	182
Chili con carne, canned, with beans	531	233
Chocolate, bitter or baking	4	830
Chocolate syrup, fudge type	89	284
Chop suey, with meat, canned	551	138
Chow mein, chicken (without noodles), canned	290	167
Citron, candied	290	120
Clams, raw		
soft, meat only	36	235
hard or round, meat only	205	311
Clams, canned, including hard, soft, razor, and unspecified solids and liquid	—	140
Cocoa and chocolate-flavored beverage powders		
cocoa powder with non-fat dry milk	525	800
mix for hot chocolate	382	605
Cocoa, dry powder		
high-fat or breakfast		
plain	6	1,522
processed with alkali	717	651
Coconut cream (liquid expressed from grated coconut meat)	4	324
Coconut meat, fresh	23	256
Cod		
cooked, broiled	110	407
dehydrated, lightly salted	8,100	160
Coffee, instant, water-soluble solids		
dry powder	72	3,256
beverage	1	36
Coleslaw, made with French dressing (commercial)	268	205
Collards, cooked, boiled, drained, leaves, including stems, cooked in small amount of water	25	234
Cookies		
assorted, packaged, commercial	365	67
butter, thin, rich	418	60
gingersnaps	571	462
molasses	386	138
oatmeal with raisins	162	370
sandwich type	483	38
vanilla wafer	252	72
Cookie dough, plain, chilled in roll, baked	548	48
Corn, sweet		
cooked, boiled, drained, white and yellow, kernels, cut off cob before cooking	Trace	165

Food and description	Sodium (mg.)	Potassium (mg.)
Corn, sweet—cont'd		
canned		
regular pack, cream style, white and yellow, solids and liquid	236[2]	(97)
special dietary pack (low-sodium), cream style, white and yellow, solids and liquid	2	(97)
frozen, kernels cut off cob, cooked, boiled, drained	1	184
Corn fritters	477	133
Corn grits, degermed, enriched, dry form	1	80
Corn products used mainly as ready-to-eat breakfast cereals		
corn flakes, added nutrients	1,005	120
corn, puffed, added nutrients	1,060	—
corn, rice, and wheat flakes, mixed, added nutrients	950	—
Cornbread, baked from home recipes, southern style, made with degermed cornmeal, enriched	591	157
Cornbread mix and cornbread baked from mix, cornbread, made with egg, milk	744	127
Cornmeal, white or yellow, degermed, enriched, dry form	1	120
Cornstarch	Trace	Trace
Cowpeas, including blackeye peas		
immature seeds, canned, solids and liquid	236[2]	352
young pods, with seeds, cooked, boiled, drained	3	196
Crab, canned	1,000	110
Crackers		
butter	1,092	113
graham, plain	670	384
saltines	(1,100)	(120)
sandwich type, peanut-cheese	992	226
soda	1,100	120
Cranberries, raw	2	82
Cranberry juice cocktail, bottled (approx. 33% cranberry juice)	1	10
Cranberry sauce, sweetened, canned, strained	1	30
Cream, fluid, light, coffee, or table, 20% fat	43	122
Cream substitutes, dried, containing		
cream, skim milk (calcium reduced), and lactose	575	—
Cream puffs with custard filling	83	121
Cress, garden, raw	14	606
Croaker, Atlantic, cooked, baked	120	323
Cucumbers, raw, pared	6	160
Custard, baked	79	146
Dates, domestic, natural and dry	1	648
Doughnuts, cake type	501	90
Duck, domesticated, raw, flesh only	74	285
Eggs, chicken		
raw		
whole, fresh and frozen	122	129
whites, fresh and frozen	146	139
yolks, fresh	52	98
Eggplant, cooked, boiled, drained	1	150
Endive (curly endive and escarole), raw	14	294
Farina		
enriched		
regular		
dry form	2	83
cooked	144	9
quick-cooking, cooked	165	10
instant-cooking, cooked	188	13
unenriched, regular, dry form	2	83

[2]Estimated average based on addition of salt in the amount of 0.6% of the finished product.

Food and description	Sodium (mg.)	Potassium (mg.)
Figs, canned, solids and liquid, syrup pack, light	2	152
Flatfishes (flounders, soles, and sand dabs), raw	78	342
Fruit cocktail, canned, solids and liquid, water pack, with or without artificial sweetener	5	168
Garlic, cloves, raw	19	529
Ginger root, fresh	6	264
Gizzard, chicken, all classes, cooked, simmered	57	211
Goose, domesticated, flesh only, cooked, roasted	124	605
Gooseberries, canned, solids and liquid, syrup pack, heavy	1	98
Grapefruit		
raw, pulp, pink, red, white, all varieties	1	135
canned, juice, sweetened	1	162
Grapefruit juice and orange juice blended, canned, sweetened	1	184
Grapes, raw, American type (slip skin) such as Concord, Delaware, Niagara, Catawba, and Scuppernong	3	158
Grapejuice, canned or bottled	2	116
Guavas, whole, raw, common	4	289
Haddock, cooked, fried	177	348
Hake, including Pacific hake, squirrel hake, and silver hake or whiting; raw	74	363
Halibut, Atlantic and Pacific, cooked, broiled	134	525
Ham croquette	342	83
Heart, beef, lean, cooked, braised	104	232
Herring		
raw, Pacific	74	420
smoked, hard	6,231	157
Honey, strained or extracted	5	51
Horse-radish, prepared	96	290
Ice cream and frozen custard		
regular, approximately 10% fat	63[8]	181
Ice cream cones	232	244
Ice milk	68[8]	195
Jams and preserves	12	88
Kale, cooked, boiled, drained, leaves including stems	43	221
Kingfish; southern, gulf, and northern (whiting); raw	83	250
Lake herring (cisco), raw	47	319
Lamb, retail cuts	70	290
Lemon juice, canned or bottled, unsweetened	1	141
Lettuce, raw crisphead varieties such as Iceberg, New York, and Great Lakes strains	9	175
Lime juice, canned or bottled, unsweetened	1	104
Liver, beef, cooked, fried	184	380
Lobster, northern, canned or cooked	210	180
Loganberries, canned, solids and liquid, syrup pack, light	1	111
Macadamia nuts	—	164
Macaroni, unenriched, dry form	2	197
Macaroni and cheese, canned	304	58
Margarine[9]	987	23
Marmalade, citrus	14	33
Milk, cow		
fluid (pasteurized and raw)		
whole, 3.7% fat	50	144
skim	52	145
canned, evaporated (unsweetened)	118	303

[8]Value for product without added salt.

[9]Values apply to salted margarine. Unsalted margarine contains less than 10 mg. per 100 grams of either sodium or potassium. Vitamin A value based on the minimum required to meet federal specifications for margarine with vitamin A added, namely 15,000 I.U. of vitamin A per pound.

Food and description	Sodium (mg.)	Potassium (mg.)
Milk, cow—cont'd		
dry, skim (non-fat solids), regular	532	1,745
malted		
dry powder	440	720
beverage	91	200
chocolate drink, fluid, commercial		
made with skim milk	46	142
made with whole (3.5% fat) milk	47	146
Molasses, cane		
first extraction or light	15	917
third extraction or blackstrap	96	2,927
Muffin mixes, corn, and muffins baked from mixes		
muffins, made with egg, milk	479	110
muffins, made with egg, water	346	104
Mushrooms		
raw	15	414
canned, solids and liquid	400	197
Muskmelons, raw, cantaloupes, other netted varieties	12	251
Mussels, Atlantic and Pacific, raw, meat only	289	315
Mustard greens, cooked, boiled, drained	18	220
Mustard, prepared		
brown	1,307	130
yellow	1,252	130
Nectarines, raw	6	294
New Zealand spinach, cooked, boiled, drained	92	463
Noodles, egg noodles, enriched, cooked	2	44
Oat products used mainly as hot breakfast cereals		
oatmeal or rolled oats		
dry form	2	352
cooked	218	61
Oat products used mainly as ready-to-eat breakfast cereals		
oats (with or without corn), puffed, added nutrients	1,267	—
Ocean perch, Atlantic (redfish)		
raw	79	269
cooked, fried	153	284
Ocean perch, Pacific, raw	63	390
Oils, salad or cooking	0	0
Okra		
raw	3	249
cooked, boiled, drained	2	174
Olives, pickled; canned or bottled		
green	2,400	55
ripe, Ascolano (extra large, mammoth, giant jumbo)	813	34
ripe, salt-cured, oil-coated, Greek style	3,288	—
Onions, mature (dry), raw	10	157
Onions, young green (bunching varieties), raw		
bulb and entire top	5	231
Oranges, raw, peeled fruit, all commercial varieties	1	200
Orange juice		
raw, all commercial varieties	1	200
canned, unsweetened	1	199
frozen concentrate, unsweetened, diluted with 3 parts water, by volume	1	186
Oysters		
raw, meat only, Eastern	73	121
cooked, fried	206	203
frozen, solids and liquid	380	210

Food and description	Sodium (mg.)	Potassium (mg.)
Oyster stew, commercial frozen, prepared with equal volume of milk	366	176
Pancake and waffle mixes and pancakes baked from mixes		
plain and buttermilk, made with egg, milk	564	154
Parsnips, cooked, boiled, drained	8	379
Peaches		
raw	1	202
canned, solids and liquid, water pack, with or without artificial sweetener	2	137
frozen, sliced, sweetened, not thawed	2	124
Peanuts		
roasted with skins	5	701
roasted and salted	418	674
Peanut butters made with small amounts of added fat, salt	607	670
Pears		
raw, including skin	2	130
canned, solids and liquid, syrup pack, light	1	85
Peas, green, immature		
cooked, boiled, drained	1	196
canned, Alaska (Early or June peas)		
regular pack, solids and liquid	236[2]	96
special dietary pack (low-sodium), solids and liquid	3	96
frozen, cooked, boiled, and drained	115	135
Peas, mature seeds, dry, whole, raw	35	1,005
Peas and carrots, frozen, cooked, boiled, drained	84	157
Pecans	Trace	603
Peppers, hot, chili, mature, red, raw, pods excluding seeds	25	564
Peppers, sweet, garden varieties, immature, green, raw	13	213
Perch, yellow, raw	68	230
Pickles, cucumber, dill	1,428	200
Pies		
baked, piecrust made with unenriched flour		
apple	301	80
cherry	304	105
mince	448	178
pumpkin	214	160
Piecrust or plain pastry, made with enriched flour, baked	611	50
Pike, walleye, raw	51	319
Pineapple		
raw	1	146
frozen chunks, sweetened, not thawed	2	100
Pizza, with cheese, from home recipe, baked		
with cheese topping	702	130
with sausage topping	729	168
Plate dinners, frozen, commercial, unheated		
beef pot roast, whole oven-browned potatoes, peas, and corn	259	244
chicken, fried; mashed potatoes; mixed vegetables (carrots, peas, corn, beans)	344	112
meat loaf with tomato sauce, mashed potatoes, and peas	393	115
turkey, sliced; mashed potatoes; peas	400	176
Plums		
raw, Damson	2	299
canned, solids and liquid, purple (Italian prunes), syrup pack, light	1	145
Popcorn, popped		
plain	(3)	—
oil and salt added	1,940	—

[2]Estimated average based on addition of salt in the amount of 0.6% of the finished product.

Food and description	Sodium (mg.)	Potassium (mg.)
Pork, fresh		
retail cuts, trimmed to retail level		
loin	65	390
Pork, cured, light-cure, commercial, ham, medium-fat class, separable		
lean, cooked, roasted	930	326
Pork, cured, canned		
ham, contents of can	(1,100)	(340)
Potatoes		
cooked, boiled in skin	3[10]	407
dehydrated mashed		
flakes without milk		
dry form	89	1,600
prepared, water, milk, table fat added	231	286
Pretzels	1,680[11]	130
Prunes		
dried, "softenized," cooked (fruit and liquid), with added sugar	3	262
Pudding mixes and puddings made from mixes		
with starch base		
pudding made with milk, cooked	129	136
pudding made with milk, without cooking	124	129
Pumpkin, canned	2	240
Radishes, raw, common	18	322
Raisins, natural (unbleached)		
cooked, fruit and liquid, added sugar	13	355
Raspberries		
canned, solids and liquid, water pack, with or without artificial		
sweetener, red	1	114
frozen, red, sweetened, not thawed	1	100
Rennin products		
tablet (salts, starch, rennin enzyme)	22,300	—
dessert mixes and desserts prepared from mixes		
chocolate, dessert made with milk	52	125
other flavors (vanilla, caramel, fruit flavorings)		
mix, dry form	6	—
dessert, made with milk	46	128
Rhubarb, cooked, added sugar	2	203
Rice		
brown		
raw	9	214
cooked	282	70
white (fully milled or polished)		
enriched		
common commercial varieties, all types		
raw	5	92
cooked	374	28
Rice products used mainly as ready-to-eat breakfast cereals		
rice flakes, added nutrients	987	180
rice, puffed; added nutrients, without salt	2	100
rice, puffed or open-popped, presweetened, honey and added		
nutrients	706	—
Rockfish, including black, canary, yellowtail, rasphead, and bocaccio,		
cooked, oven-steamed	68	446

[10]Applies to product without added salt. If salt is added, an estimated average value for sodium is 236 mg. per 100 grams.

[11]Sodium content is variable. For example, very thin pretzel sticks contain about twice the average amount listed.

Food and description	Sodium (mg.)	Potassium (mg.)
Roe, cooked, baked or broiled, cod and shad[12]	73	132
Rolls and buns		
commercial		
ready-to-serve		
Danish pastry	366	112
hard rolls, enriched	625	97
plain (pan rolls), enriched	506	95
sweet rolls	389	124
Rusk	246	161
Rutabagas, cooked, boiled, drained	4	167
Rye, flour, medium	(1)	203
Rye wafers, whole-grain	882	600
Salad dressings, commercial[13]		
Blue and Roquefort cheese		
regular	1,094	37
special dietary (low-calorie)		
low-fat (approx. 5 cal. per tsp.)	1,108	34
French		
regular	1,370	79
special dietary (low-calorie)		
low-fat (approx. 5 cal. per tsp.)	787	79
mayonnaise	597	34
Thousand island		
regular	700	113
special dietary (low-calorie, approx. 10 cal. per tsp.)	700	113
Salmon		
Coho (silver)		
raw	48[15]	421
canned, solids and liquid	351[14]	339
Salt pork, raw	1,212	42
Salt sticks, regular type	1,674	92
Sandwich spread (with chopped pickle)		
regular	626	92
special dietary (low-calorie, approx. 5 cal. per tsp.)	626	92
Sardines, Atlantic, canned in oil, drained solids	823	590
Sardines, Pacific, in tomato sauce, solids and liquid	400	320
Sauerkraut, canned, solids and liquid	747[16]	140
Sausage, cold cuts, and luncheon meats		
bologna, all samples	1,300	230
frankfurters, raw, all samples	1,100	220
luncheon meat, pork, cured ham or shoulder, chopped, spiced or		
unspiced, canned	1,234	222
pork sausage, links or bulk, cooked	958	269
Scallops, bay and sea, cooked, steamed	265	476
Soups, commercial, canned		
beef broth, bouillon, and consomme, prepared with equal volume		
of water	326	54
chicken noodle, prepared with equal volume of water	408	23
tomato		
prepared with equal volume of water	396	94
prepared with equal volume of milk	422	167
vegetable beef, prepared with equal volume of water	427	66

[12]Prepared with butter or margarine, lemon juice or vinegar.

[13]Values apply to products containing salt. For those without salt, sodium content is low, ranging from less than 10 mg. to 50 mg. per 100 grams; the amount usually is indicated on the label.

[14]For product canned without added salt, value is approximately the same as for raw salmon.

[15]Sample dipped in brine contained 215 mg. sodium per 100 grams.

[16]Values for sauerkraut and sauerkraut juice are based on salt content of 1.9 and 2.0 per cent, respectively, in the finished products. The amounts in some samples may vary significantly from this estimate.

Food and description	Sodium (mg.)	Potassium (mg.)
Soy sauce	7,325	366
Spaghetti, enriched, cooked, tender stage	1	61
Spaghetti, in tomato sauce with cheese, canned	382	121
Spinach		
cooked, boiled, drained	50	324
canned		
regular pack, drained solids	236[2]	250
special dietary pack (low-sodium), solids and liquid	34	250
frozen, chopped, cooked, boiled, drained	52	333
Squash, summer, all varieties, cooked, boiled, drained	1	141
Squash, frozen		
summer, yellow crookneck, cooked, boiled, drained	3	167
winter, heated	1	207
Strawberries		
raw	1	164
frozen, sweetened, not thawed, sliced	1	112
Sturgeon, cooked, steamed	108	235
Succotash (corn and lima beans), frozen		
cooked, boiled, drained	38	246
Sugars, beet or cane, brown	30	344
Sweet potatoes		
cooked, all, baked in skin	12	300
canned, liquid pack, solids and liquid, regular pack in syrup	48	(120)
dehydrated flakes, prepared with water	45	140
Tangerines, raw (Dancy variety)	2	126
Tapioca, dry	3	18
Tapioca desserts, tapioca cream pudding	156	135
Tartar sauce, regular	707	78
Tea, instant (water-soluble solids), carbohydrate added		
dry powder	—	4,530
beverage	—	25
Tomatoes, ripe		
raw	3	244
canned, solids and liquid, regular pack	130	217
Tomato catsup, bottled	1,042[17]	363
Tomato juice		
canned or bottled		
regular pack	200	227
special dietary pack (low-sodium)	3	227
Tomtato juice cocktail, canned or bottled	200	221
Tomtato puree, canned		
regular pack	399	426
special dietary pack (low-sodium)	6	426
Tongue, beef, medium-fat, cooked, braised	61	164
Tuna, canned		
in oil, solids and liquid	800	301
in water, solids and liquid	41[18]	279[18]
Turkey, all classes		
light meat, cooked, roasted	82	411
dark meat, cooked, roasted	99	398
Turkey potpie, commercial, frozen, unheated	369	114
Turnips, cooked, boiled, drained	34	188

[2]Estimated average based on addition of salt in the amount of 0.6% of the finished product.
[17]Applies to regular pack. For special dietary pack (low sodium), values range from 5 to 35 mg. per 100 grams.
[18]One sample with salt added contained 875 mg. of sodium per 100 grams and 275 mg. of potassium.

Food and description	Sodium (mg.)	Potassium (mg.)
Turnip greens, leaves, including stems		
canned, solids and liquid	236[2]	243
frozen, cooked, boiled, drained	17	149
Veal, retail cuts, untrimmed	80	500
Vinegar, cider	1	100
Waffles, frozen, made with enriched flour	644	158
Walnuts		
black	3	460
Persian or English	2	450
Watercress leaves including stems, raw	52	282
Watermelon, raw	1	100
Wheat flours		
whole (from hard wheats)	3	370
patent		
all-purpose or family flour, enriched	2	95
self-rising flour, enriched (anhydrous monocalcium phosphate used as a baking acid)[19]	1,079	— [20]
Wild rice, raw	7	220
Yeast		
baker's, compressed	16	610
brewer's, debittered	121	1,894
Yogurt, made from whole milk	47	132
Zweiback	250	150

[2]Estimated average based on addition of salt in the amount of 0.6% of the finished product.

[19]The acid ingredient most commonly used in self-rising flour. When sodium acid pyrophosphate in combination with either anhydrous monocalcium phosphate or calcium carbonate is used, the value for calcium is approximately 120 mg. per 100 grams; for phosphorus, 540 mg.; for sodium, 1,360 mg.

[20]90 mg. of potassium per 100 grams contributed by flour. Small quantities of additional potassium may be provided by other ingredients.

APPENDIX **D**

Cholesterol content of foods[1]

Item	Amount of cholesterol in		
	100 grams edible portion[2] (mg.)	Edible portion of 1 pound as purchased (mg.)	Refuse from item as purchased (percent)
Beef, raw			
with bone[3]	70	270	15
without bone[3]	70	320	0
Brains, raw	> 2,000	> 9,000	0
Butter	250	1,135	0
Cavier or fish roe	> 300	> 1,300	0
Cheese			
cheddar	100	455	0
cottage, creamed	15	70	0
cream	120	545	0
other (25% to 30% fat)	85	385	0
Cheese spread	65	295	0
Chicken, flesh only, raw	60	—	0
Crab			
in shell[3]	125	270	52
meat only[3]	125	565	0
Egg, whole	550	2,200	12
Egg white	0	0	0
Egg yolk			
fresh	1,500	6,800	0
frozen	1,280	5,800	0
dried	2,950	13,380	0
Fish			
steak[3]	70	265	16
fillet[3]	70	320	0
Heart, raw	150	680	0
Ice cream	45	205	0
Kidney, raw	375	1,700	0
Lamb, raw			
with bone[3]	70	265	16
without bone[3]	70	320	0
lard and other animal fat	95	430	0

[1]From Watt, B. K., and Merrill, A. L.: Composition of foods—raw, processed, prepared, U. S. Department of Agriculture, Agriculture Handbook, No. 8, December, 1963.
[2]Data apply to 100 grams of edible portion of the item, although it may be purchased with the refuse indicated and described or implied in the first column.
[3]Designate items that have the same chemical composition for the edible portion but differ in the amount of refuse.

	Amount of Cholesterol in		
Item	100 grams edible portion[2] (mg.)	Edible portion of 1 pound as purchased (mg.)	Refuse from item as purchased (percent)
Liver, raw	300	1,360	0
Lobster			
whole[3]	200	235	74
meat only[3]	200	900	0
Margarine			
all vegetable fat	0	0	0
two-thirds animal fat, one-third vegetable fat	65	295	0
Milk			
fluid, whole	11	50	0
dried, whole	85	385	0
fluid, skim	3	15	0
Mutton			
with bone[3]	65	250	16
without bone[3]	65	295	0
Oysters			
in shell[3]	> 200	> 90	90
meat only[3]	> 200	> 900	0
Pork			
with bone[3]	70	260	18
without bone[3]	70	320	0
Shrimp			
in shell[3]	125	390	31
flesh only[3]	125	565	0
Sweetbreads (thymus)	250	1,135	0
Veal			
with bone[3]	90	320	21
without bone[3]	90	410	0

[3]Designates items that have the same chemical composition for the edible portion but differ in the amount of refuse.

Calorie values of some common snack foods

Food	Weight gm.	Approximate measure	Calories
Beverages			
Carbonated, cola type	180	1 bottle, 6 ounces	70
Malted milk	405	1 regular (1½ cups)	420
Chocolate milk (made with skim milk)	250	1 cup	190
Cocoa	200	1 cup	235
Soda, vanilla ice cream	242	1 regular	260
Cake			
Angel food	40	2-inch sector	110
Cupcake, chocolate, iced	50	1 cake, 2¾ inches in diameter	185
Fruit cake	30	1 piece, 2 by 2 by ½ inch	115
Candy and popcorn			
Butterscotch	15	3 pieces	60
Candy bar, plain	57	1 bar	295
Caramels	30	3 medium	120
Chocolate coated creams	30	2 average	130
Fudge	28	1 piece	115
Peanut brittle	30	1 ounce	125
Popcorn with oil added	14	1 cup	65
Cheese			
Camembert	28	1 ounce	85
Cheddar	28	1 ounce	105
Cream	28	1 ounce	105
Swiss (domestic)	28	1 ounce	105
Cookies			
Brownies	30	1 piece, 2 by 2 by ¾ inch	140
Cookies, plain and assorted	25	1 cooky, 3 in. in diameter	120
Crackers			
Cheese	18	5 crackers	85
Graham	14	2 medium	55
Saltines	16	4 crackers	70
Rye	13	2 crackers	45
Dessert type cream puff and doughnuts			
Cream puff—custard filling	105	1 average	245
Doughnut, cake type, plain	32	1 average	125
Doughnut, jelly	65	1 average	225
Doughnut, raised	30	1 average	120

Food	Weight gm.	Approximate measure	Calories
Miscellaneous			
Hamburger and bun	96	1 average	330
Ice cream, vanilla	62	3½ ounce container	130
Sherbet	96	½ cup	120
Jams, jellies, marmalades, preserves	20	1 tablespoon	55
Syrup, blended	80	¼ cup	240
Waffles	75	1 waffle, 4½ by 5½ by ½ inch	210
Nuts			
Mixed, shelled	15	8-12	95
Peanut butter	16	1 tablespoon	95
Peanuts, shelled, roasted	144	1 cup	840
Pie			
Apple	135	4-inch sector	345
Cherry	135	4-inch sector	355
Custard	130	4-inch sector	280
Lemon meringue	120	4-inch sector	305
Mince	135	4-inch sector	365
Pumpkin	130	4-inch sector	275
Potato chips			
Potato chips	20	10 chips, 2 inches in diameter	115
Sandwiches			
Bacon, lettuce, tomato	150	1 sandwich	280
Egg salad	140	1 sandwich	280
Ham	80	1 sandwich	280
Liverwurst	90	1 sandwich	250
Peanut butter	85	1 sandwich	330
Soups, commercial canned			
Bean with pork	250	1 cup	170
Beef noodle	250	1 cup	70
Chicken noodle	250	1 cup	65
Cream (mushroom)	240	1 cup	135
Tomato	245	1 cup	90
Vegetable with beef broth	250	1 cup	80

APPENDIX **F**

Composition of beverages—alcoholic and carbonated non-alcoholic per 100 grams[1]

	Food energy	Protein	Carbo-hydrate	Calcium	Phos-phorus	Iron	Thiamine	Ribo-flavin	Niacin
Beverages, alcoholic and carbonated non-alcoholic									
Alcoholic									
Beer, alcohol 4.5% by volume (3.6% by weight)	42	.3	3.8	5	30	Trace	Trace	.03	.6
Gin, rum, vodka, whisky:									
80-proof (33.4% alcohol by weight)	231	—	Trace	—	—	—	—	—	—
86-proof (36.0% alcohol by weight)	249	—	Trace	—	—	—	—	—	—
90-proof (37.9% alcohol by weight)	263	—	Trace	—	—	—	—	—	—
94-proof (39.7% alcohol by weight)	275	—	Trace	—	—	—	—	—	—
100-proof (42.5% alcohol by weight)	295	—	Trace	—	—	—	—	—	—
Wines									
Dessert, alcohol 18.8% by volume (15.3% by weight)	137	.1	7.7	8	—	—	.01	.02	.2
Table, alcohol 12.2% by volume (9.9% by weight)	85	.1	4.2	9	10	.4	Trace	.01	.1
Carbonated, non-alcoholics									
Carbonated waters:									
sweetened (quinine sodas)	31	—	8	—	—	—	—	—	—
unsweetened (club sodas)	—	—	—	—	—	—	—	—	—
Cola type	39	—	10	—	—	—	—	—	—
Cream sodas	43	—	11	—	—	—	—	—	—
Fruit-flavored sodas (citrus, cherry, grape, strawberry, Tom Collins mixer, other) (10%-13% sugar)	46	—	12	—	—	—	—	—	—
Ginger ale, pale dry and golden	31	—	8	—	—	—	—	—	—
Root beer	41	—	10.5	—	—	—	—	—	—
Special dietary drinks with artificial sweetener (less than 1 calorie per ounce)	—	—	—	—	—	—	—	—	—

[1]From Watt, B. K., and Merrill, A. L.: Composition of foods—raw, processed, prepared, U. S. Department of Agriculture, Agriculture Handbook, No. 8, December, 1963.

APPENDIX **G**

Suggested patterns of daily food intake to supply adequate nutrition in various groups[1]

	Age years	Weight kg.	Weight lb.	Height cm.	Height in.	Milk	Veg. A	Veg. B	Fruit	Bread	Meat	Fat
									Basic foods in exchange list portions			
Children	1-3	12	27	87	34	3	1	1	3	5	1	2
	4-6	18	40	109	43	3	1	1	3	6	2	2
	7-9	27	60	129	51	3	1	1	3	8	3	3
	10-12	36	79	144	57	3	1	1	4	10	4	4
Boys	13-15	49	108	163	64	3	1	1	4	12	5	5
	16-19	63	139	175	69	3	1	1	4	16	6	6
Girls	13-15	49	108	160	63	3	1	1	4	8	6	4
	16-19	54	120	162	64	3	1	1	4	8	5	3
Men	20-34	70	154	175	69	2	1	1	4	12	6	6
	35-54	70	154	175	69	2	1	1	4	10	5	5
	55-74	70	154	175	69	2	1	1	4	10	5	5
	75-	68	150	175	69	2	1	1	4	8	5	4
Women	20-34	58	128	163	64	2	1	1	4	6	5	4
	35-54	58	128	163	64	2	1	1	4	6	5	4
	55-74	58	128	163	64	2	1	1	4	5	5	3
	75-	56	123	163	64	2	1	1	4	4	4	3
Pregnant (second half)						3	1	1	5	6	6	4
Lactating						4	1	1	5	10	6	4

[1]Based on the Recommended Daily Allowances, National Research Council (1964 rev.), Family Food Plan at Moderate Cost, U. S. Department of Agriculture, 1964, and the Basic Food Exchange Groups (see p. 483). These patterns are adequate in protein, minerals and vitamins, but relatively low in carbohydrate, fat, and total calories. When more calories are needed, bread or fruit exchanges may be added. Many authorities recommend keeping the fat intake near the minimum. (Reprinted from Church, C. F., and Church, H. N.: Food values of portions commonly used, ed. 9, Philadelphia, 1963, J. B. Lippincott Co., p. 122.)

APPENDIX **H**

Height and weight tables for adults

Desirable Weights for Persons Age 25 and Over[1]

Weight in pounds according to frame (in indoor clothing)

Men

Height (with shoes on) 1-inch heels Feet Inches		Small Frame lbs.	Medium Frame lbs.	Large Frame lbs.
5	2	112-120	118-129	126-141
5	3	115-123	121-133	129-144
5	4	118-126	124-136	132-148
5	5	121-129	127-139	135-152
5	6	124-133	130-143	138-156
5	7	128-137	134-147	142-161
5	8	132-141	138-152	147-166
5	9	136-145	142-156	151-170
5	10	140-150	146-160	155-174
5	11	144-154	150-165	159-179
6	0	148-158	154-170	164-184
6	1	152-162	158-175	168-189
6	2	156-167	162-180	173-194
6	3	160-171	167-185	178-199
6	4	164-175	172-190	182-204

Women[2]

Height (with shoes on) 2-inch heels Feet Inches		Small Frame lbs.	Medium Frame lbs.	Large Frame lbs.
4	10	92- 98	96-107	104-119
4	11	94-101	98-110	106-122
5	0	96-104	101-113	109-125
5	1	99-107	104-116	112-128
5	2	102-110	107-119	115-131
5	3	105-113	110-122	118-134
5	4	108-116	113-126	121-138
5	5	111-119	116-130	125-142
5	6	114-123	120-135	129-146
5	7	118-127	124-139	133-150
5	8	122-131	128-143	137-154
5	9	126-135	132-147	141-158
5	10	130-140	136-151	145-163
5	11	134-144	140-155	149-168
6	0	138-148	144-159	153-173

[1]Metropolitan Life Insurance Company, New York.
[2]For girls between 18 and 25, subtract 1 pound for each year under 25.

Normal constituents of the blood in the adult

Physical measurements		
Specific gravity		1.025-1.029
Viscosity (water as unity)		4.5
Bleeding time (capillary)	min.	1-3
Prothrombin time (plasma) (Quick)	sec.	10-20
Sedimentation rate (Wintrobe method)		
Men	mm. in 1 hr.	0-9
Women	mm. in 1 hr.	0-20
Hematologic studies		
Cell volume	percent	39-50
Red blood cells	million per cu. mm.	4.25-5.25
White blood cells	per cu. mm.	5000-9000
Lymphocytes	percent	25-30
Neutrophils	percent	60-65
Monocytes	percent	4-8
Eosinophils	percent	0.5-4
Basophils	percent	0-1.5
Platelets	per cu. mm.	125,000-300,000
Proteins		
Total protein (serum)	gm. per 100 ml.	6.5-7.5
Albumin (serum)	gm. per 100 ml.	4.5-5.5
Globulin (serum)	gm. per 100 ml.	1.5-2.5
Albumin: globulin ratio		1.8-2.5
Fibrinogen (plasma)	gm. per 100 ml.	0.2-0.5
Hemoglobin		
Males	gm. per 100 ml.	14-17
Females	gm. per 100 ml.	13-16
Nitrogen constituents		
Nonprotein N (serum)	mg. per 100 ml.	20-36
(whole blood)	mg. per 100 ml.	25-40
Urea (whole blood)	mg. per 100 ml.	18-38
Urea N (whole blood)	mg. per 100 ml.	8-18
Creatinine (whole blood)	mg. per 100 ml.	1-2
Uric acid (whole blood)	mg. per 100 ml.	2.5-5.0
Amino acid N (whole blood)	mg. per 100 ml.	3-6
Carbohydrates and lipids		
Glucose (whole blood)	mg. per 100 ml.	70-90
Ketones—as acetone (whole blood)	mg. per 100 ml.	1.5-2

Carbohydrates and lipids—cont'd

Fats (total lipids) (serum)	mg. per 100 ml.	570-820
Cholesterol (serum)	mg. per 100 ml.	100-230
Bilirubin (serum)	mg. per 100 ml.	0.1-0.25
Icteric index (serum)	units	4-6

Blood gases

CO_2 content (serum)	volumes percent	55-75
	mM. per liter	(24.5-33.5)
CO_2 content (whole blood)	volumes percent	40-60
	mM. per liter	(18.0-27.0)
Oxygen capacity (whole blood)		
Males	volumes percent	18.7-22.7
Females	volumes percent	17.0-21.0
Oxygen saturation		
Arterial blood	percent	94-96
Venous blood	percent	60-85

Acid-base constituents

Base, total fixed (serum)	mEq. per liter	142-150
Sodium (serum)	mg. per 100 ml.	320-335
	mEq. per liter	(139-146)
Potassium (serum)	mg. per 100 ml.	16-22
	mEq. per liter	(4.1-5.6)
Calcium (serum)	mg. per 100 ml.	9.0-11.5
	mEq. per liter	(4.5-5.8)
Magnesium (serum)	mg. per 100 ml.	1.0-3.0
	mEq. per liter	(1.0-2.5)
Phosphorus, inorganic (serum)	mg. per 100 ml.	3.0-5.0
	mEq. per liter	(1.0-1.6)
Chlorides, expressed as Cl (serum)	mg. per 100 ml.	352-383
	mEq. per liter	(99-108)
As NaCl (serum)	mg. per 100 ml.	580-630
	mEq. per liter	(99-108)
Sulfates, inorganic as SO_4 (serum)	mg. per 100 ml.	2.5-5.0
	mEq. per liter	0.5-1.0)
Lactic acid (venous blood)	mg. per 100 ml.	10-20
	mEq. per liter	(1.1-2.2)
Serum protein base binding power	mEq. per liter	(15.5-18.0)
Base bicarbonate HCO_3 (serum)	mEq. per liter	(19-30)
pH (blood or plasma at 38°C)		7.3-7.45

Miscellaneous

Phosphatase (serum)	Bodansky units per 100 ml.	5
Iron (whole blood)	mg. per 100 ml.	46-55
Ascorbic acid (whole blood)	mg. per 100 ml.	0.75-1.50
Carotene (serum)	μg. per 100 ml.	75-125

Abbreviations and conversion factors:

ml. = milliliters
mg. = milligrams
μg. = micrograms
mEq. = milliequivalents

gm. = grams
cu. mm. = cubic millimeters

$$\text{mEq. per liter} = \frac{\text{mg. per liter}}{\text{equivalent weight}}$$

$$\text{mM. (millimoles) per liter} = \frac{\text{mg. per liter}}{\text{molecular weight}}$$

$$\text{equivalent weight} = \frac{\text{atomic weight}}{\text{valence of element}}$$

$$\text{volumes percent} = \text{mM. per liter} \times 2.24$$

Normal constituents of the urine of the adult

Urine constituents	*Gm. per 24 hr.*
Total solids	55-70
Nitrogenous constituents	
Total nitrogen	10-17
Ammonia	0.5-1.0
Amino acid N	0.4-1
Creatine	none
Creatinine	1-1.5
Protein	none
Purine bases	0.016-0.060
Urea	20-35
Uric acid	0.5-0.7
Acetone bodies	0.003-0.015
Bile	none
Calcium	0.2-0.4
Chloride (as NaCl)	10-15
Glucose	none
Indican	0-0.030
Iron	0.001-0.005
Magnesium (as MgO)	0.15-0.30
Phosphate, total (as phosphoric acid)	2.5-3.5
Potassium (as K_2O)	2.0-3.0
Sodium (as Na_2O)	4.0-5.0
Sulfates, total (as sulfuric acid)	1.5-3.0
Physical measurements	
Specific gravity	1.010-1.025
Reaction (pH)	5.5-8.0
Volume (ml. per 24 hr.)	800-1600

Tools for use in calculating diets and planning meals for children with phenylketonuria

RECOMMENDED ALLOWANCES FOR PHENYLALANINE, PROTEIN, AND CALORIES FOR PKU CHILDREN OF VARIOUS AGES[1]

Age	Phenylalanine mg. per lb. body weight	Protein gm.	Calories per lb. body weight
Birth—3 months	20-22	1¾-2 gm./lb.	60-65
4-12 months	18-20	1½ gm./lb.	55-60
1-3 years	16-18	40 gm.	50-55
4-7 years	10-16	50 gm.	40-50

[1]A low-phenylalanine formula preparation (Lofenalac) is given to infants. Solid foods as permitted on the diet, chosen from the low-phenylalanine food lists, are introduced at the usual ages.

Lefenalac

Lofenalac (Mead Johnson and Company, Evansville, Indiana)—a balanced low-phenylalanine food—has the following composition:

		Powder	Normal dilution
Total nitrogen (equivalent to approximately 15% protein)		2.4%	0.36%
Fat		18.0	2.7
Carbohydrate		57.0	8.5
Minerals (ash)		5.0	0.75
including:	Calcium	0.65%	0.1%
	Phosphorus	0.50	0.07
	Iron	0.01	0.0015
	Sodium	0.4 (17.4 mEq.)	0.06
	Potassium	1.0 (25.6 mEq.)	0.15
	Chlorine	0.65	0.1
Moisture		2.0	86.0

Caloric distribution

15% of the calories of Lofenalac are derived from protein, 35% from fat, and 50% from carbohydrate.

Phenylalanine content

Lofenalac powder contains not more than 0.1% nor less than 0.06% phenylalanine (average, about 0.08%).

Vitamin content

A qt. of Lofenalac formula in normal dilution (1 measure to 2 oz. water) contains the following vitamins: Vitamin A, 1500 U.S.P. units; Vitamin D, 400 U.S.P. units; Vitamin E, 5 I.U.; ascorbic acid, 30 mg.; thiamine hydrochloride, 0.46 mg.; riboflavin, 1.8 mg., niacinamide, 4 mg.; pyridoxine hydrochloride, 0.5 mg.; calcium pantothenate, 3.2 mg.; Vitamin B_{12}, 4.5 μg.; folic acid, 0.5 mg.; biotin, 0.03 mg., and choline chloride, 150 mg.

CALORIES, PROTEIN, AND PHENYLALANINE SUPPLIED BY TYPICAL QUANTITIES OF LOFENALAC

Lofenalac	Approx. calories	Approx. protein equiv. gm.	Average phenylalanine mg.
100 gm. (2/3 cup)	450	15	80
1 packed level measure (9.5 gm.)	43	1.4	7.5
1 standard 8 oz. measuring cup (150 gm.:			
16 packed level measures)	680	22	120
1 fl. oz. of normal dilution	20	0.6	3.5
4 fl. oz. of normal dilution	80	2.4	14
8 fl. oz. of normal dilution	160	5	28
32 fl. oz. of normal dilution	640	19	110

Directions for mixing Lofenalac

Make a paste of the Lofenalac with a small amount of boiling water before adding the total water. Sprinkle the Lofenalac on top of the water and beat with an eggbeater or mix in a blender.

PHENYLALANINE, PROTEIN, AND CALORIE CONTENT OF SERVING LISTS OF FOODS USED ON RESTRICTED PHENYLALANINE DIETS[1]

Food	Measure	Phenylalanine mg.	Protein gm.	Calories
Lofenalac	1 measure (1 tablespoon)	7.5	1.5	43
Vegetables	1 serving	15	0.3	5
Fruits	1 serving	15	0.2	80
Breads, cereals	1 serving	30	0.5	20
Fats	1 serving	5	0.1	45
Desserts (special recipes)	1 serving	30	2.0	270
Free foods		0	0.0	varies
Milk	1 ounce	55	1.1	20

[1]Acosta, P. B.: Nutritional aspects of phenylketonuria. In The clinical team looks at phenylketonuria, rev., Children's Bureau, U. S. Department of Health, Education, and Welfare, 1964, p. 40. (See p. 412 of this text for listings of these Food Exchange Groups for use with the Low Phenylalanine Diet.)

GUIDELINES FOR LOW PHENYLALANINE DIETS FOR INFANTS AND CHILDREN[1]

Weight, lbs.	1 month 8 lbs.	8 months 18 lbs.	2 years 26 lbs.	4 years 36 lbs.
Diet prescription				
Phenylalanine, mg.	160-176	324-360	416-468	360-576
Protein, gm.	14-16	27	32	40
Calories	440	810	1300	1700
Lofenalac, measures	10	18	19	23
Water to make, oz.	24	32	24	24
Milk as necessary, oz.	1½	1	—	—
Vegetables, servings	—	2	4	4
Fruits, servings	1	1	4	4
Breads, servings	—	3	5	4
Fats, servings	—	—	1	1
Desserts (special recipes)	—	—	—	1
Free foods	—	—	as desired	as desired
Nutritive values				
Phenylalanine, mg.	172	325	417	447
Protein, gm.	16.8	30.4	33.1	40.6
Calories	540	944	1302	1724

[1]Acosta, P. B.: Nutritional aspects of phenylketonuria. In The clinical team looks at phenylketonuria, rev., Children's Bureau, U.S. Department of Health, Education, and Welfare, 1964, p. 52. (1 measure of Lofenalac equals 1 tablespoon. Special recipes are required for the desserts. Excess amounts of the free foods should be avoided so the child will consume proper amounts of other foods.)

APPENDIX

L

Food and Nutrition Board, National Academy of Sciences —National Research Council recommended daily dietary allowances[1] (revised 1968)

DESIGNED FOR THE MAINTENANCE OF GOOD NUTRITION OF PRACTICALLY ALL HEALTHY PEOPLE IN THE U.S.A.

Age[2] (years)	Weight (kg)	Weight (lbs)	Height (cm)	Height (in.)	kcal	Protein (gm)	Fat-soluble vitamins			Water-soluble vitamins							Minerals				
							Vitamin A activity (IU)	Vitamin D (IU)	Vitamin E activity (mg)	Ascorbic acid (mg)	Folacin[3] (mg)	Niacin (mg equiv)[4]	Riboflavin (mg)	Thiamine (mg)	Vitamin B6 (mg)	Vitamin B12 (μg)	Calcium (g)	Phosphorus (g)	Iodine (μg)	Iron (mg)	Magnesium (mg)
Infants																					
0–1/6	4	9	55	22	kg × 120	kg × 2.2[5]	1,500	400	5	35	0.05	5	0.4	0.2	0.2	1.0	0.4	0.2	25	6	40
1/6–1/2	7	15	63	25	kg × 110	kg × 2.0[5]	1,500	400	5	35	0.05	7	0.5	0.4	0.3	1.5	0.5	0.4	40	10	60
1/2–1	9	20	72	28	kg × 100	kg × 1.8[5]	1,500	400	5	35	0.1	8	0.6	0.5	0.4	2.0	0.6	0.5	45	15	70
Children																					
1–2	12	26	81	32	1,100	25	2,000	400	10	40	0.1	8	0.6	0.6	0.5	2.0	0.7	0.7	55	15	100
2–3	14	31	91	36	1,250	25	2,000	400	10	40	0.2	8	0.7	0.6	0.6	2.5	0.8	0.8	60	15	150
3–4	16	35	100	39	1,400	30	2,500	400	10	40	0.2	9	0.8	0.7	0.7	3	0.8	0.8	70	10	200
4–6	19	42	110	43	1,600	30	2,500	400	10	40	0.2	11	0.9	0.8	0.9	4	0.8	0.8	80	10	200
6–8	23	51	121	48	2,000	35	3,500	400	15	40	0.2	13	1.1	1.0	1.0	4	0.9	0.9	100	10	250
8–10	28	62	131	52	2,200	40	3,500	400	15	40	0.3	15	1.2	1.1	1.2	5	1.0	1.0	110	10	250

Males																				
10–12	35	77	140	55	2,500	45	4,500	400	20	40	0.4	17	1.3	1.3	1.2	5	1.2	1.2	125	10	300
12–14	43	95	151	59	2,700	50	5,000	400	25	45	0.4	18	1.4	1.4	1.4	5	1.4	1.4	135	18	350
14–18	59	130	170	67	3,000	60	5,000	400	30	55	0.4	20	1.5	1.5	1.8	5	1.4	1.4	150	18	400
18–22	67	147	175	69	2,800	60	5,000	400	30	60	0.4	18	1.6	1.4	2.0	5	0.8	0.8	140	10	400
22–35	70	154	175	69	2,800	65	5,000	—	30	60	0.4	18	1.7	1.4	2.0	5	0.8	0.8	140	10	350
35–55	70	154	173	68	2,600	65	5,000	—	30	60	0.4	17	1.7	1.3	2.0	5	0.8	0.8	125	10	350
55–75+	70	154	171	67	2,400	65	5,000	—	30	60	0.4	14	1.7	1.2	2.0	6	0.8	0.8	110	10	350
Females																				
10–12	35	77	142	56	2,250	50	4,500	400	20	40	0.4	15	1.3	1.1	1.4	5	1.2	1.2	110	18	300
12–14	44	97	154	61	2,300	50	5,000	400	20	45	0.4	15	1.4	1.2	1.6	5	1.3	1.3	115	18	350
14–16	52	114	157	62	2,400	55	5,000	400	25	50	0.4	16	1.4	1.2	1.8	5	1.3	1.3	120	18	350
16–18	54	119	160	63	2,300	55	5,000	400	25	50	0.4	15	1.5	1.2	2.0	5	1.3	1.3	115	18	350
18–22	58	128	163	64	2,000	55	5,000	400	25	55	0.4	13	1.5	1.0	2.0	5	0.8	0.8	100	18	350
22–35	58	128	163	64	2,000	55	5,000	—	25	55	0.4	13	1.5	1.0	2.0	5	0.8	0.8	100	18	300
35–55	58	128	160	63	1,850	55	5,000	—	25	55	0.4	13	1.5	1.0	2.0	5	0.8	0.8	90	18	300
55–75+	58	128	157	62	1,700	55	5,000	—	25	55	0.4	13	1.5	1.0	2.0	6	0.8	0.8	80	10	300
Pregnancy					+200	65	6,000	400	30	60	0.8	15	1.8	+0.1	2.5	8	+0.4	+0.4	125	18	450
Lactation					+1,000	75	8,000	400	30	60	0.5	20	2.0	+0.5	2.5	6	+0.5	+0.5	150	18	450

[1] The allowance levels are intended to cover individual variations among most normal persons as they live in the United States under usual environmental stresses. The recommended allowances can be attained with a variety of common foods, providing other nutrients for which human requirements have been less well defined. See text for more detailed discussion of allowances and of nutrients not tabulated.

[2] Entries on lines for age range 22–35 years represent the reference man and woman at age 22. All other entries represent allowances for the midpoint of the specified age range.

[3] The folacin allowances refer to dietary sources as determined by *Lactobacillus casei* assay. Pure forms of folacin may be effective in doses less than ¼ of the RDA.

[4] Niacin equivalents include dietary sources of the vitamin itself plus 1 mg equivalent for each 60 mg of dietary tryptophan.

[5] Assumes protein equivalent to human milk. For proteins not 100 percent utilized factors should be increased proportionately.

Index